Procedures, Techniques, and Minimally Invasive Monitoring in

Intensive Care Medicine

FOURTH EDITION

Procedures, Techniques, and Minimally Invasive Monitoring in

Intensive Care Medicine

FOURTH EDITION

Richard S. Irwin, M.D., F.C.C.P.

Professor of Medicine and Nursing
University of Massachusetts
Chair, Critical Care Operations
UMass Memorial Medical Center
Worcester, Massachusetts

James M. Rippe, M.D.

Professor of Biomedical Sciences
University of Central Florida
Orlando, Florida
Associate Professor of Medicine (Cardiology)
Tufts University School of Medicine
Boston, Massachusetts
Founder and Director
Rippe Lifestyle Institute
Shrewsbury, Massachusetts
Founder and Director
Rippe Health Assessment at Florida Hospital Celebration Health
Orlando, Florida

Alan Lisbon, M.D.

Associate Professor of Anesthesia
Harvard Medical School
Vice Chair for Critical Care
Beth Israel Deaconess Medical Center
Boston, Massachusetts

Stephen O. Heard, M.D.

Professor and Chair
Department of Anesthesiology
University of Massachusetts Medical School
Worcester, Massachusetts

Wolters Kluwer | Lippincott Williams & Wilkins
Health

Philadelphia • Baltimore • New York • London
Buenos Aires • Hong Kong • Sydney • Tokyo

Acquisitions Editor: Brian Brown
Managing Editor: Nicole T. Dernoski
Developmental Editor: Annette Ferran
Marketing Manager: Angela Panetta
Production Manager: Bridgett Dougherty
Senior Manufacturing Manager: Benjamin Rivera
Design Coordinator: Stephen Druding
Compositor: Aptara, Inc.

© **2008 by Richard S. Irwin, M.D. and James M. Rippe, M.D.**

530 Walnut Street
Philadelphia, PA 19106 USA
LWW.com

3rd Edition © 2003 by Richard S. Irwin, M.D., James M. Rippe, M.D, Frederick J. Curley, M.D., and Stephen O. Heard, M.D., 2nd Edition © 1999 by Richard S. Irwin, M.D., James M. Rippe, M.D., Frank B. Cerra, M.D., Frederick J. Curley, M.D., and Stephen O. Heard, M.D., 1st Edition © 1995 by James M. Rippe, M.D., Richard S. Irwin, M.D., Mitchell P. Fink, M.D., Frank B. Cerra, M.D., Frederick J. Curley, M.D., and Stephen O. Heard, M.D.

Printed in the USA

Library of Congress Cataloging-in-Publication Data

Procedures, techniques, and minimally invasive monitoring in intensive care medicine/
[edited by] Richard S. Irwin . . . [et al.]. —4th ed.
    p.; cm.
  Rev. ed. of: Procedures and techniques in intensive care medicine. c2003.
  Includes bibliographical references and index.
  ISBN-13: 978-0-7817-7862-6 (alk. paper)
  ISBN-10: 0-7817-7862-X (alk. paper)
1. Critical care medicine.   I. Irwin, Richard S.   II. Procedures and techniques in intensive care medicine.
  [DNLM: 1. Intensive Care—methods.   WX 218 P963 2008]
  RC86.7.P757 2008
  616′.028—dc22

                                                                  2007019924

To purchase additional copies of this book, call our customer service department at (800) 638-3030 or fax orders to (301) 223-2320. International customers should call (301) 223-2300.

Visit Lippincott Williams & Wilkins on the Internet: at LWW.com. Lippincott Williams & Wilkins customer service representatives are available from 8:30 am to 6 pm, EST.

10 9 8 7 6 5 4 3 2 1

To Our Families

Diane, Rachel, Sara, Jamie, Rebecca, John, Andrew K., and Andrew M.

Stephanie, Hart, Jaelin, Devon, and Jamie

Carol, Amy, and Emily

Kelly and Mark

CONTENTS

Section **2. MINIMALLY INVASIVE MONITORING**

Section Editor: Alan Lisbon

SECTION EDITORS

Stephen O. Heard, M.D.
Professor and Chair
Department of Anesthesiology
University of Massachusetts Medical School
Worcester, Massachusetts
Section 1: Procedures and Techniques

Margaret M. Hudlin, M.D.
Assistant Professor
Department of Surgery
Surgical Critical Care
UMass Memorial Medical Center
Worcester, Massachusetts
Section 1: Procedures and Techniques

Alan Lisbon, M.D.
Associate Professor of Anesthesia
Harvard Medical School
Vice Chair for Critical Care
Beth Israel Deaconess Medical Center
Boston, Massachusetts
Section 2: Minimally Invasive Monitoring

CONTRIBUTING AUTHORS

Maria E. Abruzzo, M.D.
Worcester, Massachusetts
Chapter 19

Sergio R. Acchiardo, M.D.
Professor of Medicine
University of Tennessee Health Science Center
Memphis, Tennessee
Chapter 25

Suresh Agarwal, M.D.
Assistant Professor of Surgery
Associate Surgery Residency Program Director
Boston University School of Medicine
Boston, Massachusetts
Chapter 32

Philip J. Ayvazian, M.D.
Associate Professor
Department of Anesthesiology
UMass Memorial Health Care
Worcester, Massachusetts
Chapter 18

Ruben J. Azocar, M.D.
Assistant Professor of Anesthesiology
Associate Residing Program Director
Department of Anesthesiology
Boston University Medical Center
Boston, Massachusetts
Chapter 32

Ednan K. Bajwa, M.D.
Clinical Fellow in Medicine
Harvard Medical School
Graduate Assistant in Medicine
Massachusetts General Hospital
Boston, Massachusetts
Chapter 29

Richard C. Becker, M.D.
Professor of Medicine
Director, Cardiovascular Thrombosis Center
Duke University School of Medicine
Durham, North Carolina
Chapter 7

Eric A. Bedell, M.D.
Associate Professor
Department of Anesthesiology
The University of Texas Medical Branch
Galveston, Texas
Chapter 30

Bonnie J. Bidinger, M.D.
Assistant Professor of Clinical Medicine
Department of Medicine
Division of Rheumatology
UMass Memorial Health Care
Worcester, Massachusetts
Chapter 19

Naomi F. Botkin, M.D.
Assistant Professor of Medicine
Division of Cardiology
UMass Memorial Health Care
Worcester, Massachusetts
Chapter 6

Scott A. Celinski, M.D.
Critical Care Fellow
Deparment of Surgery
The George Washington University
Washington, D.C.
Chapters 2, 3

Frederick J. Curley, M.D.
Associate Professor of Medicine
University of Massachusetts Medical School
Medical Director
Department of Pulmonary and Critical Care
Milford–Whitinsville Regional Hospital
Milford, Massachusetts
Chapters 27, 28

Seth T. Dahlberg, M.D.
Assistant Professor of Medicine and Radiology
University of Massachusetts Medical School
Physician, Division of Cardiology and
    Nuclear Medicine
UMass Memorial Health Care
Worcester, Massachusetts
Chapter 5

Mario De Pinto, M.D.
Acting Assistant Professor
Department of Anesthesiology
University of Washington
Seattle, Washington
Chapter 23

Mark Dershwitz, M.D., Ph.D.
Professor and Vice Chair of Anesthesiology
Professor of Biochemistry and Molecular
    Pharmacology
Department of Anesthesiology
UMass Memorial Health Care
Worcester, Massachusetts
Chapter 20

Alexander J. Eckardt, M.D.
Fellow, Division of Gastroenterology
UMass Memorial Health Care
Worcester, Massachusetts
Chapter 13

W. Thomas Edwards, M.D., Ph.D.
Director, Fellowship in Pain Medicine
Associate Professor of Anesthesiology
Department of Anesthesiology
University of Washington
Harborview Medical Center
Seattle, Washington
Chapter 23

Khaldoun Faris, M.D.
Associate Director of Surgical Intensive Care Unit
University of Massachusetts Medical School
Worcester, Massachusetts
Chapter 24

Andrew J. Goodwin, M.D.
Resident, Department of Medicine
Massachusetts General Hospital
Boston, Massachusetts
Chapter 29

Stephen O. Heard, M.D.
Professor and Chair
Department of Anesthesiology
University of Massachusetts Medical School
Worcester, Massachusetts
Chapter 1

Michael D. Howell, M.D.
Instructor in Medicine
Harvard Medical School
Director of Critical Care Quality
Associate Director of Medical Critical Care
Beth Israel Deaconess Medical Center
Boston, Massachusetts
Chapter 27

Richard S. Irwin, M.D., F.C.C.P.
Professor of Medicine and Nursing
University of Massachusetts
Chair, Critical Care Operations
UMass Memorial Medical Center
Worcester, Massachusetts
Chapters 9–11

Eric W. Jacobson, M.D.
Associate Professor of Medicine
University of Massachusetts Medical School
Worcester, Massachusetts
Chapter 19

Shubjeet Kaur, M.D.
Medical Director of Perioperative Service
Clinical Associate Professor
Vice Chair Anesthesiology
UMass Memorial Health Care
Worcester, Massachusetts
Chapter 1

Ducksoo Kim, M.D.
Professor of Radiology and Section Head
    of Vascular Intervention
UMass Memorial Health Care
University of Massachusetts Medical School
Worcester, Massachusetts
Chapter 21

Young H. Kim, M.D.
Assistant Professor of Radiology
UMass Memorial Health Care
University of Massachusetts Medical School
Worcester, Massachusetts
Chapter 21

Scott E. Kopec, M.D.
Assistant Professor of Medicine
Medical Director, Department of Respiratory Therapy
UMass Memorial Health Care
University of Massachusetts Medical School
Worcester, Massachusetts
Chapter 12

Stephen J. Krinzman, M.D.
Assistant Professor of Medicine
Department of Medicine
Division of Pulmonary, Allergy, and Critical
    Care Medicine
University of Massachusetts Medical School
Worcester, Massachusetts
Chapter 9

Robert A. Lancey, M.D.
Chief of Cardiac Surgery
Bassett Healthcare
Cooperstown, New York
Chapter 8

Ishaq Lat, Pharm.D., B.C.P.S.
Clinical Pharmacy Specialist
University of Chicago Hospital
Chicago, Illinois
Chapter 32

Adam B. Lerner, M.D.
Instructor, Anesthesiology
Harvard Medical School
Director, Cardiac and Transplant Anesthesia Member
    of Harvard Medical Faculty Physicians
Beth Israel Deaconess Medical Center
Boston, Massachusetts
Chapter 31

Michael Linenberger, M.D.
Associate Professor, Division of Hematology
University of Washington
Medical Director
Apheresis and Cellular Therapy
Seattle Cancer Care Alliance
University of Washington
Seattle, Washington
Chapter 26

Atul Malhotra, M.D.
Assistant Professor of Medicine
Harvard Medical School
Pulmonary and Critical Care and Sleep Divisions
Brigham and Women's Hospital
Boston, Massachusetts
Chapter 29

Deborah H. Markowitz, M.D.
Intensive Care Unit Medical Director
Leonard Morse Hospital
Framingham, Massachusetts
Medical Director
Northeast Specialty Hospital
Natick, Massachusetts
Kindred Healthcare Long Term Acute Care
Framingham, Massachusetts
Chapter 11

Raimis Matulionis, M.D.
Assistant Professor of Anesthesiology and Critical
    Care Medicine
Department of Anesthesiology
UMass Memorial Health Care
Worcester, Massachusetts
Chapter 24

Ciaran J. McNamee, M.D.
Associate Professor of Surgery
Chief, Section of Thoracic Surgery
UMass Memorial Health Care
Worcester, Massachusetts
Chapter 12

**Lena M. Napolitano, M.D. F.A.C.S., F.C.C.P.,
F.C.C.M.**
Division Chief, Acute Care Surgery
Associate Chair, Department of Surgery
Chief, Surgical Critical Care
University of Michigan
University Hospital
Ann Arbor, Michigan
Chapters 14, 16

Theresa Nester, M.D.
Assistant Professor
Department of Laboratory Medicine
University of Washington
Assistant Medical Director
Puget Sound Blood Center
Seattle, Washington
Chapter 26

Achikam Oren-Grinberg, M.D., M.S.
Resident, Department of Anesthesia and Critical Care
Beth Israel Deaconess Medical Center
Boston, Massachusetts
Chapter 31

Alan A. Orquiola, M.D.
Assistant Professor of Anesthesiology
Department of Anesthesiology
UMass Memorial Health Care
Worcester, Massachusetts
Chapter 22

William F. Owen, Jr., M.D.
Vice President of Health Affairs
Chancellor of the Health Science Center
University of Tennessee
Memphis, Tennessee
Chapter 25

John A. Paraskos, M.D.
Professor of Medicine
Director, Cardiovascular Center and Ambulatory
    Cardiology Service
UMass Memorial Health Care
Worcester, Massachusetts
Chapter 22

Marie T. Pavini, M.D., F.C.C.P.
Assistant Director
Department of Critical Care
Rutland Regional Medical Center
Rutland, Vermont
Chapter 15

Donald S. Prough, M.D.
Professor and Chair, Anesthesiology
The University of Texas Medical Branch
Galveston, Texas
Chapter 30

Juan Carlos Puyana, M.D.
Associate Professor of Surgery and Critical
    Care Medicine
University of Pittsburgh Medical Center Presbyterian
Pittsburgh, Pennsylvania
Chapter 15

Harvey Steven Reich, M.D., F.A.C.P., F.C.C.P.
Director, Critical Care Medicine
Rutland Regional Medical Center
Rutland, Vermont
Chapter 4

Ray Ritz, B.A., R.R.T., F.A.A.R.C.
Manager of Respiratory Care
Beth Israel Deaconess Medical Center
Boston, Massachusetts
Chapter 33

Kimberly A. Robinson, M.D., M.P.H.
Fellow
Division of Pulmonary, Allergy, and Critical
    Care Medicine
UMass Memorial Health Care
Worcester, Massachusetts
Chapter 11

Todd W. Sarge, M.D.
Instructor in Anaesthesia
Department of Anesthesia, Critical Care, and
    Pain Medicine
Beth Israel Deaconess Medical Center
Harvard Medical School
Boston, Massachusetts
Chapter 33

Michael G. Seneff, M.D.
Associate Professor
Critical Care Medicine Director, Intensive Care Unit
Department of Anesthesia
The George Washington University
Washington, D.C.
Chapters 2, 3

Arif Showkat, M.D.
Assistant Professor, Division of Nephrology
University of Tennessee
Memphis, Tennessee
Chapter 25

Nicholas A. Smyrnios, M.D., F.A.C.P., F.C.C.P.
Associate Professor of Medicine
Associate Chief, Division of Pulmonary, Allergy, and
    Critical Care Medicine
Director, Medical Intensive Care Units
University of Massachusetts Medical School
UMass Memorial Medical Center
Worcester, Massachusetts
Chapters 27, 28

Daniel Talmor, M.D., M.P.H.
Assistant Professor
Department of Anesthesia
Harvard Medical School
Beth Israel Deaconess Medical Center
Boston, Massachusetts
Chapters 31, 33

J. Matthias Walz, M.D.
Assistant Professor of Anesthesiology
Department of Anesthesiology
University of Massachusetts Medical School
UMass Memorial Health Care
Worcester, Massachusetts
Chapter 24

Wahid Wassef, M.D., F.A.C.G.
Associate Professor of Medicine
University of Massachusetts Medical School
Director of Endoscopy
Division of Gastroenterology
UMass Memorial Health Care
Worcester, Massachusetts
Chapter 13

John P. Weaver, M.D.
Chief, Division of Neurosurgery
UMass Memorial Health Care
Worcester, Massachusetts
Chapter 17

Mark M. Wilson, M.D.
Associate Professor
Division of Pulmonary, Allergy, and Critical
  Care Medicine
Associate Director
Medical Intensive Care Unit
University of Massachusetts Medical School
Worcester, Massachusetts
Chapter 10

PREFACE

We are pleased to offer the fourth edition of our book *Procedures, Techniques, and Minimally Invasive Monitoring in Intensive Care Medicine*. By updating all of the chapters and by adding an entirely new section on minimally invasive monitoring in the intensive care unit (ICU), we are confident that we have captured in this book all of the essential changes and advances that are needed by critical care specialists to provide state-of-the art, evidence-based care. Since the publication of the previous edition of our book, there have continued to be rapid advances occurring in every area of critical care medicine. The same can be said for the procedures, techniques, and monitoring used in our specialty, and all of these advances can be found in this edition.

Procedures, Techniques, and Minimally Invasive Monitoring in Intensive Care Medicine (fourth edition) represents an outgrowth of our textbook, *Irwin and Rippe's Intensive Care Medicine* (sixth edition). Since the initial publication of our comprehensive ICU textbook in 1985, discussion of procedures and techniques has always occupied a prominent role in the book. With each successive edition, each chapter has been updated as the procedures and techniques have been refined. During the last five years, because minimally invasive monitoring techniques have gained increasing importance, we decided to expand the subject matter of this text to include vitally important information on minimally invasive monitoring, as well as to maintain the focus on procedures and techniques. Readers of our sixth edition of *Irwin and Rippe's Intensive Care Medicine* as well as the fourth edition of this book will notice that the contents of this book mirror that of the first and second sections of our larger, comprehensive book of intensive care medicine. From previous editions, we learned that this smaller, more portable book was very useful to the critical care specialist and also emergency department physicians, surgeons, critical care nurses, residents in medicine, surgery, and anesthesia as well as medical students who either did not want to carry the larger book around with them, or who wanted a book focusing only on procedures, techniques, and noninvasive monitoring.

The fourth edition of *Procedures, Techniques, and Minimally Invasive Monitoring in Intensive Care Medicine* represents a completely updated text. Updated information with comprehensive diagrams and supporting evidence for efficacy and proper technique is contained in virtually every chapter of this book. Detailed illustrations are included that demonstrate how to perform each procedure, along with step-by-step instructions. Detailed, evidence-based discussions cover indications, contraindications, complications, equipment needed, and ongoing maintenance of equipment for common procedures, techniques, and monitoring modalities. *Every procedure and technique and minimally invasive monitoring modality that is required for certification in critical care or tested in internal medicine, surgical, or anesthesiology critical care board examinations is presented and discussed in depth.*

In this current edition, the reader will find comprehensive guidelines for most techniques and procedures performed in intensive care. Techniques such as pulmonary artery catheterization and endotracheal intubation should be mastered by all critical care physicians. Other procedures such as percutaneous cystotomy and percutaneous tracheotomy that were once performed by consulting specialists only are now increasingly performed by critical care practitioners. These have been included, along with detailed instructions. Other techniques that remain largely the domain of consulting specialists are also included because the intensivist must understand the indications, contraindications, likely results, and complications of these procedures.

New to this edition is a significant section comprising seven new chapters on minimally invasive monitoring. This includes not only routine monitoring, but such commonly employed techniques as indirect calorimetry, techniques of minimally invasive cardiology such as echocardiography, intracranial pressure monitoring, and other neurologic monitoring, as well as monitoring of the gastrointestinal tract and respiratory monitoring during mechanical ventilation. This entire section has been assembled under the expert guidance of a new member of our editorial team, Dr. Alan Lisbon.

Publication of a medical textbook is a team effort. The completion of *Procedures, Techniques, and Minimally Invasive Monitoring in Intensive Care Medicine* (fourth edition) would not have been possible without the expertise, talent, and hard work of many accomplished individuals. We continue to be blessed with wonderful friends, colleagues, and staff members who have played crucial roles at every stage of the preparation of this text. Special appreciation and thanks are due Elizabeth Grady,

Editorial Director of Dr. Rippe's laboratory. Beth embodies the principles of hard work, has superb organizational skills, and a solid background in medical publishing. She manages to retain her good humor despite the challenges of bringing multiple textbooks involving numerous contributors to completion. Karen Barrell and Cynthia French, assistants to Dr. Irwin, organize a very busy schedule to allow him time to complete this and many other editorial tasks. Marguerite Eckhouse, Administrative Assistant to Dr. Heard, helped facilitate every aspect of this project. We also appreciate the continued help of our Editor at Lippincott Williams & Wilkins, Brian Brown, who coordinates this and our other ICU book projects with guidance and great skill throughout the editorial process. Annette Ferran,

Nicole Dernoski, and Pamela Kilstein have all been instrumental in getting this book, as well as our textbook, published.

Finally, we wish to express our gratitude to our colleagues, students, and families, who continue to inspire, teach, and support us. We hope that this fourth edition of *Procedures, Techniques, and Minimally Invasive Monitoring in Intensive Care Medicine* will continue to guide the dedicated physicians who practice critical care and will advance the field of critical care medicine.

Richard S. Irwin, M.D., F.C.C.P.
James M. Rippe, M.D.
Alan Lisbon, M.D.
Stephen O. Heard, M.D.

Procedures, Techniques, and Minimally Invasive Monitoring in

Intensive Care Medicine

F O U R T H   E D I T I O N

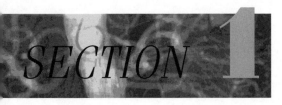

SECTION 1

PROCEDURES AND TECHNIQUES

Stephen O. Heard
Margaret M. Hudlin

Shubjeet Kaur
Stephen O. Heard

CHAPTER **1**

Airway Management and Endotracheal Intubation

In the emergency room and critical care environment, management of the airway to ensure optimal ventilation and oxygenation is of prime importance. Although initial efforts should be directed toward improving oxygenation and ventilation without intubating the patient [1], these interventions may fail and the placement of an endotracheal tube may be required. Although endotracheal intubation is best left to the trained specialist, emergencies often require that the procedure be performed before a specialist arrives. Because intubated patients are commonly seen in the intensive care unit (ICU) and coronary care unit, all physicians who work in these environments should be skilled in the techniques of airway management, endotracheal intubation, and management of intubated patients.

ANATOMY

An understanding of the techniques of endotracheal intubation and potential complications is based on knowledge of the anatomy of the respiratory passages [2]. Although a detailed anatomic description is beyond the scope of this book, an understanding of some features and relationships is essential to performing intubation.

NOSE

The roof of the nose is partially formed by the cribriform plate. The anatomic proximity of the roof to intracranial structures dictates that special caution be exercised during nasotracheal intubations. This is particularly true in patients with significant maxillofacial injuries.

The mucosa of the nose is provided with a rich blood supply from branches of the ophthalmic and maxillary arteries, which allow air to be warmed and humidified. Because the conchae provide an irregular, highly vascularized surface, they are particularly susceptible to trauma and subsequent hemorrhage. The orifices from the paranasal sinuses and nasolacrimal duct open onto the lateral wall. Blockage of these orifices by prolonged nasotracheal intubation may result in sinusitis [3].

MOUTH AND JAW

The mouth is formed inferiorly by the tongue, alveolar ridge, and mandible. The hard and soft palates compose the superior surface, and the oropharynx forms the posterior surface.

Assessment of the anatomic features of the mouth and jaw is essential before orotracheal intubation. A clear understanding of the anatomy is also essential when dealing with a patient who has a difficult airway and when learning how to insert newer airway devices such as the laryngeal mask airway (LMA; discussed in the section Management of the Difficult Airway).

NASOPHARYNX

The base of the skull forms the roof of the nasopharynx, and the soft palate forms the floor. The roof and the posterior walls of the nasopharynx contain lymphoid tissue (adenoids), which may become enlarged and compromise nasal airflow or become injured during nasal intubation, particularly in children. The eustachian tubes enter the nasopharynx on the lateral walls and may become blocked secondary to swelling during prolonged nasotracheal intubation.

OROPHARYNX

The soft palate defines the beginning of the oropharynx, which extends inferiorly to the epiglottis. The palatine tonsils protrude from the lateral walls and in children occasionally become so enlarged that exposure of the larynx for intubation becomes difficult. A large tongue can also cause oropharyngeal obstruction. Contraction of the genioglossus muscle normally moves the tongue forward to open the oropharyngeal passage during inspiration. Decreased tone of this muscle (e.g., in the anesthetized state) can cause obstruction. The oropharynx connects the posterior portion of the oral cavity to the hypopharynx.

HYPOPHARYNX

The epiglottis defines the superior border of the hypopharynx, and the beginning of the esophagus forms the inferior boundary. The larynx is anterior to the hypopharynx. The pyriform sinuses that extend around both sides of the larynx are part of the hypopharynx.

LARYNX

The larynx (Fig. 1-1) is bounded by the hypopharynx superiorly and is continuous with the trachea inferiorly. The thyroid, cricoid, epiglottic, cuneiform, corniculate, and arytenoid cartilages compose the laryngeal skeleton. The thyroid and cricoid

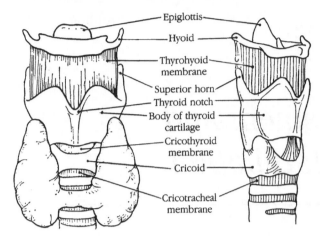

FIGURE 1-1. Anatomy of the larynx, anterior and lateral aspects. [From Ellis H: *Anatomy for Anaesthetists.* Oxford, Blackwell Scientific, 1963, with permission.]

cartilages are readily palpated in the anterior neck. The cricoid cartilage articulates with the thyroid cartilage and is joined to it by the cricothyroid ligament. When the patient's head is extended, the cricothyroid ligament can be pierced with a scalpel or large needle to provide an emergency airway (see Chapter 12). The cricoid cartilage completely encircles the airway. It is attached to the first cartilage ring of the trachea by the cricotracheal ligament. The anterior wall of the larynx is formed by the epiglottic cartilage, to which the arytenoid cartilages are attached. Fine muscles span the arytenoid and thyroid cartilages, as do the vocal cords. The true vocal cords and space between them are collectively termed the *glottis* (Fig. 1-2). The glottis is the narrowest space in the adult upper airway. In children, the cricoid cartilage defines the narrowest portion of the airway. Because normal phonation relies on the precise apposition of the true vocal cords, even a small lesion can cause hoarseness. Lymphatic drainage to the true vocal cords is sparse. Inflammation or swelling caused by tube irritation or trauma may take considerable time to resolve. The superior and recurrent laryngeal nerve branches of the vagus nerve innervate the structures of the larynx. The superior laryngeal nerve supplies sensory innervation from the inferior surface of the epiglottis to the superior surface of the vocal cords. From its takeoff from the vagus nerve, it passes deep to both branches of the carotid artery. A large internal branch pierces the thyrohyoid membrane just inferior to the greater cornu of the hyoid. This branch can be blocked with

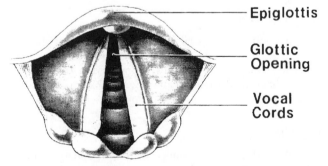

— **Epiglottis**

— **Glottic Opening**

— **Vocal Cords**

FIGURE 1-2. Superior view of the larynx (inspiration). [From Stoelting RH, Miller RD: *Basics of Anesthesia.* 2nd ed. New York, Churchill Livingstone, 1989, with permission.]

local anesthetics for oral or nasal intubations in awake patients. The recurrent laryngeal branch of the vagus nerve provides sensory innervation below the cords. It also supplies all the muscles of the larynx except the cricothyroid, which is innervated by the external branch of the superior laryngeal nerve.

TRACHEA

The adult trachea averages 15 cm long. Its external skeleton is composed of a series of C-shaped cartilages. It is bounded posteriorly by the esophagus and anteriorly for the first few cartilage rings by the thyroid gland. The trachea is lined with ciliated cells that secrete mucus; through the beating action of the cilia, foreign substances are propelled toward the larynx. The carina is located at the fourth thoracic vertebral level (of relevance when judging proper endotracheal tube positioning on chest radiograph). The right main bronchus takes off at a less acute angle than the left, making right main bronchial intubation more common if the endotracheal tube is in too far.

EMERGENCY AIRWAY MANAGEMENT

In an emergency situation, establishing adequate ventilation and oxygenation assumes primary importance [4]. Too frequently, inexperienced personnel believe that this requires immediate intubation; however, attempts at intubation may delay establishment of an adequate airway. Such efforts are time consuming, can produce hypoxemia and arrhythmias, and may induce bleeding and regurgitation, making subsequent attempts to intubate significantly more difficult and contributing to significant patient morbidity and even mortality [5,6]. Some simple techniques and principles of emergency airway management can play an important role until the arrival of an individual who is skilled at intubation.

AIRWAY OBSTRUCTION

Compromised ventilation often results from upper airway obstruction by the tongue, by substances retained in the mouth, or by laryngospasm. Relaxation of the tongue and jaw leading to a reduction in the space between the base of the tongue and the posterior pharyngeal wall is the most common cause of upper airway obstruction. Obstruction may be partial or complete. The latter is characterized by total lack of air exchange. The former is recognized by inspiratory stridor and retraction of neck and intercostal muscles. If respiration is inadequate, the head-tilt–chin-lift or jaw-thrust maneuver should be performed. In patients with suspected cervical spine injuries, the jaw-thrust maneuver (without the head tilt) may result in the least movement of the cervical spine. To perform the head-tilt maneuver, place a palm on the patient's forehead and apply pressure to extend the head about the atlantooccipital joint. To perform the chin lift place several fingers of the other hand in the submental area and lift the mandible. Care must be taken to avoid airway obstruction by pressing too firmly on the soft tissues in the submental area. To perform the jaw thrust lift up on the angles of the mandible [4] (Figure 1-3). Both of these maneuvers open the oropharyngeal passage. Laryngospasm can be treated by maintaining positive airway pressure using a face mask and bag valve device (see the following section). If the patient resumes spontaneous breathing, establishing this head position may constitute

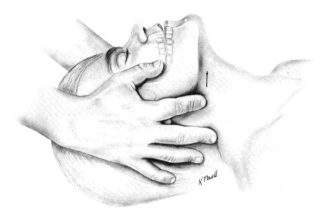

FIGURE 1-3. In an obtunded or comatose patient, the soft tissues of the oropharynx become relaxed and may obstruct the upper airway. Obstruction can be alleviated by placing the thumbs on the maxilla with the index fingers under the ramus of the mandible and rotating the mandible forward with pressure from the index fingers *(arrow)*. This maneuver brings the soft tissues forward and therefore frequently reduces the airway obstruction.

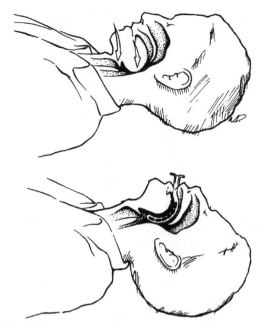

FIGURE 1-5. The mechanism of upper airway obstruction and the proper position of the oropharyngeal airway. [From *Textbook of Advanced Cardiac Life Support*. Dallas, American Heart Association, 1997, with permission.]

sufficient treatment. If obstruction persists, a check for foreign bodies, emesis, or secretions should be performed [7].

USE OF FACE MASK AND BAG VALVE DEVICE

If an adequate airway has been established and the patient is not breathing spontaneously, oxygen can be delivered via face mask and a bag valve device. It is important to establish a tight fit with the face mask, covering the patient's mouth and nose. To perform this procedure apply the mask initially to the bridge of the nose and draw it downward toward the mouth, using both hands. The operator stands at the patient's head and presses the mask onto the patient's face with the left hand. The thumb should be on the nasal portion of the mask, the index finger near the oral portion, and the rest of the fingers spread on the left side of the patient's mandible so as to pull it slightly forward. The bag is then alternately compressed and released with the right hand. A good airway is indicated by the rise and fall of the chest; moreover, lung-chest wall compliance can be estimated from the amount of pressure required to compress the bag. The minimum effective insufflation pressure should be

used to decrease the risk of insufflating the stomach with gas and subsequently increase the risk of aspiration.

AIRWAY ADJUNCTS

If proper positioning of the head and neck or clearance of foreign bodies and secretions fails to establish an adequate airway, several airway adjuncts may be helpful if an individual who is skilled in intubation is not immediately available. An oropharyngeal or nasopharyngeal airway occasionally helps to establish an adequate airway when proper head positioning alone is insufficient (Figs. 1-4 and 1-5). The oropharyngeal airway is semicircular and made of plastic or hard rubber. The two types are the Guedel airway, with a hollow tubular design, and the Berman airway, with airway channels along the sides. Both

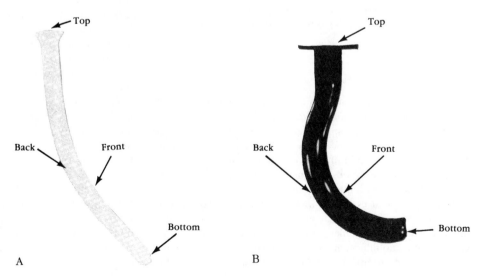

FIGURE 1-4. Nasopharyngeal **(A)** or oropharyngeal **(B)** airways can be used to relieve soft tissue obstruction if elevating the mandible proves ineffective.

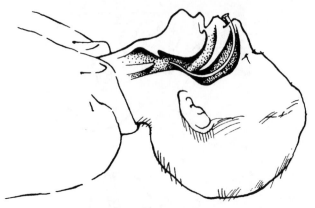

FIGURE 1-6. The proper position of the nasopharyngeal airway. [From *Textbook of Advanced Cardiac Life Support*. Dallas, American Heart Association, 1997, with permission.]

types are most easily inserted by turning the curved portion toward the palate as it enters the mouth. It is then advanced beyond the posterior portion of the tongue and rotated downward into the proper position (Fig. 1-5). Often, depressing the tongue or moving it laterally with a tongue blade helps to position the oropharyngeal airway. Care must be exercised not to push the tongue into the posterior pharynx, causing or exacerbating obstruction. Because insertion of the oropharyngeal airway can cause gagging or vomiting, or both, it should be used only in unconscious patients.

The nasopharyngeal airway is a soft tube approximately 15 cm long that is made of rubber or plastic (Figs. 1-4 and 1-6). It is inserted through the nostril into the posterior pharynx. Before insertion, the airway should be lubricated with an anesthetic gel, and, preferably, a vasoconstrictor should be administered into the nostril. The nasopharyngeal airway should not be used in patients with extensive facial trauma or cerebrospinal rhinorrhea, as it could be inserted through the cribriform plate into the brain.

INDICATIONS FOR INTUBATION

The indications for endotracheal intubation can be divided into four broad categories: (a) acute airway obstruction, (b) excessive pulmonary secretions or inability to clear secretions adequately, (c) loss of protective reflexes, and (d) respiratory failure [Table 1-1].

PREINTUBATION EVALUATION

Even in the most urgent situation, a rapid assessment of the patient's airway anatomy can expedite the choice of the proper route for intubation, the appropriate equipment, and the most useful precautions to be taken. In the less emergent situation, several minutes of preintubation evaluation can decrease the likelihood of complications and increase the probability of successful intubation with minimal trauma.

Anatomic structures of the upper airway, head, and neck must be examined, with particular attention to abnormalities that might preclude a particular route of intubation. Evaluation of cervical spine mobility, temporomandibular joint function, and dentition is important. Any abnormalities that might prohibit

TABLE 1-1. Indications for Endotracheal Intubation

Acute Airway Obstruction
  Trauma
    Mandible
    Larynx (direct or indirect injury)
  Inhalation
    Smoke
    Noxious chemicals
    Foreign bodies
  Infection
    Acute epiglottitis
    Croup
    Retropharyngeal abscess
  Hematoma
  Tumor
  Congenital anomalies
    Laryngeal web
    Supraglottic fusion
  Laryngeal edema
  Laryngeal spasm (anaphylactic response)
Access for suctioning
  Debilitated patients
  Copious Secretions
Loss of Protective Reflexes
  Head injury
  Drug overdose
  Cerebrovascular accident
Respiratory Failure
  Hypoxemia
    Acute respiratory distress syndrome
    Hypoventilation
    Atelectasis
    Secretions
    Pulmonary edema
  Hypercapnia
    Hypoventilation
    Neuromuscular failure
    Drug overdose

alignment of the oral, pharyngeal, and laryngeal axes should be noted.

Cervical spine mobility is assessed by flexion and extension of the neck (performed only after ascertaining that no cervical spine injury exists). The normal range of neck flexion-extension varies from 165 to 90 degrees, with the range decreasing approximately 20% by age 75 years. Conditions associated with decreased range of motion include any cause of degenerative disk disease (e.g., rheumatoid arthritis, osteoarthritis, ankylosing spondylitis), previous trauma, or age older than 70 years. Temporomandibular joint dysfunction can occur in any form of degenerative arthritis (particularly rheumatoid arthritis), in any condition that causes a receding mandible, and in rare conditions such as acromegaly.

Examination of the oral cavity is mandatory. Loose, missing, or chipped teeth and permanent bridgework are noted, and removable bridgework and dentures should be taken out. Mallampati et al. [8] (Fig. 1-7) developed a clinical indicator based on the size of the posterior aspect of the tongue relative to the size of the oral pharynx. The patient should be sitting, with the head fully extended, protruding the tongue and phonating [9]. When the faucial pillars, the uvula, the soft palate, and the posterior pharyngeal wall are well visualized, the airway is classified as class I, and a relatively easy intubation can be anticipated. When the faucial pillars and soft palate (class II) or soft palate only (class III) are visible, there is a greater chance of problems

L   Look externally
Look at the patient externally for characteristics that are known to cause difficult laryngoscopy, intubation or ventilation.

E   Evaluate the 3-3-2 rule
In order to allow alignment of the pharyngeal, laryngeal, and oral axes and therefore simple intubation, the following relationships should be observed. The distance between the patient's incisor teeth should be at least 3 finger breadths (3), the distance between the hyoid bone and the chin should be at least 3 finger breadths (3), and the distance between the thyroid notch and the floor of the mouth should be at least 2 finger breadths (2).

1 – Inter-incisor distance in fingers
2 – Hyoid mental distance in fingers
3 – Thyroid to floor of mouth in
    fingers

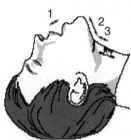

M   Mallampati
The hypopharynx should be visualized adequately. This has been done traditionally by assessing the Mallampati classification. The patient is sat upright, told to open the mouth fully and protrude the tongue as far as possible. The examiner then looks into the mouth with a light torch to assess the degree of hypopharynx visible. In the case of a supine patient, Mallampati score can be estimated by getting the patient to open the mouth fully and protrude the tongue and a laryngoscopy light can be shone into the hypopharynx from above.

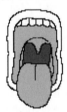 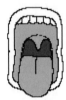 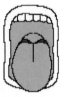

Class I: soft palate, uvula, fauces, pillars visible | Class II: soft palate, uvula, fauces visible | Class III: soft palate, base of uvula visible | Class IV: hard palate only visible

O   Obstruction?
Any condition that can cause obstruction of the airway will make laryngoscopy and ventilation difficult. Such conditions are epiglottis, peritonsillar abscesses, and trauma.

N   Neck mobility
This is a vital requirement for successful intubation. It can be assessed easily by getting the patient to place his or her chin down onto the chest and then to extend the neck so the patient is looking towards the ceiling. Patients in hard collar neck immobilization obviously have no neck movement and are therefore harder to intubate.

FIGURE 1-7.   The LEMON airway assessment method. [From Reed MJ, Dunn MJ, McKeown DW: Can an airway assessment score predict difficulty at intubation in the emergency department? *Emerg Med J* 2005;22(2): 99–102, 2005, with permission.]

visualizing the glottis during direct laryngoscopy. Difficulties in orotracheal intubation may also be anticipated if (a) the patient is an adult and cannot open his or her mouth more than 40 mm (two finger breadths), (b) the distance from the thyroid notch to the mandible is less than three finger breadths (less than or equal to 7 cm), (c) the patient has a high arched palate, or (d) the normal range of flexion-extension of the neck is decreased (less than or equal to 80 degrees) [10]. The positive predictive values of these tests alone or in combination are not particularly high; however, a straightforward intubation can be anticipated if the test results are negative [11]. However, in the emergency setting, only about 30% of airways can be assessed in this fashion [12]. A different evaluation method (LEMON) has been devised by Murphy and Walls [13]. LEMON stands for *l*ook, *e*valuate, *M*allampati class, *o*bstruction, and *n*eck mobility (Fig. 1-7). In the emergency setting, there are still limitations with the use of LEMON. However, using elements of LEMON that could be incorporated into the emergency evaluation of patients, Reed et al. [14] found that large incisors, a reduced interincisor distance, and a reduced distance between the thyroid and floor of the mouth were associated with a limited laryngoscopic view in emergency department patients.

EQUIPMENT FOR INTUBATION

Assembly of all appropriate equipment before attempted intubation can prevent potentially serious delays in the event of an unforeseen complication. Most equipment and supplies are readily available in the ICU but must be gathered so they are immediately at hand. A supply of 100% oxygen and a well-fitting mask with attached bag valve device are mandatory, as is suctioning equipment, including a large-bore tonsil suction attachment (Yankauer) and suction catheters. Adequate lighting facilitates airway visualization. The bed should be at the proper height, with the headboard removed and the wheels locked. Other necessary supplies include gloves, Magill forceps, oral and nasal airways, laryngoscope handle and blades (straight and curved), endotracheal tubes of various sizes, stylet, tongue depressors, a syringe for cuff inflation, and tape for securing the endotracheal tube in position. Table 1-2 is a checklist of supplies needed.

It is particularly important that an adequate number of personnel be available to assist the operator. Endotracheal intubation and emergency airway management are not one-person jobs. While the operator is performing a rapid preintubation assessment, ICU personnel should be gathering equipment. During and before intubation, a respiratory therapist should be present whose sole concerns should be assisting in airway control before intubation and providing adequate oxygenation. It is helpful to have another assistant present who is familiar with the procedure and equipment and who should be ready to hand items to the operator on request.

LARYNGOSCOPES

The two-piece laryngoscope has a handle containing batteries that power the bulb in the blade. The blade snaps securely into the top of the handle, making the electrical connection. Failure of the bulb to illuminate suggests improper blade positioning, bulb failure, a loose bulb, or dead batteries. Modern laryngoscope blades with fiberoptic lights obviate the problem of bulb failure. Many blade shapes and sizes are available. The two most commonly used blades are the curved (MacIntosh) and straight

TABLE 1-2. Equipment Needed for Intubation

Supply of 100% oxygen
Face mask
Bag valve device
Suction equipment
   Suction catheters
   Large-bore tonsil suction apparatus (Yankauer)
Stylet
Magill forceps
Oral airways
Nasal airways
Laryngoscope handle and blades (curved, straight; various sizes)
Endotracheal tubes (various sizes)
Tongue depressors
Syringe for cuff inflation
Headrest
Supplies for vasoconstriction and local anesthesia
Tape
Tincture of benzoin

(Miller) blades (Fig. 1-8). Although pediatric blades are available for use with the adult-sized handle, most anesthesiologists prefer a smaller handle for better control in the pediatric population. The choice of blade shape is a matter of personal preference and experience; however, one study has suggested that less force and head extension are required when performing direct laryngoscopy with a straight blade [15].

ENDOTRACHEAL TUBES

The internal diameter of the endotracheal tube is measured using both millimeters and French units. This number is stamped on the tube. Tubes are available in 0.5-mm increments, starting at 2.5 mm. Lengthwise dimensions are also marked on the tube in centimeters, beginning at the distal tracheal end.

Selection of the proper tube diameter is of utmost importance and is a frequently underemphasized consideration. The resistance to airflow varies with the fourth power of the radius of the endotracheal tube. Thus, selection of an inappropriately small tube can significantly increase the work of breathing. Moreover, certain diagnostic procedures (e.g., bronchoscopy) done through endotracheal tubes require appropriately large tubes (see Chapter 9). In general, the larger the patient, the larger the endotracheal tube that should be used. Approximate guidelines for tube sizes and lengths by age are summarized in Table 1-3. Most adults should be intubated with an endotracheal tube that has an inner diameter of at least 8.0 mm, although occasionally nasal intubation in a small adult requires a 7.0-mm tube.

ENDOTRACHEAL TUBE CUFF

Endotracheal tubes have low-pressure, high-volume cuffs to reduce the incidence of ischemia-related complications. Tracheal ischemia can occur any time cuff pressure exceeds capillary pressure (approximately 32 mm Hg), thereby causing inflammation, ulceration, infection, and dissolution of cartilaginous rings. Failure to recognize this progressive degeneration sometimes results in erosion through the tracheal wall (into the innominate artery if the erosion was anterior or the esophagus if the erosion was posterior) or long-term sequelae of tracheomalacia or tracheal stenosis. With cuff pressures of 15 to 30 mm Hg, the low-pressure, high-volume cuffs conform well to the tracheal wall and provide an adequate seal during positive-pressure ventilation. Although low cuff pressures can cause some damage (primarily ciliary denudation), major complications are rare. Nevertheless, it is important to realize that a low-pressure, high-volume cuff can be converted to a high-pressure cuff if sufficient quantities of air are injected into the cuff.

ANESTHESIA BEFORE INTUBATION

Because patients who require intubation often have a depressed level of consciousness, anesthesia is usually not required. If intubation must be performed on the alert, responsive patient, sedation or general anesthesia exposes the individual to potential pulmonary aspiration of gastric contents because protective reflexes are lost. This risk is a particularly important consideration if the patient has recently eaten and must be weighed against the risk of various hemodynamic derangements that may occur secondary to tracheal intubation and initiation of positive-pressure

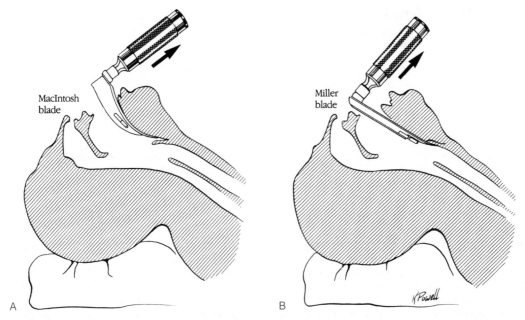

FIGURE 1-8.   The two basic types of laryngoscope blades, MacIntosh **(A)** and Miller **(B)**. The MacIntosh blade is curved. The blade tip is placed in the vallecula and the handle of the laryngoscope pulled forward at a 45-degree angle. This allows visualization of the epiglottis. The Miller blade is straight. The tip is placed posterior to the epiglottis, pinning the epiglottis between the base of the tongue and the straight laryngoscope blade. The motion on the laryngoscope handle is the same as that used with the MacIntosh blade.

ventilation. Laryngoscopy in an inadequately anesthetized patient can result in tachycardia and an increase in blood pressure. This may be well tolerated in younger patients but may be detrimental in a patient with coronary artery disease or raised ·intracranial pressure. Sometimes laryngoscopy and intubation may result in a vasovagal response, leading to bradycardia and hypotension. Initiation of positive-pressure ventilation in a hypovolemic patient can lead to hypotension from diminished venous return.

TABLE 1-3.   Dimensions of Endotracheal Tubes Based on Patient Age

Age	Internal Diameter (mm)	French Unit	Distance Between Lips and Location in Midtrachea of Distal End (cm)[a]
Premature	2.5	10–12	10
Full term	3.0	12–14	11
1–6 mo	3.5	16	11
6–12 mo	4.0	18	12
2 yr	4.5	20	13
4 yr	5.0	22	14
6 yr	5.5	24	15–16
8 yr	6.5	26	16–17
10 yr	7.0	28	17–18
12 yr	7.5	30	18–20
≥14 yr	8.0–9.0	32–36	20–24

[a]Add 2 to 3 cm for nasal tubes.
From Stoelting RK: Endotracheal intubation, in Miller RD (ed): *Anesthesia.* 2nd ed. New York, Churchill Livingstone, 1986, p 531, with permission.

Some of these responses can be attenuated by providing local anesthesia to the nares, mouth, and/or posterior pharynx before intubation. Topical lidocaine (1% to 4%) with phenylephrine (0.25%) or cocaine (4%, 200 mg total dose) can be used to anesthetize the nasal passages and provide local vasoconstriction. This allows the passage of a larger endotracheal tube with less likelihood of bleeding. Aqueous lidocaine-phenylephrine or cocaine can be administered via atomizer, nose dropper, or long cotton-tipped swabs inserted into the nares. Alternatively, viscous 2% lidocaine can be applied via a 3.5-mm endotracheal tube or small nasopharyngeal airway inserted into the nose. Anesthesia of the tongue and posterior pharynx can be accomplished with lidocaine spray (4% to 10%) administered via an atomizer or an eutectic mixture of local anesthetics (EMLA) cream applied on a tongue blade and oral airway [16]. Alternatively, the glossopharyngeal nerve can be blocked bilaterally with an injection of a local anesthetic, but this should be performed by experienced personnel.

Anesthetizing the larynx below the vocal cords before intubation is controversial. The cough reflex can be compromised, increasing the risk of aspiration. However, tracheal anesthesia may decrease the incidence of arrhythmias or untoward circulatory responses to intubation and improve patient tolerance of the endotracheal tube. Clinical judgment in this situation is necessary. Several methods can be used to anesthetize these structures. Transtracheal lidocaine (4%, 160 mg) is administered by cricothyroid membrane puncture with a small needle to anesthetize the trachea and larynx below the vocal cords. Alternatively, after exposure of the vocal cords with the laryngoscope, the cords can be sprayed with lidocaine via an atomizer. Aerosolized lidocaine (4%, 6 mL) provides excellent anesthesia to the mouth, pharynx, larynx, and trachea [17]. The superior laryngeal nerve can be blocked with 2 mL of 1.0% to 1.5%

TABLE 1-4. Drugs Used to Facilitate Intubation

Drug	IV Dose (mg/kg)	Onset of Action (sec)	Side Effects
Induction drugs			
Thiopental	2.5–4.5	20–50	Hypotension
Propofol	1.0–2.5	<60	Pain on injection
			Hypotension
Midazolam	0.02–0.20	30–60	Hypotension
Ketamine	0.5–2.0	30–60	Increases in intracranial pressure
			Increase in secretions
			Emergence reactions
Etomidate	0.2–0.3	20–50	Adrenal insufficiency
			Pain on injection
Muscle relaxants			
Succinylcholine	1–2	45–60	Hyperkalemia
			Increased intragastric pressure
			Increased intracranial pressure
Rocuronium	0.6–1.0	60–90	—

lidocaine injected just inferior to the greater cornu of the hyoid bone. The rate of absorption of lidocaine differs by method, being greater with the aerosol and transtracheal techniques. The patient should be observed for signs of lidocaine toxicity (circumoral paresthesia, agitation, and seizures).

If adequate topical anesthesia cannot be achieved or if the patient is not cooperative, general anesthesia may be required for intubation. Table 1-4 lists common drugs and doses that are used to facilitate intubation. Ketamine and etomidate are two drugs that are used commonly because cardiovascular stability is maintained. Use of opioids such as morphine, fentanyl, sufentanil, alfentanil, or remifentanil allow the dose of the induction drugs to be reduced and may attenuate the hemodynamic response to laryngoscopy and intubation. Muscle relaxants can be used to facilitate intubation, but unless the practitioner has extensive experience with these drugs and airway management, alternative means of airway control and oxygenation should be used until an anesthesiologist arrives to administer the anesthetic and perform the intubation.

Recent reviews have extolled the virtue of rapid sequence intubation (RSI) [18]: The process by which a drug such as etomidate, thiopental, ketamine, or propofol (Table 1-4) is administered to the patient to induce anesthesia and is followed immediately by a muscle relaxant to facilitate intubation. Although numerous studies exist in the emergency medicine literature attesting to the safety and efficacy of this approach, the practitioner who embarks on this route to intubation in the intensive care unit must be knowledgeable about the pharmacology and side effects of the agents used *and* the use of rescue methods should attempt(s) at intubation fail.

TECHNIQUES OF INTUBATION

In a true emergency, some of the preintubation evaluation is necessarily neglected in favor of rapid control of the airway. Attempts at tracheal intubation should not cause or exacerbate hypoxia. Whenever possible, an oxygen saturation monitor should be used. Preoxygenation (denitrogenation), which replaces the nitrogen in the patient's functional residual capacity with oxygen, can maximize the time available for intubation. During laryngoscopy, apneic oxygenation can occur from this reservoir. Preoxygenation is achieved by providing 100% oxygen at a high flow rate via a tight-fitting face mask for 3.5 to 4.0 minutes. In

patients who are being intubated for airway control, preoxygenation is usually efficacious; whereas, the value of preoxygenation in patients with acute lung injury is less certain [19]. In obese patients, use of the 25-degree head-up position improves the effectiveness of preoxygenation [20].

Just before intubation, the physician should assess the likelihood of success for each route of intubation, the urgency of the clinical situation, the likelihood that intubation will be prolonged, and the prospect of whether diagnostic or therapeutic procedures such as bronchoscopy will eventually be required. Factors that can affect patient comfort should also be weighed. In the unconscious patient in whom a secure airway must be established immediately, orotracheal intubation with direct visualization of the vocal cords is generally the preferred technique. In the conscious patient, blind nasotracheal intubation is often favored because it affords greater patient comfort. Nasotracheal intubation should be avoided in patients with coagulopathies or those who are anticoagulated for medical indications. In the trauma victim with extensive maxillary and mandibular fractures and inadequate ventilation or oxygenation, cricothyrotomy may be mandatory (see Chapter 12). In the patient with cervical spine injury or decreased neck mobility, intubation using the flexible bronchoscope or specialized laryngoscope (Bullard) may be necessary. Many of these techniques require considerable skill and should be performed only by those who are experienced in airway management [21].

SPECIFIC TECHNIQUES AND ROUTES OF ENDOTRACHEAL INTUBATION

Orotracheal Intubation

Orotracheal intubation is the technique most easily learned and most often used for emergency intubations in the ICU. Traditional teaching dictates that successful orotracheal intubation requires alignment of the oral, pharyngeal, and laryngeal axes by putting the patient in the "sniffing position" in which the neck is flexed and the head is slightly extended about the atlanto-occipital joint. However, a magnetic resonance imaging study has called this concept into question, as the alignment of these three axes could not be achieved in any of the three positions tested: neutral, simple extension, and the "sniffing position" [22]. In addition, a randomized study in elective surgery patients examining the utility of the sniffing position as a means to

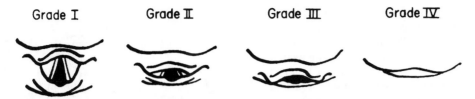

FIGURE 1-9.   The four grades of laryngeal view during direct laryngoscopy. Grade I: the entire glottis is seen. Grade II: only the posterior aspect of the glottis is seen. Grade III: only the epiglottis is seen. Grade IV: the epiglottis is not visualized. [From Cormack RS, Lehane J: Difficult tracheal intubation in obstetrics. *Anaesthesia* 39:1105–1111, 1984, with permission.]

facilitate orotracheal intubation failed to demonstrate that such positioning was superior to simple head extension [23].

In a patient with a full stomach, compressing the cricoid cartilage posteriorly against the vertebral body can occlude the esophagus. This technique, known as *Sellick's maneuver*, may prevent passive regurgitation of stomach contents into the trachea during intubation [24]. However, a recent magnetic resonance imaging (MRI) study of awake volunteers demonstrated that the esophagus was lateral to the larynx in more than 50% of the subjects. Moreover, cricoid pressure *increased* the incidence of an unopposed esophagus by 50% and caused airway compression of greater than 1 mm in 81% of the volunteers [25]. These findings are difficult to reconcile with data from cadaver studies demonstrating the efficacy of cricoid pressure [26] and clinical studies showing that gastric insufflation with gas during mask ventilation is reduced when cricoid pressure is applied [27]. Until more MRI studies are performed in anesthetized and/or paralyzed volunteers or patients, it is prudent to continue to use cricoid pressure in patients suspected of having full stomachs. In addition, placing the patient in the partial recumbent or reverse Trendelenburg position may reduce the risk of regurgitation and aspiration.

The laryngoscope handle is grasped in the left hand while the patient's mouth is opened with the gloved right hand. Often, when the head is extended in the unconscious patient, the mouth opens; if not, the thumb and index finger of the right hand are placed on the lower and upper incisors, respectively, and moved past each other in a scissorlike motion. The laryngoscope blade is inserted on the right side of the mouth and advanced to the base of the tongue, pushing it toward the left. If the straight blade is used, it should be extended below the epiglottis. If the curved blade is used, it is inserted in the vallecula.

With the blade in place, the operator should lift forward in a plane 45 degrees from the horizontal to expose the vocal cords (Figs. 1-2 and 1-8). This motion decreases the risk of the blade striking the upper incisors and either chipping or dislodging teeth. Both lips should be swept away from between the teeth and blade to avoid soft tissue damage. The endotracheal tube is then held in the right hand and inserted at the right corner of the patient's mouth in a plane that intersects with the laryngoscope blade at the level of the glottis. This prevents the endotracheal tube from obscuring the view of the vocal cords. The endotracheal tube is advanced through the vocal cords until the cuff just disappears from sight. The cuff is inflated with enough air to prevent a leak during positive-pressure ventilation with a bag valve device.

A classification grading the view of the laryngeal aperture during direct laryngoscopy has been described [28] and is depicted in Figure 1-9. Occasionally, the vocal cords cannot be seen entirely; only the corniculate and cuneiform tubercles, interarytenoid incisure, and posterior portion of the vocal cords or only the epiglottis is visualized (grades II to IV view, Fig. 1-9). In this situation, it is helpful to insert the soft metal stylet into the endotracheal tube and bend it into a hockey-stick configuration. The stylet should be bent or coiled at the proximal end to prevent the distal end from extending beyond the endotracheal tube and causing tissue damage. The stylet should be lubricated to ensure easy removal. The BURP maneuver (*b*ackward-*u*pward-*r*ightward *p*ressure on the larynx) improves the view of the laryngeal aperture [29]. Alternatively, a control-tip endotracheal tube can be used. This tube has a nylon cord running the length of the tube attached to a ring at the proximal end, which allows the operator to direct the tip of the tube anteriorly. Another aid is a stylet with a light (light wand). With the room lights dimmed, the endotracheal tube containing the lighted stylet is inserted into the oropharynx and advanced in the midline. When it is just superior to the larynx, a glow is seen over the anterior neck. The stylet is advanced into the trachea, and the tube is threaded over it. The light intensity is diminished if the wand enters the esophagus [30]. The gum elastic bougie (flexible stylet) is another alternative device that can be passed into the larynx; once in place, the endotracheal tube is advance over it and the stylet is removed. Endotracheal tubes and stylets are now available that have a fiberoptic bundle intrinsic to the tube or the stylet that can be attached to a video monitor. If the attempt to intubate is still unsuccessful, the algorithm that is described in the Management of the Difficult Airway section should be followed.

Proper depth of tube placement is clinically ascertained by observing symmetric expansion of both sides of the chest and auscultating equal breath sounds in both lungs. The stomach should also be auscultated to ensure that the esophagus has not been entered. If the tube has been advanced too far, it will lodge in one of the main bronchi (particularly the right bronchus), and only one lung will be ventilated. If this error goes unnoticed, the nonventilated lung may collapse. A useful rule of thumb for tube placement in adults of average size is that the incisors should be at the 23-cm mark in men and the 21-cm mark in women [31]. Alternatively, proper depth (5 cm above the carina) can be estimated using the following formula: (height in cm/5) minus 13 [32]. Palpation of the anterior trachea in the neck may detect cuff inflation as air is injected into the pilot tube and can serve as a means to ascertain correct tube position. Measurement of end-tidal carbon dioxide by standard capnography if available or by means of a calorimetric chemical detector of end-tidal carbon dioxide (e.g., Easy Cap II, Nellcor, Inc, Pleasanton, CA), can be used to verify correct endotracheal tube placement or detect esophageal intubation. The latter device is attached to the proximal end of the endotracheal tube and changes color on exposure to carbon dioxide. An additional method to detect esophageal intubation uses a bulb that attaches to the proximal end of the endotracheal tube [33]. The bulb is squeezed. If the tube is in the trachea, the bulb reexpands, and if the tube is in the esophagus, the bulb remains collapsed. It must be remembered that none of these techniques is foolproof. Bronchoscopy is the only method to be absolutely sure the tube is in the trachea. After estimating proper tube placement clinically, it should be confirmed by chest radiograph or bronchoscopy because the tube may be malpositioned. The tip of the endotracheal tube should be several centimeters above the carina (T-4 level). It must be remembered that flexion or extension of the head can advance or withdraw the tube 2 to 5 cm, respectively.

Nasotracheal Intubation

Many of the considerations concerning patient preparation and positioning outlined for orotracheal intubation apply to nasal intubation as well. Blind nasal intubation is more difficult to perform than oral intubation, because the tube cannot be observed directly as it passes between the vocal cords. However, nasal intubation is usually more comfortable for the patient and is generally preferable in the awake, conscious patient. Nasal intubation should not be attempted in patients with abnormal bleeding parameters, nasal polyps, extensive facial trauma, cerebrospinal rhinorrhea, sinusitis, or any anatomic abnormality that would inhibit atraumatic passage of the tube.

As previously discussed in the section Airway Adjuncts, after the operator has alternately occluded each nostril to ascertain that both are patent, a topical vasoconstrictor and anesthetic are applied to the nostril that will be intubated. The nostril may be dilated with lubricated nasal airways of increasing size to facilitate atraumatic passage of the endotracheal tube. The patient should be monitored with a pulse oximeter, and supplemental oxygen should be given as necessary. The patient may be either supine or sitting with the head extended in the sniffing position. The tube is guided slowly but firmly through the nostril to the posterior pharynx. Here the tube operator must continually monitor for the presence of air movement through the tube by listening for breath sounds with the ear near the open end of the tube. The tube must never be forced or pushed forward if breath sounds are lost, because damage to the retropharyngeal mucosa can result. If resistance is met, the tube should be withdrawn 1 to 2 cm and the patient's head repositioned (extended further or turned to either side). If the turn still cannot be negotiated, the other nostril or a smaller tube should be tried. Attempts at nasal intubation should be abandoned and oral intubation performed if these methods fail.

Once positioned in the oropharynx, the tube should be advanced to the glottis while listening for breath sounds through the tube. If breath sounds cease, the tube is withdrawn several centimeters until breath sounds resume, and the plane of entry is adjusted slightly. Passage through the vocal cords should be timed to coincide with inspiration. Entry of the tube into the larynx is signaled by an inability to speak. The cuff should be inflated and proper positioning of the tube ascertained as previously outlined.

Occasionally, blind nasal intubation cannot be accomplished. In this case, after adequate topical anesthesia, laryngoscopy can be used to visualize the vocal cords directly and Magill forceps used to grasp the distal end of the tube and guide it through the

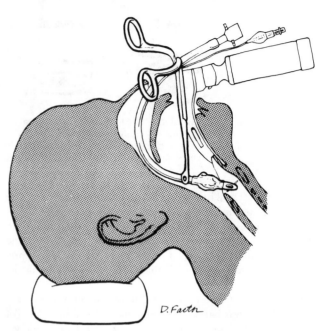

FIGURE 1-10.   Magill forceps may be required to guide the endotracheal tube into the larynx during nasotracheal intubation. [From Barash PG, Cullen BF, Stoelting RK: *Clinical Anesthesia.* 2nd ed. Philadelphia, JB Lippincott Co, 1992, with permission.]

vocal cords (Fig. 1-10). Assistance in pushing the tube forward is essential during this maneuver, so that the operator merely guides the tube. The balloon on the tube should not be grasped with the Magill forceps.

Occasionally, one may not be able to successfully place the endotracheal tube in the trachea. The technique of managing a difficult airway is detailed below.

MANAGEMENT OF THE DIFFICULT AIRWAY

A difficult airway may be recognized (anticipated) or unrecognized at the time of the initial preintubation airway evaluation. Difficulty managing the airway may be the result of abnormalities such as congenital hypoplasia, hyperplasia of the mandible or maxilla, or prominent incisors; injuries to the face or neck; acromegaly; tumors; and previous head and neck surgery. Difficulties ventilating the patient with a mask can be anticipated if two of the following factors are present: age older than 55 years, body mass index greater than 26 kg per m^2, beard, lack of teeth, and a history of snoring [34]. When a difficult airway is encountered, the algorithm as detailed in Figure 1-11 should be followed [35].

When a difficult airway is recognized before the patient is anesthetized, an awake tracheal intubation is usually the best option. Multiple techniques can be used and include (after adequate topical or local anesthesia) direct laryngoscopy, LMA (or variants), blind or bronchoscopic oral or nasal intubation, retrograde technique, rigid bronchoscopy, lighted stylet, or a surgical airway.

Flexible Bronchoscopic Intubation

Flexible bronchoscopy is an efficacious method of intubating the trachea in difficult cases. It may be particularly useful when the upper airway anatomy has been distorted by tumors, trauma,

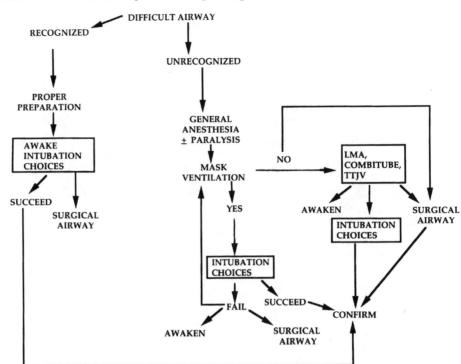

FIGURE 1-11. Modification of the difficult airway algorithm. Awake intubation choices include direct laryngoscopy with topical or local anesthesia, blind nasal intubation, flexible-assisted oral or nasal intubation, intubation through a laryngeal mask airway (LMA), or the retrograde technique. TTJV, transtracheal jet ventilation. [Adapted from Benumof JL: Laryngeal mask airway and the ASA difficult airway algorithm. *Anesthesiology* 84:686–699, 1996, with permission.]

endocrinopathies, or congenital anomalies. This technique is sometimes valuable in accident victims in whom a question of cervical spine injury exists and the patient's neck cannot be manipulated. An analogous situation exists in patients with severe degenerative disk disease of the neck or rheumatoid arthritis with markedly impaired neck mobility. After adequate topical anesthesia is obtained as described in the section Anesthesia before Intubation, the bronchoscope can be used to intubate the trachea via either the nasal or oral route. An appropriately sized warmed and lubricated endotracheal tube that has been preloaded onto the bronchoscope is advanced through the vocal cords into the trachea and positioned above the carina under direct vision. The flexible bronchoscope has also been used as a stent over which endotracheal tubes are exchanged and as a means to assess tracheal damage periodically during prolonged intubations. (A detailed discussion of bronchoscopy is found in Chapter 9.) Intubation by this technique requires skill and experience and is best performed by a fully trained operator.

If the operator is able to maintain mask ventilation in a patient with an unrecognized difficult airway, a call for experienced help should be initiated (Fig. 1-11). If mask ventilation cannot be maintained, a cannot ventilate–cannot intubate situation exists and immediate lifesaving rescue maneuvers are required. Options include an emergency cricothyrotomy or insertion of specialized airway devices, such as an LMA or a Combitube. (Puritan Bennett, Pleasanton, CA.)

Other Airway Adjuncts

The LMA is composed of a plastic tube attached to a shallow mask with an inflatable rim (Fig. 1-12). When properly inserted, it fits over the laryngeal inlet and allows positive-pressure ventilation of the lungs. Although aspiration can occur around the mask, the LMA can be lifesaving in a cannot ventilate–cannot

intubate situation. An intubating LMA (LMA-Fastrach, LMA North America, Inc, San Diego, CA) has a shorter plastic tube and can be used to provide ventilation as well as to intubate the trachea with or without the aid of a flexible bronchoscope (Fig. 1-13). The Combitube (Puritan Bennett, Pleasanton, CA, Fig. 1-14) combines the features of an endotracheal tube and an esophageal obturator airway and reduces the risk of aspiration. Personnel who are unskilled in airway management can easily learn how to use the LMA and the Combitube together [36].

Special rigid fiberoptic laryngoscopes (Bullard Elite Laryngoscope, ACMI Circon, Stamford, CT (Fig. 1-15) or the Upsher Laryngoscope, Mercury Medical, Clearwater, FL; see video at http://www.mercurymedical.com/images/mmp/icu_start.swf) are useful in patients with difficult airways. In addition, cervical spine extension appears to be reduced with their use [37]. The use of these laryngoscopes requires much more training and skill than the use of either the LMA or Combitube.

Cricothyrotomy

In a truly emergent situation, when intubation is unsuccessful, a cricothyrotomy may be required. The technique is described in detail in Chapter 12. The quickest method, needle cricothyrotomy, is accomplished by introducing a large-bore (i.e., 14-gauge) catheter into the airway through the cricothyroid membrane while aspirating with a syringe attached to the needle of the catheter. When air is aspirated, the needle is in the airway and the catheter is passed over the needle into the trachea. The needle is attached to a high-frequency jet ventilation apparatus. Alternatively, a 3-mL syringe barrel can be connected to the catheter. Following this, a 7-mm inside diameter endotracheal tube adapter is fitted into the syringe and is connected to a high-pressure gas source or a high-frequency jet ventilator (Fig. 1-16).

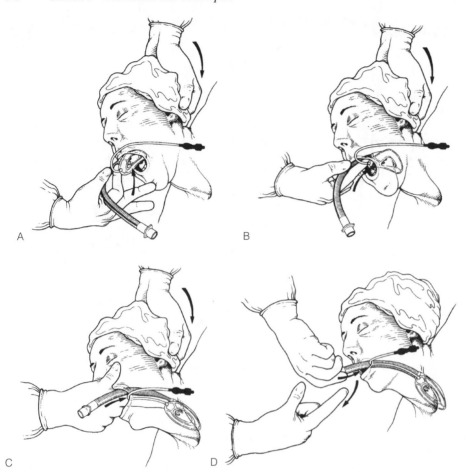

FIGURE 1-12. Technique for insertion of the laryngeal mask airway. [From Civetta JM, Taylor RW, Kirby RR: *Critical Care.* 3rd ed. Philadelphia, Lippincott–Raven Publishers, 1997, with permission.]

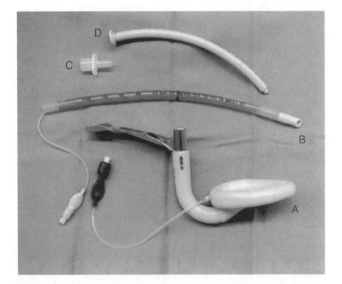

FIGURE 1-13. The laryngeal mask airway (LMA)-Fastrach **(A)** has a shorter tube than a conventional LMA. A special endotracheal tube **(B)** [without the adapter **(C)**] is advanced through the LMA-Fastrach into the trachea. The extender **(D)** is attached to the endotracheal tube, and the LMA-Fastrach is removed. After the extender is removed, the adapter is placed back on the tube.

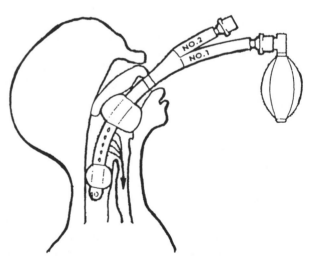

FIGURE 1-14. The proper placement of the Combitube. [Courtesy of Puritan Bennett, Pleasanton, CA, with permission.]

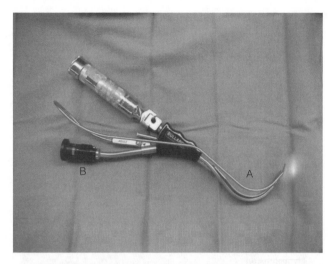

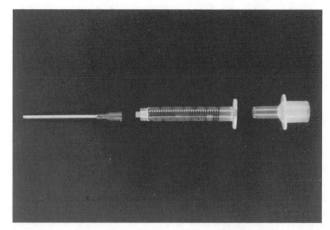

FIGURE 1-16. A needle cricothyrotomy set. A large-bore (14-gauge) catheter is inserted through the cricothyroid membrane. The needle is removed, and the catheter is attached to a 3-mL syringe barrel. A 7-mm endotracheal tube adapter is then attached to the syringe barrel. Alternatively, a 3-mm endotracheal tube adapter can be attached directly to the catheter.

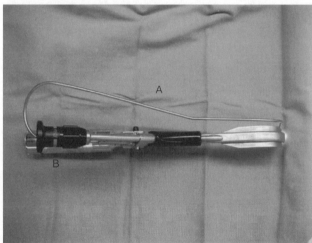

FIGURE 1-15. The Bullard laryngoscope. The endotracheal tube is loaded onto the stylet **(A)** and advanced into the trachea under visualization via the eyepiece **(B)**.

Management of the Airway in Patients with Suspected Cervical Spine Injury

Any patient with multiple trauma who requires intubation should be treated as if cervical spine injury were present. In the absence of severe maxillofacial trauma or cerebrospinal rhinorrhea, nasal intubation can be considered. However, in the profoundly hypoxemic or apneic patient, the orotracheal approach should be used. If oral intubation is required, an assistant should maintain the neck in the neutral position by ensuring axial stabilization of the head and neck as the patient is intubated [38]. A cervical collar also assists in immobilizing the cervical spine. In a patient with maxillofacial trauma and suspected cervical spine injury, retrograde intubation can be performed by puncturing the cricothyroid membrane with an 18-gauge catheter and threading a 125-cm Teflon-coated (0.025-cm diameter) guidewire through the catheter. The wire is advanced into the oral cavity, and the endotracheal tube is then advanced over the wire into the trachea. Alternatively, the wire can be threaded through the suction port of a 3.9-mm bronchoscope.

AIRWAY MANAGEMENT IN THE INTUBATED PATIENT

Securing the Tube

Properly securing the endotracheal tube in the desired position is important for three reasons: (a) to prevent accidental extubation, (b) to prevent advancement into one of the main bronchi, and (c) to minimize damage to the upper airway, larynx, and trachea caused by patient motion. The endotracheal tube is usually secured in place with adhesive tape wrapped around the tube and applied to the patient's cheeks. Tincture of benzoin sprayed on the skin provides greater fixation. Alternatively, tape, intravenous (IV) tubing, or umbilical tape can be tied to the endotracheal tube and brought around the patient's neck to secure the tube. Care must be taken to prevent occlusion of neck veins. Other products (e.g., Velcro straps) to secure the tube are available. A bite block can be positioned in patients who are orally intubated to prevent them from biting down on the tube and occluding it. Once the tube has been secured and its proper position verified, it should be plainly marked on the portion protruding from the patient's mouth or nose so that advancement can be noted.

Cuff Management

Although low-pressure cuffs have markedly reduced the incidence of complications related to tracheal ischemia, monitoring cuff pressures remains important. The cuff should be inflated just beyond the point where an audible air leak occurs. Maintenance of intracuff pressures between 17 and 23 mm Hg should allow an adequate seal to permit mechanical ventilation under most circumstances while not compromising blood flow to the tracheal mucosa. The intracuff pressure should be checked periodically by attaching a pressure gauge and syringe to the cuff port via a three-way stopcock. The need to add air continually to the cuff to maintain its seal with the tracheal wall indicates that (a) the cuff or pilot tube has a hole in it, (b) the pilot tube valve is broken or cracked, or (c) the tube is positioned incorrectly, and the cuff is between the vocal cords. The tube position should be reevaluated to exclude the latter possibility. If the valve is broken, attaching a three-way stopcock to it will solve the problem. If the valve housing is cracked, cutting the pilot tube and inserting a blunt needle with a stopcock into the lumen of the pilot tube can maintain a competent system. A hole in the cuff necessitates a change of tube.

Tube Suctioning

Routine suctioning should not be performed in patients in whom secretions are not a problem. Suctioning can produce a variety of complications, including hypoxemia, elevations in intracranial pressure, and serious ventricular arrhythmias. Preoxygenation should reduce the likelihood of arrhythmias. Closed ventilation suction systems (Stericath) may reduce the risk of hypoxemia and infection.

Humidification

Intubation of the trachea bypasses the normal upper airway structures responsible for heating and humidifying inspired air. It is thus essential that inspired air be heated and humidified.

Tube Replacement

At times, endotracheal tubes may need to be replaced because of an air leak, obstruction, or other problems. Before attempting to change an endotracheal tube, one should assess how difficult it will be. After obtaining appropriate topical anesthesia or IV sedation and achieving muscle relaxation, direct laryngoscopy can be performed to ascertain whether there will be difficulties in visualizing the vocal cords. If the cords can be seen, the defective tube is removed under direct visualization and reintubation performed using the new tube. If the cords cannot be seen on direct laryngoscopy, the tube can be changed over a long, plastic stylet (gum elastic bougie [Eschmann stylet]), an airway exchange catheter, or flexible bronchoscope. The airway exchange catheter (Cook Critical Care, Bloomington, IN) allows insufflation of oxygen via either standard oxygen tubing or a bag valve device [39]. The disadvantage to using the bronchoscope is that the old tube must be cut away with a scalpel before the new tube can be advanced into the trachea. In a patient with a large intrapulmonary shunt, severe hypoxemia might develop while the old tube is being replaced. Alternatively, the bronchoscope (with the new tube on it) can be advanced into the trachea next to (rather than through) the old endotracheal tube after deflating the cuff. The old tube is then withdrawn and the new tube positioned over the bronchoscope.

COMPLICATIONS OF ENDOTRACHEAL INTUBATION

Table 1-5 is a partial listing of the complications associated with endotracheal intubation. Factors implicated in the etiology of complications include tube size, characteristics of the tube and cuff, trauma during intubation, duration and route of intubation, metabolic or nutritional status of the patient, tube motion, and laryngeal motor activity.

During endotracheal intubation, traumatic injury can occur to any anatomic structure from the lips to the trachea. Possible complications include aspiration; damage to teeth and dental work; corneal abrasions; perforation or laceration of

TABLE 1-5.   Complications of Endotracheal Intubation

Complications during intubation
  Spinal cord injury
  Excessive delay of cardiopulmonary resuscitation
  Aspiration
  Damage to teeth and dental work
  Corneal abrasions
  Perforation or laceration of
    Pharynx
    Larynx
    Trachea
  Dislocation of an arytenoid cartilage
  Passage of endotracheal tube into cranial vault
  Epistaxis
  Cardiovascular problems
    Ventricular premature contractions
    Ventricular tachycardia
    Bradyarrhythmias
    Hypotension
    Hypertension
    Hypoxemia
  Complications while tube is in place
    Blockage or kinking of tube
    Dislodgment of tube
    Advancement of tube into a bronchus
    Mechanical damage to any upper airway structure
    Problems related to mechanical ventilation
Complications following extubation
  Immediate complications
    Laryngospasm
    Aspiration
  Intermediate and long-term complications
    Sore throat
    Ulcerations of lips, mouth, pharynx, or vocal cords
    Tongue numbness (hypoglossal nerve compression)
    Laryngitis
    Vocal cord paralysis (unilateral or bilateral)
    Laryngeal edema
    Laryngeal ulcerations
    Laryngeal granuloma
    Vocal cord synechiae
    Tracheal stenosis

the pharynx, larynx, or trachea; dislocation of an arytenoid cartilage; retropharyngeal perforation; epistaxis; hypoxemia; myocardial ischemia; laryngospasm with noncardiogenic pulmonary edema; and death [6,40]. Many of these complications can be avoided by paying careful attention to technique and ensuring that personnel with the greatest skill and experience perform the intubation.

COMPLICATIONS DURING INTUBATION

A variety of cardiovascular complications can accompany intubation. Ventricular arrhythmias have been reported in 5% to 10% of intubations. Ventricular tachycardia and ventricular fibrillation are uncommon but have been reported. Patients with myocardial ischemia are susceptible to ventricular arrhythmias, and lidocaine prophylaxis (100 mg IV bolus) before intubation may be warranted in such individuals. Bradyarrhythmias can also be observed and are probably caused by stimulation of the laryngeal branches of the vagus nerve. They may not require therapy but usually respond to IV atropine (1 mg IV bolus). Hypotension or hypertension can occur during intubation. In the patient with myocardial ischemia, short-acting agents to control blood pressure (nitroprusside) and heart rate (esmolol) during intubation may be needed.

COMPLICATIONS WHILE THE TUBE IS IN PLACE

Despite adherence to guidelines designed to minimize damage from endotracheal intubation, the tube can damage local structures. Microscopic alterations to the surface of the vocal cords can occur within 2 hours after intubation. Evidence of macroscopic damage can occur within 6 hours. As might be expected, clinically significant damage typically occurs when intubation is prolonged. The sudden appearance of blood in tracheal secretions suggests anterior erosion into overlying vascular structures, and the appearance of gastric contents suggests posterior erosion into the esophagus. Both situations require urgent bronchoscopy, and it is imperative that the mucosa underlying the cuff be examined. Other complications include tracheomalacia and stenosis and damage to the larynx. Failure to secure the endotracheal tube properly or patient agitation can contribute to mechanical damage.

Another complication is blockage or kinking of the tube, resulting in compromised ventilation. Placing a bite block in the patient's mouth can minimize occlusion of the tube caused by the patient biting down on it. Suctioning can usually solve blockage from secretions, although changing the tube may be necessary.

Unplanned extubation and endobronchial intubation are potentially life threatening. Judicious use of sedatives and analgesics and appropriately securing and marking the tube should minimize these problems. Daily chest radiographs with the head always in the same position can be used to assess the position of the tube. Other complications that occur while the tube is in position relate to mechanical ventilation (e.g., pneumothorax).

COMPLICATIONS AFTER EXTUBATION

Sore throat occurs after 40% to 100% of intubations. Using a smaller endotracheal tube may decrease the incidence of postextubation sore throat and hoarseness. Ulcerations of the lips, mouth, or pharynx can occur and are more common if the initial intubation was traumatic. Pressure from the endotracheal tube can traumatize the hypoglossal nerve, resulting in numbness of the tongue that can persist for 1 to 2 weeks. Irritation of the larynx appears to be due to local mucosal damage and occurs in as many as 45% of individuals after extubation. Unilateral or bilateral vocal cord paralysis is an uncommon but serious complication following extubation.

Some degree of laryngeal edema accompanies almost all endotracheal intubations. In adults, this is usually clinically insignificant. In children, however, even a small amount of edema can compromise the already small subglottic opening. In a newborn, 1 mm of laryngeal edema results in a 65% narrowing of the airway. Laryngeal ulcerations are commonly observed after extubation. They are more commonly located at the posterior portion of the vocal cords, where the endotracheal tube tends to rub. Ulcerations become increasingly common the longer the tube is left in place. The incidence of ulceration is decreased by the use of endotracheal tubes that conform to the anatomic shape of the larynx. Laryngeal granulomas and synechiae of the vocal cords are extremely rare, but these complications can se-

riously compromise airway patency. Surgical treatment is often required to treat these problems.

A feared late complication of endotracheal intubation is tracheal stenosis. This occurs much less frequently now that high-volume, low-pressure cuffs are routinely used. Symptoms can occur weeks to months after extubation. In mild cases, the patient may experience dyspnea or ineffective cough. If the airway is narrowed to less than 5 mm, the patient presents with stridor. Dilation may provide effective treatment, but in some instances surgical intervention is necessary.

EXTUBATION

The decision to extubate a patient is based on (a) a favorable clinical response to a carefully planned regimen of weaning from mechanical ventilation, (b) recovery of consciousness following anesthesia, or (c) sufficient resolution of the initial indications for intubation.

TECHNIQUE OF EXTUBATION

The patient should be alert, lying with the head of the bed elevated to at least a 45-degree angle. The posterior pharynx must be thoroughly suctioned. The procedure is explained to the patient. The cuff is deflated, and positive pressure is applied to expel any foreign material that has collected above the cuff as the tube is withdrawn. Supplemental oxygen is then provided.

In situations in which postextubation difficulties are anticipated, equipment for emergency reintubation should be assembled at the bedside. Some clinicians have advocated the "leak test" as a means to predict the risk of stridor after extubation. The utility of this procedure is limited in routine practice, but for patients with certain risk factors (e.g., traumatic intubation, prolonged intubation, previous accidental extubation), a leak volume of greater than 130 mL or 12% of the tidal volume has a sensitivity and specificity of 85% and 95% respectively for the development of postextubation stridor [41]. Probably the safest means to extubate the patient if there are concerns about airway edema or the potential need to reintubate a patient with a difficult airway is to use an airway exchange catheter (Cook Critical Care, Bloomington, IN) [39]. This device is inserted through the endotracheal tube, and then the tube is removed over the catheter. Supplemental oxygen can be provided via the catheter to the patient, and the catheter can be used as a stent for reintubation if necessary.

One of the most serious complications of extubation is laryngospasm, and it is more likely to occur if the patient is not fully conscious. The application of positive pressure can sometimes relieve laryngospasm. If this maneuver is not successful, a small dose of succinylcholine (by the IV or intramuscular route) can be administered. Succinylcholine can cause severe hyperkalemia in a variety of clinical settings; therefore, only clinicians who are experienced with its use should administer it. Ventilation with a mask and bag unit is needed until the patient has recovered from the succinylcholine.

TRACHEOSTOMY

In the past it was common to perform a tracheostomy to replace the endotracheal tube as soon as the need for prolonged airway control became apparent. Improvements in cuff design have permitted progressively longer periods of translaryngeal intubation. The optimal time of conversion from an endotracheal tube to a tracheostomy remains controversial, and decisions regarding the timing of tracheostomy should be based on the overall clinical situation. The reader is referred to Chapter 12 for details on tracheostomy.

REFERENCES

1. Caples SM, Gay PC: Noninvasive positive pressure ventilation in the intensive care unit: a concise review. *Crit Care Med* 33(11):2651–2658, 2005.
2. Snell RS, Katz J: *Clinical Anatomy for Anesthesiologists.* Norwalk, CT, Appleton and Lange, 1988.
3. Fassoulaki A, Pamouktsoglou P: Prolonged nasotracheal intubation and its association with inflammation of paranasal sinuses. *Anesth Analg* 69(1):50–52, 1989.
4. Fowler RA, Pearl RG: The airway: emergent management for nonanesthesiologists. *West J Med* 176(1):45–50, 2002.
5. Mort TC: The incidence and risk factors for cardiac arrest during emergency tracheal intubation: a justification for incorporating the ASA Guidelines in the remote location. *J Clin Anesth* 16(7):508–516, 2004.
6. Mort TC: Emergency tracheal intubation: complications associated with repeated laryngoscopic attempts. *Anesth Analg* 99(2):607–613, 2004.
7. 2005 American Heart Association guidelines for cardiopulmonary resuscitation and emergency cardiovascular care. *Circulation* 112(24):IV1–IV5, 2005.
8. Mallampati SR, Gatt SP, Gugino LD, et al: A clinical sign to predict difficult tracheal intubation: a prospective study. *Can Anaesth Soc J* 32(4):429–434, 1985.
9. Lewis M, Keramati S, Benumof JL, et al: What is the best way to determine oropharyngeal classification and mandibular space length to predict difficult laryngoscopy? *Anesthesiology* 81(1):69–75, 1994.
10. Gal TJ: Airway management, in Miller RD (ed): *Anesthesia.* 6th ed. Philadelphia, Churchill Livingstone, 2005, pp 1617–1652.
11. Tse JC, Rimm EB, Hussain A: Predicting difficult endotracheal intubation in surgical patients scheduled for general anesthesia: a prospective blind study. *Anesth Analg* 81(2):254–258, 1995.
12. Levitan RM, Everett WW, Ochroch EA: Limitations of difficult airway prediction in patients intubated in the emergency department. *Ann Emerg Med* 44(4):307–313, 2004.
13. Murphy MF, Walls RM: *Manual of Emergency Airway Management.* Chicago, Lippincott Williams & Wilkins, 2000.
14. Reed MJ, Dunn MJ, McKeown DW: Can an airway assessment score predict difficulty at intubation in the emergency department? *Emerg Med J* 22(2):99–102, 2005.
15. Hastings RH, Hon ED, Nghiem C, et al: Force, torque, and stress relaxation with direct laryngoscopy. *Anesth Analg* 82(3):456–461, 1996.
16. Larijani GE, Cypel D, Gratz I, et al: The efficacy and safety of EMLA cream for awake fiberoptic endotracheal intubation. *Anesth Analg* 91(4):1024–1026, 2000.
17. Venus B, Polassani V, Pham CG: Effects of aerosolized lidocaine on circulatory responses to laryngoscopy and tracheal intubation. *Crit Care Med* 12(4):391–394, 1984.
18. Reynolds SF, Heffner J: Airway management of the critically ill patient: rapid-sequence intubation. *Chest* 127(4):1397–1412, 2005.
19. Mort TC: Preoxygenation in critically ill patients requiring emergency tracheal intubation. *Crit Care Med* 33(11):2672–2675, 2005.
20. Dixon BJ, Dixon JB, Carden JR, et al: Preoxygenation is more effective in the 25 degrees head-up position than in the supine position in severely obese patients: a randomized controlled study. *Anesthesiology* 102(6):1110–1105; discussion 5A, 2005.
21. Hastings RH, Marks JD: Airway management for trauma patients with potential cervical spine injuries. *Anesth Analg* 73(4):471–482, 1991.
22. Adnet F, Borron SW, Dumas JL et al: Study of the "sniffing position" by magnetic resonance imaging. *Anesthesiology* 94(1):83–86, 2001.
23. Adnet F, Baillard C, Borron SW, et al: Randomized study comparing the "sniffing position" with simple head extension for laryngoscopic view in elective surgery patients. *Anesthesiology* 95(4):836–841, 2001.
24. Sellick BA: Cricoid pressure to control regurgitation of stomach contents during induction of anesthesia. *Lancet* 2:404, 1961.
25. Smith KJ, Dobranowski J, Yip G, et al: Cricoid pressure displaces the esophagus: an observational study using magnetic resonance imaging. *Anesthesiology* 99(1):60–64, 2003.
26. Salem MR, Joseph NJ, Heyman HJ, et al: Cricoid compression is effective in obliterating the esophageal lumen in the presence of a nasogastric tube. *Anesthesiology* 63(4):443–446, 1985.
27. Lawes EG, Campbell I, Mercer D: Inflation pressure, gastric insufflation and rapid sequence induction. *Br J Anaesth* 59(3):315–318, 1987.
28. Cormack RS, Lehane J: Difficult tracheal intubation in obstetrics. *Anaesthesia* 39(11):1105–1111, 1984.
29. Ulrich B, Listyo R, Gerig HJ, et al: The difficult intubation. The value of BURP and 3 predictive tests of difficult intubation. *Anaesthetist* 47(1):45–50, 1998.
30. Agro F, Hung OR, Cataldo R, et al: Lightwand intubation using the Trachlight: a brief review of current knowledge. *Can J Anaesth* 48(6):592–599, 2001.
31. Owen RL, Cheney FW: Endobronchial intubation: a preventable complication. *Anesthesiology* 67(2):255–257, 1987.
32. Cherng CH, Wong CS, Hsu CH, et al: Airway length in adults: estimation of the optimal endotracheal tube length for orotracheal intubation. *J Clin Anesth* 14(4):271–274, 2002.
33. Kasper CL, Deem S: The self-inflating bulb to detect esophageal intubation during emergency airway management. *Anesthesiology* 88(4):898–902, 1998.
34. Langeron O, Masso E, Huraux C, et al: Prediction of difficult mask ventilation. *Anesthesiology* 92(5):1229–1236, 2000.
35. Benumof JL: Laryngeal mask airway and the ASA difficult airway algorithm. *Anesthesiology* 84(3):686–699, 1996.
36. Yardy N, Hancox D, Strang T: A comparison of two airway aids for emergency use by unskilled personnel. The Combitube and laryngeal mask. *Anaesthesia* 54(2):181–183, 1999.
37. Watts AD, Gelb AW, Bach DB, et al: Comparison of the Bullard and Macintosh laryngoscopes for endotracheal intubation of patients with a potential cervical spine injury. *Anesthesiology* 87(6):1335–1342, 1997.
38. Criswell JC, Parr MJ, Nolan JP: Emergency airway management in patients with cervical spine injuries. *Anaesthesia* 49(10):900–903, 1994.
39. Loudermilk EP, Hartmannsgruber M, Stoltzfus DP, et al: A prospective study of the safety of tracheal extubation using a pediatric airway exchange catheter for patients with a known difficult airway. *Chest* 111(6):1660–1665, 1997.
40. Schwartz DE, Matthay MA, Cohen NH: Death and other complications of emergency airway management in critically ill adults. A prospective investigation of 297 tracheal intubations. *Anesthesiology* 82(2):367–376, 1995.
41. Jaber S, Chanques G, Matecki S, et al: Post-extubation stridor in intensive care unit patients. Risk factors evaluation and importance of the cuff-leak test. *Intensive Care Med* 29(1):69–74, 2003.

Scott A. Celinski
Michael G. Seneff

CHAPTER **2**

Central Venous Catheterization

Placement of central venous catheters (CVC) remains one of the most commonly performed procedures in the intensive care unit (ICU). Since the publication of the previous edition of this textbook, a significant milestone in CVC management was achieved with the report of a sustained zero incidence of catheter-related infection (CRI) in a clinical setting of a complicated medical-surgical ICU [1]. That experience was duplicated by several other medical-surgical ICUs across the state of Michigan participating in the Keystone Project. Of significant note, this zero incidence of CRI was primarily achieved not through new catheter technology but rather by adherence to strict catheter insertion and maintenance protocols. The implication is that any ICU can duplicate these experiences, independent of budget or specialty, using appropriate management and empowerment of bedside caregivers. Inexplicably, many ICUs still have not incorporated these protocols into standardized daily practices. In this chapter, we review the techniques and complications of the various routes available for central venous catheterization and present a strategy for catheter management that incorporates all of the recent advances.

INDICATIONS AND SITE SELECTION

Technical advances and a better understanding of anatomy have made insertion of central venous catheters easier and safer, but there is still an underappreciation of the inherent risks. Like any medical procedure, central venous catheterization has specific indications and should be reserved for the patient who has potential to benefit from it. After determining that CVC is necessary, physicians often proceed with catheterization at the site they are most experienced with, which might not be the most appropriate route in that particular patient. Table 2-1 lists general priorities in site selection for different indications of CVC; the final choice of site in a particular patient should vary based on individual institutional and operator experiences.

Volume resuscitation alone is not an indication for CVC. A 2.5-inch, 16-gauge catheter used to cannulate a peripheral vein can infuse twice the amount of fluid as an 8-inch, 16-gauge central venous catheter [2]. However, peripheral vein cannulation can be impossible in the hypovolemic, shocked individual. In this instance, the subclavian vein (SV) is the most reliable central site because it remains patent due to its fibrous attachments to the clavicle. Depending on the clinical situation, the femoral vein (FV) is a reasonable alternative, but the risk of deep venous thrombosis always needs to be considered [3–6].

Central venous access is often required for the infusion of irritant medications (concentrated potassium chloride) or va-soactive agents, certain diagnostic or therapeutic radiologic procedures, and in any patient for whom peripheral access is not possible.

Long-term total parenteral nutrition is best administered through SV catheters, which should be surgically implanted if appropriate. The internal jugular vein (IJV) is the preferred site for acute hemodialysis, and the SV should be avoided because of the relatively high incidence of subclavian stenosis following temporary dialysis, which then limits options for an AV fistula should long-term dialysis become necessary [7,8]. The FV is also suitable for acute short-term hemodialysis or plasmapheresis in nonambulatory patients [9].

Emergency transvenous pacemakers and flow-directed pulmonary artery catheters are best inserted through the right IJV because of the direct path to the right ventricle. This route is associated with the fewest catheter tip malpositions. For patients with coagulopathy, the external jugular vein (EJV) is an acceptable alternative, but we rarely find it necessary. The SV is an alternative second choice for pulmonary artery catheterization, even in many patients with coagulopathy [10], but the left SV is preferred to the right SV because of the less acute turns required to reach the heart. The reader is referred to Chapter 4 for additional information on the insertion and care of pulmonary artery catheters.

Preoperative CVC is desirable in a wide variety of clinical situations. One specific indication for preoperative right ventricular catheterization is the patient undergoing a posterior craniotomy or cervical laminectomy in the sitting position. These patients are at risk for air embolism, and the catheter can be used to aspirate air from the right ventricle [11]. Neurosurgery is the only common indication for an antecubital approach, as IJV catheters are in the operative field and theoretically can obstruct blood return from the cranial vault and increase intracranial pressure. Subclavian catheters are an excellent alternative for preoperative neurosurgical patients if pneumothorax is ruled out prior to induction of general anesthesia.

Venous access during cardiopulmonary resuscitation warrants special comment. Peripheral vein cannulation in circulatory arrest may prove impossible, and circulation times of drugs administered peripherally are prolonged when compared to central injection [12]. Drugs injected through femoral catheters also have a prolonged circulation time unless the catheter tip is advanced beyond the diaphragm, although the clinical significance of this is debated. Effective drug administration is an extremely important element of successful cardiopulmonary resuscitation; venous access should be established as quickly as possible, either peripherally or centrally if qualified personnel

TABLE 2-1. Indications for Central Venous Catheterization

Indication	Site Selection		
	1st	*2nd*	*3rd*
1. Pulmonary artery catheterization	RIJV	LSV	LIJV or LSV
with coagulopathy	EJV	IJV	FV
with pulmonary compromise or high-level positive end-expiratory pressure (PEEP)	RIJV	LIJV	EJV
2. Total parenteral nutrition (TPN)	SV	IJV	
Long term	SV (surgically implanted)	PICC	
3. Acute hemodialysis/plasmapheresis	IJV	FV	SV
4. Cardiopulmonary arrest	FV	SV	IJV
5. Emergency transvenous pacemaker	RIJV	SV	
6. Hypovolemia, inability to perform peripheral catheterization	SV or FV	IJV	
7. Preoperative preparation	IJV	SV	AV/PICC (Neurosurgical procedure)
8. General purpose venous access, vasoactive agents, caustic medications, radiologic procedures	SV	IJV/EJV	FV
with coagulopathy	FV	EJV	IJV
9. Emergency airway management	FV	SV	IJV
10. Inability to lie supine	FV	EJV	AV/PICC
11. Central venous oxygen satuation monitoring	SV	IJV	EJV
12. Fluid management of ARDS (CVP monitoring)	IJV	EJV	SV

AV, antecubital vein; CVP, central venous pressure; EJV, external jugular vein; FV, femoral vein; IJV, internal jugular vein; L, left; PICC, peripherally inserted central venous catheter; R, right; SV, subclavian vein.

are present. Prolonged attempts at arm vein cannulation are not warranted, and under these circumstances the FV is a good alternative because, despite the potential of longer drug circulation times, cardiopulmonary resuscitation (CPR) is interrupted the least with its placement. If circulation is not restored after administration of appropriate drugs and defibrillation, central access should be obtained by the most experienced operator available with a minimum interruption of CPR [13].

The placement of central venous catheters is now also specifically indicated for patients with severe sepsis, septic shock, or acute respiratory distress syndrome (ARDS), in order to monitor central venous oxygen saturation ($ScvO_2$) [14] and central venous pressure (CVP) [15]. Rivers et al. [14] showed a 16% absolute reduction of in-hospital mortality with early goal directed therapy for patients with severe sepsis, which included keeping the $ScvO_2$ greater than 70%. Early goal-directed therapy was subsequently shown to be achievable in "real world" settings [16]. For these patients, the relationship between superior vena caval and inferior vena caval oxygen saturations has not been elucidated; therefore, at this time we recommend superior vena caval catheterization through the SV, IJV, or EJV for this patient population. Likewise, the ARDS network recently reported that CVP monitoring utilizing a CVC is as effective as a pulmonary artery catheter in managing patients with acute lung injury and ARDS [15,17]. Since many of these patients are on high levels of positive end expiratory pressure (PEEP) and at high risk for complications from pneumothorax, the IJV or EJV represents the safest approach, especially in the absence of an experienced operator.

GENERAL CONSIDERATIONS AND COMPLICATIONS

General considerations for CVC independent of the site of insertion are catheter tip location, vascular erosions, catheter-associated thrombosis, air and catheter embolism, and coagulopathy, which are discussed below. Catheter-associated infection is discussed separately.

CATHETER TIP LOCATION

Catheter tip location is a very important consideration in CVC. The ideal location for the catheter tip is the distal innominate or proximal superior vena cava (SVC), 3 to 5 cm proximal to the caval-atrial junction. Positioning of the catheter tip within the right atrium or right ventricle should be avoided. Cardiac tamponade secondary to catheter tip perforation of the cardiac wall is uncommon, but two thirds of patients suffering this complication die [18]. Perforation likely results from vessel wall damage from infused solutions combined with catheter tip migration that occurs from the motion of the beating heart as well as patient arm and neck movements. Migration of catheter tips can be impressive: 5 to 10 cm with antecubital catheters and 1 to 5 cm with IJV or SV catheters [19,20]. Other complications from intracardiac catheter tip position include provocation of arrhythmias from mechanical irritation and infusion of caustic medications or unwarmed blood [21].

Correct placement of the catheter tip is relatively simple, beginning with an appreciation of anatomy. The caval-atrial junction is approximately 16 to 18 cm from right-sided skin punctures and 19 to 21 cm from left-sided insertions and is relatively independent of patient gender and body habitus [22,23]. Insertion of a standard triple-lumen catheter to its full 20 cm frequently places the tip within the heart, especially following right-sided insertions. A chest radiograph should be obtained following every initial central venous catheter insertion to ascertain catheter tip location and to detect complications. The right tracheobronchial angle is the most reliable landmark on plain film chest radiograph for the upper margin of the SVC and is always at least 2.9 cm above the caval-atrial junction. The catheter tip should lie about 1 cm below this landmark, and above the right upper cardiac silhouette to ensure placement outside of the pericardium [24].

VASCULAR EROSIONS

Large-vessel perforations secondary to central venous catheters are uncommon and often not immediately recognized. Vessel perforation typically occurs 1 to 7 days after catheter insertion. Patients usually present with sudden onset of dyspnea and often with new pleural effusions on chest radiograph [25]. Catheter stiffness, position of the tip within the vessel, and the site of insertion are important factors causing vessel perforation. The relative importance of these variables is unknown. Repeated irritation of the vessel wall by a stiff catheter tip or infusion of hyperosmolar solutions may be the initiating event. Vascular erosions are more common with left IJV and EJV catheters, because for anatomical reasons the catheter tip is more likely to be positioned laterally under tension against the SVC wall [26]. Positioning of the catheter tip within the vein parallel to the vessel wall must be confirmed on chest radiograph. Free aspiration of blood from one of the catheter ports is not always sufficient to rule out a vascular perforation.

AIR AND CATHETER EMBOLISM

Significant air and catheter embolism are rare and preventable complications of CVC. Catheter embolism can occur at the time of insertion when a catheter-through- or over-needle technique is used and the operator withdraws the catheter without simultaneously retracting the needle. It more commonly occurs with antecubital or femoral catheters after insertion, because they are prone to breakage when the agitated patient vigorously bends an arm or leg. Prevention, recognition, and management of catheter embolism are covered in detail elsewhere [27].

Air embolism is of greater clinical importance, often goes undiagnosed, and may prove fatal [28,29]. This complication is totally preventable with compulsive attention to proper catheter insertion and maintenance. Factors resulting in air embolism during insertion are well known, and methods to increase venous pressure, such as use of the Trendelenburg position, should not be forgotten. In modern ICUs, catheter disconnect or passage of air through a patent tract *after* catheter removal are more common causes of catheter-associated air embolism. An air embolus should be suspected in any patient with an indwelling or

recently discontinued CVC who develops sudden unexplained hypoxemia or cardiovascular collapse, often after being moved out of bed or to a stretcher. A characteristic mill wheel sound may be auscultated over the precordium. Treatment involves placing the patient in the left lateral decubitus position and using the catheter to aspirate air from the right ventricle. Hyperbaric oxygen therapy to reduce bubble size has a controversial role in treatment [28]. The best treatment is prevention, and prevention can be most effectively achieved through comprehensive nursing and physician-in-training educational modules and proper supervision of inexperienced operators [29]. Discontinuation of catheters should always be done with the patient supine.

COAGULOPATHY

Central venous access in the patient with a bleeding diathesis is problematic. The SV and IJV routes have increased risks in the presence of coagulopathy, but it is not known at what degree of abnormality the risk becomes unacceptable. A coagulopathy is generally defined as an international normalization ratio (INR) greater than 1.5 or platelet count less than 50,000. Thrombocytopenia is probably a greater risk than prolonged coagulation times. Although it is clear that safe venipuncture is possible with greater degrees of coagulopathy [10,30], even with the subclavian approach, the literature is also fraught with case reports of serious hemorrhagic complications. In patients with severe coagulopathy, the EJV is an alternative for central venous access, especially pulmonary artery catheterization, while the FV offers a safe alternative for general-purpose venous access. In appropriate patients, peripherally inserted central venous catheter (PICC) is useful. If these sites cannot be used, the IJV is the best alternative.

THROMBOSIS

Catheter-related thrombosis is very common but usually of little clinical significance. The spectrum of thrombotic complications includes a fibrin sleeve surrounding the catheter from its point of entry into the vein distal to the tip, to mural thrombus, a clot that forms on the wall of the vein secondary to mechanical or chemical irritation, or occlusive thrombus, which blocks flow and may result in collateral formation. All of these lesions are usually clinically silent; therefore, studies that do not use venography or color flow Doppler imaging to confirm the diagnosis underestimate its incidence. Using venography, fibrin sleeve formation can be documented in a majority of catheters, mural thrombi in 10% to 30%, and occlusive thrombi in 0% to 10% [31–37]. In contrast, clinical symptoms of thrombosis occur in only 0% to 3% of patients [6,32]. The incidence of thrombosis probably increases with duration of catheterization but does not appear reliably related to the site of insertion [6,31–37]. However, femoral vein catheter-associated thrombosis in the lower extremity is almost certainly more clinically important than upper extremity thrombosis caused by IJ and SV catheters [3–5]. The presence of catheter-associated thrombosis is also associated with a higher incidence of infection [36,37].

Catheter design and composition impact the frequency of thrombotic complications. The ideal catheter material is nonthrombogenic and relatively stiff at room temperature to facilitate percutaneous insertion, yet soft and pliable at body temperature to minimize intravascular mechanical trauma. Not all studies are consistent, but polyurethane, especially when coated with hydromer, appears to be the best material available for bedside catheter insertions [32,38,39]. Silastic catheters have low thrombogenicity but must be surgically implanted, and pressure monitoring may not be possible. Heparin bonding of catheters decreases thrombogenicity and also appears to decrease the rate of catheter related infections [40]. Low dose heparin infused through the catheter or administered subcutaneously and very-low-dose warfarin therapy also decrease the incidence of venogram-proven and clinically apparent thrombosis [41].

ROUTES OF CENTRAL VENOUS CANNULATION

ANTECUBITAL APPROACH

The antecubital veins are used in the ICU for CVC with PICC and midline catheters. Use of PICCs in critically ill adults is limited by lack of surface anatomy in obese and edematous patients, lack of technological versatility (i.e., limited pressure monitoring [42], small lumens, and no triple-lumen capability), and increased time and decreased predictability of bedside insertion. PICCs are potentially useful in highly selected ICU patients undergoing neurosurgery, with coagulopathy, or in the rehabilitative phase of critical illness for whom general purpose central venous access is required for parenteral nutrition or long-term medication access (see Table 2-1) [43,44]. The technique of percutaneous insertion of these catheters using the basilic, cephalic, or brachial vein is described below.

Anatomy

The basilic vein is formed at the ulnar aspect of the dorsal venous network of the hand (Fig. 2-1). It may be found in the medial part of the antecubital fossa, where it is usually joined by the median basilic vein. It then ascends in the groove between the biceps brachii and pronator teres on the medial aspect of the arm to perforate the deep fascia distal to the midportion of the arm, where it joins the brachial vein to become the axillary vein. The basilic vein is preferred for CVC because it is almost always of substantial size and the anatomy is predictable; since the axillary vein is a direct continuation of it, the basilic vein provides an unimpeded path to the central venous circulation [45,46].

The cephalic vein begins in the radial aspect of the dorsal venous network of the hand and ascends around the radial border of the forearm (see Fig. 2-1). In the lateral aspect of the antecubital fossa, it forms an anastomosis with the median basilic vein and then ascends the lateral part of the arm in the groove along the lateral border of the biceps brachii. It pierces the clavipectoral fascia in the deltopectoral triangle and empties into the proximal part of the axillary vein caudal to the clavicle. The variability of the cephalic vein anatomy renders it less suitable than the basilic vein for CVC. It joins the axillary vein at nearly a right angle, which can be difficult for a catheter to traverse. Instead of passing beneath the clavicle, the cephalic vein may pass through the clavicle, compressing the vein and making catheter passage impossible. Furthermore, in a significant percentage of cases, the cephalic does not empty into the axillary vein but divides into smaller branches or a venous plexus, which empties

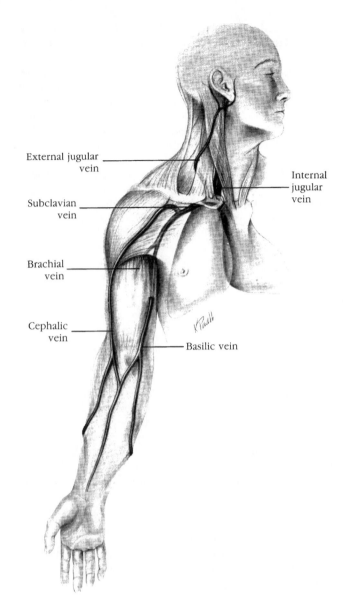

FIGURE 2-1. Venous anatomy of the upper extremity. The internal jugular, external jugular, and subclavian veins are also shown.

into the ipsilateral EJV. The cephalic vein may also simply terminate or become attenuated just proximal to the antecubital fossa [45,46].

Technique of Cannulation

Several kits are available for antecubital CVC. The PICC and midline catheters are made of silicone or polyurethane and, depending on catheter stiffness and size, are usually placed through an introducer. The method described below is for a PICC catheter inserted through a tear-away introducer.

The right basilic vein should be selected for the initial attempt at CVC because of the above anatomical considerations and clinical studies that confirm a higher success rate with the basilic than the cephalic vein [47]. The success rates from either arm are comparable, though the catheter must traverse a greater distance from the left. With the patient's arm at his or her side, the antecubital fossa is prepared and draped, adhering to strict aseptic technique. A tourniquet is placed proximally and if an appropriate vein is not part of the surface anatomy, we use a portable ultrasound device to identify the basilic or its main branches. After local anesthesia, venipuncture is performed with the thin-wall entry needle proximal to the antecubital crease to avoid catheter breakage and embolism. When free backflow of venous blood is confirmed, the tourniquet is released and the guidewire carefully threaded into the vein for a distance of 15 to 20 cm. Leaving the guidewire in place, the thin-wall needle is withdrawn and the puncture site enlarged with a scalpel blade. The sheath-introducer assembly is then threaded over the guidewire with a twisting motion, and the guidewire is removed. Next, leaving the sheath in place, the dilator is removed, and the introducer is now ready for PICC insertion. The length of insertion is estimated by measuring the distance along the predicted vein path from the venipuncture site to the manubriosternal junction, using the measuring tape provided in the kit. The PICC is supplied with an inner obturator that provides stiffness for insertion, which must be inserted into the PICC after it has been flushed and before insertion. After measurement, the PICC is trimmed to the desired length, and the obturator is inserted into the PICC and advanced until the tips are equal. The PICC/obturator is then inserted through the introducer to the appropriate distance, the introducer peeled away, and the obturator removed. The PICC is then secured in place and a chest radiograph is obtained to determine tip position.

If resistance to advancing the PICC is met, options are limited. Techniques such as abducting the arm are of limited value. If a catheter-through or over-needle device has been used, the catheter must never be withdrawn without simultaneously retracting the needle to avoid catheter shearing and embolism. If the catheter cannot be advanced easily, another site should be chosen.

Success Rate and Complications

Using the above technique the PICC has a 75% to 95% successful placement rate, and success is increased with operator experience, identification of a large vein, or the use of fluoroscopy [43,44,48]. Overall, PICCs appear to be at least as safe as CVCs, but frequent occlusions and impaired flow are a significant limitation. Important complications include sterile phlebitis, thrombosis (especially of the SV and IJV), infection, limb edema, and pericardial tamponade. Phlebitis may be more common with antecubital central venous catheters, probably due to less blood flow in these veins as well as the proximity of the venipuncture site to the skin [49,50]. The risk of pericardial tamponade may also be increased if the catheter tip is inserted too deep because of greater catheter tip migration occurring with arm movements [51]. Complications are minimized by strict adherence to recommended techniques for catheter placement and care.

INTERNAL-EXTERNAL JUGULAR APPROACH

Pediatricians used the IJV for venous access long before Hermosura et al. [52] described the technique and advocated its use in adults in 1966. The first large series on IJV catheterization appeared in 1969, when English et al. [53] reported on 500 percutaneous IJV catheterizations. Reports confirming this route's efficiency and low complication rate followed, and it has remained a popular site for central venous access.

Anatomy

The IJV emerges from the base of the skull through the jugular foramen and enters the carotid sheath dorsally with the internal carotid artery (ICA) (see Fig. 2-1). It then courses posterolaterally to the artery and runs beneath the sternocleidomastoid (SCM) muscle. The vein lies medial to the anterior portion of the SCM muscle superiorly, then runs beneath the triangle formed by the two heads of the muscle in its medial portion before entering the SV near the medial border of the anterior scalene muscle at the sternal border of the clavicle. The junction of the right IJV (which averages 2 to 3 cm in diameter) with the right SV forming the innominate vein follows a straight path to the SVC. As a result, malpositions and looping of a catheter inserted through the right IJV are unusual. In contrast, a catheter passed through the left IJV must negotiate a sharp turn at the left jugulosubclavian junction, which results in a greater percentage of catheter malpositions [54]. This sharp turn may also produce tension and torque at the catheter tip, resulting in a higher incidence of vessel erosion [25,26].

Knowledge of the structures neighboring the IJV is essential as they may be compromised by a misdirected needle. The ICA runs medial to the IJV but, rarely, may lie directly posterior or anterior. Behind the ICA, just outside the sheath, lie the stellate ganglion and the cervical sympathetic trunk. The dome of the pleura, which is higher on the left, lies caudal to the junction of the IJV and SV. Posteriorly, at the root of the neck, course the phrenic and vagus nerves [45,46]. The thoracic duct lies behind the left IJV and enters the superior margin of the SV near the jugulosubclavian junction. The right lymphatic duct has the same anatomical relationship but is much smaller, and chylous effusions typically occur only with left-sided IJV cannulations.

Techniques of Cannulation

Internal jugular venipuncture may be accomplished by a variety of methods; all methods use the same landmarks but differ in the site of venipuncture or orientation of the needle. Defalque [55] grouped the methods into three general approaches: anterior, central, and posterior (Fig. 2-2). We prefer the central approach for the initial attempt, but the method chosen varies with the institution and the operator's experience. All approaches require identical equipment, and the operator may choose from many different catheters and prepackaged kits.

Standard triple-lumen catheter kits include the equivalent of a 7-French (Fr) triple-lumen catheter with 15 (recommended), 20, or 30 cm of usable length, a 0.032-inch diameter guidewire with straight and J tip, an 18-gauge thin-wall needle, an 18-gauge catheter-over-needle, a 7-Fr vessel dilator, a 22-gauge "finder" needle, and appropriate syringes and suture material. Preparation of the guidewire and catheter prior to insertion is important; all lumina should be flushed with saline and the cap to the distal lumen removed. The patient is placed in a 15-degree Trendelenburg position to distend the vein and minimize the risk of air embolism, with the head turned gently to the contralateral side. The surface anatomy is identified, especially the angle of the mandible, the two heads of the SCM, the clavicle, the EJV, and the trachea (see Fig. 2-2). The neck is then prepared with chlorhexidine and fully draped, with the operator wearing a hat, mask, sterile gown, and gloves. It is recommended that all

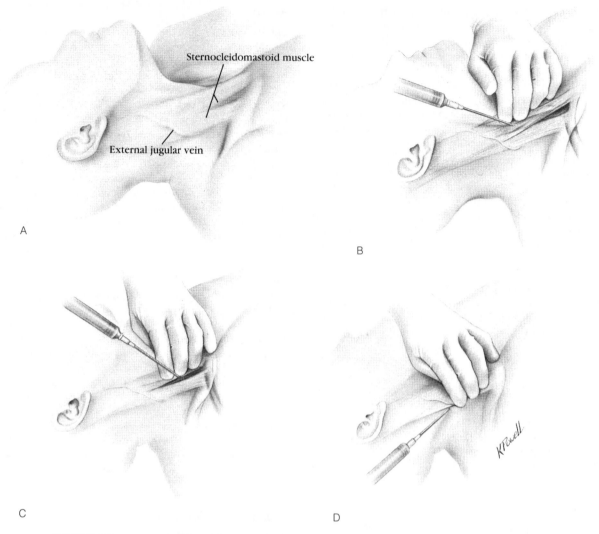

FIGURE 2-2.   Surface anatomy and various approaches to cannulation of the internal jugular vein. **A:** Surface anatomy. **B:** Anterior approach. **C:** Central approach. **D:** Posterior approach.

catheter preparation be performed prior to draping the patient, as they often develop a sense of claustrophobia with draping.

For the central approach [55], skin puncture is at the apex of the triangle formed by the two muscle bellies of the SCM and the clavicle. The ICA pulsation is usually felt 1 to 2 cm medial to this point, beneath or just medial to the sternal head of the SCM. The skin at the apex of the triangle is infiltrated with 1% lidocaine using the smallest needle available. Use of a small-bore finder needle to locate the IJV should prevent unintentional ICA puncture and unnecessary probing with a larger-bore needle. To avoid collapsing the IJV, the operator should maintain minimal to no pressure on the ICA with the left hand and insert the finder needle with the right hand at the apex of the triangle at a 45-degree angle with the frontal plane, directed at the ipsilateral nipple. The needle is advanced steadily with constant negative pressure in the syringe, and venipuncture occurs within 1 to 5 cm. If venipuncture does not occur on the initial forward thrust, negative pressure should be maintained and the needle slowly withdrawn, as often, the needle will compress the vein on the forward thrust, penetrating the back wall without

blood return. Once the needle is pulled back past the posterior wall of the vessel, it achieves free flow of blood from the vessel. If the first attempt is unsuccessful, the operator should reassess patient position, landmarks, and techniques to ensure that he or she is not doing anything to decrease IJV lumen size (see below). Subsequent attempts may be directed slightly laterally or medially to the initial thrust, as long as the plane of the ICA is not violated. If venipuncture does not occur after three to five attempts, further attempts are unlikely to be successful and only increase complications [56–58].

When venipuncture has occurred with the finder needle, the operator can either withdraw the finder needle and introduce the large-bore needle in the identical plane or leave the finder needle in place and introduce the larger needle directly above it. Leaving the finder needle in place has been shown to facilitate successful puncture with the introducer needle [59]. Many kits provide both an 18-gauge thin-wall needle through which a guidewire can be directly introduced and a 16-gauge catheter-over-needle device. With the latter apparatus, the catheter is threaded over the needle into the vein, the needle withdrawn, and the guidewire inserted through the catheter. Both techniques are effective; the choice is strictly a matter of operator preference. Regardless of which large-bore needle is used, once venipuncture has occurred, the syringe is removed after ensuring that the backflow of blood is not pulsatile and the hub is then occluded with a finger to prevent air embolism or excessive bleeding. The guidewire, with the J-tip oriented appropriately, is then inserted and should pass freely up to 20 cm, at which point the thin-wall needle or catheter is withdrawn. The tendency to insert the guidewire deeper than 15 to 20 cm should be avoided, as it is the most common cause of ventricular arrhythmias during insertion and also poses a risk for cardiac perforation. Occasionally, the guidewire does not pass easily beyond the tip of the thin-wall needle. The guidewire should then be withdrawn, the syringe attached, and free backflow of blood reestablished and maintained while the syringe and needle are brought to a more parallel plane with the vein. The guidewire should then pass easily. If resistance is still encountered, rotation of the guidewire during insertion often allows passage, but extensive manipulation and force only lead to complications.

With the guidewire in place, a scalpel is used to make two 90-degree stab incisions at the skin entry site to facilitate passage of the 7-Fr vessel dilator. The dilator is inserted down the wire to a depth that ensures that the soft tissues are sufficiently dilated to accept the catheter while maintaining control and sterility of the guidewire. Except in obese or edematous patients where the distance from the skin to the vessel may be large, the dilator should not be inserted to the hub in order to avoid vessel damage. The dilator is then withdrawn and pressure used at the puncture site to control oozing and prevent air embolism down the needle tract. The triple-lumen catheter is then inserted over the guidewire, ensuring that the operator has control of the guidewire, either proximal or distal to the catheter, at all times to avoid intravascular loss of the wire. The catheter is then advanced 15 to 17 cm (17 to 19 cm for left IJV) into the vein, the guidewire withdrawn, and the distal lumen capped. The catheter is sutured securely to limit tip migration and bandaged in a standard manner. A chest radiograph should be obtained to detect complications and tip location.

Alternative Approaches

The anterior and posterior approaches are identical in technique, differing only in venipuncture site and plane of insertion. For the anterior approach (see Fig. 2-2) [55,60,61], the important landmark is the midpoint of the sternal head of the SCM, approximately 5 cm from both the angle of the mandible and the sternum. At this point, the carotid artery can be palpated 1 cm inside the lateral border of the sternal head. The index and middle fingers of the left hand gently palpate the artery, and the needle is introduced 0.5 to 1 cm lateral to the pulsation. The needle should form a 45-degree angle with the frontal plane and be directed caudally parallel to the carotid artery toward the ipsilateral nipple. Venipuncture occurs within 2 to 4 cm, sometimes only while the needle is slowly withdrawn. If the initial attempt is unsuccessful, the next attempt should be at a 5-degree lateral angle, followed by a cautious attempt more medially, never crossing the plane of the carotid artery.

The posterior approach (see Fig. 2-2) [55,62–64] uses the EJV as a surface landmark. The needle is introduced 1 cm dorsally to the point where the EJV crosses the posterior border of the SCM or 5 cm cephalad from the clavicle along the clavicular head of the SCM. The needle is directed caudally and ventrally toward the suprasternal notch at an angle of 45 degrees to the sagittal plane, with a 15-degree upward angulation. Venipuncture occurs within 5 to 7 cm. If this attempt is unsuccessful, the needle should be aimed slightly more cephalad on the next attempt.

Success Rates

Internal jugular vein catheterization is associated with a high rate of successful catheter placement regardless of the approach used. Elective procedures are successful more than 90% of the time, generally within the first three attempts, and catheter malposition is rare [54,55,57,60]. Operator experience does not appear to be as important a factor in altering the success rate of venipuncture as it is in increasing the number of complications [57,65]. Emergent IJV catheterization is less successful and is not the preferred technique during airway emergencies or other situations that may make it difficult to identify landmarks in the neck.

Ultrasound studies have been useful in delineating factors that improve the efficiency of IJV cannulation. The ability to perform IJV venipuncture is directly proportional to its cross-sectional lumen area (CSLA); thus, these factors increase or decrease the vein's caliber impact on the success rate [66,67]. Factors that decrease the CSLA include hypovolemia, carotid artery palpation, and excessive tension on a finder needle. Predictably, the Valsalva maneuver and Trendelenburg position increase CSLA, as does high-level PEEP. There is also a progressive increase in CSLA as the IJV nears the SV. Overrotation of the neck may place the vein beneath the SCM muscle belly [66].

Often, cannulation is successful on the first attempt by optimizing CLSA through attention to the above measures. If the IJV is still not punctured after one or two attempts, it is usually because of anatomical variation, not because of the absence of jugular flow [67,68]. In this situation, we use a portable ultrasound device to locate the IJV [69]. Whatever technique is employed, prolonged attempts at catheterization after optimization of IJV CSLA are only likely to increase complications.

Complications

The incidence and types of complications are similar regardless of the approach. Operator inexperience appears to increase the number of complications, but to an undefined extent, and probably does not have as great an impact as it does on the incidence of pneumothorax in subclavian venipuncture [55,70].

The overall incidence of complications in IJV catheterization is 0.1% to 4.2% [53,55,62]. Important complications include ICA puncture, pneumothorax, vessel erosion, thrombosis, and infection. By far the most common complication is ICA puncture, which constitutes 80% to 90% of all complications. In the absence of a bleeding diathesis, arterial punctures are usually benign and are managed conservatively without sequelae by applying local pressure for 10 minutes. Even in the absence of clotting abnormalities, a sizable hematoma may form, frequently preventing further catheterization attempts or, rarely, exerting pressure on vital neck structures [71,72]. Unrecognized arterial puncture can lead to catheterization of the ICA with a large-bore catheter or introducer and can have disastrous consequences, especially if heparin is subsequently administered [73]. Management of carotid cannulation with a large-bore catheter, such as a 7-Fr introducer, is controversial. Options include pulling the catheter and applying pressure, percutaneous closure devices, internal stent grafting, or surgical repair [74,75]. Some experts advise administration of anticoagulants to prevent thromboembolic complications, while others advise the opposite. Our approach is to remove small-bore catheters and avoid heparinization if possible, as hemorrhage appears to be a greater risk than thromboembolism [73]. For larger bore catheters and complicated cases, we involve interventional radiology and vascular surgery before removal and individualize the management based on the circumstances.

Coagulopathy is a relative contraindication to IJV catheterization, but extensive experience suggests that it is generally safe [56]. In patients with clinical bleeding abnormalities, it is prudent to first proceed with EJV or FV catheterization, but if the IJV is considered most appropriate, a finder needle should always be used in an attempt to avoid ICA puncture with a larger needle, and ultrasound localization of the vessel is recommended.

Pneumothorax and hemothorax are considered unusual adverse consequences of IJV cannulation, but with an incidence of 1.3% in a large meta-analysis, statistically the same as 1.5% found for subclavian puncture [76]. It usually results from a skin puncture too close to the clavicle or, rarely, from other causes [56]. Pneumothorax may be complicated by heme, infusion of intravenous fluid, or tension.

An extraordinary number of case reports indicate that any complication from IJV catheterization is possible, even the intrathecal insertion of a Swan-Ganz catheter [77]. In reality, this route is reliable, with a low incidence of major complications. Operator experience is not as important a factor as in SV catheterization; the incidence of catheter tip malposition is low, and patient acceptance is high. It is best suited for acute, short-term hemodialysis and for elective or urgent catheterizations in volume-replete patients, especially pulmonary artery catheterizations and insertion of temporary transvenous pacemakers. It is not the preferred site during airway emergencies, for parenteral nutrition, or for long-term catheterization because infectious complications are higher with IJV compared to SCV catheterizations.

EXTERNAL JUGULAR VEIN APPROACH

Motivated by the search for a "golden route" [78], Nordlund and Thoren [79] performed EJV catheterization and advocated a more extensive use of this approach. In 1974, Blitt et al. [80] described a technique of CVC via the EJV employing a J-wire. Although the success rate of this route is lower than with the IJV, a "central" venipuncture is avoided, and in selected cases catheterization via the EJV remains an excellent alternative. The main advantages to the EJV route for CVC are that it is part of the surface anatomy, it may be cannulated in the presence of clotting abnormalities, and the risk of pneumothorax is all but eliminated. The main disadvantage is the unpredictability of passage of the catheter to the central compartment. We rarely use this approach anymore, primarily because of greater experience with the IJV and SV in patients with coagulopathy.

Anatomy

The EJV is formed anterior and caudal to the ear at the angle of the mandible by the union of the posterior auricular and retromandibular veins (Fig. 2-3). It courses obliquely across the anterior surface of the SCM, then pierces the deep fascia just posterior to the SCM and joins the SV behind the medial third of the clavicle. In 5% to 15% of patients, the EJV is not a distinct structure but a venous plexus, in which case it may receive the ipsilateral cephalic vein. The EJV varies in size and contains valves throughout its course. Its junction with the SV may be at a severe, narrow angle that can be difficult for a catheter to traverse.

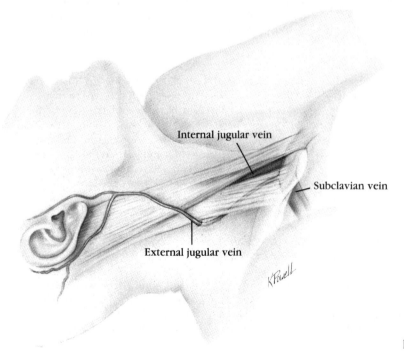

FIGURE 2-3.   External jugular vein.

Technique

The EJV should be cannulated using the 16-gauge catheter-over-needle, since guidewire manipulations are often necessary and secure venous access with a catheter is preferable. The patient is placed in a slight Trendelenburg position, with arms to the side and head turned gently to the contralateral side. The right EJV should be chosen for the initial attempt and can be identified where it courses over the anterior portion of the clavicular belly of the SCM. After sterile preparation, venipuncture is performed with the 16-gauge catheter-over-needle using the left index finger and thumb to distend and anchor the vein. Skin puncture should be well above the clavicle and the needle advanced in the axis of the vein at 20 degrees to the frontal plane. The EJV may be more difficult to cannulate than expected because of its propensity to roll and displace rather than puncture in response to the advancing needle. A firm, quick thrust is often required to effect venipuncture. When free backflow of blood is established, the needle tip is advanced a few millimeters further into the vein and the catheter is threaded over the needle. The catheter may not thread its entire length because of valves, tortuosity, or the SV junction, but should be advanced at least 3 to 5 cm to secure venous access. The syringe and needle can then be removed and the guidewire, J-tip first, threaded up to 20 cm and the catheter removed. Manipulation and rotation of the guidewire, especially when it reaches the SV junction, may be necessary but should not be excessive. Various arm and head movements are advocated to facilitate guidewire passage; abduction of the ipsilateral arm and anterior-posterior pressure exerted on the clavicle may be helpful. Once the guidewire has advanced 20 cm, two 90-degree skin stabs are made with a scalpel, and the vein dilator is inserted to the appropriate depth, maintaining control of the guidewire. The triple-lumen catheter is then inserted an appropriate length (16 to 17 cm on the right, 18 to 20 cm on the left). The guidewire is withdrawn, the catheter bandaged, and a chest radiograph obtained to screen for complications and tip placement.

Success Rates and Complications

Central venous catheterization via the EJV is successful in 80% of patients (range 75% to 95%) [80–82]. Inability to perform venipuncture accounts for up to 10% of failures [81,83,84] and the remainder are a result of catheter tip malpositioning. Failure to position the catheter tip is usually due to inability to negotiate the EJV-SV junction, loop formation, or retrograde passage down the ipsilateral arm.

Serious complications arising from the EJV approach are rare and almost always associated with catheter maintenance rather than venipuncture. A local hematoma forms in 1% to 5% of patients at the time of venipuncture [81,84,85] but has little consequence unless it distorts the anatomy leading to catheterization failure. External jugular venipuncture is safe in the presence of coagulopathy. Infectious, thrombotic, and other mechanical complications are no more frequent than with other central routes.

FEMORAL VEIN APPROACH

The FV has many practical advantages for CVC; it is directly compressible, it is remote from the airway and pleura, the technique is relatively simple, and the Trendelenburg position is not required during insertion. During the mid-1950s percutaneous catheterization of the IVC via a femoral vein approach became popular until 1959 when Moncrief [86] and Bansmer et al. [87] reported a high incidence of complications, especially infection and thrombosis, after which it was largely abandoned. In the subsequent two decades, FV cannulation was restricted to specialized clinical situations. Interest in short-term (less than 48 hours) FV catheterization was renewed by positive experiences during the Vietnam conflict and with patients in the emergency department [88]. Recent reports on long-term FV catheterization [6,89,90] suggest an overall complication rate no higher than that with other routes, although deep vein thrombosis and infection remain a legitimate concern.

Anatomy

The FV (Fig. 2-4) is a direct continuation of the popliteal vein and becomes the external iliac vein at the inguinal ligament. At the inguinal ligament the FV lies within the femoral sheath a few centimeters from the skin surface. The FV lies medial to the femoral artery, which in turn lies medial to the femoral branch of the genitofemoral nerve. The medial compartment contains lymphatic channels and Cloquet's node. The external iliac vein courses cephalad from the inguinal ligament along the anterior surface of the iliopsoas muscle to join its counterpart from the other leg and form the (IVC) anterior to and to the right of the fifth lumbar vertebra [45,46].

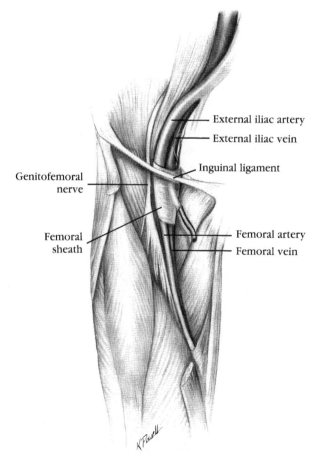

FIGURE 2-4. Anatomy of the femoral vein.

Technique

Femoral vein cannulation is the easiest of all central venous procedures to learn and perform. Either side is suitable, and the side chosen is based on operator convenience. The patient is placed in the supine position (if tolerated) with the leg extended and slightly abducted at the hip. Excessive hair should be clipped with scissors and the skin prepped in standard fashion. The FV lies 1 to 1.5 cm medial to the arterial pulsation, and the overlying skin is infiltrated with 1% lidocaine. In a patient without femoral artery pulsations, the FV can be located by dividing the distance between the anterior-superior iliac spine and the pubic tubercle into three equal segments. The femoral artery is usually found where the medial segment meets the two lateral ones, and the FV lies 1 to 1.5 cm medial. An 18-gauge thin-wall needle is inserted at this point, 2 to 3 cm inferior to the inguinal ligament, ensuring that venipuncture occurs caudal to the inguinal ligament, which minimizes the risk of retroperitoneal hematoma in the event of arterial puncture. While maintaining constant back pressure on the syringe, the needle, tip pointed cephalad, is advanced at a 45-degree angle to the frontal plane. Insertion of the needle to its hub is sometimes required in obese patients. Blood return may not occur until slow withdrawal. If the initial attempt is unsuccessful, landmarks should be reevaluated and subsequent attempts oriented slightly more medial or lateral. A common error is to direct the needle tip too medially, toward the umbilicus. The femoral vessels lie in the sagittal plane at the inguinal ligament (see Fig. 2-4), and the needle should be directed accordingly. If unintentional arterial puncture occurs, pressure is applied for 5 to 10 minutes.

When venous blood return is established, the syringe angle is depressed slightly and free aspiration of blood reconfirmed. The syringe is removed, ensuring that blood return is not pulsatile. The guidewire should pass easily and never be forced, although rotation and minor manipulation are sometimes required. The needle is then withdrawn, two scalpel blade stab incisions made at 90 degrees at the guidewire insertion site, and the vein dilator inserted over the wire to the appropriate depth. The dilator is then withdrawn and a catheter appropriate to clinical requirements inserted, taking care never to lose control of the guidewire. The catheter is secured with a suture and bandage applied.

Success Rate and Complications

FV catheterization is successful in 90% to 95% of patients, including those in shock or cardiopulmonary arrest [91,92]. Unsuccessful catheterizations are usually a result of venipuncture failure, hematoma formation, or inability to advance the guidewire into the vein. Operator inexperience may increase the number of attempts and complication rate but does not appear to significantly decrease the overall success rate [91].

Three complications occur regularly with FV catheterization: arterial puncture with or without local bleeding, infection, and thromboembolic events. Other reported complications are rare and include scrotal hemorrhage, right lower quadrant bowel perforation, retroperitoneal hemorrhage, puncture of the kidney, and perforation of IVC tributaries. These complications occur when skin puncture sites are cephalad to the inguinal ligament or when long catheters are threaded into the FV.

Femoral artery puncture occurs in 5% to 10% of adults [91,92]. Most arterial punctures are uncomplicated, but major hematomas may form in 1% of patients, especially in the presence of anticoagulants, fibrinolytics, or antithrombotic agents [91]. Even in the presence of coagulopathy, arterial puncture with the 18-gauge thin-wall needle is usually of minor consequence, but there is a potential for life-threatening thigh or retroperitoneal hemorrhage [93]. Arteriovenous fistula and pseudoaneurysm are rare chronic complications of arterial puncture; the former is more likely to occur when both femoral vessels on the same side are cannulated concurrently [94].

Infectious complications with FV catheters are probably more frequent than SV catheters but comparable to IJV catheters [3,95,96]. Recent series involving both short- and long-term FV catheterization in adults and children have reported significant catheter-related infection rates of about 5% or less [91,97]. Further evidence that the inguinal site is not inherently "dirty" is provided by experience with femoral artery catheters, which have an infection rate comparable to that with radial artery catheters [98]. More recent reports are suggesting that a catheter properly placed and cared for has a similar rate of infection regardless of venipuncture site [90].

Two reports in 1958 [86,87] highlighted the high incidence of FV catheter-associated deep venous thrombosis (DVT), but these studies were primarily autopsy based and prior to modern technological advances. Catheter-associated thrombosis is a risk of all central venous catheters, regardless of the site of insertion, and comparative studies using contrast venography, impedance plethysmography, or Doppler ultrasound suggest that FV catheters are no more prone to thrombosis than upper extremity catheters [6,31,32,33,35]. Pulmonary emboli have been reported following CVC-associated upper extremity thrombosis [35], and the relative risk of femoral catheter-related thrombosis is unknown. Clearly, the potential thromboembolic complications of FV catheters cannot be discounted [99], but they do not warrant total abandonment of this approach.

In summary, available evidence supports the view that the FV may be cannulated safely in critically ill adults. It is particularly useful for inexperienced operators because of the high rate of success and lower incidence of major complications. FV catheterizations may be performed during airway emergencies and cardiopulmonary arrest, in patients with coagulopathy, and in patients who are unable to lay flat. The most common major complication during venipuncture is arterial puncture, which is usually easily managed. Infection is no more common than with IJV catheters. Catheter-associated thrombosis occurs with similar frequency as with IJ and SV catheters, but is likely more clinically relevant.

SUBCLAVIAN VEIN APPROACH

The first published description of infraclavicular subclavian venipuncture in humans is credited to Aubaniac in 1952 [100]. Subsequently, Yoffa [101] reported his experience with supraclavicular subclavian venipuncture, claiming a lower incidence of complications, but his results were not uniformly reproduced. An important development occurred in 1959, when Hughes and Magovern [102] described the clinical use of CVP measurements in humans undergoing thoracotomy. In 1962, Wilson et al. [103]

extended the practicality of CVP monitoring by using percutaneous infraclavicular SV catheterization. Experienced operators have a pneumothorax rate of 1% or less and can justify use of the SV as primary central venous access in almost all patients. Inexperienced operators have a far greater rate of pneumothorax; therefore, in settings where relatively inexperienced physicians perform the majority of CVC, the SV should be used selectively [104]. The advantages of this route include consistent identifiable landmarks, easier long-term catheter maintenance with a comparably lower rate of infection, and relatively high patient comfort. Assuming an experienced operator is available, the SV is the preferred site for CVC in patients with hypovolemia, for long-term total parenteral nutrition (TPN), and in patients with elevated intracranial pressure who require hemodynamic monitoring. It should not be considered the primary choice in the presence of thrombocytopenia (platelets less than 150,000), for acute hemodialysis, or in patients with high PEEP (i.e., greater than 12 cm H_2O).

Anatomy

The SV is a direct continuation of the axillary vein, beginning at the lateral border of the first rib, extending 3 to 4 cm along the undersurface of the clavicle and becoming the brachiocephalic vein where it joins the ipsilateral IJV at Pirogoff's confluence behind the sternoclavicular articulation (Fig. 2-5) [45,46]. The vein is 1 to 2 cm in diameter, contains a single set of valves just distal to the EJV junction, and is fixed in position directly beneath the clavicle by its fibrous attachments. These attachments prevent collapse of the vein, even with severe volume depletion. Anterior to the vein throughout its course lie the subclavius muscle, clavicle, costoclavicular ligament, pectoralis muscles, and epidermis. Posteriorly, the SV is separated from the subclavian artery and brachial plexus by the anterior scalenus muscle, which is 10 to 15 mm thick in the adult. Posterior to the medial portion of the SV are the phrenic nerve and internal mammary artery as they pass into the thorax. Superiorly, the relationships are the skin, platysma, and superficial aponeurosis. Inferiorly, the vein rests on the first rib, Sibson's fascia, the cupola of the pleura (0.5 cm behind the vein), and the pulmonary apex [105]. The thoracic duct on the left and right lymphatic duct cross the anterior scalene muscle to join the superior aspect of the SV near its union with the IJV.

Technique

Although there are many variations, the SV may be cannulated by two basic techniques: the infraclavicular [78,100,103, 105,106] or supraclavicular [107,108] approach (Fig. 2-6). The differences in success rate, catheter tip malposition, and complications between the two approaches are negligible, although catheter tip malposition and pneumothorax may be less likely with supraclavicular cannulation [109,110]. In general, when discussing the success rate and incidence of complications of SV catheterization, there is no need to specify the approach used.

The 18-gauge thin-wall needle is preferable for SV cannulation [111]. The patient is placed in a 15- to 30-degree Trendelenburg position, with a small bedroll between the shoulder blades. The head is turned gently to the contralateral side and the arms are kept to the side. The pertinent landmarks are the clavicle, the two muscle bellies of the SCM, the suprasternal notch, the deltopectoral groove, and the manubriosternal junction. For the infraclavicular approach (see Fig. 2-6), the operator is positioned next to the patient's shoulder on the side to be cannulated. For reasons cited earlier, the left SV should be chosen for pulmonary artery catheterization; otherwise, the success rate appears to be equivalent regardless of the side chosen. Skin puncture is 2 to 3 cm caudal to the clavicle at the deltopectoral groove, corresponding to the area where the clavicle turns from the shoulder to the manubrium. Skin puncture should be distant enough from the clavicle to avoid a downward angle of the needle in clearing the inferior surface of the clavicle, which also obviates any need to bend the needle. The path of the needle is toward the suprasternal notch. After skin infiltration and liberal injection of the clavicular periosteum with 1% lidocaine,

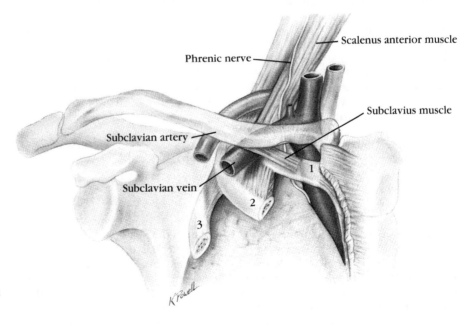

Phrenic nerve

Scalenus anterior muscle

Subclavius muscle

Subclavian artery

Subclavian vein

1

2

3

K. Powell

FIGURE 2-5.   Anatomy of the subclavian vein and adjacent structures.

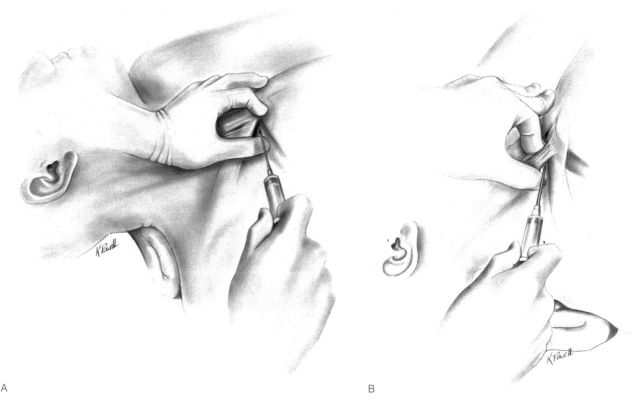

A   B

FIGURE 2-6.   A: Patient positioning for subclavian cannulation. **B:** Cannulation technique for supraclavicular approach.

the 18-gauge thin-wall needle is mounted on a 10-mL syringe. Skin puncture is accomplished with the needle bevel up, and the needle is advanced in the plane described above until the tip abuts the clavicle. The needle is then "walked" down the clavicle until the inferior edge is cleared. In order to avoid pneumothorax, it is imperative the needle stay parallel to the floor and not angle down toward the chest. This is accomplished by using the operator's left thumb to provide downward displacement in the vertical plane during needle advancement, until the needle advances under the clavicle.

As the needle is advanced further, the inferior surface of the clavicle should be felt hugging the needle. This ensures that the needle tip is as superior as possible to the pleura. The needle is advanced toward the suprasternal notch during breath holding or expiration, and venipuncture occurs when the needle tip lies beneath the medial end of the clavicle. This may require insertion of the needle to its hub. Blood return may not occur until slow withdrawal of the needle. If venipuncture is not accomplished on the initial effort, the next attempt should be directed slightly more cephalad. If venipuncture does not occur by the third or fourth attempt, another site should be chosen, as additional attempts are unlikely to be successful and may result in complications [104].

When blood return is established, the bevel of the needle is rotated 90 degrees toward the heart. The needle is anchored firmly with the left hand while the syringe is detached with the right. Blood return should not be pulsatile, and air embolism prophylaxis is necessary at all times. The guidewire is then advanced through the needle to 15 cm and the needle withdrawn. To increase the success rate of proper placement of the catheter,

the J-wire tip should point inferiorly [112]. The remainder of the procedure is as previously described. Triple-lumen catheters should be sutured at 15 to 16 cm on the right and 17 to 18 cm on the left to avoid intracardiac tip placement [22–24,113].

For the supraclavicular approach (see Fig. 2-6), the important landmarks are the clavicular insertion of the SCM muscle and the sternoclavicular joint. The operator is positioned at the head of the patient on the side to be cannulated. The site of skin puncture is the claviculosterno-cleidomastoid angle, just above the clavicle and lateral to the insertion of the clavicular head of the SCM. The needle is advanced toward or just caudal to the contralateral nipple just under the clavicle. This corresponds to a 45-degree angle to the sagittal plane, bisecting a line between the sternoclavicular joint and clavicular insertion of the SCM [108]. The depth of insertion is from just beneath the SCM clavicular head at a 10- to 15-degree angle below the coronal plane. The needle should enter the jugulosubclavian venous bulb after 1 to 4 cm, and the operator may then proceed with catheterization.

Success and Complication Rates

Subclavian vein catheterization is successful in 90% to 95% of cases, generally on the first attempt [104,106,114]. The presence of shock does not alter the success rate as significantly as it does during IJV catheterization [114]. Unsuccessful catheterizations are a result of venipuncture failure or inability to advance the guidewire or catheter [54,107]. Catheter tip malposition occurs in 5% to 20% of cases [54,106,109,114] and tends to be more frequent with the infraclavicular approach [54,106]. Malposition occurs most commonly to the ipsilateral IJV and contralateral SV and is usually correctable without repeat venipuncture.

The overall incidence of noninfectious complications varies depending on the operator's experience and the circumstances under which the catheter is inserted. Large series involving several thousand SV catheters have reported an incidence of major complications of 1% to 3%, with an overall rate of 5% [105,106]. In smaller, probably more clinically relevant studies, the major complication rate has ranged from 1% to 10% [54,104,114–116]. Factors resulting in a higher complication rate are operator inexperience, multiple attempts at venipuncture, emergency conditions, variance from standardized technique, and body mass index [104]. Major noninfectious complications include pneumothorax, arterial puncture, and thromboembolism. There are many case reports of isolated major complications involving neck structures or the brachial plexus; the reader is referred elsewhere for a complete listing of reported complications [117].

Pneumothorax accounts for one fourth to one half of reported complications, with an incidence of about 1.5% [76]. The incidence varies inversely with the operator's experience and the number of "breaks" in technique [65,104,109,110,114–116]. There is no magic figure whereby an operator matures from inexperienced to experienced. Fifty catheterizations is cited frequently as a cutoff number, but it is reasonable to expect an operator to be satisfactorily experienced after having performed fewer. For the experienced operator, a pneumothorax incidence of less than 1% is expected. Most pneumothoraces are a result of lung puncture at the time of the procedure, but late-appearing pneumothoraces have been reported.

Most pneumothoraces will require thoracostomy tube drainage with a small chest tube and a Heimlich valve, but some can be managed conservatively with 100% oxygen and serial radiographs or needle aspiration only [105,114,118]. Rarely a pneumothorax is complicated by tension, heme, infusion of intravenous fluid (immediately or days to weeks after catheter placement), chyle, or massive subcutaneous emphysema. Bilateral pneumothoraces can occur from unilateral attempts at venipuncture. Pneumothorax can result in death, especially when it goes unrecognized [119].

Subclavian artery puncture occurs in 0.5% to 1.0% of cases, constituting one fourth to one third of all complications [54,106,116]. Arterial puncture is usually managed easily by applying pressure above and below the clavicle. Bleeding can be catastrophic in patients with coagulopathy, especially thrombocytopenia. As with other routes, arterial puncture may result in arteriovenous fistula or pseudoaneurysm.

Clinical evidence of central venous thrombosis, including SVC syndrome, development of collaterals around the shoulder girdle, and pulmonary embolism, occurs in 0% to 3% of SV catheterizations [6,30,31,32,33,35], but routine phlebography performed at catheter removal reveals a much higher incidence of thrombotic phenomena. The importance of the discrepancy between clinical symptoms and radiologic findings is unknown, but it exists for all routes of CVC. Duration of catheterization, catheter material, and patient condition probably impact the frequency of thrombosis, but to an uncertain degree.

In summary, the SV is an extremely reliable and useful route for CVC, and it is the recommended site for catheterization of most patients. It should not be the primary choice in patients at high risk for bronchopleural fistula after lung puncture, patients who cannot tolerate a pneumothorax (severe lung disease, one lung), or in patients with severe coagulopathy. Inexperienced operators should be closely supervised and not allowed to perform SV catheterization independently.

ULTRASOUND GUIDANCE

The role of routine portable ultrasound in the placement of CVCs has been debated. The use of ultrasound localization to aid in IJV catheterization improves success rate and decreases the need for multiple attempts, but it has not been widely adopted, probably because of cost and training issues. The time saved by improved first attempt success may be offset by the time required for mobilization and setup of the ultrasound machine. Most studies examine ultrasound for IJV cannulation, with mixed results. Additionally, one must choose between dynamic and static US, with the latter requiring more training and experience. At our institution, ultrasound is not routinely used, but is often employed in high-risk patients (maximal ventilator support, severe coagulopathy), and those in whom landmarks are difficult to assess (obese or edematous patients). In special circumstances, ultrasound or Doppler localization is helpful in performing difficult or previously unsuccessful IJV catheterization [68].

INFECTIOUS COMPLICATIONS

Tremendous advances in the understanding of the pathophysiology, causes, and prevention of catheter-related infection (CRI) have occurred in recent years and have led to corresponding dramatic improvements in catheter technology, insertion, and management. In our ICU, we have achieved a reduction in CRIs by implementing an annual comprehensive standardized catheter educational seminar designed for the housestaff and other interested physicians [120], as well as incorporating some of the newer technological advances. Table 2-2 summarizes current recommendations or interventions that have been shown to reduce the risk of CRI. This section reviews these recommendations, focusing on the epidemiology, pathogenesis, diagnosis, management, and prevention of central CRI.

DEFINITIONS AND EPIDEMIOLOGY

Consensus regarding the definition and diagnosis of CRI is a necessary initial step in discussing CRI complications. The semiquantitative culture method described by Maki et al. [121] for culturing catheter segments is the most accepted technique for diagnosing catheter-related infection. Which catheter segment to culture (the tip or intradermal segment) is still controversial; out of convenience most centers routinely culture the catheter tip. If semiquantitative methods are used, catheter contamination (probably occurring at time of withdrawal) is defined as less than 15 colony-forming units (CFUs) per culture plate. CRI is defined as greater than 15 CFUs and is identified as colonization (all other cultures negative and no clinical symptoms); local or exit-site infection (skin site with erythema, cellulitis, or purulence); catheter-related bacteremia (systemic blood cultures positive for identical organism on catheter segment and no other source); and catheter-related sepsis or septic shock. Alternative methods to diagnose CRI include differential time to positivity [122] and direct Gram [123] or acridine-orange

TABLE 2-2.   Steps to Minimize CVC-Related Infection

1. Institution-supported standardized education, with knowledge assessment, of all physicians involved in CVC insertion and care
2. Site preparation with approved chlorhexidine-based preparation
3. Maximal barrier precautions during catheter insertion
4. Use of mobile procedure carts, safety checklist, empowerment of staff
5. Strict protocols for catheter maintenance (including bandage and tubing changes), preferably by dedicated IV catheter team
6. Appropriate site selection, avoiding heavily colonized or anatomically abnormal areas; use of SV for anticipated CVC of greater than 4 days
7. For anticipated duration of catheterization exceeding 96 hours, use of silver-impregnated cuff, sustained release chlorhexidine gluconate patch, and/or antibiotic/antiseptic-impregnated catheters
8. Prompt removal of any catheter which is no longer required
9. Remove pulmonary artery catheters and introducers after 5 days
10. Replace any catheter not placed with sterile precautions within 48 hours (i.e., catheter placed in emergency)
11. Use multilumen catheters only when indicated; remove when no longer needed
12. Avoid "routine" guidewire exchanges
13. Use surgically implanted catheters or PICCs for long term (i.e., greater than 3 weeks) or permanent CVC

CVC, central venous catheterization; PICC, peripherally inserted central catheter; SV, subclavian vein.

staining [124] of catheters. Using the differential time to positivity, blood cultures are drawn from the catheter and peripherally. If the time to positive culture was greater than 120 minutes longer for the peripheral cultures, a diagnosis of CRI is made. This method has good sensitivity, specificity and the advantage of faster diagnosis.

The morbidity and mortality associated with CRI is truly impressive. Estimates vary, mainly because the overall incidence of CRI is impacted by so many independent variables, including type of ICU, catheter type and composition, duration of catheterization, and site of insertion. Overall more than 5 million CVCs are inserted annually in the United States, accounting for 15 million central venous catheter days. Various estimates cite the overall risk of CRI as 3% to 9% of catheters, and the National Nosocomial Infection Surveillance (NNIS) system reports rates of CVC-related bloodstream infection averaging 3.2 to 4.0 per 1,000 catheter days in medical-surgical ICUs [125]. These figures translate into as many as 850,000 total episodes of CRI with at least 60,000 to 80,000 associated with bacteremia [126,127]. The attributable mortality of catheter-related bloodstream infection is approximately 14% to 28% [128–131], with an added duration of hospitalization of 7 days and a cost as high as $40,000 per survivor [129].

An analysis of the data by Wenzel and Edmond [132] is especially startling. They report that of the 200,000 total nosocomial bloodstream infections (NBSI) annually, 70% occur from CVCs. Assuming an attributable mortality of 10% to 30%, NBSI represent the *fourth to thirteenth* leading cause of death in the United States, a large percentage of these directly a result of CVCs. They also highlight the importance of measures proven to reduce the frequency of CRI, estimating that the routine use of new antiinfective catheter technologies could result in 4,000 to 9,000 lives saved, and increased handwashing could save between 1,000 to 2,000 lives annually [132,133]. These figures are a powerful impetus and render it indefensible for critical care physicians not to implement everything possible to minimize CRI.

PATHOPHYSIOLOGY OF CATHETER INFECTION

Assuming that they are not contaminated during insertion, catheters can become infected from four potential sources: the skin insertion site, the catheter hub(s), hematogenous seeding, and infusated contamination. Animal and human studies have shown that catheters are most commonly infected by bacteria colonizing the skin site, followed by invasion of the intradermal catheter tract. Once the external surface of the intradermal catheter is infected, bacteria can quickly traverse the entire length and infect the catheter tip, sometimes encasing the catheter in a slime layer known as a biofilm (coagulase-negative staph) [134]. From the catheter tip, bacteria may shed into the bloodstream, potentially creating metastatic foci of infection [126]. This pathophysiology of catheter infections explains why guidewire exchanges are not effective in preventing or treating catheter-related infection: the colonized tract and, in many cases, biofilm, remain intact and quickly reinfect the new catheter [135].

The catheter hub(s) also becomes colonized but contributes to catheter-related infectious complications less frequently than the insertion site [136,137]. Hub contamination may be relatively more important as a source of infection the longer the catheter remains in place [138]. Hematogenous seeding of catheters from bacteremia is an infrequent cause of CRI.

SITE PREPARATION AND CATHETER MAINTENANCE

That the majority of catheter-related infections are caused by skin flora highlights the importance of site sterility during insertion and catheter maintenance. Organisms that colonize the insertion site originate from the patient's own skin flora or the hands of operators. Catheters are frequently contaminated at the time of insertion, and thorough hand washing and scrupulous attention to aseptic technique are mandatory. A prospective study proved that a nonsterile cap and mask, sterile gown, and a large drape covering the patient's head and body (maximal sterile barriers, compared to sterile gloves and small drape) reduced the catheter-related bloodstream infection rate sixfold, and were highly cost effective [139]. If a break in sterile technique occurs during insertion, termination of the procedure and replacement of contaminated equipment is mandatory.

Chlorhexidine demonstrated superiority as a disinfectant and should be used instead of iodine-based solutions [140,141]. Proper application includes liberally scrubbing the site using expanding concentric circles. Excessive hair should be clipped with scissors prior to application of the antiseptic, as shaving can cause minor skin lacerations and disruption of the epidermal barrier to infection.

Care of the catheter after insertion is extremely important in minimizing infection, and all medical personnel should follow standardized protocols [142]. The number of piggyback infusions and medical personnel handling tubing changes and manipulation of the catheter site should be minimized. Replacement of administration sets every 72 to 96 hours is safe and cost-efficient [143], unless there are specific recommendations for the infusate (e.g., propofol). Transparent polyurethane dressings have become more popular than gauze and tape, but have not been found to be superior. It is recommended that gauze be changed every 2 days and transparent dressing changed every 7 days. Either dressing should be changed when damp or soiled [144]. Addition of a chlorhexidine impregnated sponge (BIOPATCH) has been shown to reduce the rate of CRI in a multicenter study and is cost effective [127]. Application of iodophor or polymicrobial ointments to the skin site at the time of insertion or during dressing changes does not convincingly reduce the overall incidence of catheter infection, and certain polymicrobial ointments may increase the proportion of *Candida* infections [127,145].

FREQUENCY OF CATHETER-RELATED INFECTION

Observing the above recommendations for catheter insertion and maintenance will minimize catheter-associated infection. Colonization of the insertion site can begin within 24 hours and increases with duration of catheterization; 10% to 40% of catheters eventually become colonized [136,137,139,140,146]. Catheter-associated bacteremia and sepsis occurs in 3% to 8% of catheters [3,60,95,136,137,139,140,146–149], although some studies incorporating newer catheter technologies and procedures have demonstrated rates of catheter-associated bacteremia of 2% or less [136,139,150–152]. Bacteremia is a significant complication, extending hospitalization, adding to cost, and resulting in metastatic infection and death in a significant percentage of patients [128–131,147,153]. Gram-positive organisms, especially *Staphylococcus* species, are the most common infecting agents, but gram-negative enteric organisms are not rare. *Candida* species are more likely in certain clinical situations, such as the diabetic patient with prolonged catheterization on broad-spectrum antibiotics.

TYPE OF CATHETER

The data presented above are derived from large studies and are not necessarily applicable to any given catheter because of variations in definitions, types of catheters, site of insertion, duration of catheterization, types of fluid infused, and policies regarding routine guidewire changes, all of which have been implicated at some point as important factors in the incidence of CRI. The duration of catheterization in combination with the type of catheter are major factors; the site of insertion is less important. Guidewire changes have an important role in evaluation of the febrile catheterized patient, but routine guidewire changes do not prevent infection. Under ideal conditions, all of these factors are less important. Long-term TPN catheters can be maintained for months with low rates of infection, and there is no cutoff time at which colonization and clinical infection accelerate. Today, when the need for long-term catheterization is anticipated, surgically implanted catheters should be used. These catheters have low infection rates and are never changed routinely [154]. PICCs also appear to be an acceptable option for patients requiring long-term CVC [48–50].

Catheters inserted percutaneously in the critical care unit, however, are not subject to ideal conditions and have a finite lifespan. For practical purposes, multilumen catheters have replaced single-lumen catheters for many indications for central venous access. Since catheter hubs are a potential source of infection and triple-lumen catheters can require 3 times the number of tubing changes, it was widely believed that they would have a higher infection rate. Studies have presented conflicting results, but overall the data support the view that triple-lumen catheters have a modestly higher rate of infection [146,155–157]. If used efficiently, however, they provide greater intravascular access per device and can decrease the total number of catheter days and exposure to central venipuncture. A slight increase in infection rate per catheter is therefore justifiable from an overall risk-benefit analysis, if multilumen catheters are used only when multiple infusion ports are truly indicated.

Finally, it was hoped that routine subcutaneous tunneling of short-term central venous catheters, similar to long-term catheters, might be an effective way to minimize CRI. This approach is rational since the long subcutaneous tract acts to stabilize the catheter and perhaps act as a barrier to bacterial invasion, and great technical skill is not required. A recently completed meta-analysis did not support the routine practice of tunneling all percutaneously inserted CVCs, and it is not a common practice. However, further studies of the tunneling of short-term IJV and FV catheters is warranted, since these sites have a higher infection rate and past studies have generally favored this approach [158].

DURATION OF CATHETERIZATION

The length of catheterization should be based solely on the need for continued catheterization of the patient. No catheter should be left in longer than absolutely necessary. Most data suggest that the daily risk of infection remains relatively constant, and routine replacement of CVCs without a clinical indication does not reduce the rate of CRI [159,160]. Multiple clinical and experimental studies have also demonstrated that guidewire exchanges neither decrease nor increase infectious risk [135,159–161].

The above recommendations do not necessarily apply to other special-use catheters, which can be exposed to different clinical situations and risk. Pulmonary artery catheters (PACs) and the introducer should be removed after 96 to 120 hours because of the increased risk of infection after this time [146,153,162]. These catheters are at greater risk for infection because patients are sicker, the introducer used for insertion is shorter, and catheter manipulations are frequent [153].

Catheters inserted for acute temporary hemodialysis historically have had a higher rate of infection than other percutaneously placed catheters. Factors contributing to the increased rate have not been completely elucidated, but logically patient factors probably influence the incidence of infection more than the type of catheter or site of insertion. For acutely ill, hospitalized patients, temporary dialysis catheters should be managed similarly to other multilumen catheters. For ambulatory outpatients, long-term experience with double-lumen, Dacron-cuffed, silicone CVCs inserted in the IJV has been positive [163].

SITE OF INSERTION

The condition of the site is more important than the location. Whenever possible, sites involved by infection, burns, or other dermatologic processes, or in close proximity to a heavily colonized area (e.g., tracheostomy) should not be used as primary access. Data tend to support that PICC and SV catheters are associated with the lowest rate of CRI, and IJV and FV catheters the highest [3,95,121,126,127].

GUIDEWIRE EXCHANGES

Guidewire exchanges have always been theoretically flawed as a form of infection control, because although a new catheter is placed, the site, specifically the intradermal tract, remains the same. Studies have shown that when the tract and old catheter are colonized, the new catheter invariably also becomes infected [135]. Alternatively, if the initial catheter is not colonized, there is no reason the new catheter will be more resistant to subsequent infection than the original one. In neither situation will a guidewire change prevent infection [159,160]. However, guidewire changes continue to have a valuable role for replacing defective catheters, exchanging one type of catheter for another, and in the evaluation of a febrile patient with an existing central catheter. In the latter situation, the physician can assess the sterility of the catheter tract without subjecting the patient to a new venipuncture. However one decides to use guidewire exchanges, they must be performed properly. Using maximal barriers, the catheter should be withdrawn until an intravascular segment is exposed, transected sterilely, and the guidewire inserted through the distal lumen. The catheter fragment can then be removed (always culture the tip) and a new catheter threaded over the guidewire. To ensure sterility, most operators should reprep the site and change gloves before inserting the new catheter or introducer over the guidewire. Insertion of the guidewire through the distal hub of the existing catheter is not appropriate.

NEW CATHETER TECHNOLOGIES

Improvements in catheter technology continue to play an important role in minimizing catheter complications. Catheter material is an important factor in promoting thrombogenesis and adherence of organisms. Most catheters used for CVC are composed of flexible silicone (for surgical implantation) and polyurethane (for percutaneous insertion), because research has shown these materials are less thrombogenic. Knowledge of the pathogenesis of most CRI has stimulated improvements designed to interrupt bacterial colonization of the skin site, catheter, and intradermal tract, and migration to the catheter tip. Antibiotic and antiseptic coated and impregnated catheters represent a major advance in catheter management. The catheters differ from one another in that one is coated with the antiseptics silver sulfadiazine and chlorhexidine (Arrowguard Blue, Arrow International), while the other two are impregnated with the antibiotics minocycline and rifampin (Cook Spectrum, Cook Critical Care) or silver, carbon, and platinum (Vantex Catheter with Oligon, Edwards Lifesciences), which also protects the inner lumens. Clinical results with these commercially available catheters have been impressive, with a significant reduction in colonization and bacteremia [40,95,148,149,151,152,164]. Good randomized controlled trials comparing these catheters are lacking, but current evidence supports use of one of the above catheters decreases the rate of CRI and prolongs the duration of safe catheterization [95,148,165,166]. The emergence of resistant organisms and allergic reactions has not yet been a problem, but ongoing surveillance is needed.

SYSTEMS-BASED MEASURES

As stated in the introduction to this chapter, evidence is pointing to systems-based factors, not new catheter technology for making the jump to a zero CRI rate in the ICU. At Johns Hopkins, the addition of five systems-based changes reduced the CRI rate from 11.3 to 0 per 1,000 catheter days [1]. These simple interventions were: education of physicians and nurses of evidence-based infection control practices, creation of a central catheter insertion cart that contained every item needed for insertion of a catheter, daily questioning of whether catheters could be removed, a bedside checklist for insertion of catheters, and empowering nurses to stop procedures where the infection control guidelines were not being followed. Similar interventions in Pennsylvania reduced their CRI rate from 4.31 to 1.36 per 1,000 catheter days [167]. A statewide initiative in Michigan, the Keystone Project, is implementing the strategies used in the previous reports on a large scale over the entire state. Though no data have been published in peer-reviewed journals to date, preliminary press releases are suggesting that the project is accomplishing its goal of significant reductions in the CRI rate in participating ICUs.

MANAGEMENT OF THE FEBRILE PATIENT

Patients with a central venous catheter frequently develop fever. Removal of the catheter in every febrile patient is neither feasible nor clinically indicated, as the fever is often unrelated to the catheter. Management must be individualized and depends on the type of catheter, duration of catheterization, anticipated need for continued central venous access, risk of establishing new central venous access, and underlying medical condition and prognosis. All critical care units must have protocols for managing the febrile, catheterized patient. Decisions to remove, change over a guidewire, or leave catheters in place must be based on a fundamental knowledge of risks and benefits for catheters inserted at each site.

Catheter sites in the febrile patient should always be examined. Clinical infection of the site mandates removal of the catheter and institution of antibiotics. Surgically implanted catheters are not easily removed or replaced and can often be left in place while the infection is cleared with antibiotics, unless tunnel infection is present [154]. Percutaneously inserted CVCs are relatively easily removed, and the risks of leaving a catheter in place through an infected site outweigh the risk of replacement at a new site, except in very unusual circumstances.

In patients with severe sepsis or septic shock, CVCs should be considered a possible source. If all catheter sites appear normal and a noncatheter source of infection is implicated, appropriate antibiotics are initiated and the catheters left in place. The usual guidelines for subsequent catheter management should be followed, and this rarely results in treatment failure. In contrast, if a noncatheter source cannot be identified, then central catheters in place more than 3 days should be managed individually, with attention to duration of catheterization (Table 2-3). For patients with excessive risks for new catheter placement (i.e., severe coagulopathy), guidewire exchange of the catheter is justifiable after obtaining blood cultures through the catheter and a peripheral site and semiquantitative culture of a catheter segment. If within the next 24 hours an alternative source for sepsis is found, or if the catheter segment culture is negative and the

TABLE 2-3.   Approach to the Febrile Patient with a Central Venous Catheter

1. Catheter no longer needed; remove and culture tip
2. Patient with severe sepsis or septic shock (catheter greater than 72 hours); promptly remove catheter and culture tip
3. Patient with severe sepsis or septic shock (catheter less than 72 hours); initiate antibiotics, remove catheter if no improvement in 12 to 24 hours and no other source identified
4. Stable patient (catheter greater than 72 hours); guidewire exchange with tip culture, if culture with greater than 15 CFU, remove catheter

patient improves and stabilizes, the guidewire catheter can be left in place and the risk of catheter insertion avoided. Alternatively, if the catheter culture becomes positive, especially if the same organism is identified on peripheral blood cultures, the cutaneous tract is also infected and the guidewire catheter should be removed and alternative access achieved.

The most common situation is the stable febrile patient with a CVC in place. As above, if a noncatheter source for fever is identified, appropriate antibiotics are given and the catheter left in place, assuming it is still needed and the site is clinically uninvolved. In the patient with no obvious source of fever, indications for the central venous catheters should be reviewed and the catheter withdrawn if it is no longer required. Otherwise, the physician must decide between observation, potential premature withdrawal, or a guidewire change of the catheter. If the catheter is less than 72 hours old, observation is reasonable, as it is very unlikely that the catheter is already infected unless breaks in sterile technique occurred during insertion. For catheters that are at least 72 hours old, guidewire exchanges are rational. An appropriately performed guidewire change allows comparison of catheter segment cultures to other clinical cultures without subjecting the patient to repeat venipuncture. If within the next 24 hours an alternative source for fever is identified and/or the initial catheter segment culture is negative, then the guidewire catheter can be left in place.

When catheter-related bacteremia does develop, antibiotic therapy is necessary for a period of 7 to 14 days. Even in patients treated for 14 days, metastatic infection can develop. Catheter-related fever, infection, and septicemia is a complicated disease, and the expertise of an infectious disease consultant may be required to assist with the decision on how long to continue antibiotic therapy [153].

REFERENCES

1. Berenholtz SM, Pronovost PJ, Lipsett PA, et al: Eliminating catheter-related bloodstream infections in the intensive care unit. *Crit Care Med* 32:2014, 2004.
2. Graber D, Dailey RH: Catheter flow rates updated. *JACEP* 6:518, 1977.
3. Merrer J, De Jonghe B, Golliot F, et al: Complications of femoral and subclavian venous catheterization in critically ill patients: a randomized controlled trial. *JAMA* 286:700, 2001.
4. Trottier SJ, Veremakis C, O'Brien J, et al: Femoral deep vein thrombosis associated with central venous catheterization: results from a prospective, randomized trial. *Crit Care Med* 23:52, 1995.
5. Joynt GM, Kew J, Gomersall CD, et al: Deep venous thrombosis caused by femoral venous catheters in critically ill adult patients. *Chest* 117:178, 2000.
6. Durbec O, Viviand X, Potie F, et al: A prospective evaluation of the use of femoral venous catheters in critically ill adults. *Crit Care Med* 25:1986, 1997.
7. Huijbregts HJ, Blankestijn PJ: Dialysis access-guidelines for current practice. *Eur J Vasc Endo Surg* 31:284–247, 2006.
8. Cimochowski G, Sartain J, Worley E, et al: Clear superiority of internal jugular access over subclavian vein for temporary dialysis. *Kidney Int* 33:230, 1987.
9. Firek AF, Cutler RE, St. John Hammond PG. Reappraisal of femoral vein cannulation for temporary hemodialysis vascular access. *Nephron* 47:227, 1987.
10. Doerfler ME, Kaufman B, Goldenberg AS: Central venous catheter placement in patients with disorders of hemostasis. *Chest* 110:185, 1996.
11. Dripps RD, Eckenhoff JE, Vandam LD: *Introduction to Anesthesia: The Principles of Safe Practice.* 6th ed. Philadelphia, WB Saunders, 1982.
12. Emerman CL, Pinchak AC, Hancock D, et al: Effect of injection site on circulation times during cardiac arrest. *Crit Care Med* 16:1138, 1988.
13. ECC Committee, Subcommittees and Task Forces of the American Heart Association: 2005 American Heart Association guidelines for cardiopulmonary resuscitation and emergency cardiovascular care. *Circulation* 112:1, 2005.
14. Rivers E, Nguyen B, Havstad S, et al: Early goal-directed therapy in the treatment of severe sepsis and septic shock. *N Engl J Med* 345:1368, 2001.
15. The National Heart, Lung, and Blood Institute Acute Respiratory Distress Syndrome (ARDS) Clinical Trials Network. Pulmonary-artery versus central venous catheters to guide treatment of acute lung injury. *New Engl J Med* 354:2213, 2006.
16. Trzeciak S, Dellinger RP, Abate NL, et al: Translating research to clinical practice: a 1-year experience with implementing early goal-directed therapy for septic shock in the emergency department. *Chest* 129:225, 2006.
17. The National Heart, Lung, and Blood Institute Acute Respiratory Distress Syndrome (ARDS) Clinical Trials Network: Comparison of two fluid management strategies in acute lung injury. *New Engl J Med* 354:1, 2006.
18. Long R, Kassum D, Donen N, et al: Cardiac tamponade complicating central venous catheterization for total parenteral nutrition: a review. *J Crit Care* 2:39, 1987.
19. Curelaru I, Linder LE, Gustavsson B: Displacement of catheters inserted through internal jugular veins with neck flexion and extension. A preliminary study. *Intensive Care Med* 6:179, 1980.
20. Wojciechowski J, Curelaru I, Gustavsson B, et al: "Half-way" venous catheters. III. Tip displacements with movements of the upper extremity. *Acta Anaesthesiol Scand* 81:36, 1985.
21. Marx GF: Hazards associated with central venous pressure monitoring. *NY State J Med* 69:955, 1969.
22. Andrews RT, Bova DA, Venbrux AC: How much guidewire is too much? Direct measurement of the distance from subclavian and internal jugular vein access sites to the superior vena cava-atrial junction during central venous catheter placement. *Crit Care Med* 28:138, 2000.
23. Czepizak CA, O'Callaghan JM, Venus B: Evaluation of formulas for optimal positioning of central venous catheters. *Chest* 107:1662, 1995.
24. Aslamy Z, Dewald CL, Heffner JE: MRI of central venous anatomy: implications for central venous catheter insertion. *Chest* 114:820, 1998.
25. Robinson JF, Robinson WA, Cohn A, et al: Perforation of the great vessels during central venous line placement. *Arch Intern Med* 155:1225, 1995.
26. Duntley P, Siever J, Korwes ML, et al: Vascular erosion by central venous catheters. Clinical features and outcome. [Review] [44 refs]. *Chest* 101:1633, 1992.
27. Doering RB, Stemmer EA, Connolly JE: Complications of indwelling venous catheters, with particular reference to catheter embolus. *Am J Surg* 114:259, 1967.
28. Orebaugh SL: Venous air embolism: clinical and experimental considerations. [Review] [94 refs]. *Crit Care Med* 20:1169, 1992.
29. Ely EW, Hite RD, Baker AM, et al: Venous air embolism from central venous catheterization: a need for increased physician awareness. *Crit Care Med* 27:2113, 1999.
30. Mumtaz H, Williams V, Hauer-Jensen M, et al: Central venous catheter placement in patients with disorders of hemostasis. *Am J Surg* 180:503, 2000.
31. Brismar B, Hardstedt C, Jacobson S: Diagnosis of thrombosis by catheter phlebography after prolonged central venous catheterization. *Ann Surg* 194:779, 1981.
32. Rooden CJ, Tesselaar ME, Osanto S, et al: Deep vein thrombosis associated with central venous catheters-a review. *J Thromb Haemost* 3:2409, 2005.
33. Axelsson CK, Efsen F: Phlebography in long-term catheterization of the subclavian vein. A retrospective study in patients with severe gastrointestinal disorders. *Scand J Gastroenterol* 13:933, 1978.
34. Bonnet F, Loriferne JF, Texier JP, et al: Evaluation of Doppler examination for diagnosis of catheter-related deep vein thrombosis. *Intensive Care Med* 15:238, 1989.
35. Prandoni P, Polistena P, Bernardi E, et al: Upper-extremity deep vein thrombosis. Risk factors, diagnosis, and complications. *Arch Intern Med* 157:57, 1997.
36. Raad II, Luna M, Khalil SA, et al: The relationship between the thrombotic and infectious complications of central venous catheters. *JAMA* 271:1014, 1994.
37. Timsit JF, Farkas JC, Boyer JM, et al: Central vein catheter-related thrombosis in intensive care patients: incidence, risks factors, and relationship with catheter-related sepsis. *Chest* 114:207, 1998.
38. Linder LE, Curelaru I, Gustavsson B, et al: Material thrombogenicity in central venous catheterization: a comparison between soft, antebrachial catheters of silicone elastomer and polyurethane. *JPEN: J Parenter Enteral Nutrition* 8:399, 1984.
39. Madan M, Alexander DJ, McMahon MJ: Influence of catheter type on occurrence of thrombophlebitis during peripheral intravenous nutrition. *Lancet* 339:101, 1992.
40. Marin MG, Lee JC, Skurnick JH: Prevention of nosocomial bloodstream infections: effectiveness of antimicrobial-impregnated and heparin-bonded central venous catheters. *Crit Care Med* 28:3332, 2000.
41. Randolph AG, Cook DJ, Gonzales CA, et al: Benefit of heparin in peripheral venous and arterial catheters: systematic review and meta-analysis of randomised controlled trials. *BMJ* 316:969, 1998.
42. Black IH, Blosser SA, Murray WB: Central venous pressure measurements: peripherally inserted catheters versus centrally inserted catheters. *Crit Care Med* 28:3833, 2000.
43. Ng PK, Ault MJ, Maldonado LS: Peripherally inserted central catheters in the intensive care unit. *J Intensive Care Med* 11:49, 1996.
44. Robinson MK, Mogensen KM, Grudinskas GF, et al: Improved care and reduced costs for

patients requiring peripherally inserted central catheters: the role of bedside ultrasound and a dedicated team. *JPEN: J Parenter Enteral Nutrition* 29:374, 2005.
45. Netter FH: *Atlas of Human Anatomy.* Summit, NJ, Cibn-Geigy, 1989.
46. Williams PL, Warwick R. *Gray's Anatomy.* 8th ed. Philadelphia, WB Saunders, 1980.
47. Lumley J, Russell WJ. Insertion of central venous catheters through arm veins. *Anaesth Intensive Care* 3:101, 1975.
48. Cardella JF, Cardella K, Bacci N, et al: Cumulative experience with 1,273 peripherally inserted central catheters at a single institution. *J Vasc Interv Radiol* 7:5, 1996.
49. Raad I, Davis S, Becker M, et al: Low infection rate and long durability of nontunneled silastic catheters. A safe and cost-effective alternative for long-term venous access. *Arch Intern Med* 153:1791, 1993.
50. Duerksen DR, Papineau N, Siemens J, et al: Peripherally inserted central catheters for parenteral nutrition: a comparison with centrally inserted catheters. *JPEN: J Parenter Enteral Nutrition* 23:85, 1999.
51. Gustavsson B, Curelaru I, Hultman E, et al: Displacements of the soft, polyurethane central venous catheters inserted by basilic and cephalic veins. *Acta Anaesthesiol Scand* 27:102, 1983.
52. Hermosura B, Vanags L, Dickey NW: Measurement of pressure during intravenous therapy. *JAMA* 195:321, 1966.
53. English IC, Frew RM, Pigott JF, et al: Percutaneous cannulation of the internal jugular vein. *Thorax* 24:496, 1969.
54. Malatinsky J, Faybik M, Griffith M, et al: Venepuncture, catheterization and failure to position correctly during central venous cannulation. *Resuscitation* 10:259, 1983.
55. Defalque RJ: Percutaneous catheterization of the internal jugular vein. [Review] [30 refs]. *Anesth Analg* 53:116, 1974.
56. Goldfarb G, Lebrec D: Percutaneous cannulation of the internal jugular vein in patients with coagulopathies: an experience based on 1,000 attempts. *Anesthesiology* 56:321, 1982.
57. Johnson FE: Internal jugular vein catheterization. *NY State J Med* 78:2168, 1978.
58. Sznajder JI, Zveibil FR, Bitterman H, et al: Central vein catheterization. Failure and complication rates by three percutaneous approaches. *Arch Intern Med* 146:259, 1986.
59. Tripathi M, Pandey M: Anchoring of the internal jugular vein with a pilot needle to facilitate its puncture with a wide bore needle: a randomised, prospective, clinical study. *Anaesthesia* 61:15, 2006.
60. Civetta JM, Gabel JC, Gemer M: Internal-jugular-vein puncture with a margin of safety. *Anesthesiology* 36:622, 1972.
61. Petty C: An alternate method for internal jugular venipuncture for monitoring central venous pressure. *Anesth Analg* 54:157, 1975.
62. Jernigan WR, Gardner WC, Mahr MM, et al: Use of the internal jugular vein for placement of central venous catheter. *Surg Gynecol Obstet* 130:520, 1970.
63. Brinkman AJ, Costley DO: Internal jugular venipuncture. *JAMA* 223:182, 1973.
64. Kaiser CW, Koornick AR, Smith N, et al: Choice of route for central venous cannulation: subclavian or internal jugular vein? A prospective randomized study. *J Surg Oncol* 17:345, 1981.
65. Bo-Linn GW, Anderson DJ, Anderson KC, et al: Percutaneous central venous catheterization performed by medical house officers: a prospective study. *Catheter Cardiovasc Diagn* 8:23, 1982.
66. Bazaral M, Harlan S: Ultrasonographic anatomy of the internal jugular vein relevant to percutaneous cannulation. *Crit Care Med* 9:307, 1981.
67. Mallory DL, Shawker T, Evans RG, et al: Effects of clinical maneuvers on sonographically determined internal jugular vein size during venous cannulation. *Crit Care Med* 18:1269, 1990.
68. Denys BG, Uretsky BF: Anatomical variations of internal jugular vein location: impact on central venous access. *Crit Care Med* 19:1516, 1991.
69. Gilbert TB, Seneff MG, Becker RB: Facilitation of internal jugular venous cannulation using an audio-guided Doppler ultrasound vascular access device: results from a prospective, dual-center, randomized, crossover clinical study. *Crit Care Med* 23:60, 1995.
70. Eisenhauer ED, Derveloy RJ, Hastings PR: Prospective evaluation of central venous pressure (CVP) catheters in a large city-county hospital. *Ann Surg* 196:560, 1982.
71. Klineberg PL, Greenhow DE, Ellison N: Hematoma following internal jugular vein cannulation. *Anesth Intensive Care* 8:94, 1980.
72. Briscoe CE, Bushman JA, McDonald WI: Extensive neurological damage after cannulation of internal jugular vein. *Br Med J* 1:314, 1974.
73. Schwartz AJ, Jobes CR, Greenhow DE, et al: Carotid artery puncture with internal jugular cannulation. *Anesthesiology* 51:S160, 1980.
74. Nicholson T, Ettles D, Robinson G: Managing inadvertent arterial catheterization during central venous access procedures. *Cardiovasc Interv Radiol* 27:21, 2004.
75. Shah PM, Babu SC, Goyal A, et al: Arterial misplacement of large-caliber cannulas during jugular vein catheterization: case for surgical management. *J Am Coll Surg* 198:939, 2004.
76. Ruesch S, Walder B, Tramer MR: Complications of central venous catheters: internal jugular versus subclavian access—a systematic review. [Review] [53 refs]. *Crit Care Med* 30:454, 2002.
77. Nagai K, Kemmotsu O: An inadvertent insertion of a Swan-Ganz catheter into the intrathecal space. *Anesthesiology* 62:848, 1985.
78. Linos DA, Mucha P Jr, van Heerden JA: Subclavian vein. A golden route. *Mayo Clin Proc* 55:315, 1980.
79. Nordlund S, Thoren L: Catheter in the superior vena cava for parenteral feeding. *Acta Chir Scand* 127:39, 1964.
80. Blitt CD, Wright WA, Petty WC, et al: Central venous catheterization via the external jugular vein. A technique employing the J-wire. *JAMA* 229:817, 1974.
81. Schwartz AJ, Jobes DR, Levy WJ, et al: Intrathoracic vascular catheterization via the external jugular vein. *Anesthesiology* 56:400, 1982.
82. Blitt CD, Carlson GL, Wright WA, et al: J-wire versus straight wire for central venous system cannulation via the external jugular vein. *Anesth Analg* 61:536, 1982.
83. Giesy J: External jugular vein access to central venous system. *JAMA* 219:1216, 1972.
84. Riddell GS, Latto IP, Ng WS: External jugular vein access to the central venous system—a trial of two types of catheter. *Br J Anaesth* 54:535, 1982.
85. Jobes DR, Schwartz AJ, Greenhow DE, et al: Safer jugular vein cannulation: recognition of arterial puncture and preferential use of the external jugular route. *Anesthesiology* 59:353, 1983.
86. Moncrief JA: Femoral catheters. *Ann Surg* 147:166, 1958.
87. Bansmer G, Keith D, Tesluk H: Complications following use of indwelling catheters of inferior vena cava. *JAMA* 167:1606, 1958.
88. Dailey RH: "Code Red" protocol for resuscitation of the exsanguinated patient. *J Emerg Med* 2:373, 1985.
89. Kruse JA, Carlson RW: Infectious complications of femoral vs. internal jugular and subclavian vein central venous catheterization. *Crit Care Med* 19:843, 1991.
90. Deshpande KS, Hatem C, Ulrich HL, et al: The incidence of infectious complications of central venous catheters at the subclavian, internal jugular, and femoral sites in an intensive care unit population. *Crit Care Med* 33:13, 2005.
91. Williams JF, Friedman BC, Mcgrath BJ, et al: The use of femoral venous catheters in critically ill adults: a prospective study. *Crit Care Med* 17:584, 1989.
92. Dailey RH: Femoral vein cannulation: a review. [Review] [26 refs]. *J Emerg Med* 2:367, 1985.
93. Sharp KW, Spees EK, Selby LR, et al: Diagnosis and management of retroperitoneal hematomas after femoral vein cannulation for hemodialysis. *Surgery* 95:90, 1984.
94. Fuller TJ, Mahoney JJ, Juncos LI, et al: Arteriovenous fistula after femoral vein catheterization. *JAMA* 236:2943, 1976.
95. Norwood S, Wilkins HE 3rd, Vallina VL, et al: The safety of prolonging the use of central venous catheters: a prospective analysis of the effects of using antiseptic-bonded catheters with daily site care. *Crit Care Med* 28:1376, 2000.
96. Goetz AM, Wagener MM, Miller JM, et al: Risk of infection due to central venous catheters: effect of site of placement and catheter type. *Infect Control Hosp Epidemiol* 19:842, 1998.
97. Stenzel JP, Green TP, Fuhrman BP, et al: Percutaneous femoral venous catheterizations: a prospective study of complications. *J Pediatr* 114:411, 1989.
98. Russell JA, Joel M, Hudson RJ, et al: Prospective evaluation of radial and femoral artery catheterization sites in critically ill adults. *Crit Care Med* 11:936, 1983.
99. Lynn KL, Maling TM: A major pulmonary embolus as a complication of femoral vein catheterization. *Br J Radiol* 50:667, 1977.
100. Aubaniac R: L'injection intraveneuse sousclaviculare advantage et technique. *Presse Med* 60:1456, 1952.
101. Yoffa D: Supraclavicular subclavian venepuncture and catheterisation. *Lancet* 2:614, 1965.
102. Hughes RE, Magovern GJ: The relationship between right atrial pressure and blood volume. *Arch Surg* 79:238, 1959.
103. Wilson JN, Grow JB, Demong CV, et al: Central venous pressure in optimal blood volume maintenance. *Arch Surg* 85:55, 1962.
104. Mansfield PF, Hohn DC, Fornage BD, et al: Complications and failures of subclavian-vein catheterization. *N Engl J Med* 331:1735, 1994.
105. Moosman DA: The anatomy of infraclavicular subclavian vein catheterization and its complications. *Surg Gynecol Obstet* 136:71, 1973.
106. Eerola R, Kaukinen L, Kaukinen S: Analysis of 13 800 subclavian vein catheterizations. *Acta Anaesthesiol Scand* 29:193, 1985.
107. James PM Jr, Myers RT: Central venous pressure monitoring: misinterpretation, abuses, indications and a new technic. *Ann Surg* 175:693, 1972.
108. MacDonnell JE, Perez H, Pitts SR, et al: Supraclavicular subclavian vein catheterization: modified landmarks for needle insertion. *Ann Emerg Med* 21:421, 1992.
109. Dronen S, Thompson B, Nowak R, et al: Subclavian vein catheterization during cardiopulmonary resuscitation. A prospective comparison of the supraclavicular and infraclavicular percutaneous approaches. *JAMA* 247:3227, 1982.
110. Sterner S, Plummer DW, Clinton J, et al: A comparison of the supraclavicular approach and the infraclavicular approach for subclavian vein catheterization. *Ann Emerg Med* 15:421, 1986.
111. Seneff MG: Central venous catheterization: A comprehensive review. *J Intensive Care Med* 2:218, 1987.
112. Park HP, Jeon Y, Hwang JW, et al: Influence of orientations of guidewire tip on the placement of subclavian venous catheters. *Acta Anaesthesiol Scand* 49:1460, 2005.
113. McGee WT, Ackerman BL, Rouben LR, et al: Accurate placement of central venous catheters: a prospective, randomized, multicenter trial. *Crit Care Med* 21:1118, 1993.
114. Simpson ET, Aitchison JM: Percutaneous infraclavicular subclavian vein catheterization in shocked patients: a prospective study in 172 patients. *J Trauma-Injury Infect Crit Care* 22:781, 1982.
115. Herbst CA Jr: Indications, management, and complications of percutaneous subclavian catheters. An audit. *Arch Surgery* 113:1421, 1978.
116. Bernard RW, Stahl WM: Subclavian vein catheterizations: a prospective study. I. Non-infectious complications. *Ann Surg* 173:184, 1971.
117. McGoon MD, Benedetto PW, Greene BM: Complications of percutaneous central venous catheterization: a report of two cases and review of the literature. *Johns Hopkins Med J* 145:1, 1979.
118. Despars JA, Sassoon CS, Light RW: Significance of iatrogenic pneumothoraces. *Chest* 105:1147, 1994.
119. Matz R: Complications of determining the central venous pressure. *N Engl J Med* 273:703, 1965.
120. Sherertz RJ, Ely EW, Westbrook DM, et al: Education of physicians-in-training can decrease the risk for vascular catheter infection. *Ann Intern Med* 132:641, 2000.
121. Maki DG, Weise CE, Sarafin HW: A semiquantitative culture method for identifying intravenous-catheter-related infection. *N Engl J Med* 296:1305, 1977.
122. Raad I, Hanna HA, Alakech B, et al: Differential time to positivity: a useful method for diagnosing catheter-related bloodstream infections. [see comment] [summary for pa-

tients in *Ann Intern Med Jan* 6;140(1):I39, 2004; PMID: 14706995]. *Ann Intern Med* 140:18, 2004.

123. Cooper GL, Hopkins CC: Rapid diagnosis of intravascular catheter-associated infection by direct Gram staining of catheter segments. *N Engl J Med* 312:1142, 1985.

124. Zufferey J, Rime B, Francioli P, et al: Simple method for rapid diagnosis of catheter-associated infection by direct acridine orange staining of catheter tips. *J Clin Microbiol* 26:175, 1988.

125. National Nosocomial Infections Surveillance System: National Nosocomial Infections Surveillance (NNIS) system report, data summary from January 1992 through June 2004; issued October 2004. *Am J Infect Control* 32:470, 2004.

126. Raad I: Intravascular-catheter-related infections. *Lancet* 351:893, 1998.

127. O'Grady NP, Alexander M, Dellinger EP, et al: Guidelines for the prevention of intravascular catheter-related infections. *Am J Infect Control* 30:476, 2002.

128. Martin MA, Pfaller MA, Wenzel RP: Coagulase-negative staphylococcal bacteremia. Mortality and hospital stay. *Ann Intern Med* 110:9, 1989.

129. Smith RL, Meixler SM, Simberkoff MS: Excess mortality in critically ill patients with nosocomial bloodstream infections. *Chest* 100:164, 1991.

130. Pittet D, Tarara D, Wenzel RP: Nosocomial bloodstream infection in critically ill patients. Excess length of stay, extra costs, and attributable mortality. *JAMA* 271:1598, 1994.

131. Rello J, Ochagavia A, Sabanes E, et al: Evaluation of outcome of intravenous catheter-related infections in critically ill patients. *Am J Respir Crit Care Med* 162:1027–1030, 2000.

132. Wenzel RP, Edmond MB: The impact of hospital-acquired bloodstream infections. *Emerg Infect Dis* 7:172, 2001.

133. Doebbeling BN, Stanley GL, Sheetz CT, et al: Comparative efficacy of alternative handwashing agents in reducing nosocomial infections in intensive care units. *N Engl J Med* 327:88, 1992.

134. Passerini L, Lam K, Costerton JW, et al: Biofilms on indwelling vascular catheters. *Crit Care Med* 20:665, 1992.

135. Olson ME, Lam K, Bodey GP, et al: Evaluation of strategies for central venous catheter replacement. *Crit Care Med* 20:797, 1992.

136. Maki DG, Cobb L, Garman JK, et al: An attachable silver-impregnated cuff for prevention of infection with central venous catheters: a prospective randomized multicenter trial. *Am J Med* 85:307, 1988.

137. Moro ML, Vigano EF, Cozzi Lepri A: Risk factors for central venous catheter-related infections in surgical and intensive care units. The Central Venous Catheter-Related Infections Study Group. [erratum appears in *Infect Control Hosp Epidemiol* 15(8):508–509, 1994]. *Infect Control Hosp Epidemiol* 15:253, 1994.

138. Raad I, Costerton W, Sabharwal U, et al: Ultrastructural analysis of indwelling vascular catheters: a quantitative relationship between luminal colonization and duration of placement. *J Infect Dis* 168:400, 1993.

139. Raad II, Hohn DC, Gilbreath BJ, et al: Prevention of central venous catheter-related infections by using maximal sterile barrier precautions during insertion. *Infect Control Hosp Epidemiol* 15:231, 1994.

140. Mimoz O, Pieroni L, Lawrence C, et al: Prospective, randomized trial of two antiseptic solutions for prevention of central venous or arterial catheter colonization and infection in intensive care unit patients. *Crit Care Med* 24:1818, 1996.

141. Maki DG, Ringer M, Alvarado CJ: Prospective randomised trial of povidone-iodine, alcohol, and chlorhexidine for prevention of infection associated with central venous and arterial catheters. *Lancet* 338:339, 1991.

142. Parras F, Ena J, Bouza E, et al: Impact of an educational program for the prevention of colonization of intravascular catheters. *Infect Control Hosp Epidemiol* 15:239, 1994.

143. Maki DG, Botticelli JT, LeRoy ML, et al: Prospective study of replacing administration sets for intravenous therapy at 48- vs. 72-hour intervals. 72 hours is safe and cost-effective. *JAMA* 258:1777, 1987.

144. Hoffmann KK, Weber DJ, Samsa GP, et al: Transparent polyurethane film as an intravenous catheter dressing. A meta-analysis of the infection risks. *JAMA* 267:2072, 1992.

145. Hill RL, Fisher AP, Ware RJ, et al: Mupirocin for the reduction of colonization of internal jugular cannulae—a randomized controlled trial. *J Hosp Infect* 15:311, 1990.

146. Miller JJ, Venus B, Mathru M: Comparison of the sterility of long-term central venous catheterization using single lumen, triple lumen, and pulmonary artery catheters. *Crit Care Med* 12:634, 1984.

147. Arnow PM, Quimosing EM, Beach M: Consequences of intravascular catheter sepsis. *Clin Infect Dis* 16:778, 1993.

148. Veenstra DL, Saint S, Sullivan SD: Cost-effectiveness of antiseptic-impregnated central venous catheters for the prevention of catheter-related bloodstream infection. *JAMA* 282:554, 1999.

149. Hanley EM, Veeder A, Smith T, et al: Evaluation of an antiseptic triple-lumen catheter in an intensive care unit. *Crit Care Med* 28:366, 2000.

150. Flowers RH 3rd, Schwenzer KJ, Kopel RF, et al: Efficacy of an attachable subcutaneous cuff for the prevention of intravascular catheter-related infection. A randomized, controlled trial. *JAMA* 261:878, 1989.

151. Kamal GD, Pfaller MA, Rempe LE, et al: Reduced intravascular catheter infection by antibiotic bonding. A prospective, randomized, controlled trial. *JAMA* 265:2364, 1991.

152. Collin GR: Decreasing catheter colonization through the use of an antiseptic-impregnated catheter: a continuous quality improvement project. *Chest* 115:1632, 1999.

153. Mermel LA, Farr BM, Sherertz RJ, et al: Guidelines for the management of intravascular catheter-related infections. *Infect Control Hosp Epidemiol* 22:222, 2001.

154. Clarke DE, Raffin TA: Infectious complications of indwelling long-term central venous catheters. *Chest* 97:966, 1990.

155. McCarthy MC, Shives JK, Robison RJ, et al: Prospective evaluation of single and triple lumen catheters in total parenteral nutrition. *JPEN: J Parenter Enteral Nutrition* 11:259, 1987.

156. Clark-Christoff N, Watters VA, Sparks W, et al: Use of triple-lumen subclavian catheters for administration of total parenteral nutrition. *JPEN: J Parenter Enteral Nutrition* 16:403, 1992.

157. Farkas JC, Liu N, Bleriot JP, et al: Single- versus triple-lumen central catheter-related sepsis: a prospective randomized study in a critically ill population. *Am J Med* 93:277, 1992.

158. Randolph AG, Cook DJ, Gonzales CA, et al: Tunneling short-term central venous catheters to prevent catheter-related infection: a meta-analysis of randomized, controlled trials. *Crit Care Med* 26:1452, 1998.

159. Eyer S, Brummitt C, Crossley K, et al: Catheter-related sepsis: prospective, randomized study of three methods of long-term catheter maintenance. *Crit Care Med* 18:1073, 1990.

160. Cobb DK, High KP, Sawyer RG, et al: A controlled trial of scheduled replacement of central venous and pulmonary-artery catheters. *N Engl J Med* 327:1062, 1992.

161. Badley AD, Steckelberg JM, Wollan PC, et al: Infectious rates of central venous pressure catheters: comparison between newly placed catheters and those that have been changed. *Mayo Clin Proc* 71:838, 1996.

162. Rello J, Coll P, Net A, et al: Infection of pulmonary artery catheters. Epidemiologic characteristics and multivariate analysis of risk factors. [Review] [37 refs.] *Chest* 103:132, 1993.

163. Moss AH, Vasilakis C, Holley JL, et al: Use of a silicone dual-lumen catheter with a Dacron cuff as a long-term vascular access for hemodialysis patients. *Am J Kidney Dis* 16:211, 1990.

164. Sherertz RJ, Carruth WA, Hampton AA, et al: Efficacy of antibiotic-coated catheters in preventing subcutaneous Staphylococcus aureus infection in rabbits. *J Infect Dis* 167:98, 1993.

165. Mangano DT: Heparin bonding and long-term protection against thrombogenesis. *N Engl J Med* 307:894, 1982.

166. Darouiche RO, Raad II, Heard SO, et al: A comparison of two antimicrobial-impregnated central venous catheters. Catheter Study Group. *N Engl J Med* 340:1, 1999.

167. Centers for Disease Control and Prevention (CDC): Reduction in central line-associated bloodstream infections among patients in intensive care units—Pennsylvania, April 2001–March 2005. *MMWR Morb Mortal Wkly Rep* 54:1013, 2005.

Scott A. Celinski
Michael G. Seneff

CHAPTER **3**

Arterial Line Placement and Care

Arterial catheterization is the second most frequent invasive procedure performed in the intensive care unit (ICU). In nearly all institutions, the logistics of setup, maintenance, and troubleshooting of pressure monitoring equipment are now largely relegated to personnel other than physicians [1]. Unfortunately, this shift away from physician involvement has left many intensivists without an adequate working knowledge of these important systems. While historically the most common indications to place an arterial catheter have been for beat-to-beat monitoring of blood pressure in unstable patients and frequent blood gas sampling, new technologies have arisen that necessitate arterial access. For example, arterial pulse contour analysis can now be used to determine cardiac output reliably and less invasively in patients compared to the traditional thermodilution method [2,3]. Additional technological improvements will undoubtedly follow, and the need for arterial line placement may decrease as technologies such as transcutaneous PCO_2 monitoring and noninvasive systems for measuring arterial waveforms mature [4,5]. In this chapter, we review the principles of hemodynamic monitoring and discuss the indications and routes of arterial cannulation.

INDICATIONS FOR ARTERIAL CANNULATION

Arterial catheters should be inserted only when they are specifically required and removed immediately when no longer needed. Too often, they are left in place for convenience to allow easy access to blood sampling. Many studies have documented that arterial catheters are associated with an increased number of laboratory blood tests, leading to greater costs and excessive diagnostic blood loss [6,7]. Protocols incorporating guidelines for arterial catheterization and alternative noninvasive monitoring, such as pulse oximetry and end tidal CO_2 monitoring, have realized significant improvements in resource utilization and cost savings, without impacting the quality of care [8].

The indications for arterial cannulation can be grouped into four broad categories (Table 3-1): (a) hemodynamic monitoring (including pulse contour cardiac output monitoring); (b) frequent arterial blood gas sampling; (c) arterial administration of drugs, such as thrombolytics; and (d) intraaortic balloon pump use.

Noninvasive, indirect blood pressure measurements determined by auscultation of Korotkoff sounds distal to an occluding cuff (Riva-Rocci method) are generally accurate, although systolic readings are consistently lower compared to a simultaneous direct measurement. In hemodynamically unstable patients, however, indirect techniques may significantly underestimate blood pressure [9]. Automated noninvasive blood pressure measurement devices can also be inaccurate, particularly in rapidly changing situations, at the extremes of blood pressure, and in patients with dysrhythmias [10]. For these reasons, direct blood pressure monitoring is usually required for unstable patients. Rapid beat-to-beat changes can easily be monitored and appropriate therapeutic modalities initiated, and variations in individual pressure waveforms may prove diagnostic. Waveform inspection can rapidly diagnose electrocardiogram (ECG) lead disconnect, indicate the presence of aortic valve disease, help determine the effect of dysrhythmias on perfusion, and reveal the impact of the respiratory cycle on blood pressure (pulsus paradoxus). Additionally, the responsiveness of cardiac output to fluid boluses may be predicted by calculating the systolic pressure variation (SPV) or pulse pressure variation (PPV) through the respiratory cycle. Using PPV has been shown to be superior to SPV, with a PPV greater than 13% predicting an increase in cardiac output (CO) greater than or equal to 15% in response to a fluid challenge [11].

Recent advances allow continuous CO monitoring using arterial pulse contour analysis. This method relies on the assumption that the contour of the arterial pressure waveform is proportional to the stroke volume [12]. This, however, does not take into consideration the differing impedances between the arteries of individuals, and therefore requires calibration with another method of determining cardiac output [13]. Calibration is usually done with lithium or transpulmonary thermal dilution methods. A new pulse contour analysis instrument has been introduced that does not require an additional method of determining CO for calibration, but instead estimates impedance based on the waveform and patient demographic data [3]. This method has significant limitations (i.e., atrial fibrillation), and further data and comparison to other methods in authentic clinical situations are required before recommendations for widespread adoption can be made.

Management of patients in critical care units typically requires multiple laboratory determinations. Unstable patients on mechanical ventilators or in whom intubation is contemplated may need frequent monitoring of arterial blood gases. In these situations, arterial cannulation prevents repeated trauma by frequent arterial punctures and permits routine laboratory tests without multiple needle sticks. In our opinion, an arterial line for blood gas determination should be placed when a patient will require three or more measurements daily.

TABLE 3-1. Indications for Arterial Cannulation

Hemodynamic monitoring
  Acutely hypertensive or hypotensive patients
  Continuous cardiac output monitoring
  Use of vasoactive drugs
Multiple blood sampling
  Ventilated patients
  Limited venous access
Arterial administration of drugs
Intraaortic balloon pump use

EQUIPMENT, MONITORING TECHNIQUES, AND SOURCES OF ERROR

The equipment necessary to display and measure an arterial waveform includes: (a) an appropriate intravascular catheter; (b) fluid-filled noncompliant tubing with stopcocks; (c) transducer; (d) a constant flush device; and (e) electronic monitoring equipment. Using this equipment, intravascular pressure changes are transmitted through the hydraulic (fluid-filled) elements to the transducer, which converts mechanical displacement into a proportional electrical signal. The signal is amplified, processed, and displayed as a waveform by the monitor. Undistorted presentation of the arterial waveform is dependent on the performance of each component. A detailed discussion of relevant pressure monitoring principles is beyond the scope of this chapter, but consideration of a few basic concepts is useful to understand the genesis of most monitoring inaccuracies.

 The major problems inherent to pressure monitoring with a catheter system are inadequate dynamic response, improper zeroing and zero drift, and improper transducer/monitor calibration [14]. Most physicians are aware of zeroing techniques but do not appreciate the importance of dynamic response in ensuring system fidelity. Catheter-tubing-transducer systems used for pressure monitoring can best be characterized as underdamped second-order dynamic systems with mechanical parameters of elasticity, mass, and friction [14]. Overall, the dynamic response of such a system is determined by its resonant frequency and damping coefficient (zeta). The resonant or natural frequency of a system is the frequency at which it oscillates when stimulated. When the frequency content of an input signal (i.e., pressure waveform) approaches the resonant frequency of a system, progressive amplification of the output signal occurs, a phenomenon known as ringing [15]. To ensure a flat frequency response (accurate recording across a spectrum of frequencies),

the resonant frequency of a monitoring system should be at least 5 times higher than the highest frequency in the input signal [14]. Physiologic peripheral arterial waveforms have a fundamental frequency of 3 to 5 Hz, and therefore the resonant frequency of a system used to monitor arterial pressure should ideally be greater than 20 Hz to avoid ringing and systolic overshoot.

The system component most likely to cause amplification of a pressure waveform is the hydraulic element. A good hydraulic system will have a resonant frequency between 10 and 20 Hz, which may overlap with arterial pressure frequencies. Thus, amplification can occur, which may require damping to accurately reproduce the waveform [16].

The damping coefficient is a measure of how quickly an oscillating system comes to rest. A system with a high damping coefficient absorbs mechanical energy well (i.e., compliant tubing), causing a diminution in the transmitted waveform. Conversely, a system with a low damping coefficient results in underdamping and systolic overshoot. Damping coefficient and resonant frequency together determine the dynamic response of a recording system. If the system's resonant frequency is less than 7.5 Hz, the pressure waveform will be distorted no matter what the damping coefficient. On the other hand, a resonant frequency of 24 Hz allows a range in the damping coefficient of 0.15 to 1.1 without resultant distortion of the pressure waveform [14,17].

Although there are other techniques [18], the easiest method to test the damping coefficient and resonant frequency of a monitoring system is the fast-flush test (also known as the square wave test). This is performed at the bedside by briefly opening and closing the continuous flush device, which produces a square wave displacement on the monitor followed by a return to baseline, usually after a few smaller oscillations (Fig. 3-1). Values for the damping coefficient and resonant frequency can be computed by printing the wave on graph paper [14], but visual inspection is usually adequate to ensure a proper frequency response. An optimum fast-flush test results in one undershoot followed by small overshoot, then settles to the patient's waveform (Fig. 3-1).

For peripheral pulse pressure monitoring, an adequate fast-flush test usually corresponds to a resonant frequency of 10 to 20 Hz coupled with a damping coefficient of 0.5 to 0.7 [17]. To ensure the continuing fidelity of a monitoring system, dynamic response validation by fast-flush test should be performed frequently: at least every 8 hours, with every significant change in patient hemodynamic status, after each opening of the system (zeroing, blood sampling, tubing change), and whenever the waveform appears damped.

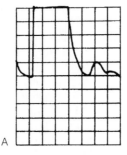
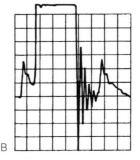
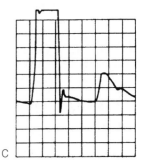

FIGURE 3-1. Fast-flush test. **A:** Overdamped system. **B:** Underdamped system. **C:** Optimal damping.

With consideration of the above concepts, components of the monitoring system are designed to optimize the frequency response of the entire system. The 18- and 20-gauge catheters used to gain vascular access are not a major source of distortion but can become kinked or occluded by thrombus, resulting in overdamping of the system. Standard, noncompliant tubing is provided with most disposable transducer kits and should be as short as possible to minimize signal amplification [15]. Air bubbles in the tubing and connecting stopcocks are a notorious source of overdamping of the tracing and can be cleared by flushing through a stopcock. Currently available disposable transducers incorporate microchip technology, are very reliable, and have relatively high resonant frequencies [19]. The transducer is attached to the electronic monitoring equipment by a cable. Modern monitors have internal calibration, filter artifacts, and print the display on request. The digital readout display is usually an average of values over time and therefore does not accurately represent beat-to-beat variability. Monitors provide the capability to freeze a display with on-screen calibration to measure beat-to-beat differences in amplitude precisely. This allows measurement of the effect of ectopic beats on blood pressure, PPV, SPV, or assessment of the severity of pulsus paradoxus.

When presented with pressure data or readings believed to be inaccurate, or which are significantly different from indirect readings, a few quick checks can ensure system accuracy. Improper zeroing of the system is the single most important source of error. Zeroing can be checked by opening the transducer stopcock to air and aligning with the midaxillary line, confirming that the monitor displays zero. Zeroing should be repeated with patient position changes, when significant changes in blood pressure occur, and routinely every 6 to 8 hours because of zero drift. Disposable pressure transducers incorporate semiconductor technology and are very small, yet rugged and reliable, and due to standardization, calibration of the system is not necessary [19]. Transducers are faulty on occasion, however, and calibration may be checked by attaching a mercury manometer to the stopcock and applying 100, 150, and/or 200 mm Hg pressure. A variation of plus or minus 5 mm Hg is acceptable. If calibration is questioned and the variation is out of range, or a manometer is not available for testing, the transducer should be replaced.

If zero referencing and calibration are correct, a fast-flush test will assess the system's dynamic response. Overdamped tracings are usually caused by air bubbles, kinks, clot formation, overly compliant tubing, loose connections, a deflated pressure bag, or anatomical factors affecting the catheter. All of these are usually correctable and should be assessed if the system is overdamped. An underdamped tracing results in systolic overshoot and can be secondary to excessive tubing length or patient factors such as increased inotropic or chronotropic state. Many monitors can be adjusted to filter out frequencies above a certain limit, which can eliminate frequencies in the input signal that causes ringing. However, this may also cause inaccurate readings if important frequencies are excluded.

TECHNIQUE OF ARTERIAL CANNULATION

SITE SELECTION

Several factors are important in selecting the site for arterial cannulation. The ideal artery has extensive collateral circulation that will maintain the viability of distal tissues if thrombosis occurs. The site should be comfortable for the patient, accessible for nursing care and insertion, and close to the monitoring equipment. Sites involved by infection or disruption in the epidermal barrier should be avoided. Certain procedures, such as coronary artery bypass grafting, may dictate preference for one site over another. Larger arteries and catheters provide more accurate (central aortic) pressure measurements. Physicians should also be cognizant of differences in pulse contour recorded at different sites. As the pressure pulse wave travels outward from the aorta, it encounters arteries that are smaller and less elastic, with multiple branch points, causing reflections of the pressure wave. This results in a peripheral pulse contour with increased slope and amplitude, causing recorded values to be artificially elevated. As a result, distal extremity artery recordings yield higher systolic values than central aortic or femoral artery recordings. Diastolic pressures tend to be less affected, and mean arterial pressures measured at the different sites are similar [20,21].

The most commonly used sites for arterial cannulation in adults are the radial, femoral, axillary, dorsalis pedis, and brachial arteries. Additional sites include the ulnar, posterior tibial, and superficial temporal arteries. Peripheral sites are cannulated percutaneously with a 2-inch, 20-gauge, nontapered Teflon catheter-over-needle and larger arteries using the Seldinger technique with a prepackaged kit, typically containing a 6-inch, 18- or 20-gauge Teflon catheter and appropriate introducer needles and guidewire.

Critical care physicians should be facile with arterial cannulation at all sites, but the radial and femoral arteries are used successfully for more than 90% of all arterial catheterizations. Although each site has unique complications, available data do not indicate a preference for any one site [22–26]. Radial artery cannulation is usually attempted initially unless the patient is in shock and/or pulses are not palpable. If this fails, femoral artery cannulation should be performed.

RADIAL ARTERY CANNULATION

A thorough understanding of normal arterial anatomy and common anatomical variants greatly facilitates insertion of catheters and management of unexpected findings at all sites. The reader is referred elsewhere for a comprehensive review of arterial anatomy [27]; only relevant anatomical considerations are presented here. The radial artery is one of two final branches of the brachial artery. It courses over the flexor digitorum sublimis, flexor pollicis longus, and pronator quadratus muscles and lies just lateral to the flexor carpi radialis in the forearm (Fig. 3-2). As the artery enters the floor of the palm, it ends in the deep volar arterial arch at the level of the metacarpal bones and communicates with the ulnar artery. A second site of collateral flow for the radial artery occurs via the dorsal arch running in the dorsum of the hand.

The ulnar artery runs between the flexor carpi ulnaris and flexor digitorum sublimis in the forearm, with a short course over the ulnar nerve. In the hand the artery runs over the transverse carpal ligament and becomes the superficial volar arch, which forms an anastomosis with a small branch of the radial artery. These three anastomoses provide excellent collateral flow to the hand. A competent superficial or deep palmar arch must be present to ensure adequate collateral flow. At least one of these arches may be absent in up to 20% of individuals.

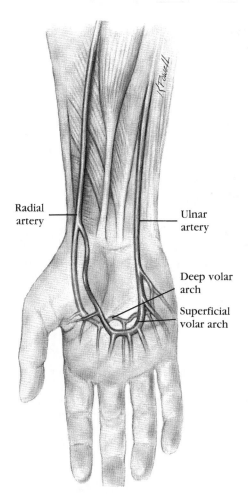

FIGURE 3-2. Anatomy of the radial artery. Note the collateral circulation to the ulnar artery through the deep volar arterial arch and dorsal arch.

Radial artery

Ulnar artery

Deep volar arch

Superficial volar arch

Modified Allen's Test

Prior to placement of a radial or ulnar arterial line, it must be demonstrated that the blood supply to the hand would not be eliminated by a catheter-induced thrombus. In 1929, Allen [28] described a technique of diagnosing occlusive arterial disease. His technique has been modified and serves as the most common screening test prior to radial artery cannulation. The examiner compresses both radial and ulnar arteries and asks the patient to clinch and unclench the fist repeatedly until pallor of the palm is produced. Hyperextension of the hand is avoided, as it may cause a false-negative result, suggesting inadequate collateral flow [29]. One artery is then released and the time to blushing of the palm noted. The procedure is repeated with the other artery. Normal palmar blushing is complete before 7 seconds (positive test); 8 to 14 seconds is considered equivocal; and 15 or more seconds abnormal (negative test).

The modified Allen's test is not an ideal screening procedure. In one study comparing the Allen's test to Doppler examination, Allen's test had a sensitivity of 87% (i.e., it detected ulnar collateral flow in 87% of cases in which Doppler study confirmed its presence) and a negative predictive value of only 0.18 (i.e., only 18% of patients with no collateral flow by Allen's test had this confirmed by Doppler study) [30]. Other studies have compared Allen's test to plethysmography, with similar results [31]. Thus, the modified Allen's test does not necessarily predict the presence of collateral circulation, and many centers, including ours, have abandoned its use as a routine screening procedure. Each institution should establish its own guidelines regarding routine Allen's testing and the evaluation and management of negative results. Hand ischemia is a significant complication that frequently results in amputation [32,33], and if the lack of collateral circulation is verified by confirmatory testing, it is advisable to avoid arterial cannulation on that hand.

Percutaneous Insertion

The hand is positioned in 30 to 60 degrees of dorsiflexion with the aid of a roll of gauze and arm band, avoiding hyperabduction of the thumb. The volar aspect of the wrist is prepared and draped using sterile technique, and approximately 0.5 mL of 1% lidocaine is infiltrated on both sides of the artery through a 25-gauge or smaller needle. Lidocaine serves to decrease patient discomfort and may decrease the likelihood of arterial vasospasm [34].

A 20-gauge, nontapered, Teflon 1.5- or 2-inch catheter-over-needle apparatus is used for puncture. Entry is made at a 30- to 60-degree angle to the skin approximately 3 to 5 cm proximal to the distal wrist crease. The needle and cannula are advanced until blood return is noted in the hub, signifying intra-arterial placement of the tip of the needle (Fig. 3-3). A small amount of further advancement is necessary for the cannula to enter the artery as well. With this accomplished, needle and cannula are brought flat to the skin and the cannula advanced to its hub with a firm, steady rotary action. Correct positioning is confirmed by pulsatile blood return on removal of the needle. If the initial attempt is unsuccessful, subsequent attempts should be more proximal, rather than closer to the wrist crease, as the artery is of greater diameter [27]. However, more proximal insertion may increase the incidence of catheters becoming kinked or occluded [35].

If difficulty is encountered when attempting to pass the catheter, carefully replacing the needle and slightly advancing the whole apparatus may remedy the problem. Alternately, a fixation technique can be attempted (Fig. 3-3). Advancing the needle and catheter through the far wall of the vessel purposely transfixes the artery. The needle is then pulled back with the cannula until vigorous arterial blood return is noted. The catheter can then be advanced into the arterial lumen, although occasionally the needle must be carefully partially reinserted (never forced, to avoid shearing the catheter) to serve as a rigid stent.

Catheters with self-contained guidewires to facilitate passage of the cannula into the artery are available. Percutaneous puncture is made in the same manner, but when blood return is noted in the catheter hub the guidewire is passed through the needle into the artery, serving as a stent for subsequent catheter advancement. The guidewire and needle are then removed and placement confirmed by pulsatile blood return. The cannula is then secured firmly, attached to transducer tubing, and the site bandaged. Video instruction for the insertion of a radial arterial line is available at the website for *New England Journal of Medicine* [36].

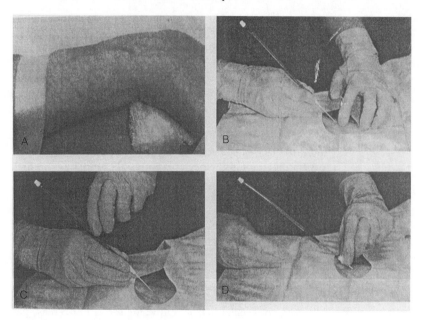

FIGURE 3-3. Cannulation of the radial artery. **A:** A towel is placed behind the wrist, and the hand is immobilized with tape. **B:** The catheter-needle-guidewire apparatus is inserted into the skin at a 30–60 degree angle. **C:** The guidewire is advanced into the artery after pulsatile blood flow is obtained. **D:** The catheter is advanced over the guidewire into the artery. [From Irwin RS, Rippe JM: *Manual of Intensive Care Medicine* 4th ed. Philadelphia, Lippincott Williams & Wilkins, 2006, p 17, with permission.]

DORSALIS PEDIS ARTERY CANNULATION

Dorsalis pedis artery catheterization is uncommon in most critical care units; compared to the radial artery, the anatomy is less predictable and the success rate is lower [37]. The dorsalis pedis artery is the main blood supply of the dorsum of the foot. The artery runs from the level of the ankle to the great toe. It lies very superficial and just lateral to the tendon of the extensor hallucis longus (Fig. 3-4). The dorsalis pedis anastomoses with branches from the posterior tibial (lateral plantar artery) and, to a lesser extent, peroneal arteries, creating an arterial arch network analogous to that in the hand. Occluding the dorsalis pedis and posterior tibial pulses and blanching the great toe by repeated flexion assess collateral circulation. Release of the posterior tibial artery should result in blushing of the toe within 10 seconds; longer blushing times may represent poor collateral circulation. Tests using Doppler probes or pneumatic cuffs around the great toe have also been proposed.

The foot is placed in plantar flexion and prepared in the usual fashion. Vessel entry is obtained approximately halfway up the dorsum of the foot; advancement is the same as with cannulation of the radial artery. Patients usually find insertion here more painful but less physically limiting. Systolic pressure readings are usually 5 to 20 mm Hg higher with dorsalis pedis catheters than radial artery catheters, but mean pressure values are generally unchanged.

BRACHIAL ARTERY CANNULATION

Cannulation of the brachial artery is infrequently performed because of concern regarding the lack of effective collateral circulation. Centers experienced in the use of brachial artery catheters, however, have reported complication rates no higher than with other routes [27,38,39]. Even when diminution of distal pulses occurs, either because of proximal obstruction or distal embolization, clinical ischemia is unlikely [38]. An additional anatomic consideration is the median nerve, which lies in close proximity to the brachial artery in the antecubital fossa

and may be punctured in 1% to 2% of cases [39]. This usually causes only transient paresthesias, but median nerve palsy has been reported. Median nerve palsy is a particular risk in patients with coagulopathy because even minor bleeding into the fascial planes can produce compression of the median nerve [40].

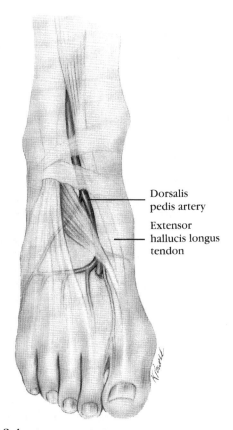

Dorsalis pedis artery

Extensor hallucis longus tendon

FIGURE 3-4. Anatomy of dorsalis pedis artery and adjacent structures.

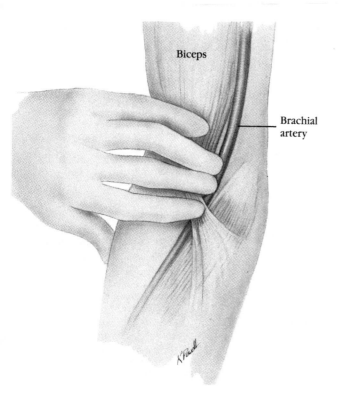

FIGURE 3-5. Palpation of the brachial artery. The arm is fully extended at the elbow and the artery palpated in the antecubital fossa as indicated. The brachial artery is then cannulated at this site.

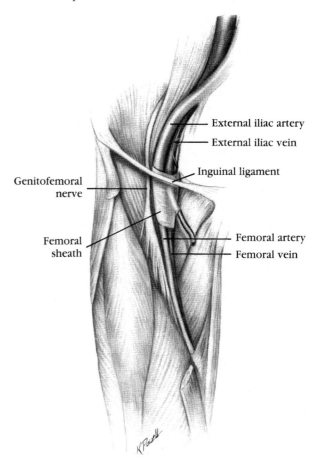

FIGURE 3-6. Anatomy of the femoral artery and adjacent structures. The artery is cannulated below the inguinal ligament.

Coagulopathy should be considered a relative contraindication to brachial artery cannulation.

Cannulation of the brachial artery can be performed with a 2-inch catheter-over-needle as described for the radial artery, but most centers use the Seldinger technique. Inserting a 6-inch catheter using the Seldinger technique (see Femoral Artery Cannulation, below) into the brachial artery places the catheter tip in the axillary artery where pressures obtained are more representative of aortic pressures, and catheter patency is improved. The brachial artery is punctured by extending the arm at the elbow and locating the pulsation in or slightly proximal to the antecubital fossa, just medial to the bicipital tendon (Fig. 3-5). Once catheterization is established, the elbow must be kept in full extension to avoid kinking or breaking the catheter. Clinical examination of the hand, and Doppler studies if indicated, should be repeated daily while the brachial catheter is in place. The catheter should be promptly removed if diminution of any pulse occurs or there is evidence of embolism.

FEMORAL ARTERY CANNULATION

The femoral artery is usually the next alternative when radial artery cannulation fails or is inappropriate [22–26]. The femoral artery is large and often palpable when other sites are not, and the technique of cannulation is easy to learn. The most common reason for failure to cannulate is severe atherosclerosis or prior vascular procedures involving both femoral arteries, in which case axillary or brachial artery cannulation is appropriate. Complications unique to this site are rare but include retroperitoneal hemorrhage and intraabdominal viscus perforation. These complications occur because of poor technique (puncture above the inguinal ligament) or in the presence of anatomical variations (i.e., large inguinal hernia). Ischemic complications from femoral artery catheters are very rare.

The external iliac artery becomes the common femoral artery at the inguinal ligament (Fig. 3-6). The artery courses under the inguinal ligament near the junction of the medial and the middle third of a straight line drawn between the pubis and the anterior superior iliac spine. The artery is cannulated using the Seldinger technique and any one of several available prepackaged kits. Kits contain the equivalent of an 18- or 19-gauge thin-wall needle, appropriate guidewire, and a 6-inch, 18- or 20-gauge Teflon catheter. The patient lies supine with the leg extended and slightly abducted. Site preparation includes clipping of pubic hair if necessary. Skin puncture should be 3 to 5 cm caudal to the inguinal ligament to minimize the risk of retroperitoneal hematoma or bowel perforation, which can occur when needle puncture of the vessel is cephalad to the inguinal ligament. The thin-wall needle is directed, bevel up, and cephalad at a 45-degree angle. When arterial blood return is confirmed, the needle and syringe may need to be brought down against the skin to facilitate guidewire passage. The guidewire should advance smoothly, but minor manipulation and rotation is sometimes required if the wire meets resistance at the needle tip or after it has advanced into the vessel. Inability to pass the guidewire may be due to an intimal flap over the needle bevel or atherosclerotic plaques in the vessel. In the latter instance, cannulation of that femoral artery may prove impossible. When the guidewire will not pass beyond the needle tip it should be withdrawn and blood return reestablished by advancing the needle or repeat vascular puncture. The guidewire is then inserted and the needle withdrawn. A stab incision made with a scalpel at the skin puncture site is usually not needed. The catheter is next threaded over the guidewire to its hub and the guidewire withdrawn. The catheter is then sutured securely and connected to the transducer tubing.

AXILLARY ARTERY CANNULATION

Axillary artery catheterization in the ICU occurs infrequently, but centers experienced with it report a low rate of complications [41]. The axillary artery is large and frequently palpable when all other sites are not and has a rich collateral circulation. The tip of a 6-inch catheter inserted through an axillary approach lies in the subclavian artery, and thus accurate central pressures are obtained. The central location of the tip makes cerebral air embolism a greater risk; therefore, left axillary catheters are preferred for the initial attempt, since air bubbles passing into the right subclavian artery are more likely to traverse the aortic arch [42]. Caution should be exercised in flushing axillary catheters, which is best accomplished manually using low pressures and small volumes.

The axillary artery begins at the lateral border of the first rib as a continuation of the subclavian artery and ends at the inferior margin of the teres major muscle, where it becomes the brachial artery. The optimal site for catheterization is the junction of the middle and lower third of the vessel, which usually corresponds to its highest palpable point in the axilla. At this point the artery is superficial and is located at the inferior border of the pectoralis major muscle. The artery is enclosed in a neurovascular bundle, the axillary sheath, with the medial, posterior, and lateral cords of the brachial plexus. Medial to the medial cord is the axillary vein. Not surprisingly, brachial plexus neuropathies have been reported from axillary artery cannulation [43]. Coagulopathy is a relative contraindication, as the axillary sheath can rapidly fill with blood from an uncontrolled arterial puncture, resulting in a compressive neuropathy.

The axillary artery is cannulated using the Seldinger technique and a prepackaged kit. The arm is abducted, externally rotated, and flexed at the elbow by having the patient place the hand under his or her head. Axillary hair should be clipped and the site prepared in standard fashion. The artery is palpated at the lower border of the pectoralis major muscle and fixed against the shaft of the humerus. After local infiltration with lidocaine, the thin-wall needle is introduced at a 30- to 45-degree angle to the vertical plane until return of arterial blood. The remainder of the catheterization proceeds as described for femoral artery cannulation.

COMPLICATIONS OF ARTERIAL CANNULATION

Arterial cannulation is a relatively safe invasive procedure. Although estimates of the total complication rate range from 15% to 40%, clinically relevant complications occur in 5% or less (Table 3-2). Risk factors for infectious and noninfectious complications have been identified [44–51] (Table 3-3), but the clinical

TABLE 3-2.   Complications Associated with Arterial Cannulation

Site	Complication
All sites	Pain and swelling
	Thrombosis
	Asymptomatic
	Symptomatic
	Embolization
	Hematoma
	Hemorrhage
	Limb ischemia
	Catheter-related infection
	Local
	Systemic
	Diagnostic blood loss
	Pseudoaneurysm
	Heparin-associated thrombocytopenia
Radial artery	Cerebral embolization
	Peripheral neuropathy
Femoral artery	Retroperitoneal hemorrhage
	Bowel perforation
	Arteriovenous fistula
Axillary artery	Cerebral embolization
	Brachial plexopathy
Brachial artery	Median nerve damage
	Cerebral embolization

impact of most of these factors is minimal, given the overall low incidence of complications.

THROMBOSIS

Thrombosis is the single most common complication of intraarterial catheters. The incidence of thrombosis varies with the site, method of detection, size of the cannula, and duration of cannulation. Thrombosis is common with radial and dorsalis pedis catheters, but very rare with femoral or axillary catheters. The incidence of radial artery thrombosis following cannulation has progressively declined due to recognition of the importance of catheter size and composition and the use of continuous versus intermittent heparin flush systems [44,46–51]. The incidence probably increases significantly with duration of cannulation [51]. When a 20-gauge nontapered Teflon catheter with a continuous 3 mL per hour heparinized saline flush is used to cannulate the radial artery for 3 to 4 days, thrombosis

TABLE 3-3.   Factors Predisposing to Complications with Arterial Cannulation

Large tapered cannulas (>20 gauge except at the large artery sites)
Hypotension
Coagulopathy
Low cardiac output
Multiple puncture attempts
Use of vasopressors
Atherosclerosis
Hypercoagulable state
Placement by surgical cutdown
Site inflammation
Intermittent flushing system
Bacteremia

of the vessel can be detected by Doppler study in 5% to 25% of cases [48,50]. Use of a flush solution containing heparin is standard and may reduce the incidence of thrombosis, but in patients with relative or absolute contraindications to heparin use, sodium citrate or saline alone may be substituted [52,53].

Thrombosis often occurs after catheter removal. Women represent a preponderance of patients who experience flow abnormalities following radial artery cannulation, probably because of smaller arteries and a greater tendency to exhibit vasospasm [35]. Most patients eventually recanalize, generally by 3 weeks after removal of the catheter. Despite the high incidence of Doppler-detected thrombosis, clinical ischemia of the hand is rare and usually resolves following catheter removal. Symptomatic occlusion requiring surgical intervention occurs in fewer than 1% of cases, but when it occurs, tissue loss is common [33]. Most patients who develop clinical ischemia have an associated contributory cause, such as prolonged circulatory failure with high-dose vasopressor therapy [49].

Regular inspection of the extremity for unexplained pain or signs of ischemia and immediate removal of the catheter minimize significant ischemic complications. If evidence of ischemia persists after catheter removal, anticoagulation, thrombolytic therapy, embolectomy, surgical bypass, or cervical sympathetic blockade are treatment options [33,49].

CEREBRAL EMBOLIZATION

Continuous flush devices used with arterial catheters are designed to deliver 3 mL per hour of heparinized saline (generally 1 to 5 units heparin/mL saline) from an infusion bag pressurized to 300 mm Hg. Lowenstein et al. [54] demonstrated that with rapid flushing of radial artery lines with relatively small volumes of radiolabeled solution, traces of the solution could be detected in the central arterial circulation in a time frame representative of retrograde flow. Chang et al. [55] demonstrated that injection of greater than 2 mL of air into the radial artery of small primates resulted in retrograde passage of air into the vertebral circulation. Factors that increase the risk for retrograde passage of air are patient size and position (air travels up in a sitting patient), injection site, and flush rate. Air embolism has been cited as a risk mainly for radial arterial catheters [55,56] but logically could occur with all arterial catheters, especially axillary and brachial artery catheters. The risk is minimized by clearing all air from tubing before flushing, opening the flush valve for no more than 2 to 3 seconds, and avoiding overaggressive manual flushing of the line.

DIAGNOSTIC BLOOD LOSS

Diagnostic blood loss (DBL) is patient blood loss that occurs due to frequent blood sampling obtained for laboratory testing. The significance of DBL is underappreciated. It is a particular problem in patients with standard arterial catheter setups that are used as the site for sampling, because 3 to 5 mL of blood is typically wasted (to avoid heparin/saline contamination) every time a sample is obtained. In patients with frequent arterial blood gas determinations, DBL can be substantial and result in a transfusion requirement [57]. There are several ways to minimize DBL, including tubing systems employing a reservoir for blood sampling [58,59], continuous intraarterial blood gas monitoring [60], point of care microchemistry analysis, and the

use of pediatric collection tubes. Given the expense and risks of blood component therapy, any or all of the above techniques should be routinely implemented in every ICU. Protocols that are designed to optimize laboratory use have resulted in significant cost savings and reduced transfusion requirements [61].

HEPARIN-ASSOCIATED THROMBOCYTOPENIA

Thrombocytopenia is very common in critically ill adults and usually not due to heparin [62]. However, when the platelet count falls below 50% of baseline, or to an absolute value of 80,000 to 100,000 per mL, it is advisable to discontinue all heparin, even the small amount contained in continuous flush devices, because of the possibility of heparin-associated thrombocytopenia (HAT) [63,64]. Heparin containing continuous flush solutions probably reduce the rate of thrombosis and occlusion of arterial catheters [65], but in the presence of thrombocytopenia, sodium citrate, saline, and lactated Ringer's solution are suitable replacements [66].

OTHER MECHANICAL AND TECHNICAL COMPLICATIONS

Other noninfectious complications reported with arterial lines are pseudoaneurysm formation [67], hematoma, local tenderness, hemorrhage, neuropathies, and catheter embolization.

Infection

Infectious sequelae are the most important clinical complications occurring because of arterial cannulation, and many of the concepts and definitions applied to central venous catheter–related infection (see Chapter 2) are also relevant to arterial catheters.

Catheter-associated infection is usually initiated by skin flora that invades the intracutaneous tract, causing colonization of the catheter, and ultimately, bacteremia. An additional source of infection from pressure-monitoring systems is contaminated infusate, which is at greater risk for infection than central venous catheters because: (a) the transducer can become colonized because of stagnant flow, (b) the flush solution is infused at a slow rate (3 mL per hour) and may hang for several days, and (c) multiple blood samples are obtained by several different personnel from stopcocks in the system, which can serve as entry sites for bacteria [68].

Appreciation of the mechanisms responsible for initiating arterial catheter–related infection is important in understanding how to minimize infection. Thorough operator and site preparation is paramount. Chlorhexidine has a broader antibacterial spectrum and longer duration of action than 10% povidone-iodine solution and has demonstrated an impressive reduction in catheter-related infection [69,70]. Operators must wash their hands and wear sterile gloves during insertion of radial artery catheters, and triple barrier precautions are appropriate for large artery cannulations. Breaks in sterile technique during insertion mandate termination of the procedure and replacement of compromised equipment. Nursing personnel should follow strict guidelines when drawing blood samples or manipulating tubing. Ideally, stopcocks are covered with diaphragms instead of caps. Blood withdrawn to clear the tubing prior to drawing samples should not be reinjected unless a specially designed system is in use [71]. Daily inspection of the site is mandatory, and the catheter should be removed promptly if abnormalities are noted. Dressings should be changed every 48 to 72 hours.

Finally, older recommendations to completely change the monitoring setup every 48 hours as a means of infection control are obsolete. Routine frequent changes of the pressure monitoring system do not reduce infectious complications and may simply be another opportunity to introduce colonization. Recent studies have documented the safety of prolonging the interval of routine changes [72]; in our institution, we change the monitoring setup every 96 hours.

These measures have contributed to an impressive decrease in arterial catheter–related infection. Arterial catheter–related infection, defined as 15 or more colonies on semiquantitative culture of a catheter segment [73], occurs in 4% to 20% of catheters but contributes to bacteremia or septicemia in 0% to 3% of cases [22,23,24,69,74–77]. The site of insertion does not appear to be an important factor impacting on the incidence of infection [23,24,37,78]; duration of catheterization continues to be important, but recommendations are changing. It is no longer necessary to change arterial catheters routinely, as studies of catheters remaining in place a week or longer have not demonstrated a higher rate of clinically important infection [77,78]. Each institution should determine its own catheter-associated infection rate so that rational policies can be formulated based on existing infection rates.

When arterial catheter infection does occur, staphylococcus species, especially *S. epidermidis*, are commonly isolated. Gram-negative organisms are less frequent, but predominate in contaminated infusate or equipment-related infection [79,80]. Candida species are a greater risk in prolonged catheterization of the glucose-intolerant patient on multiple systemic broad-spectrum antibiotics. Catheter-associated bacteremia should be treated with a 7- to 14-day course of appropriate antibiotics. In complicated cases, longer courses are sometimes necessary.

The optimal evaluation of febrile catheterized patients is a challenging problem. The decision to discontinue or change an arterial catheter differs from the approach with central venous catheters discussed in Chapter 2 in some fundamental ways. Arterial catheters are less likely to be the source of fever than central venous catheters, and changing of arterial lines is frequently not indicated. If the site appears abnormal or the patient is in septic shock with no other etiology, the catheter should be removed. More specific guidelines are difficult to recommend, and individual factors should always be considered. In general, arterial catheters in place less than 4 days will not be the source of fever unless insertion was contaminated. Catheters in place 7 days or longer should be changed to a different site given the safety of arterial cannulation and the small but measurable chance of infection. Guidewire exchanges have limited utility in the management of arterial catheters unless alternative sites are not available.

RECOMMENDATIONS

Either the radial or femoral artery is an appropriate initial site for percutaneous arterial cannulation. Most centers have more experience with radial artery cannulation, but femoral artery catheters are reliable and have a comparable incidence of complication. In more than 90% of patients, one of these two sites is adequate to achieve arterial pressure monitoring. When these sites are not appropriate, the dorsalis pedis artery is a good alternative, but cannulation is frequently not possible, especially if radial artery cannulation failed because of poor perfusion. Under these circumstances, the axillary or brachial artery can be safely cannulated unless a coagulopathy is present. The site selected for any given patient may not be of prime importance, as centers experienced in the use of alternative sites report excellent results with low rates of complication. Arterial catheters can be left in place until there is clinical indication to remove them. Iatrogenic anemia and over utilization of blood tests are real phenomena associated with arterial catheters. Consequently, these catheters should be discontinued promptly when no longer required for patient management.

REFERENCES

1. Gronbeck C 3rd, Miller EL: Nonphysician placement of arterial catheters. Experience with 500 insertions. *Chest* 104:1716, 1993.
2. Pittman J, Bar-Yosef S, SumPing J, et al: Continuous cardiac output monitoring with pulse contour analysis: a comparison with lithium indicator dilution cardiac output measurement. *Crit Care Med* 33:2015, 2005.
3. Manecke GR: Edwards FloTrac sensor and Vigileo monitor: easy, accurate, reliable cardiac output assessment using the arterial pulse wave. *Expert Rev Med Devices* 2:523, 2005.
4. Belani K, Ozaki M, Hynson J, et al: A new noninvasive method to measure blood pressure: results of a multicenter trial. *Anesthesiology* 91:686, 1999.
5. Bendjelid K, Schutz N, Stotz M, et al: Transcutaneous PCO2 monitoring in critically ill adults: clinical evaluation of a new sensor. *Crit Care Med* 33:2203, 2005.
6. Low LL, Harrington GR, Stoltzfus DP: The effect of arterial lines on blood-drawing practices and costs in intensive care units. *Chest* 108:216, 1995.
7. Zimmerman JE, Seneff MG, Sun X, et al: Evaluating laboratory usage in the intensive care unit: patient and institutional characteristics that influence frequency of blood sampling. *Crit Care Med* 25:737, 1997.
8. Clark JS, Votteri B, Ariagno RL, et al: Noninvasive assessment of blood gases. *Am Rev Respir Dis* 145:220, 1992.
9. Cohn JN: Blood pressure measurement in shock. Mechanism of inaccuracy in ausculatory and palpatory methods. *JAMA* 199:118, 1967.
10. Bur A, Hirschl MM, Herkner H, et al: Accuracy of oscillometric blood pressure measurement according to the relation between cuff size and upper-arm circumference in critically ill patients. *Crit Care Med* 28:371, 2000.
11. Michard F, Boussat S, Chemla D, et al: Relation between respiratory changes in arterial pulse pressure and fluid responsiveness in septic patients with acute circulatory failure. *Am J Respir Crit Care Med* 162:134, 2000.
12. Hirschl MM, Kittler H, Woisetschlager C, et al: Simultaneous comparison of thoracic bioimpedance and arterial pulse waveform-derived cardiac output with thermodilution measurement. *Crit Care Med* 28:1798, 2000.
13. Chaney JC, Derdak S: Minimally invasive hemodynamic monitoring for the intensivist: current and emerging technology. *Crit Care Med* 30:2338, 2002.
14. Gardner R: Direct arterial pressure monitoring. *Curr Anaesth Crit Care* 1:239, 1990.
15. Boutros A, Albert S: Effect of the dynamic response of transducer-tubing system on accuracy of direct blood pressure measurement in patients. *Crit Care Med* 11:124, 1983.
16. Rothe CF, Kim KC: Measuring systolic arterial blood pressure. Possible errors from extension tubes or disposable transducer domes. *Crit Care Med* 8:683, 1980.
17. Gardner RM: Direct blood pressure measurement—dynamic response requirements. *Anesthesiology* 54:227, 1981.
18. Billiet E, Colardyn F: Pressure measurement evaluation and accuracy validation: the Gabarith test. *Intensive Care Med* 24:1323, 1998.
19. Gardner RM: Accuracy and reliability of disposable pressure transducers coupled with modern pressure monitors. *Crit Care Med* 24:879, 1996.
20. Pauca AL, Wallenhaupt SL, Kon ND, et al: Does radial artery pressure accurately reflect aortic pressure? *Chest* 102:1193, 1992.
21. O'Rourke MF, Yaginuma T: Wave reflections and the arterial pulse. *Arch Intern Med* 144:366, 1984.
22. Soderstrom CA, Wasserman DH, Dunham CM, et al: Superiority of the femoral artery of monitoring. A prospective study. *Am J Surg* 144:309, 1982.
23. Gurman GM, Kriemerman S: Cannulation of big arteries in critically ill patients. *Crit Care Med* 13:217, 1985.
24. Russell JA, Joel M, Hudson RJ, et al: Prospective evaluation of radial and femoral artery catheterization sites in critically ill adults. *Crit Care Med* 11:936, 1983.
25. Norwood SH, Cormier B, McMahon NG, et al: Prospective study of catheter-related infection during prolonged arterial catheterization. *Crit Care Med* 16:836, 1988.
26. Gordon LH, Brown M, Brown OW, et al: Alternative sites for continuous arterial monitoring. *South Med J* 77:1498, 1984.
27. Mathers LH: Anatomical considerations in obtaining arterial access. *J Intensive Care Med* 5:110, 1990.
28. Allen EV: Thromboangiitis obliterans: method of diagnosis of chronic occlusive arterial lesions distal to the wrist with illustrative cases. *Am J Med Sci* 178:237, 1929.
29. Ejrup B, Fischer B, Wright IS: Clinical evaluation of blood flow to the hand: the false-positive Allen test. *Circulation* 33:778, 1966.

30. Glavin RJ, Jones HM: Assessing collateral circulation in the hand—four methods compared. *Anaesthesia* 44:594, 1989.

31. Fuhrman TM, Reilley TE, Pippin WD: Comparison of digital blood pressure, plethysmography, and the modified Allen's test as means of evaluating the collateral circulation to the hand. *Anaesthesia* 47:959, 1992.

32. Mangar D, Laborde RS, Vu DN: Delayed ischaemia of the hand necessitating amputation after radial artery cannulation. *Can J Anaesth* 40:247, 1993.

33. Valentine RJ, Modrall JG, Clagett GP: Hand ischemia after radial artery cannulation. *J Am Coll Surg* 201:18, 2005.

34. Giner J, Casan P, Belda J, et al: Pain during arterial puncture. *Chest* 110:1443, 1996.

35. Kaye J, Heald GR, Morton J, et al: Patency of radial arterial catheters. *Am J Critical Care* 10:104, 2001.

36. Tegtmeyer K, Brady G, Lai S, et al: Videos in clinical medicine. Placement of an arterial line. *N Engl J Med* 2006;354:e13. Video available at: www.nejm.org

37. Martin C, Saux P, Papazian L, et al: Long-term arterial cannulation in ICU patients using the radial artery or dorsalis pedis artery. *Chest* 119:901, 2001.

38. Barnes RW, Foster EJ, Janssen GA, et al: Safety of brachial arterial catheters as monitors in the intensive care unit—prospective evaluation with the Doppler ultrasonic velocity detector. *Anesthesiology* 44:260, 1976.

39. Mann S, Jones RI, Millar-Craig MW, et al: The safety of ambulatory intra-arterial pressure monitoring: a clinical audit of 1000 studies. *Int J Cardiol* 5:585, 1984.

40. Macon WL 4th, Futrell JW: Median-nerve neuropathy after percutaneous puncture of the brachial artery in patients receiving anticoagulants. *N Engl J Med* 288:1396, 1973.

41. Brown M, Gordon LH, Brown OW, et al: Intravascular monitoring via the axillary artery. *Anesth Intensive Care* 13:38, 1984.

42. Bryan-Brown CW, Kwun KB, Lumb PD, et al: The axillary artery catheter. *Heart Lung* 12:492, 1983.

43. Lipchik EO, Sugimoto H: Percutaneous brachial artery catheterization. *Radiology* 160:842, 1986.

44. Bedford RF, Wollman H: Complications of percutaneous radial-artery cannulation: an objective prospective study in man. *Anesthesiology* 38:228, 1973.

45. Puri VK, Carlson RW, Bander JJ, et al: Complications of vascular catheterization in the critically ill. A prospective study. *Crit Care Med* 8:495, 1980.

46. Gardner RM, Schwartz R, Wong HC, et al: Percutaneous indwelling radial-artery catheters for monitoring cardiovascular function. Prospective study of the risk of thrombosis and infection. *N Engl J Med* 290:1227, 1974.

47. Davis FM: Radial artery cannulation: influence of catheter size and material on arterial occlusion. *Anaesth Intensive Care* 6:49, 1978.

48. Bedford RF: Radial arterial function following percutaneous cannulation with 18- and 20-gauge catheters. *Anesthesiology* 47:37, 1977.

49. Wilkins RG: Radial artery cannulation and ischaemic damage: a review. *Anaesthesia* 40:896, 1985.

50. Weiss BM, Gattiker RI: Complications during and following radial artery cannulation: a prospective study. *Intensive Care Med* 12:424, 1986.

51. Bedford RF: Long-term radial artery cannulation: effects on subsequent vessel function. *Crit Care Med* 6:64, 1978.

52. Clifton GD, Branson P, Kelly HJ, et al: Comparison of normal saline and heparin solutions for maintenance of arterial catheter patency. *Heart Lung* 20:115, 1990.

53. Hook ML, Reuling J, Luettgen ML, et al: Comparison of the patency of arterial lines maintained with heparinized and nonheparinized infusions. The Cardiovascular Intensive Care Unit Nursing Research Committee of St. Luke's Hospital. *Heart Lung* 16:693, 1987.

54. Lowenstein E, Little JW 3rd, Lo HH: Prevention of cerebral embolization from flushing radial-artery cannulas. *N Engl J Med* 285:1414, 1971.

55. Chang C, Dughi J, Shitabata P, et al: Air embolism and the radial arterial line. *Crit Care Med* 16:141, 1988.

56. Dube L, Soltner C, Daenen S, et al: Gas embolism: an exceptional complication of radial arterial catheterization. *Acta Anaesthesiol Scand* 48:1208, 2004.

57. Smoller BR, Kruskall MS: Phlebotomy for diagnostic laboratory tests in adults. Pattern of use and effect on transfusion requirements. *N Engl J Med* 314:1233, 1986.

58. Peruzzi WT, Parker MA, Lichtenthal PR, et al: A clinical evaluation of a blood conservation device in medical intensive care unit patients. *Crit Care Med* 21:501, 1993.

59. Silver MJ, Jubran H, Stein S, et al: Evaluation of a new blood-conserving arterial line system for patients in intensive care units. *Crit Care Med* 21:507, 1993.

60. Southworth R, Sutton R, Mize S, et al: Clinical evaluation of a new in-line continuous blood gas monitor. *J Extra Corpor* 30:166, 1998.

61. Roberts DE, Bell DD, Ostryzniuk T, et al: Eliminating needless testing in intensive care—an information-based team management approach. *Crit Care Med* 21:1452, 1993.

62. Wittels EG, Siegel RD, Mazur EM: Thrombocytopenia in the intensive care unit setting. *J Intensive Care Med* 5:224, 1990.

63. Warkentin TE, Greinacher A: Heparin-induced thrombocytopenia: recognition, treatment, and prevention: the seventh ACCP Conference on Antithrombotic and Thrombolytic Therapy. *Chest* 126:311S, 2004.

64. Kelton JG: The pathophysiology of heparin-induced thrombocytopenia: biological basis for treatment. *Chest* 127:9S, 2005.

65. Randolph AG, Cook DJ, Gonzales CA, et al: Benefit of heparin in peripheral venous and arterial catheters: systematic review and meta-analysis of randomised controlled trials. *BMJ* 316:969, 1998.

66. Branson PK, McCoy RA, Phillips BA, et al: Efficacy of 1.4 percent sodium citrate in maintaining arterial catheter patency in patients in a medical ICU. *Chest* 103:882, 1993.

67. Altin RS, Flicker S, Naidech HJ: Pseudoaneurysm and arteriovenous fistula after femoral artery catheterization: association with low femoral punctures. *AJR* 152:629, 1989.

68. Shinozaki T, Deane RS, Mazuzan JE Jr, et al: Bacterial contamination of arterial lines. A prospective study. *JAMA* 249:223, 1983.

69. Maki DG, Ringer M, Alvarado CJ: Prospective randomised trial of povidone-iodine, alcohol, and chlorhexidine for prevention of infection associated with central venous and arterial catheters. *Lancet* 338:339, 1991.

70. Mimoz O, Pieroni L, Lawrence C, et al: Prospective, randomized trial of two antiseptic solutions for prevention of central venous or arterial catheter colonization and infection in intensive care unit patients. *Crit Care Med* 24:1818, 1996.

71. Peruzzi WT, Noskin GA, Moen SG, et al: Microbial contamination of blood conservation devices during routine use in the critical care setting: results of a prospective, randomized trial. *Crit Care Med* 24:1157, 1996.

72. O'Malley MK, Rhame FS, Cerra FB, et al: Value of routine pressure monitoring system changes after 72 hours of continuous use. *Crit Care Med* 22:1424, 1994.

73. Maki DG, Weise CE, Sarafin HW: A semiquantitative culture method for identifying intravenous-catheter-related infection. *N Engl J Med* 296:1305, 1977.

74. Traore O, Liotier J, Souweine B: Prospective study of arterial and central venous catheter colonization and of arterial- and central venous catheter-related bacteremia in intensive care units. *Crit Care Med* 33:1276, 2005.

75. Scheer B, Perel A, Pfeiffer UJ: Clinical review: complications and risk factors of peripheral arterial catheters used for haemodynamic monitoring in anaesthesia and intensive care medicine. *Critical Care (London)* 6:199, 2002.

76. Band JD, Maki DG: Infections caused by arterial catheters used for hemodynamic monitoring. *Am J Med* 67:735, 1979.

77. Leroy O, Billiau V, Beuscart C, et al: Nosocomial infections associated with long-term radial artery cannulation. *Intensive Care Med* 15:241, 1989.

78. Thomas F, Parker J, Burke J, et al: Prospective randomized evaluation of indwelling radial vs. femoral arterial catheters in high risk critically ill patients. *Crit Care Med* 10:226, 1982.

79. Maki DG: Nosocomial bacteremia. An epidemiologic overview. *Am J Med* 70:719, 1981.

80. Ransjo U, Good Z, Jalakas K, et al: An outbreak of Klebsiella oxytoca septicemias associated with the use of invasive blood pressure monitoring equipment. *Acta Anaesthesiol Scand* 36:289, 1992.

Harvey Steven Reich

CHAPTER **4**

Pulmonary Artery Catheterization

Since their introduction into clinical practice in 1970 by Swan et al. [1], balloon-tipped, flow-directed pulmonary artery (PA) catheters have found widespread use in the clinical management of critically ill patients. However, in recent years, both the safety and efficacy of these catheters have been brought into question. In this chapter, I review the physiologic basis for their use, some history regarding their development and use, the concerns raised about their use, and suggestions for appropriate use of the catheters and the information obtained from them.

PHYSIOLOGIC RATIONALE FOR USE OF THE PULMONARY ARTERY CATHETER

In unstable situations, during which hemodynamic changes often occur rapidly, clinical evaluation may be misleading [2]. PA catheters allow for direct and indirect measurement of several major determinants and consequences of cardiac performance—preload, afterload, cardiac output (CO)—thereby supplying additional data to aid in clinical decision making [3].

Cardiac function depends on the relationship between muscle length (preload), the load on the muscle (afterload), and the intrinsic property of contractility. Until the development of the flow-directed PA catheter, there was no way to assess all of these using one instrument in a clinically useful way at bedside. The catheter allows the reflection of right ventricular (RV) preload (right atrial pressure), RV afterload (PA pressure), left ventricular preload—PA occlusion pressure (PAOP) or pulmonary capillary wedge pressure (PCWP)—and contractility (stroke volume or CO). Left ventricular afterload is reflected by the systemic arterial pressure. This information allows the calculation of numerous parameters, including vascular resistances. No other tool allows the gathering of such a large amount of information.

CONTROVERSIES REGARDING USE OF THE PULMONARY ARTERY CATHETER

Despite all of the advantages of the PA catheter, a number of clinical studies have been published in the past decade that have shown either no benefit or an increased risk of morbidity or mortality associated with its use. (See Table 4-1 for a summary of the evidence for its utility.) Consequently, a number of clinicians have elected to minimize the use of this monitoring device.

Furthermore, the relationship of central venous (CV) pressure and PA pressure to predict ventricular filling was studied in normal volunteers by Kumar et al. [4] who found there was a poor correlation between initial CV pressure and PAOP with both respective end diastolic ventricular volume and stroke volume indices. Their data call into question the basic tenet of the theoretical benefit of the PA catheter.

INDICATIONS FOR PULMONARY ARTERY CATHETER USE

Clinicians who use a PA catheter for monitoring should understand the fundamentals of the insertion technique, the equipment used, and the data that can be generated. The Pulmonary Artery Catheter Education Program (PACEP) has been developed by seven specialty organizations, along with the NHLBI and the FDA and is available at http://www.pacep.org.

The use of the PA catheter for monitoring has four central objectives: (a) to assess left or right ventricular function, or both, (b) to monitor changes in hemodynamic status, (c) to guide treatment with pharmacologic and nonpharmacologic agents, and (d) to provide prognostic information. The conditions in which PA catheterization may be useful are characterized by a clinically unclear or rapidly changing hemodynamic status. Table 4-2 is a partial listing of the indications. Use of PA catheters in specific disease entities is discussed in other chapters.

CATHETER FEATURES AND CONSTRUCTION

The catheter is constructed from polyvinylchloride and has a pliable shaft that softens further at body temperature. Because polyvinylchloride has a high thrombogenicity, the catheters are generally coated with heparin. Heparin bonding of catheters, introduced in 1981, has been shown to be effective in reducing catheter thrombogenicity [43,44]. The standard catheter length is 110 cm, and the most commonly used external diameter is 5 or 7 French (Fr) (1 Fr = 0.0335 mm). A balloon is fastened 1 to 2 mm from the tip (Fig. 4-1); when inflated, it guides the catheter (by virtue of fluid dynamic drag) from the greater intrathoracic veins through the right heart chambers into the PA. When fully inflated in a vessel of sufficiently large caliber, the balloon protrudes above the catheter tip, thus distributing tip forces over a large area and minimizing the chances for endocardial damage or arrhythmia induction during catheter insertion (Fig. 4-2). Progression of the catheter is stopped when it impacts in a PA slightly smaller in diameter than the fully inflated balloon. From this position, the PAOP is obtained. Balloon capacity varies according to catheter size, and the operator must be aware of the individual balloon's maximal inflation volume as recommended by the manufacturer. The balloon is usually inflated with air, but filtered carbon dioxide should be used in any situation in which balloon rupture might result in access of the inflation medium to the arterial system (e.g., if a right-to-left intracardiac shunt or a pulmonary arteriovenous fistula is suspected). If carbon dioxide is used, periodic deflation and reinflation may be necessary, since carbon dioxide diffuses through the latex balloon at a rate

TABLE 4-1.   Evidence Basis for the PA Catheter

Authors	Year	N	Design	Outcomes
Lower Morbidity/Mortality				
Rao et al. [5]	1983	733/364	Historical controls/cohort	Lower mortality
Hesdorffer et al. [6]	1987	61/87	Historical controls/cohort	Lower mortality
Shoemaker et al. [7]	1988	146	RCT	Lower mortality
Berlauk et al. [8]	1991	89	RCT	Lower morbidity
Fleming et al. [9]	1992	33/34	RCT	Lower morbidity
Tuchschmidt et al. [10]	1992	26/25	RCT	Decreased LOS; trend toward lower mortality
Boyd et al. [11]	1993	53/54	RCT	Lower mortality
Bishop et al. [12]	1995	50/65	RCT	Lower mortality
Schiller et al. [13]	1997	53/33/30	Retrospective cohort	Lower mortality
Wilson et al. [14]	1999	92/46	RCT	Lower mortality
Chang et al. [15]	2000	20/39	Prospective retrospective cohort	Lower morbidity
Polonen et al. [16]	2000	196/197	RCT	Decreased morbidity
Friese et al. [155]	2006	51379 (no PAC)/ 1933 (PAC)	Retrospective analysis of National Trauma Data Bank	Improved survival in patients older than 60 or with ISS 25-75 and severe shock
No Difference				
Pearson et al. [17]	1989	226	RCT	No difference
Isaacson et al. [18]	1990	102	RCT	No difference
Joyce et al. [19]	1990	40	RCT	No difference
Yu et al. [20]	1993	35/32	RCT	No difference
Gattinoni et al. [21]	1995	252/253/257	RCT	No difference
Yu et al. [22]	1995	89	RCT	No difference
Durham et al. [23]	1996	27/31	Prospective cohort	No difference
Afessa et al. [24]	2001	751	Prospective observational	No difference
Rhodes et al. [25]	2002	201	RCT	No difference
Richard [26]	2003	676	RCT	No difference
Yu et al. [27]	2003	1,010	Prospective cohort	No difference
Sandham et al. [28]	2003	997/997	RCT	No difference in mortality; increased risk of pulmonary embolism in PA group
Sakr et al. [29]	2005	3,147	Observational cohort	No difference
Harvey et al. [30]	2005	519/522	RCT	No difference in mortality
Binanay et al. [31]	2005	433	RCT	No difference in mortality
The National Heart, Lung and Blood Institute ARDS Clinical Trials Network [71]	2006	513/487	RCT	No difference in mortality or organ function
Higher or Worse Morbidity/Mortality				
Tuman et al. [32]	1989	1094	Controlled prospective cohort	Increased ICU stay with PAC
Guyatt [33]	1991	33/148	RCT	Higher morbidity
Hayes et al. [34]	1994	50	RCT	Higher mortality
Connors et al. [35]	1996	5,735	Prospective cohort	Higher mortality
Valentine et al. [36]	1998	60	RCT	Increased morbidity
Stewart et al. [37]	1998	133/61	Retrospective cohort	Increased morbidity
Ramsey et al. [38]	2000	8,064/5,843	Retrospective cohort	Higher mortality
Polanczyk et al. [39]	2001	215/215	Prospective cohort	Increased morbidity
Chittock et al. [40]	2004	7,310	Observational cohort	Increased mortality in low severity; decreased mortality in high severity
Peters et al. [41]	2003	360/690	Retrospective case control	Increased risk of death
Cohen et al. [42]	2005	26,437/735	Retrospective cohort	Increased mortality

ICU, intensive care unit; ISS, injury security score; LOS, length of stay; PA, pulmonary artery; PAC, pulmonary artery catheter; RCT, randomized control trial.

of approximately 0.5 cc per minute. Liquids should never be used as the inflation medium.

A variety of catheter constructions is available, each designed for particular clinical applications. Double-lumen catheters allow balloon inflation through one lumen, and a distal opening at the tip of the catheter is used to measure intravascular pressures and sample blood. Triple-lumen catheters have a proximal port terminating 30 cm from the tip of the catheter, allowing si-

multaneous measurement of right atrial and PA or occlusion pressures. The most commonly used PA catheter in the ICU setting is a quadruple-lumen catheter, which has a lumen containing electrical leads for a thermistor positioned at the catheter surface 4 cm proximal to its tip (Fig. 4-1) [45]. The thermistor measures PA blood temperature and allows thermodilution CO measurements. A five-lumen catheter is also available, with the fifth lumen opening 40 cm from the tip of the

TABLE 4-2.   General Indications for Pulmonary Artery Catheterization

Management of complicated myocardial infarction
    Hypovolemia vs. cardiogenic shock
    Ventricular septal rupture vs. acute mitral regurgitation
    Severe left ventricular failure
    Right ventricular infarction
    Unstable angina
    Refractory ventricular tachycardia
Assessment of respiratory distress
    Cardiogenic vs. noncardiogenic (e.g., acute respiratory distress
      syndrome) pulmonary edema
    Primary vs. secondary pulmonary hypertension
Assessment of shock
    Cardiogenic
    Hypovolemic
    Septic
    Pulmonary embolism
Assessment of therapy in selected individuals
    Afterload reduction in patients with severe left ventricular function
    Inotropic agent
    Vasopressors
    Beta-blockers
    Temporary pacing (ventricular vs. atrioventricular)
    Intraaortic balloon counterpulsation
    Mechanical ventilation (e.g., with positive end-expiratory pressure)
Management of postoperative open heart surgical patients
Assessment of cardiac tamponade/constriction
Assessment of valvular heart disease
Perioperative monitoring of patients with unstable cardiac status
  during noncardiac surgery
Assessment of fluid requirements in critically ill patients
    Gastrointestinal hemorrhage
    Sepsis
    Acute renal failure
    Burns
    Decompensated cirrhosis
    Advanced peritonitis
Management of severe preeclampsia[a]

---

[a]Isner JM, Horton J, Ronan JAS: Systolic click from a Swan-Ganz catheter: phonoechocardiographic depiction of the underlying mechnasim. *Am J Cardiol* 42:1046, 1979.
Adapted from JM Gore, JS Alpert, JR Benotti, et al: *Handbook of Hemodynamic Monitoring.* Boston, Little, Brown, 1984.

---

catheter. The fifth lumen provides additional central venous access for fluid or medication infusions when peripheral access is limited or when drugs requiring infusion into a large vein (e.g., dopamine, epinephrine) are used. Figure 4-2 shows the balloon on the tip inflated.

Several special-purpose PA catheter designs are available. Pacing PA catheters incorporate two groups of electrodes on the catheter surface, enabling intracardiac electrocardiographic (ECG) recording or temporary cardiac pacing [46]. These catheters are used for emergency cardiac pacing, although it is often difficult to position the catheter for reliable simultaneous cardiac pacing and PA pressure measurements. A 5-lumen catheter allows passage of a specially designed 2.4-Fr bipolar pacing electrode (probe) through the additional lumen (located 19 cm from the catheter tip) and allows emergency temporary intracardiac pacing without the need for a separate central venous puncture. The pacing probe is Teflon coated to allow easy introduction through the pacemaker port lumen; the intracavitary part of the probe is heparin impregnated to reduce the risk

of thrombus formation. One report demonstrated satisfactory ventricular pacing in 19 of 23 patients using this catheter design (83% success rate) [47]. When a pacing probe is not in use, the fifth lumen may be used for additional central venous access or continuous RV pressure monitoring.

Continuous mixed venous oxygen saturation measurement is clinically available using a fiberoptic 5-lumen PA catheter [48]. Segal et al. [49] described a catheter that incorporates Doppler technology for continuous CO determinations. Catheters equipped with a fast-response (95 milliseconds) thermistor and intracardiac ECG monitoring electrodes are also available. These catheters allow determination of the RV ejection fraction and RV systolic time intervals in critically ill patients [50–53]. The calculated RV ejection fraction has correlated well with simultaneous radionuclide first-pass studies [52].

Aside from the intermittent determination of CO by bolus administration of cold injectate, PA catheters have been adapted to determine near continuous CO by thermal pulses generated by a heating filament on the catheter to produce temperature changes [54]. The accuracy and reliability of CO determination by this heating-cooling cycle have been confirmed by several studies [55–58].

PRESSURE TRANSDUCERS

Hemodynamic monitoring requires a system able to convert changes in intravascular pressure into electrical signals suitable for interpretation. The most commonly used hemodynamic monitoring system is a catheter-tubing–transducer system. A fluid-filled intravascular catheter is connected to a transducer by a fluid-filled tubing system. (For more details, see the discussion in Chapter 3.)

INSERTION TECHNIQUES

GENERAL CONSIDERATIONS

Manufacturers' recommendations should be carefully followed. All catheter manufacturers have detailed insertion and training materials.

PA catheterization can be performed in any hospital location where continuous ECG and hemodynamic monitoring are possible and where equipment and supplies needed for cardiopulmonary resuscitation are readily available. Fluoroscopy is not essential, but it can facilitate difficult placements. Properly constructed beds and protective aprons are mandatory for safe use of fluoroscopic equipment. Meticulous attention to sterile technique is of obvious importance; all involved personnel must wear sterile caps, gowns, masks, and gloves, and the patient must be fully protected by sterile drapes.

The catheter should be inserted percutaneously (not by cutdown) into the basilic, brachial, femoral, subclavian, or internal jugular veins using techniques described in Chapter 2. Threading the catheter into the pulmonary artery is more difficult from the basilica, brachial, or femoral vein.

TYPICAL CATHETER INSERTION PROCEDURE

The procedures for typical catheter insertion are as follows:

  1. Prepare and connect pressure tubing, manifolds, stopcocks, and transducers. Remove the sterile balloon-tipped

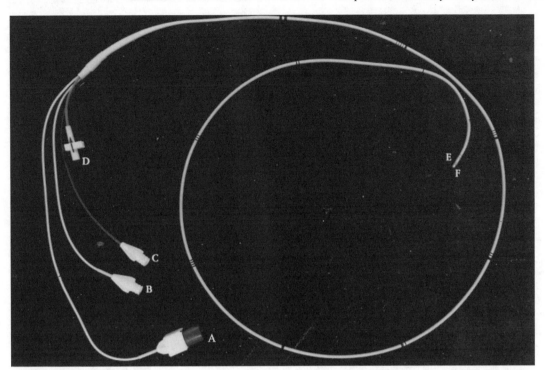

FIGURE 4-1. Quadruple-lumen pulmonary artery catheter. **A:** Connection to thermodilution cardiac output computer. **B:** Connection to distal lumen. **C:** Connection to proximal lumen. **D:** Stopcock connected to balloon at the catheter tip for balloon inflation. **E:** Thermistor. **F:** Balloon. Note that the catheter is marked in 10-cm increments.

catheter from its container. Balloon integrity may be tested by submerging the balloon in a small amount of fluid and checking for air leaks as the balloon is inflated (using the amount of air recommended by the manufacturer). Deflate the balloon.

2. Insert a central venous cannula or needle into the vein as described in Chapter 2. Using the Seldinger technique, thread the guidewire contained in the catheter kit into the vein and remove the catheter or needle (Figs. 4-3 and 4-4).

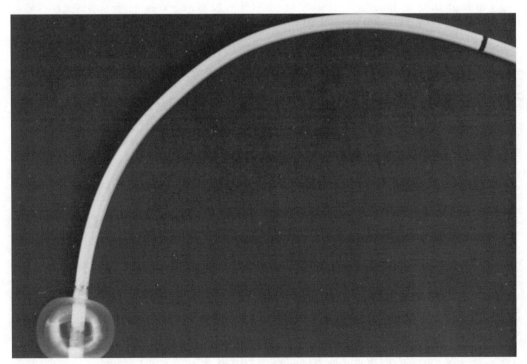

FIGURE 4-2. Balloon properly inflated at the tip of a pulmonary artery catheter. Note that the balloon shields the catheter tip and prevents it from irritating cardiac chambers on its passage to the pulmonary artery.

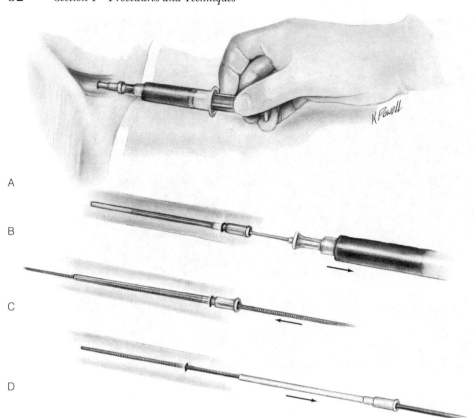

A

B

C

D

FIGURE 4-3. **A:** Easy blood aspiration has been demonstrated using the guidewire introducer needle. **B:** The inner needle is removed. **C:** The spring guidewire is advanced, soft end first, through the cannula into the vessel. **D:** With the guidewire held in place, the cannula is withdrawn from the vessel by being pulled over and off the length of the guidewire.

3. Make a small incision with a scalpel to enlarge the puncture site (Fig. 4-5). While holding the guidewire stationary, thread a vessel dilator-sheath apparatus (the size should be 8 Fr if a 7-Fr catheter is to be used) over the guidewire and advance it into the vessel, using a twisting motion to get through the puncture site (Fig. 4-6). The dilator and sheath should only be advanced until the tip of the sheath is in the vessel—estimated by the original

depth of the cannula or needle required to access the vein. At that point, the dilator and guidewire are held stationary and the sheath is advance off the dilator into the vessel. Advancing the dilator further may cause great vessel or cardiac damage.

4. Remove the guidewire and vessel dilator, leaving the introducer sheath in the vessel (Fig. 4-7). Suture the sheath in place.

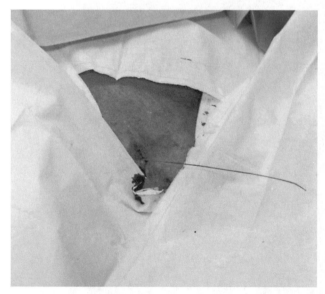

FIGURE 4-4. The spring guidewire, stiff end protruding, is now located in the subclavian vein.

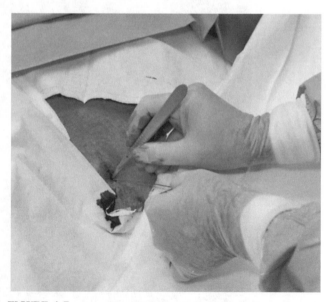

FIGURE 4-5. A small incision is made with a scalpel to enlarge the puncture site.

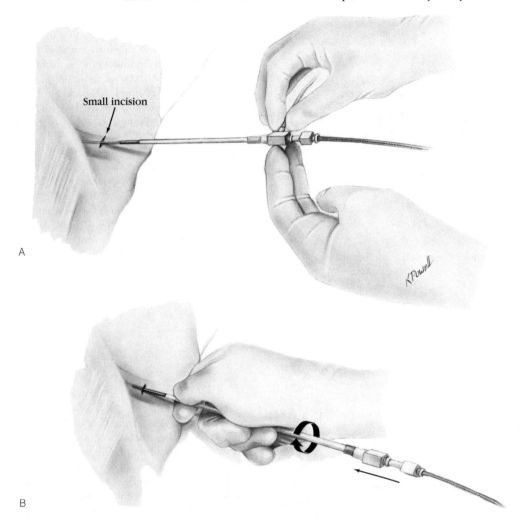

FIGURE 4-6.   A: The vessel dilator-sheath apparatus is threaded over the guidewire and advanced into the vessel. **B:** A twisting motion is used to thread the apparatus into the vessel.

5. Attach stopcocks to the right atrium and PA ports of the PA catheter and fill the proximal and distal catheter lumens with flush solution. Close the stopcocks to keep flush solution within the lumens and to avoid introduction of air into the circulation.

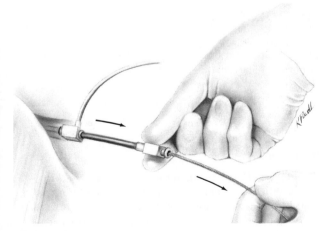

FIGURE 4-7.   The guidewire and vessel dilator are removed, leaving the introducer sheath in the vessel.

6. If a sterile sleeve adapter is to be used, insert the catheter through it and pull the adapter proximally over the catheter to keep it out of the way. Once the catheter is advanced to its desired intravascular location, attach the distal end of the sleeve adapter to the introducer sheath hub.

7. Pass the catheter through the introducer sheath into the vein (Fig. 4-8). Advance it, using the marks on the catheter shaft indicating 10-cm distances from the tip, until the tip is in the right atrium. This requires advancement of approximately 35 to 40 cm from the left antecubital fossa, 10 to 15 cm from the internal jugular vein, 10 cm from the subclavian vein, and 35 to 40 cm from the femoral vein. A right atrial waveform on the monitor, with appropriate fluctuations accompanying respiratory changes or cough, confirms proper intrathoracic location (Fig. 4-9, center). If desired, obtain right atrial blood for oxygen saturation from the distal port. Flush the distal lumen with heparinized saline and record the right atrial pressures. (Occasionally, it is necessary to inflate the balloon to keep the tip from adhering to the atrial wall during blood aspiration.)

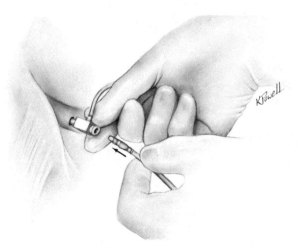

FIGURE 4-8. The catheter is passed through the introducer sheath into the vein.

8. With the catheter tip in the right atrium, inflate the balloon with the recommended amount of air or carbon dioxide (Fig. 4-9A). Inflation of the balloon should be associated with a slight feeling of resistance—if it is not, suspect balloon rupture and do not attempt further inflation or advancement of the catheter before properly reevaluating balloon integrity. If significant resistance to balloon inflation is encountered, suspect malposition of the catheter in a small vessel; withdraw the catheter and readvance it to a new position. Do not use liquids to inflate the balloon, as they might be irretrievable and could prevent balloon deflation.

9. With the balloon inflated, advance the catheter until a RV pressure tracing is seen on the monitor (Fig. 4-9, center). Obtain and record RV pressures. Catheter passage into and through the RV is an especially risky time in terms of arrhythmias. Maintaining the balloon inflated in the RV minimizes ventricular irritation (Fig. 4-9B), but it is important to monitor vital signs and ECG throughout the entire insertion procedure. Elevating the head of the bed to 5 degrees and a right tilt position will facilitate the passage of the catheter through the right ventricle and minimize the generation of arrhythmias [59].

10. Continue advancing the catheter until the diastolic pressure tracing rises above that in the RV (Fig. 4-9, center), indicating PA placement (Fig. 4-9C). If a RV trace still appears after the catheter has been advanced 15 cm beyond the original distance needed to reach the right atrium, suspect curling in the ventricle; deflate the balloon, withdraw it to the right atrium, then reinflate it and try again. Advancement beyond the PA position results in a fall on the pressure tracing from the levels of systolic pressure noted in the RV and PA. When this is noted, record the PAOP (Fig. 4-9, center, D) and deflate the balloon. Phasic PA pressure should reappear on the pressure tracing when the balloon is deflated. If it does not, pull back the catheter with the deflated balloon until the PA tracing appears. With the balloon deflated, blood may be aspirated for oxygen saturation measurement. Watch for intermittent RV tracings indicating slippage of the catheter backward into the ventricle.

11. Carefully record the balloon inflation volume needed to change the PA pressure tracing to the PAOP tracing. If PAOP is recorded with an inflation volume significantly lower than the manufacturer's recommended volume, or if subsequent PAOP determinations require decreasing amounts of balloon inflation volume as compared to an initial appropriate amount, the catheter tip has migrated too far peripherally and should be pulled back immediately.

12. Secure the catheter in the correct PA position by suturing or taping it to the skin to prevent inadvertent advancement. Apply a germicidal agent and dress appropriately.

13. Order a chest radiograph to confirm catheter position; the catheter tip should appear no more than 3 to 5 cm from the midline. To assess whether peripheral catheter migration has occurred, daily chest radiographs are recommended to supplement pressure monitoring and checks on balloon inflation volumes. An initial cross-table lateral radiograph may be obtained in patients on positive end-expiratory pressure (PEEP) to rule out superior placements.

SPECIAL CONSIDERATIONS

In certain disease states (right atrial or RV dilatation, severe pulmonary hypertension, severe tricuspid insufficiency, low CO syndromes), it may be difficult to position a flow-directed catheter properly. These settings may require fluoroscopic guidance to aid in catheter positioning. Infusion of 5 to 10 mL of cold saline through the distal lumen may stiffen the catheter and aid in positioning. Alternatively, a 0.025-cm guidewire 145 cm long may be used to stiffen the catheter when placed through the distal lumen of a 7-Fr PA catheter. This manipulation should be performed only under fluoroscopic guidance by an experienced operator. Rarely, nonflow-directed PA catheters (e.g., Cournand catheters) may be required. Because of their rigidity, these catheters have the potential to perforate the right heart and must be placed only under fluoroscopy by a physician experienced in cardiac catheterization techniques.

PHYSIOLOGIC DATA

Measurement of a variety of hemodynamic parameters and oxygen saturations is possible using the PA catheter. A summary of normal values for these parameters is found in Tables 4-3 and 4-4.

PRESSURES

Right Atrium

With the tip of the PA catheter in the right atrium (Fig. 4-9A), the balloon is deflated and a right atrial waveform recorded (Fig. 4-10). Normal resting right atrial pressure is 0 to 6 mm Hg. Two major positive atrial pressure waves, the a wave and v wave, can usually be recorded. On occasion, a third positive wave, the c wave, can also be seen. The a wave is due to atrial contraction and

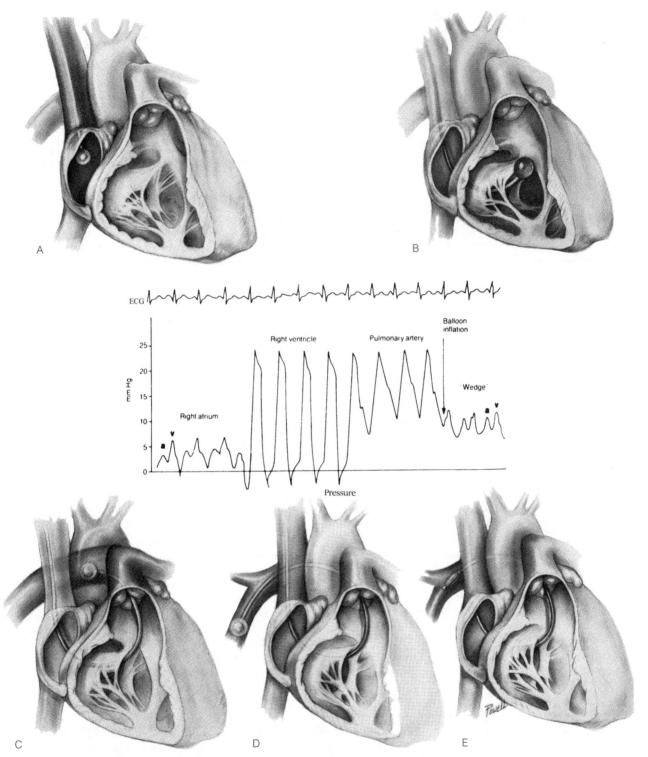

FIGURE 4-9. **A:** With the catheter tip in the right atrium, the balloon is inflated. **B:** The catheter is advanced into the right ventricle with the balloon inflated, and right ventricle pressure tracings are obtained. (*Center*): Waveform tracings generated as the balloon-tipped catheter is advanced through the right heart chambers into the pulmonary artery. [Adapted from Wiedmann HP, Matthay MA, Matthey RA: Cardiovascular pulmonary monitoring in the intensive care unit (Part 1) *Chest* 85:537;1984, with permission.] **C:** The catheter is advanced through the pulmonary valve into the pulmonary artery. A rise in diastolic pressure should be noted. **D:** The catheter is advanced to the pulmonary artery occlusion pressure position. A typical pulmonary artery occlusion pressure tracing should be noted with a and v waves. **E:** The balloon is deflated. Phasic pulmonary artery pressure should reappear on the monitor. (See text for details.)

TABLE 4-3. Normal Resting Pressures Obtained during Right Heart Catheterization

Cardiac Chamber	Pressure (mm Hg)
Right atrium	
Range	0–6
Mean	3
Right ventricle	
Systolic	17–30
Diastolic	0–6
Pulmonary artery	
Systolic	15–30
Diastolic	5–13
Mean	10–18
Pulmonary artery occlusion (mean)	2–12

Adapted from JM Gore, JS Alpert, JR Benotti, et al: *Handbook of Hemodynamic Monitoring.* Boston, Little, Brown, 1984.

follows the simultaneously recorded ECG P wave [60,61]. The a wave peak generally follows the peak of the electrical P wave by approximately 80 milliseconds [62]. The v wave represents the pressure generated by venous filling of the right atrium while the tricuspid valve is closed. The peak of the v wave occurs at the end of ventricular systole when the atrium is maximally filled, corresponding to the point near the end of the T wave on the ECG. The c wave is due to the sudden motion of the atrioventricular valve ring toward the right atrium at the onset of ventricular systole. The c wave follows the a wave by a time equal to the ECG P-R interval. The c wave is more readily visible in cases of P-R prolongation [62]. The x descent follows the c wave and reflects atrial relaxation. The y descent is due to rapid emptying of the atrium after opening of the tricuspid valve. The mean right atrial pressure decreases during inspiration with spontaneous respiration (secondary to a decrease in intrathoracic pressure), whereas the a and v waves and the x and y descents become more prominent. Once a multilumen PA catheter is in position, right atrial blood can be sampled and pressure monitored using the proximal lumen. It should be noted that the pressures obtained via the proximal lumen may not accurately reflect right atrial pressure, due to positioning of the lumen against the atrial wall or within the introducer sheath. The latter problem is more frequently encountered in shorter patients [63].

TABLE 4-4. Approximate Normal Oxygen Saturation and Content Values

Chamber Sampled	Oxygen Content (vol %)	Oxygen Saturation (%)
Superior vena cava	14.0	70
Inferior vena cava	16.0	80
Right atrium	15.0	75
Right ventricle	15.0	75
Pulmonary artery	15.0	75
Pulmonary vein	20.0	98
Femoral artery	19.0	96
Atrioventricular oxygen content difference	3.5–5.5	—

Adapted from JM Gore, JS Alpert, JR Benotti, et al: *Handbook of Hemodynamic Monitoring.* Boston, Little, Brown, 1984.

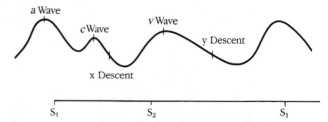

FIGURE 4-10. Stylized representation of a right atrial waveform in relation to heart sounds. (See text for discussion of a, c, and v waves and x and y descents.) S_1, first heart sound; S_2, second heart sound.

Right Ventricle

The normal resting RV pressure is 17 to 30/0 to 6 mm Hg, recorded when the PA catheter crosses the tricuspid valve (Fig. 4-9B). The RV systolic pressure should equal the PA systolic pressure (except in cases of pulmonic stenosis or RV outflow tract obstruction). The RV diastolic pressure should equal the mean right atrial pressure during diastole when the tricuspid valve is open. Introduction of the catheter with a pacing lumen allows continuous monitoring of RV hemodynamics when the pacing wire is not in place. Using special catheters, RV end-diastolic volume index and RV ejection fraction can be accurately measured [64–67].

Pulmonary Artery

With the catheter in proper position and the balloon deflated, the distal lumen transmits PA pressure (Fig. 4-9E). Normal resting PA pressure is 15 to 30/5 to 13 mm Hg, with a mean pressure of 10 to 18 mm Hg. The PA waveform is characterized by a systolic peak and diastolic trough with a dicrotic notch due to closure of the pulmonic valve. The peak PA systolic pressure occurs in the T wave of a simultaneously recorded ECG.

Since the pulmonary vasculature is normally a low-resistance circuit, PA diastolic pressure (PADP) is closely related to mean PAOP (PADP is usually 1 to 3 mm Hg higher than mean PAOP) and thus can be used as an index of left ventricle filling pressure in patients in whom an occlusion pressure is unobtainable or in whom PADP and PAOP have been shown to correlate closely. However, if pulmonary vascular resistance is increased, as in pulmonary embolic disease, pulmonary fibrosis, or reactive pulmonary hypertension, PADP may markedly exceed mean PAOP and thus become an unreliable index of left heart function [62]. Similar provisos apply when using PA mean pressure as an index of left ventricular function.

Pulmonary Artery Occlusion Pressure

An important application of the balloon flotation catheter is the recording of PAOP. This measurement is obtained when the inflated balloon impacts a slightly smaller branch of the PA (Fig. 4-9D). In this position, the balloon stops the flow, and the catheter tip senses pressure transmitted backward through the static column of blood from the next active circulatory bed—the pulmonary veins. Pulmonary venous pressure is a prime determinant of pulmonary congestion and thus of the tendency for fluid to shift from the pulmonary capillaries into the interstitial tissue and alveoli. Also, pulmonary venous pressure and PAOP closely reflect left atrial pressure (except in rare instances, such as pulmonary venocclusive disease, in which there is obstruction in the small pulmonary veins), and serve as indices of left ventricular filling pressure [68,69]. The PAOP is required to assess left ventricular filling pressure, since multiple studies have demonstrated that right atrial (e.g., central venous) pressure correlates poorly with PAOP [70].

The PAOP is a phase-delayed, amplitude-dampened version of the left atrial pressure. The normal resting PAOP is 2 to 12 mm Hg and averages 2 to 7 mm Hg below the mean PA pressure. The PAOP waveform is similar to that of the right atrium, with a, c, and v waves and x and y descents (Fig. 4-10). However, in contradistinction to the right atrial waveform, the PAOP waveform demonstrates a v wave that is slightly larger than the a wave [14]. Due to the time required for left atrial mechanical events to be transmitted through the pulmonary vasculature, PAOP waveforms are further delayed when recorded with a simultaneous ECG. The peak of the a wave follows the peak of the ECG P wave by approximately 240 milliseconds, and the peak of the v wave occurs after the ECG T wave has been inscribed. Occlusion position is confirmed by withdrawing a blood specimen from the distal lumen and measuring oxygen saturation. Measured oxygen saturation of 95% or more is satisfactory [69]. The lung segment from which the sample is obtained will be well ventilated if the patient breathes slowly and deeply.

A valid PAOP measurement requires a patent vascular channel between the left atrium and catheter tip. Thus, the PAOP approximates pulmonary venous pressure (and therefore left atrial pressure) only if the catheter tip lies in zone 3 of the lungs [60,72]. (The lung is divided into three physiologic zones, dependent on the relationship of PA, pulmonary venous, and alveolar pressures. In zone 3, the PA and pulmonary venous pressure exceed the alveolar pressure, ensuring an uninterrupted column of blood between the catheter tip and the pulmonary veins.) If, on portable lateral chest radiograph, the catheter tip is below the level of the left atrium (posterior position in supine patients), it can be assumed to be in zone 3. This assumption holds if applied PEEP is less than 15 cm H_2O and the patient is not markedly volume depleted. Whether the catheter is positioned in zone 3 may also be determined by certain physiologic characteristics (Table 4-5). A catheter occlusion outside zone 3 shows marked respiratory variation, an unnaturally smooth vascular waveform, and misleading high pressures.

With a few exceptions [73], estimates of capillary hydrostatic filtration pressure from PAOP are acceptable [74]. It should

TABLE 4-5. Checklist for Verifying Position of Pulmonary Artery Catheter

	Zone 3	Zone 1 or 2
PAOP contour	Cardiac ripple (A + V waves)	Unnaturally smooth
PAD vs. PAOP	PAD > PAOP	PAD < PAOP
PEEP trial	ΔPAOP $<\frac{1}{2}$ ΔPEEP	ΔPAOP $>\frac{1}{2}$ ΔPEEP
Respiratory variation of PAOP	$<\frac{1}{2}$ P_{ALV}	$\geq\frac{1}{2}$ ΔP_{ALV}
Catheter tip location	LA level or below	Above LA level

LA, left atrium; PAD, pulmonary artery diastolic pressure; P_{ALV}, alveolar pressure; PAOP, pulmonary artery occlusion pressure; PEEP, positive end-expiratory pressure.
Adapted from RJ Schultz, GF Whitfield, JJ LaMura, et al: The role of physiologic monitoring in patients with fractures of the hip. *J Trauma* 1985,25:309.

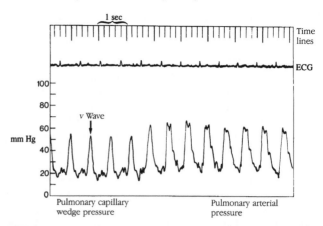

FIGURE 4-11. Pulmonary artery and pulmonary artery occlusion tracings with giant v waves distorting with pulmonary artery recording. ECG, electrocardiogram.

be noted that measurement of PAOP does not take into account capillary permeability, serum colloid osmotic pressure, interstitial pressure, or actual pulmonary capillary resistance [74,75]. These factors all play roles in the formation of pulmonary edema, and the PAOP should be interpreted in the context of the specific clinical situation.

Mean PAOP correlates well with left ventricular end-diastolic pressure (LVEDP), provided the patient has a normal mitral valve and normal left ventricular function. In myocardial infarction, conditions with decreased left ventricular compliance (e.g., ischemia, left ventricular hypertrophy), and conditions with markedly increased left ventricular filling pressure (e.g., dilated cardiomyopathy), the contribution of atrial contraction to left ventricular filling is increased. Thus, the LVEDP may be significantly higher than the mean left atrial pressure or PAOP [60].

The position of the catheter can be misinterpreted in patients with the presence of giant v waves. The most common cause of these v waves is mitral regurgitation. During this condition, left ventricular blood floods a normal-sized, noncompliant left atrium during ventricular systole, causing giant v waves in the occlusion pressure tracing (Fig. 4-11). The giant v wave of mitral regurgitation may be transmitted to the PA tracing, yielding a bifid PA waveform composed of the PA systolic wave and the v wave. As the catheter is occluded, the PA systolic wave is lost, but the v wave remains. It is important to note that the PA systolic wave occurs earlier in relation to the QRS of a simultaneously recorded ECG (between the QRS and T waves) than does the v wave (after the T wave).

Although a large v wave is not diagnostic of mitral regurgitation and is not always present in this circumstance, acute mitral regurgitation remains the most common cause of giant v waves in the PAOP tracing. Prominent v waves may occur whenever the left atrium is distended and noncompliant due to left ventricular failure from any cause (e.g., ischemic heart disease, dilated cardiomyopathy) [76,77] or secondary to the increased pulmonary blood flow in acute ventricular septal defect [78]. Acute mitral regurgitation is the rare instance when the PA end-diastolic pressure may be lower than the computer-measured mean occlusion pressure [62].

End expiration provides a readily identifiable reference point for PAOP interpretation because pleural pressure returns to baseline at the end of passive deflation (approximately equal to atmospheric pressure). Pleural pressure can exceed the normal resting value with active expiratory muscle contraction or use of PEEP. How much PEEP is transmitted to the pleural space cannot be estimated easily, since it varies depending on lung compliance and other factors. When normal lungs deflate passively, end-expiratory pleural pressure increases by approximately one-half the applied PEEP. In patients with reduced lung compliance (e.g., patients with acute respiratory distress syndrome; ARDS), the transmitted fraction may be one-fourth or less of the PEEP value. In the past, PEEP levels greater than 10 mm Hg were thought to interrupt the column of blood between the left atrium and PA catheter tip, causing the PAOP to reflect alveolar pressure more accurately than left atrial pressure. However, two studies suggest that this may not hold true in all cases. Hasan et al. [79] concluded that the PAOP left atrial fluid column was protected by lung injury, and Teboul et al. [80] could find no significant discrepancy between PAOP and simultaneously measured LVEDP at PEEP levels of 0, 10, and 16 to 20 cm H_2O in patients with ARDS. They hypothesize that (a) a large intrapulmonary right-to-left shunt may provide a number of microvessels shielded from alveolar pressure, allowing free communication from PA to pulmonary veins, or (b) in ARDS, both vascular and lung compliance may decrease, reducing transmission of alveolar pressure to the pulmonary microvasculature and maintaining an uninterrupted blood column from the catheter tip to the left atrium.

Although it is difficult to estimate precisely the true transmural vascular pressure in a patient on PEEP, temporarily disconnecting PEEP to measure PAOP is not recommended. Because the hemodynamics have been destabilized, these measurements will be of questionable value. Venous return increases acutely after discontinuation of PEEP [80], and abrupt removal of PEEP will cause hypoxia, which may not reverse quickly on reinstitution of PEEP [81].

CARDIAC OUTPUT

Thermodilution Technique

A catheter equipped with a thermistor 4 cm from its tip allows calculation of CO using the thermodilution principle [45,82]. The thermodilution principle holds that if a known quantity of cold solution is introduced into the circulation and adequately mixed (passage through two valves and a ventricle is adequate), the resultant cooling curve recorded at a downstream site allows calculation of net blood flow. CO is inversely proportional to the integral of the time-versus-temperature curve.

In practice, a known amount of cold or room temperature solution (typically 10 mL of 0.9% saline in adults and 5 mL of 0.9% saline in children) is injected into the right atrium via the catheter's proximal port. The thermistor allows recording of the baseline PA blood temperature and subsequent temperature change. The resulting curve is usually analyzed by computer, although it can be analyzed manually by simple planimetric methods. Correction factors are added by catheter manufacturers to account for the mixture of cold indicator with warm residual fluid in the catheter injection lumen and the heat transfer from the catheter walls to the cold indicator.

Reported coefficients of variation using triplicate determinations, using 10 mL of cold injectate and a bedside computer, are

TABLE 4-6.   Selected Hemodynamic Variables Derived from Right Heart Catheterization

Hemodynamic Variable	Normal Range
Arterial-venous content difference	3.5-5.5 mL/100 mL
Cardiac index	2.5–4.5 L/min/m^2
Cardiac output	3.0–7.0 L/min
Left ventricular stroke work index	45–60 g/beat/m^2
Mixed venous oxygen content	18.0 mL/100 mL
Mixed venous saturation	75% (approximately)
Oxygen consumption	200–250 mL/min
Pulmonary vascular resistance	120–250 dynes/sec/cm^{-5}
Stroke volume	70–130 mL/contraction
Stroke volume index	40–50 mL/contraction/m^2
Systemic vascular resistance	1,100–1,500 dynes/sec/cm^2

Adapted from JM Gore, JS Alpert, JR Benotti, et al: *Handbook of Hemodynamic Monitoring.* Boston, Little, Brown, 1984.

approximately 4% or less. Variations in the rate of injection can also introduce error into CO determinations, and it is thus important that the solution be injected as rapidly as possible. Careful attention must be paid to the details of this procedure; even then, changes of less than 10% to 15% above or below an initial value may not truly establish directional validity. Thermodilution CO is inaccurate in low-output states, tricuspid regurgitation, and in cases of atrial or ventricular septal defects [83].

Normal values for arterial-venous oxygen content difference, mixed venous oxygen saturation, and CO can be found in Table 4-6.

Analysis of Mixed Venous Blood

CO can be approximated merely by examining mixed venous (PA) oxygen saturation. Theoretically, if CO rises, then the mixed venous oxygen partial pressure will rise, since peripheral tissues need to exact less oxygen per unit of blood. Conversely, if CO falls, peripheral extraction from each unit will increase to meet the needs of metabolizing tissues. Serial determinations of mixed venous oxygen saturation may display trends in CO. Normal mixed venous oxygen saturation is 70% to 75%; values of less than 60% are associated with heart failure and values of less than 40% with shock [84]. Potential sources of error in this determination include extreme low-flow states where poor mixing may occur, contamination of desaturated mixed venous blood by saturated pulmonary capillary blood when the sample is aspirated too quickly through the nonwedged catheter [85] or in certain disease states (e.g., sepsis) where microcirculatory shunting may occur. Fiberoptic reflectance oximetry PA catheters can continuously measure and record mixed venous oxygen saturations in appropriate clinical situations [48,86].

DERIVED PARAMETERS

Useful hemodynamic parameters that can be derived using data with PA catheters include the following:

1. Cardiac index = CO (L/minute)/BSA (m^2)
2. Stroke volume = CO (L/minute)/heart rate (beats/minute)

TABLE 4-7. Hemodynamic Parameters in Commonly Encountered Clinical Situations (Idealized)

	RA	RV	PA	PAOP	AO	CI	SVR	PVR
Normal	0–6	25/0–6	25/6–12	6–12	130/80	≥2.5	1,500	≤250
Hypovolemic shock	0–2	15–20/0–2	15–20/2–6	2–6	≤90/60	<2.0	>1,500	≤250
Cardiogenic shock	8	50/8	50/35	35	≤90/60	<2.0	>1,500	≤250
Septic shock								
Early	0–2	20–25/0–2	20–25/0–6	0–6	≤90/60	≥2.5	<1,500	<250
Late[a]	0–4	25/4–10	25/4–10	4–10	≤90/60	<2.0	>1,500	>250
Acute massive pulmonary embolism	8–12	50/12	50/12–15	≤12	≤90/60	<2.0	>1,500	>450
Cardiac tamponade	12–18	25/12–18	25/12–18	12–18	≤90/60	<2.0	>1,500	≤250
AMI without LVF	0–6	25/0–6	25/12–18	≤18	140/90	≤2.5	1,500	≤250
AMI with LVF	0–6	30–40/0–6	30–40/18–25	>18	140/90	>2.0	>1,500	>250
Biventricular failure secondary to LVF	>6	50–60/>6	50–60/25	18–25	120/80	~2.0	>1,500	>250
RVF secondary to RVI	12–20	30/12–20	30/12	<12	≤90/60	<2.0	>1,500	>250
Cor pulmonale	>6	80/>6	80/35	<12	120/80	~2.0	>1,500	>400
Idiopathic pulmonary hypertension	0–6	80–100/0–6	80–100/40	<12	100/60	<2.0	>1,500	>500
Acute ventricular septal rupture[b]	6	60/6–8	60/35	30	≤90/60	<2.0	>1,500	>250

AMI, acute myocardial infarction; AO, aortic; CI, cardiac index; LVF, left ventricular failure; PA, pulmonary artery; PAOP, pulmonary artery occlusion pressure; PVR, pulmonary vascular resistance; RA, right atrium; RV, right ventricle; RVF, right ventricular failure; RVI, right ventricular infarction; SVR, systemic vascular resistance.
[a]Hemodynamic profile seen in approximately one third of patients in late septic shock.
[b]Confirmed by appropriate RA–PA oxygen saturation step-up. See text for discussion.
Adapted from JM Gore, JS Alpert, JR Benotti, et al: *Handbook of Hemodynamic Monitoring.* Boston, Little, Brown, 1984.

3. Stroke index = CO (L/minute)/heart rate (beats/minute) × BSA (m^2)
4. Mean arterial pressure (mm Hg) = (2 × diastolic) + systolic/3
5. Systemic vascular resistance (dyne/second/cm^{-5}) = mean arterial pressure – mean right atrial pressure (mm Hg)/CO (L/minute) × 80
6. Pulmonary arteriolar resistance (dyne/second/cm^{-5}) = mean PA pressure − PAOP (mm Hg)/CO (L/minute) × 80
7. Total pulmonary resistance (dyne/second/cm^{-5}) = mean PA pressure (mm Hg)/CO (L/minute) × 80
8. Left ventricular stroke work index = 1.36 (mean arterial pressure – PAOP) × stroke index/100
9. Do_2 (mL/minute/m^2) = cardiac index × arterial O_2 content

Normal values are listed in Table 4-6.

CLINICAL APPLICATIONS OF THE PULMONARY ARTERY CATHETER

NORMAL RESTING HEMODYNAMIC PROFILE

The finding of normal CO associated with normal left and right heart filling pressures is useful in establishing a noncardiovascular basis to explain abnormal symptoms or signs and as a baseline to gauge a patient's disease progression or response to therapy. Right atrial pressures of 0 to 6 mm Hg, PA systolic pressures of 15 to 30 mm Hg, PADPs of 5 to 12 mm Hg, PA mean pressures of 9 to 18 mm Hg, PAOP of 5 to 12 mm Hg, and a cardiac index exceeding 2.5 L per minute per m^2 characterize a normal cardiovascular state at rest.

Table 4-7 summarizes specific hemodynamic patterns for a variety of disease entities in which PA catheters have been indicated and provide clinical information that can impact patient care.

COMPLICATIONS

Minor and major complications associated with bedside balloon flotation PA catheterization have been reported (Table 4-8). During the 1970s, in the first 10 years of clinical catheter

TABLE 4-8. Complications of Pulmonary Artery Catheterization

Associated with central venous access
Balloon rupture
Knotting
Pulmonary infarction
Pulmonary artery perforation
Thrombosis, embolism
Arrhythmias
Intracardiac damage
Infections
Miscellaneous complications

use, a number of studies reported a relatively high incidence of certain complications. Consequent revision of guidelines for PA catheter use and improved insertion and maintenance techniques resulted in a decreased incidence of these complications in the 1980s [87]. The majority of complications are avoidable by scrupulous attention to detail in catheter placement and maintenance.

COMPLICATIONS ASSOCIATED WITH CENTRAL VENOUS ACCESS

The insertion techniques and complications of central venous cannulation are discussed in Chapter 2. Reported local vascular complications include local arterial or venous hematomas, unintentional entry of the catheter into the carotid system, atrioventricular fistulas, and pseudoaneurysm formation [88–90]. Adjacent structures, such as the thoracic duct, can be damaged, with resultant chylothorax formation. Pneumothorax can be a serious complication of insertion, although the incidence is relatively low (1% to 2%) [62,88,91]. The incidence of pneumothorax is higher with the subclavian approach than with the internal jugular approach in some reports [92], but other studies demonstrate no difference between the two sites [93,94]. The incidence of complications associated with catheter insertion is generally considered to be inversely proportional to the operator's experience.

BALLOON RUPTURE

Balloon rupture occurred more frequently in the early 1970s than it does now and was generally related to exceeding recommended inflation volumes. The main problems posed by balloon rupture are air emboli gaining access to the arterial circulation and balloon fragments embolizing to the distal pulmonary circulation. If rupture occurs during catheter insertion, the loss of the balloon's protective cushioning function can predispose to endocardial damage and attendant thrombotic and arrhythmic complications.

KNOTTING

Knotting of a catheter around itself is most likely to occur when loops form in the cardiac chambers and the catheter is repeatedly withdrawn and readvanced [95]. Knotting is avoided if care is taken not to advance the catheter significantly beyond the distances at which entrance to the ventricle or PA would ordinarily be anticipated. Knotted catheters usually can be extricated transvenously; guidewire placement [96], venotomy, or more extensive surgical procedures are occasionally necessary.

Knotting of PA catheters around intracardiac structures [97] or other intravascular catheters [98] has been reported. Rarely, entrapment of a PA catheter in cardiac sutures after open-heart surgery has been reported, requiring varying approaches for removal [99].

PULMONARY INFARCTION

Peripheral migration of the catheter tip (caused by catheter softening and loop tightening over time) with persistent, undetected wedging in small branches of the PA is the most common mechanism underlying pulmonary ischemic lesions attributable

to PA catheters [100]. These lesions are usually small and asymptomatic, often diagnosed solely on the basis of changes in the chest radiograph demonstrating an occlusion-shaped pleural-based density with a convex proximal contour [101].

Severe infarctions are usually produced if the balloon is left inflated in the occlusion position for an extended period, thus obstructing more central branches of the PA, or if solutions are injected at relatively high pressure through the catheter lumen in an attempt to restore an apparently damped pressure trace. Pulmonary embolic phenomena resulting from thrombus formation around the catheter or over areas of endothelial damage can also result in pulmonary infarction.

The reported incidence of pulmonary infarction secondary to PA catheters in 1974 was 7.2% [100], but recently reported rates of pulmonary infarction are much lower. Boyd et al. [102] found a 1.3% incidence of pulmonary infarction in a prospective study of 528 PA catheterizations. Sise et al. [103] reported no pulmonary infarctions in a prospective study of 319 PA catheter insertions. Use of continuous heparin flush solution and careful monitoring of PA waveforms are important reasons for the decreased incidence of this complication.

PULMONARY ARTERY PERFORATION

A serious and feared complication of PA catheterization is rupture of the PA leading to hemorrhage, which can be massive and sometimes fatal [104–106]. Rupture may occur during insertion or may be delayed a number of days [106]. PA rupture or perforation has been reported in approximately 0.1% to 0.2% of patients [92,107,108], although recent pathologic data suggest the true incidence of PA perforation is somewhat higher [109]. Proposed mechanisms by which PA rupture can occur include: (a) an increased pressure gradient between PAOP and PA pressure brought about by balloon inflation and favoring distal catheter migration, where perforation is more likely to occur; (b) an occluded catheter tip position favoring eccentric or distended balloon inflation with a spearing of the tip laterally and through the vessel; (c) cardiac pulsation causing shearing forces and damage as the catheter tip repeatedly contacts the vessel wall; (d) presence of the catheter tip near a distal arterial bifurcation where the integrity of the vessel wall against which the balloon is inflated may be compromised; and (e) simple lateral pressure on vessel walls caused by balloon inflation (this tends to be greater if the catheter tip was occluded before inflation began). Patient risk factors for PA perforation include pulmonary hypertension, mitral valve disease, advanced age, hypothermia, and anticoagulant therapy. In patients with these risk factors and in whom PADP reflects PAOP reasonably well, avoidance of subsequent balloon inflation altogether constitutes prudent prophylaxis.

Another infrequent but life-threatening complication is false aneurysm formation associated with rupture or dissection of the PA [110]. Technique factors related to PA hemorrhage are distal placement or migration of the catheter; failure to remove large catheter loops placed in the cardiac chambers during insertion; excessive catheter manipulation; use of stiffer catheter designs; and multiple overzealous or prolonged balloon inflations. Adherence to strict technique may decrease the incidence of this complication. In a prospective study reported in 1986, no cases of PA rupture occurred in 1,400 patients undergoing PA catheterization for cardiac surgery [92].

PA perforation typically presents with massive hemoptysis. Emergency management includes immediate occlusion arteriogram and bronchoscopy, intubation of the unaffected lung, and consideration of emergency lobectomy or pneumonectomy. PA catheter balloon tamponade resulted in rapid control of bleeding in one case report [111]. Application of PEEP to intubated patients may also tamponade hemorrhage caused by a PA catheter [112,113].

THROMBOEMBOLIC COMPLICATIONS

Because PA catheters constitute foreign bodies in the cardiovascular system and can potentially damage the endocardium, they are associated with an increased incidence of thrombosis. Thrombi encasing the catheter tip and aseptic thrombotic vegetations forming at endocardial sites in contact with the catheter have been reported [102,114]. Extensive clotting around the catheter tip can occlude the pulmonary vasculature distal to the catheter, and thrombi anywhere in the venous system or right heart can serve as a source of pulmonary emboli. Subclavian venous thrombosis, presenting with unilateral neck vein distention and upper extremity edema, may occur in up to 2% of subclavian placements [115,116]. Venous thrombosis complicating percutaneous internal jugular vein catheterization is fairly commonly reported, although its clinical importance remains uncertain [117]. Consistently damped pressure tracings without evidence of peripheral catheter placement or pulmonary vascular occlusion should arouse suspicion of thrombi at the catheter tip. A changing relationship of PADP to PAOP over time should raise concern about possible pulmonary emboli.

If an underlying hypercoagulable state is known to exist, if catheter insertion was particularly traumatic, or if prolonged monitoring becomes necessary, one should consider cautiously anticoagulating the patient.

Heparin-bonded catheters reduce thrombogenicity [43] and have become the most commonly used PA catheters. An important complication of heparin-bonded catheters is heparin-induced thrombocytopenia [118,119]. Routine platelet counts are recommended for patients with heparin-bonded catheters in place.

RHYTHM DISTURBANCES

Atrial and ventricular arrhythmias occur commonly during insertion of PA catheters [120]. Premature ventricular contractions occurred during 11% of the catheter insertions originally reported by Swan et al. [1].

Studies have reported advanced ventricular arrhythmias (three or more consecutive ventricular premature beats) in approximately 30% to 60% of patients undergoing right heart catheterization [92,116,121–123]. Most arrhythmias are self-limited and do not require treatment, but sustained ventricular arrhythmias requiring treatment occur in 0% to 3% of patients [102,122,123]. Risk factors associated with increased incidence of advanced ventricular arrhythmias are acute myocardial ischemia or infarction, hypoxia, acidosis, hypocalcemia, and hypokalemia [122,124]. Prophylactic use of lidocaine in higher-risk patients may reduce the incidence of this complication [125]. A right lateral tilt position (5-degree angle) during PA catheter insertion is associated with a lower incidence of malig-nant ventricular arrhythmias than is the Trendelenburg position [59].

Although the majority of arrhythmias occur during catheter insertion, arrhythmias may develop at any time after the catheter has been correctly positioned. These arrhythmias are due to mechanical irritation of the conducting system and may be persistent. Ventricular ectopy may also occur if the catheter tip falls back into the RV outflow tract. Evaluation of catheter-induced ectopy should include a portable chest radiograph to evaluate catheter position and assessment of the distal lumen pressure tracing to ensure that the catheter has not slipped into the RV. Lidocaine may be used but is unlikely to ablate the ectopy because the irritant is not removed [125]. If the arrhythmia persists after lidocaine therapy or is associated with hemodynamic compromise, the catheter should be removed. Catheter removal should be performed by physicians under continuous ECG monitoring, since the ectopy occurs almost as frequently during catheter removal as during insertion [126,127].

Right bundle branch block (usually transient) can also complicate catheter insertion [128]. Patients undergoing anesthesia induction, those in the early stages of acute anteroseptal myocardial infarction, and those with acute pericarditis appear particularly susceptible to this complication. Patients with pre-existing left bundle branch block are at risk for developing complete heart block during catheter insertion, and some have advocated the insertion of a temporary transvenous pacing wire, a PA catheter with a pacing lumen, or pacing PA catheter with the pacing leads on the external surface of the catheter [129]. However, use of an external transthoracic pacing device should be sufficient to treat this complication.

INTRACARDIAC DAMAGE

Damage to the right heart chambers, tricuspid valve, pulmonic valve, and their supporting structures as a consequence of PA catheterization has been reported [130–133]. The reported incidence of catheter-induced endocardial disruption detected by pathologic examination varies from 3.4% [114] to 75% [134], but most studies suggest a range of 20% to 30% [116,131,132]. These lesions consist of hemorrhage, sterile thrombus, intimal fibrin deposition, and nonbacterial thrombotic endocarditis. Their clinical significance is not clear, but there is concern that they may serve as a nidus for infectious endocarditis.

Direct damage to the cardiac valves and supporting chordae occurs primarily by withdrawal of the catheters while the balloon is inflated [1]. However, chordal rupture has been reported despite balloon deflation [112]. The incidence of intracardiac and valvular damage discovered on postmortem examination is considerably higher than that of clinically significant valvular dysfunction.

INFECTIONS

Catheter-related septicemia (the same pathogen growing from blood and the catheter tip) was reported in up to 2% of patients undergoing bedside catheterization in the 1970s [135]. However, the incidence of septicemia related to the catheter appears to have declined in recent years, with a number of studies suggesting a septicemia rate of 0% to 1% [92,136,137]. In situ time of more than 72 to 96 hours significantly increases the risk of catheter-related sepsis. Right-sided septic endocarditis has been reported [133,138], but the true incidence of this complication is unknown. Becker et al. [130] noted two cases of left ventricular abscess formation in patients with PA catheters and *S. aureus septicemia*. Incidence of catheter colonization or contamination varies from 5% to 20%, depending on the duration of catheter placement and the criteria used to define colonization [137–139]. In situ catheter-related bloodstream infection may be diagnosed by either differential time to positivity or by quantitative blood cultures [140]. With the former method, paired blood cultures are drawn from a peripheral vein and the catheter. If the catheter blood culture turns positive two or more hours sooner than the peripheral blood culture, the catheter is the likely cause of the bacteremia. With the other method, positive quantitative blood cultures drawn from the catheter are sensitive, specific, and predictive of catheter-related bacteremia [141].

Pressure transducers have also been identified as an occasional source of infection [142]. The chance of introducing infection into a previously sterile system is increased during injections for CO determinations and during blood withdrawal. Approaches to reduce the risk of catheter-related infection include use of a sterile protective sleeve and antibiotic bonding to the catheter [93,143,144]. Scheduled changes of catheters do not reduce the rate of infection [145].

OTHER COMPLICATIONS

Rare miscellaneous complications that have been reported include: (a) hemodynamically significant decreases in pulmonary blood flow caused by balloon inflation in the central PA in postpneumonectomy patients with pulmonary hypertension in the remaining lung [146], (b) disruption of the catheter's intraluminal septum as a result of injecting contrast medium under pressure [147], (c) artifactual production of a midsystolic click caused by a slapping motion of the catheter against the interventricular septum in a patient with RV strain and paradoxic septal motion [148], (d) thrombocytopenia secondary to heparin-bonded catheters [118,119], and (e) dislodgment of pacing electrodes [149]. Multiple unusual placements of PA catheters have also been reported, including in the left pericardiophrenic vein, via the left superior intercostal vein into the abdominal vasculature, and from the superior vena cava through the left atrium and left ventricle into the aorta after open-heart surgery [150–152].

GUIDELINES FOR SAFE USE OF PULMONARY ARTERY CATHETERS

Multiple revisions and changes in emphasis to the original recommended techniques and guidelines have been published [87,153,154]. These precautions are summarized as follows:

1. Avoiding complications associated with catheter insertion.
   a. Inexperienced personnel performing insertions must be supervised. Many hospitals require that PA catheters be inserted by a fully trained intensivist, cardiologist, or anesthesiologist.
   b. Keep the patient as still as possible. Restraints or sedation may be required.
   c. Strict sterile technique is mandatory.
   d. Examine the postprocedure chest radiograph for pneumothorax (especially after subclavian or internal jugular venipuncture) and for catheter tip position.
2. Avoiding balloon rupture.
   a. Always inflate the balloon gradually. Stop inflation if no resistance is felt.
   b. Do not exceed recommended inflation volume. At the recommended volume, excess air will automatically be expelled from a syringe with holes bored in it that is constantly attached to the balloon port. Maintaining recommended volume also helps prevent the accidental injection of liquids.
   c. Keep the number of inflation-deflation cycles to a minimum.
   d. Do not reuse catheters designed for single usage, and do not leave catheters in place for prolonged periods.
   e. Use carbon dioxide as the inflation medium if communication between the right and left sides of the circulation is suspected.
3. Avoiding knotting. Discontinue advancement of the catheter if entrance to right atrium, RV, or PA has not been achieved at distances normally anticipated from a given insertion site. If these distances have already been significantly exceeded, or if the catheter does not withdraw easily, use fluoroscopy before attempting catheter withdrawal. Never pull forcefully on a catheter that does not withdraw easily.
4. Avoiding damage to pulmonary vasculature and parenchyma.
   a. Keep recording time of PAOP to a minimum, particularly in patients with pulmonary hypertension and other risk factors for PA rupture. Be sure the balloon is deflated after each PAOP recording. There is never an indication for continuous PAOP monitoring.
   b. Constant pressure monitoring is required each time the balloon is inflated. It should be inflated slowly, in small increments, and must be stopped as soon as the pressure tracing changes to PAOP or damped.
   c. If an occlusion is recorded with balloon volumes significantly less than the inflation volume recommended on the catheter shaft, withdraw the catheter to a position where full (or nearly full) inflation volume produces the desired trace.
   d. Anticipate catheter tip migration. Softening of the catheter material with time, repeated manipulations, and cardiac motion make distal catheter migration almost inevitable.
      i. Continuous PA pressure monitoring is mandatory, and the trace must be closely watched for changes from characteristic PA pressures to those indicating a PAOP or damped tip position.
      ii. Decreases over time in the balloon inflation volumes necessary to attain occlusion tracings should raise suspicion regarding catheter migration.
      iii. Confirm satisfactory tip position with chest radiographs immediately after insertion and at least daily.
   e. Do not use liquids to inflate the balloon. They may prevent deflation, and their relative incompressibility may increase lateral forces and stress on the walls of pulmonary vessels.

f. Hemoptysis is an ominous sign and should prompt an urgent diagnostic evaluation and rapid institution of appropriate therapy.

g. Avoid injecting solutions at high pressure through the catheter lumen on the assumption that clotting is the cause of the damped pressure trace. First, aspirate from the catheter. Then consider problems related to catheter position, stopcock position, transducer dome, transducers, pressure bag, flush system, or trapped air bubbles. Never flush the catheter in the occlusion position.

5. Avoiding thromboembolic complications.
   a. Minimize trauma induced during insertion.
   b. Use heparin-bonded catheters if there are no clinical contraindications.
   c. Consider the judicious use of anticoagulants in patients with hypercoagulable states or other risk factors.
   d. Avoid flushing the catheter under high pressure.
   e. Watch for a changing PADP-PAOP relationship, as well as for other clinical indicators of pulmonary embolism.

6. Avoiding arrhythmias.
   a. Constant ECG monitoring during insertion and maintenance, as well as ready accessibility of all supplies for performing cardiopulmonary resuscitation, defibrillation, and temporary pacing, are mandatory.
   b. Use caution when catheterizing patients with an acutely ischemic myocardium or preexisting left bundle branch block.
   c. When the balloon is deflated, do not advance the catheter beyond the right atrium.
   d. Avoid overmanipulation of the catheter.
   e. Secure the introducer in place at the insertion site.
   f. Watch for intermittent RV pressure tracings when the catheter is thought to be in the PA position. An unexplained ventricular arrhythmia in a patient with a PA catheter in place indicates the possibility of catheter-provoked ectopy.

7. Avoiding valvular damage.
   a. Avoid prolonged catheterization and excessive manipulation.
   b. Do not withdraw the catheter when the balloon is inflated.

8. Avoiding infections.
   a. Use meticulously sterile technique on insertion.
   b. Avoid excessive number of CO determinations and blood withdrawals.
   c. Avoid prolonged catheterization.
   d. Remove the catheter if signs of phlebitis develop. Culture the tip and use antibiotics as indicated.

SUMMARY

Hemodynamic monitoring enhances the understanding of cardiopulmonary pathophysiology in critically ill patients. Nonetheless, the risk-to-benefit profile of PA catheterization in various clinical circumstances remains uncertain. Recent large trials have concluded that there may be no outcome benefit to patients with PA catheters used as part of clinical decision making. There is increasing concern that PA catheterization may be overused and that the data obtained may not be optimally used, or perhaps in specific groups may increase morbidity and mortality.

Currently there is one additional clinical trial involving the pulmonary catheter and involves evaluating the effectiveness of a computer application in improving PA catheter waveform interpretation [156].

Until the results of this and future studies are available, clinicians using hemodynamic monitoring should carefully assess the risk-to-benefit ratio on an individual patient basis. The operator should understand the indications, insertion techniques, equipment, and data that can be generated before undertaking PA catheter insertion. PA catheterization must not delay or replace bedside clinical evaluation and treatment.

REFERENCES

1. Swan HJC, Ganz W, Forrester J, et al: Catheterization of the heart in man with use of a flow-directed balloon-tipped catheter. *N Engl J Med* 283:447, 1970.
2. Connors AF, McCaffree DR, Gray BA: Evaluation of right heart catheterization in the critically ill patient without acute myocardial infarction. *N Engl J Med* 308:263, 1983.
3. Gorlin R: Current concepts in cardiology: practical cardiac hemodynamics. *N Engl J Med* 296:203, 1977.
4. Kumar A, Anel R, Bunnell E: Pulmonary artery occlusion pressure and central venous pressure fail to predict ventricular filling volume, cardiac performance, or the response to volume infusion in normal subjects. *Crit Care Med* 32:691, 2004.
5. Rao TK, Jacobs KH, El-Etr AA: Reinfarction following anesthesia in patients with myocardial infarction. *Anesthesiology* 59:499, 1983.
6. Hesdorffer CS, Milne JF, Meyers AM, et al: The value of Swan-Ganz catheterization and volume loading in preventing renal failure in patients undergoing abdominal aneurysmectomy. *Clin Nephrol* 28:272, 1987.
7. Shoemaker WC, Appel PL, Kram HB, et al: Prospective trial of supranormal values of survivors as therapeutic goals in high-risk surgical patients. *Chest* 94:1176, 1988.
8. Berlauk JF, Abrams JH, Gilmour IL, et al: Preoperative optimization of cardiovascular hemodynamics improves outcome in peripheral vascular surgery: a prospective, randomized clinical trial. *Ann Surg* 214:289, 1991.
9. Fleming A, Bishop M, Shoemaker W, et al: Prospective trial of supernormal values as goals of resuscitation in severe trauma. *Arch Surg* 127:1175, 1992.
10. Tuchschmidt J, Fried J, Astiz M, et al: Elevation of cardiac output and oxygen delivery improves outcome in septic shock. *Chest* 102:216, 1992.
11. Boyd O, Grounds RM, Bennett ED: A randomized clinical trial or the effect of deliberate perioperative increase of oxygen delivery on mortality in high-risk surgical patients. *JAMA* 270:2699, 1993.
12. Bishop MH, Shoemaker WC, Appel PL, et al: Prospective randomized trial of survivor values of cardiac index, oxygen delivery, and oxygen consumption as resuscitation endpoints in severe trauma. *J Trauma* 38:780, 1995.
13. Schiller WR, Bay RC, Garren RL, et al: Hyperdynamic resuscitation improves in patients with life-threatening burns. *J Burn Care Rehabil* 18:10, 1997.
14. Wilson J, Woods I, Fawcett J, et al: Reducing the risk of major elective surgery: randomized controlled trial of preoperative optimization of oxygen delivery. *BMJ* 318:1099, 1999.
15. Chang MC, Meredith JW, Kincaid EH, et al: Maintaining survivors' of left ventricular power output during shock resuscitation: a prospective pilot study. *J Trauma* 49:26, 2000.
16. Polonen P, Ruokonen E, Hippelainen M, et al: A prospective, randomized study of goal-oriented hemodynamic therapy in cardiac surgical patients. *Anesth Analg* 90:1052, 2000.
17. Pearson KS, Gomez MN, Moyers, JR, et al: A cost/benefit analysis of randomized invasive monitoring for patients undergoing cardiac surgery. *Anesth Analg* 69:336, 1989.
18. Isaacson IJ, Lowdon JD, Berry AJ, et al: The value of pulmonary artery and central venous monitoring in patients undergoing abdominal aortic reconstructive surgery: a comparative study of two selected, randomized groups. *J Vasc Surg* 12:754, 1990.
19. Joyce WP, Provan JL, Ameli FM, et al: The role of central hemodynamic monitoring in abdominal aortic surgery: a prospective randomized study. *Eur J Vasc Surg* 4:633, 1990.
20. Yu M, Levy M, Smith P: Effect of maximizing oxygen delivery on morbidity and mortality rates in critically ill patients. *Crit Care Med* 21:830, 1993.
21. Gattinoni L, Brazzi L, Pelosi P, et al: A trial of goal-oriented hemodynamic therapy in critically ill patients. *N Engl J Med* 333:1025, 1995.
22. Yu M, Takanishi D, Myers SA, et al: Frequency of mortality and myocardial infarction during maximizing oxygen delivery: a prospective, randomized trial. *Crit Care Med* 23:1025, 1995.
23. Durham RM, Neunaber K, Mazuski JE, et al: The use of oxygen consumption and delivery as endpoints for resuscitation in critically ill patients. *J Trauma* 41:32, 1996.
24. Afessa B, Spenser S, Khan W, et al: Association of pulmonary artery catheter use with in-hospital mortality. *Crit Care Med* 29:1145, 2001.
25. Rhodes A, Cusack RJ, Newman PJ et al: A randomized, controlled trial of the pulmonary artery catheter in critically ill patients. *Intensive Care Med* 28:256, 2002.

26. Richard C: Early use of the pulmonary artery catheter and outcomes in patients with shock and acute respiratory distress syndrome: a randomized controlled trial. *JAMA* 290:2713, 2003.

27. Yu DT, Platt R, Lanken PN, et al: Relationship of pulmonary artery catheter use to mortality and resource utilization in patients with severe sepsis. *Crit Care Med* 31:2734, 2003.

28. Sandham JD, Hull RD, Brant RF, et al: A randomized, controlled trial of the use of pulmonary-artery catheters in high-risk surgical patients. *N Engl J Med* 348:5, 2003.

29. Sakr Y, Vincent JL, Reinhart K, et al: Use of the pulmonary artery catheter is not associated with worse outcome in the ICU. *Chest* 128:2722, 2005.

30. Harvey S, Harrison DA, Singer M, et al: Assessment of the clinical effectiveness of pulmonary-artery catheters in management of patients in intensive care (PAC-Man): a randomized controlled trial. *Lancet* 366:472, 2005.

31. Binanay C, Califf RM, Hasselblad V, et al: Evaluation study of congestive heart failure and pulmonary artery catheterization effectiveness: the ESCAPE trial. *JAMA* 294:1625, 2005.

32. Tuman KJ, McCarthy RJ, Spiess BD, et al: Effect of pulmonary artery catheterization on outcome in patients undergoing coronary artery surgery. *Anesthesiology* 70:199, 1989.

33. Guyatt G: A randomized control trial of right heart catheterization in critically ill patients. Ontario Intensive Care Study Group. *J Intensive Care Med* 6:91, 1991.

34. Hayes MA, Timmins AC, Yau H, et al: Elevation of systemic oxygen delivery in the treatment of critically ill patients. *N Eng J Med* 330:1717, 1994.

35. Connors AF, Speroff T, Dawson NV, et al: The effectiveness of right heart catheterization in the initial care of critically ill patients. *JAMA* 276:889, 1996.

36. Valentine RJ, Duke ML, Inman MH, et al: Effectiveness of pulmonary artery catheters in aortic surgery: a randomized trial. *J Vasc Surg* 27:203, 1998.

37. Stewart RD, Psyhojos T, Lahey SJ, et al: Central venous catheter use in low risk coronary artery bypass grafting. *Ann Thorac Surg* 66:1306, 1998.

38. Ramsey SD, Saint S, Sullivan SD, et al: Clinical and economic effects of pulmonary artery catheterization in nonemergent coronary artery bypass graft surgery. *J Cardiothorac Vasc Anesth* 14:113, 2000.

39. Polanczyk CA, Rohde LE, Goldman L, et al: Right heart catheterization and cardiac complications in patients undergoing noncardiac surgery: an observational study. *JAMA* 286:348, 2001.

40. Chittock DR, Dhingra VK, Ronco JJ, et al: Severity of illness and risk of death associated with pulmonary artery catheter use. *Crit Care Med* 32:911, 2004.

41. Peters SG, Afessa B, Decker PA, et al: Increased risk associated with pulmonary artery catheterization in the medical intensive care unit. *J Crit Care* 18:166, 2003.

42. Cohen MG, Kelley RV, Kong DF, et al: Pulmonary artery catheterization in acute coronary syndromes: insights from the GUSTO IIb and GUSTO III trials. *Am J Med* 118:482, 2005.

43. Hoar PF, Wilson RM, Mangano DT, et al: Heparin bonding reduces thrombogenicity of pulmonary-artery catheters. *N Engl J Med* 305:993, 1981.

44. Mangano DT: Heparin bonding long-term protection against thrombogenesis. *N Engl J Med* 307:894, 1982.

45. Forrester JS, Ganz W, Diamond G, et al: Thermodilution cardiac output determination with a single flow-directed catheter. *Am Heart J* 83:306, 1972.

46. Chatterjee K, Swan JHC, Ganz W, et al: Use of a balloon-tipped flotation electrode catheter for cardiac monitoring. *Am J Cardiol* 36:56, 1975.

47. Simoons ML, Demey HE, Bossaert LL, et al: The Paceport catheter: a new pacemaker system introduced through a Swan-Ganz catheter. *Cathet Cardiovasc Diagn* 15:66, 1988.

48. Baele PL, McMechan JC, Marsh HM, et al: Continuous monitoring of mixed venous oxygen saturation in critically ill patients. *Anesth Analg* 61:513, 1982.

49. Segal J, Pearl RG, Ford AJ, et al: Instantaneous and continuous cardiac output obtained with a Doppler pulmonary artery catheter. *J Am Coll Cardiol* 13:1382, 1989.

50. Vincent JL, Thirion M, Bumioulle S, et al: Thermodilution measurement of right ventricular ejection fraction with a modified pulmonary artery catheter. *Intensive Care Med* 12:33, 1986.

51. Guerrero JE, Munoz J, De Lacalle B, et al: Right ventricular systolic time intervals determined by means of a pulmonary artery catheter. *Crit Care Med* 20:1529, 1992.

52. Dhainaut JF, Brunet F, Monsallier JF, et al: Bedside evaluation of right ventricular performance using a rapid computerized thermodilution mode. *Crit Care Med* 15:148, 1987.

53. Vincent JL: Measurement of right ventricular ejection fraction. *Intensive Care World* 7:133, 1990.

54. Nelson, LD: The new pulmonary arterial catherers: Right ventricular ejection fraction and continuous cardiac output. *Critical Care Clin* 12:795, 1996.

55. Boldt J, Mendes T, Wollbruck M, et al: Is continuous cardiac output measurement using thermodilution reliable in the critically ill patient? *Crit Care Med* 22:1913, 1994.

56. Haller M, Zollner C, Briegel J, et al: Evaluation of a new continuous thermodilution cardiac output monitor in critically ill patients: a prospective criterion standard study. *Crit Care Med* 23:860, 1995.

57. Mihaljevic T, von Segesser L, Tonz M, et al: Continuous verses bolus thermodilution cardiac output measurements: a comparative study. *Crit Care Med* 23:944, 1995.

58. Munro H, Woods C, Taylor B, et al: Continuous invasive cardiac output monitoring: The Baxter/Edwards Critical-Care Swan Ganz IntelliCath and Vigilance system. *Clin Intensive Care* 5:52, 1994.

59. Keusch DJ, Winters S, Thys DM: The patient's position influences the incidence of dysrhythmias during pulmonary artery catheterization. *Anesthesiology* 70:582, 1989.

60. Marini JJ: Hemodynamic monitoring with the pulmonary artery catheter. *Crit Care Clin* 2:551, 1986.

61. Barry WA, Grossman W: Cardiac catheterization, in Braunwald E (ed): *Heart Disease: A Textbook of Cardiovascular Medicine*. Philadelphia, WB Saunders, 1988; p 287 (vol 1).

62. Sharkey SW: Beyond the occlusion: clinical physiology and the Swan-Ganz catheter. *Am J Med* 83:111, 1987.

63. Bohrer H, Fleischer F: Errors in biochemical and haemodynamic data obtained using introducer lumen and proximal port of Swan-Ganz catheter. *Intensive Care Med* 15:330, 1989.

64. Huford WE, Zapol WM: The right ventricle and critical illness: a review of anatomy, physiology, and clinical evaluation of its function. *Intensive Care Med* 14:448, 1988.

65. Diebel LN, Wilson RF, Tagett MG, et al: End diastolic volume: a better indicator of preload in the critically ill. *Arch Surg* 127:817, 1992.

66. Martyn JA, Snider MT, Farago LF, et al: Thermodilution right ventricular volume: a novel and better predictor of volume replacement in acute thermal injury. *J Trauma* 21:619, 1981.

67. Reuse C, Vincent JL, Pinsky MR, et al: Measurements of right ventricular volumes during fluid challenge. *Chest* 98:1450, 1990.

68. Lange RA, Moore DM, Cigarroa RG, et al: Use of pulmonary capillary occlusion pressure to assess severity of mitral stenosis: is true left atrial pressure needed in this condition? *J Am Coll Cardiol* 13:825, 1989.

69. Alpert JS: The lessons of history as reflected in the pulmonary capillary occlusion pressure. *J Am Coll Cardiol* 13:830, 1989.

70. Forrester JS, Diamond G, McHugh TJ, et al: Filling pressures in the right and left sides of the heart in acute myocardial infarction. *N Engl J Med* 285:190, 1971.

71. The National Heart, Lung and Blood Institute ARDS Clinical Trials Network: Pulmonary artery versus central venous catheter to guide treatment of acute lung injury. *New Engl J Med* 354:2213, 2006.

72. O'Quin R, Marini JJ: Pulmonary artery occlusion pressure: clinical physiology, measurement, and interpretation. *Am Rev Respir Dis* 128:319, 1983.

73. Timmis AD, Fowler MB, Burwood RJ, et al: Pulmonary edema without critical increase in left atrial pressure in acute myocardial infarction. *BMJ* 283:636, 1981.

74. Holloway H, Perry M, Downey J, et al: Estimation of effective pulmonary capillary pressure in intact lungs. *J Appl Physiol* 54:846, 1983.

75. Dawson CA, Linehan JH, Rickaby DA: Pulmonary microcirculatory hemodynamics. *Ann NY Acad Sci* 384:90, 1982.

76. Pichard AD, Kay R, Smith H, et al: Large V waves in the pulmonary occlusion pressure tracing in the absence of mitral regurgitation. *Am J Cardiol* 50:1044, 1982.

77. Ruchs RM, Heuser RR, Yin FU, et al: Limitations of pulmonary occlusion V waves in diagnosing mitral regurgitation. *Am J Cardiol* 49:849, 1982.

78. Bethen CF, Peter RH, Behar VS, et al: The hemodynamic simulation of mitral regurgitation in ventricular septal defect after myocardial infarction. *Cathet Cardiovasc Diagn* 2:97, 1976.

79. Hasan FM, Weiss WB, Braman SS, et al: Influence of lung injury on pulmonary occlusion-left atrial pressure correlation during positive end-expiratory pressure ventilation. *Annu Rev Respir Dis* 131:246, 1985.

80. Teboul JL, Zapol WM, Brun-Buisson C, et al: A comparison of pulmonary artery occlusion pressure and left ventricular end diastolic pressure during mechanical ventilation with PEEP in patients with severe ARDS. *Anesthesiology* 70:261, 1989.

81. DeCampo T, Civetta JM: The effect of short-term discontinuation of high-level PEEP in patients with acute respiratory failure. *Crit Care Med* 7:47, 1979.

82. Ganz W, Swan HJC: Measurement of blood flow by thermodilution. *Am J Cardiol* 29:241, 1972.

83. Grossman W: Blood flow measurement: the cardiac output, in Grossman W (ed): *Cardiac Catheterization and Angiography*. Philadelphia, Lea & Febiger, 1985; p 116.

84. Goldman RH, Klughaupt M, Metcalf T, et al: Measurement of central venous oxygen saturation in patients with myocardial infarction. *Circulation* 38:941, 1968.

85. Pace NL: A critique of flow-directed pulmonary artery catheterization. *Anesthesiology* 47:455, 1977.

86. Rayput MA, Rickey HM, Bush BA, et al: A comparison between a conventional and a fiberoptic flow-directed thermal dilution pulmonary artery catheter in critically ill patients. *Arch Intern Med* 149:83, 1989.

87. Matthay MA, Chatterjee K: Bedside catheterization of the pulmonary artery: risks compared with benefits. *Ann Intern Med* 109:826, 1988.

88. McNabb TG, Green CH, Parket FL: A potentially serious complication with Swan-Ganz catheter placement by the percutaneous internal jugular route. *Br J Anaesth* 47:895, 1975.

89. Hansbroyh JF, Narrod JA, Rutherford R: Arteriovenous fistulas following central venous catheterization. *Intensive Care Med* 9:287, 1983.

90. Shield CF, Richardson JD, Buckley CJ, et al: Pseudoaneurysm of the brachiocephalic arteries: a complication of percutaneous internal jugular vein catheterization. *Surgery* 78:190, 1975.

91. Patel C, LaBoy V, Venus B, et al: Acute complications of pulmonary artery catheter insertion in critically ill patients. *Crit Care Med* 14:195, 1986.

92. Damen J, Bolton D: A prospective analysis of 1,400 pulmonary artery catheterizations in patients undergoing cardiac surgery. *Acta Anaesthesiol Scand* 14:1957, 1986.

93. Senagere A, Waller JD, Bonnell BW, et al: Pulmonary artery catheterization: a prospective study of internal jugular and subclavian approaches. *Crit Care Med* 15:35, 1987.

94. Nembre AE: Swan-Ganz catheter. *Arch Surg* 115:1194, 1980.

95. Lipp H, O'Donoghue K, Resnekov L: Intracardiac knotting of a flow-directed balloon catheter. *N Engl J Med* 284:220, 1971.

96. Mond HG, Clark DW, Nesbitt SJ, et al: A technique for unknotting an intracardiac flow-directed balloon catheter. *Chest* 67:731, 1975.

97. Meister SG, Furr CM, Engel TR, et al: Knotting of a flow-directed catheter about a cardiac structure. *Cathet Cardiovasc Diagn* 3:171, 1977.

98. Swaroop S: Knotting of two central venous monitoring catheters. *Am J Med* 53:386, 1972.

99. Loggam C, Sanborn TA, Christian F: Ventricular entrapment of a Swan-Ganz catheter: a technique for nonsurgical removal. *J Am Coll Cardiol* 13:1422, 1989.

100. Foote GA, Schabel SI, Hodges M: Pulmonary complications of the flow-directed balloon-tipped catheter. *N Engl J Med* 290:927, 1974.

101. Wechsler RJ, Steiner RM, Kinori F: Monitoring the monitors: the radiology of thoracic catheters, wires and tubes. *Semin Roentgenol* 23:61, 1988.

102. Boyd KD, Thomas SJ, Gold J, et al: A prospective study of complications of pulmonary artery catheterizations in 500 consecutive patients. *Chest* 84:245, 1983.

103. Sise MJ, Hollingsworth P, Bumm JE, et al: Complications of the flow directed pulmonary artery catheter: a prospective analysis of 219 patients. *Crit Care Med* 9:315, 1981.

104. Barash PG, Nardi D, Hammond G, et al: Catheter-induced pulmonary artery perforation: mechanisms, management and modifications. *J Thorac Cardiovasc Surg* 82:5, 1981.

105. Pape LA, Haffajee CI, Markis JE, et al: Fatal pulmonary hemorrhage after use of the flow-directed balloon-tipped catheter. *Ann Intern Med* 90:344, 1979.

106. Lapin ES, Murray JA: Hemoptysis with flow-directed cardiac catheterization. *JAMA* 220:1246, 1972.

107. McDaniel DD, Stone JG, Faltas AN, et al: Catheter induced pulmonary artery hemorrhage: diagnosis and management in cardiac operations. *J Thorac Cardiovasc Surg* 82:1, 1981.

108. Shah KB, Rao TL, Laughlin S, et al: A review of pulmonary artery catheterization in 6245 patients. *Anesthesiology* 61:271, 1984.

109. Fraser RS: Catheter-induced pulmonary artery perforation: pathologic and pathogenic features. *Hum Pathol* 18:1246, 1987.

110. Declen JD, Friloux LA, Renner JW: Pulmonary artery false-aneurysms secondary to Swan-Ganz pulmonary artery catheters. *AJR Am J Roentgenol* 149:901, 1987.

111. Thoms R, Siproudhis L, Laurent JF, et al: Massive hemoptysis from iatrogenic balloon catheter rupture of pulmonary artery: successful early management by balloon tamponade. *Crit Care Med* 15:272, 1987.

112. Slacken A: Complications of invasive hemodynamic monitoring in the intensive care unit. *Curr Probl Surg* 25:69, 1988.

113. Scuderi PE, Prough DS, Price JD, et al: Cessation of pulmonary artery catheter-induced endobronchial hemorrhage associated with the use of PEEP. *Anesth Analg* 62:236, 1983.

114. Pace NL, Horton W: Indwelling pulmonary artery catheters: their relationship to aseptic thrombotic endocardial vegetations. *JAMA* 233:893, 1975.

115. Dye LE, Segall PH, Russell RO, et al: Deep venous thrombosis of the upper extremity associated with use of the Swan-Ganz catheter. *Chest* 73:673, 1978.

116. Elliot CG, Zimmerman GA, Clemmer TP: Complications of pulmonary artery catheterization in the care of critically ill patients: a prospective study. *Chest* 76:647, 1979.

117. Chastre J, Cornud F, Bouchama A, et al: Thrombosis as a complication of pulmonary artery catheterization via the internal jugular vein. *N Engl J Med* 306:278, 1982.

118. Laster JL, Nichols WK, Silver D: Thrombocytopenia associated with heparin-coated catheters in patients with heparin-associated antiplatelet antibodies. *Arch Intern Med* 149:2285, 1989.

119. Laster JL, Silver D: Heparin coated catheters and heparin-induced thrombocytopenia. *J Vasc Surg* 7:667, 1988.

120. Geha DG, Davis NJ, Lappas DG: Persistent atrial arrhythmias associated with placement of a Swan-Ganz catheter. *Anesthesiology* 39:651, 1973.

121. Spring CL, Jacobs JL, Caralis PV, et al: Ventricular arrhythmias during Swan-Ganz catheterization of the critically ill. *Chest* 79:413, 1981.

122. Spring CL, Pozen PG, Rozanski JJ, et al: Advanced ventricular arrhythmias during bedside pulmonary artery catheterization. *Am J Med* 72:203, 1982.

123. Iberti TJ, Benjamin E, Grupzi L, et al: Ventricular arrhythmias during pulmonary artery catheterization in the intensive care unit. *Am J Med* 78:451, 1985.

124. Patel C, Laboy V, Venus B, et al: Acute complications of pulmonary artery catheter insertion in critically ill patients. *Crit Care Med* 14:195, 1986.

125. Spring CL, Marical EH, Garcia AA, et al: Prophylactic use of lidocaine to prevent advanced ventricular arrhythmias during pulmonary artery catheterization: prospective, double blind study. *Am J Med* 75:906, 1983.

126. Johnston W, Royster R, Beamer W, et al: Arrhythmias during removal of pulmonary artery catheters. *Chest* 85:296, 1984.

127. Damen J: Ventricular arrhythmia during insertion and removal of pulmonary artery catheters. *Chest* 88:190, 1985.

128. Morris D, Mulvihill D, Lew WY: Risk of developing complete heart block during bedside pulmonary artery catheterization in patients with left bundle branch block. *Arch Intern Med* 147:2005, 1987.

129. Lavie CJ, Gersh BJ: Pacing in left bundle branch block during Swan-Ganz catheterization [letter]. *Arch Intern Med* 148:981, 1988.

130. Becker RC, Martin RG, Underwood DA: Right-sided endocardial lesions and flow-directed pulmonary artery catheters. *Cleve Clin J Med* 54:384, 1987.

131. Lange HW, Galliani CA, Edwards JE: Local complications associated with indwelling Swan-Ganz catheters. *Am J Cardiol* 52:1108, 1983.

132. Sage MD, Koelmeyer TD, Smeeton WMI: Evolution of Swan-Ganz catheter related pulmonary valve nonbacterial endocarditis. *Am J Forensic Med Pathol* 9:112, 1988.

133. Rowley KM, Clubb KS, Smith GJW, et al: Right sided infective endocarditis as a consequence of flow directed pulmonary artery catheterization. *N Engl J Med* 311:1152, 1984.

134. Ford SE, Manley PN: Indwelling cardiac catheters: an autopsy study of associated endocardial lesions. *Arch Pathol Lab Med* 106:314, 1982.

135. Prochan H, Dittel M, Jobst C, et al: Bacterial contamination of pulmonary artery catheters. *Intensive Care Med* 4:79, 1978.

136. Pinella JC, Ross DF, Martin T, et al: Study of the incidence of intravascular catheter infection and associated septicemia in critically ill patients. *Crit Care Med* 11:21, 1983.

137. Michel L, Marsh HM, McMichan JC, et al: Infection of pulmonary artery catheters in critically ill patients. *JAMA* 245:1032, 1981.

138. Greene JF, Fitzwater JE, Clemmer TP: Septic endocarditis and indwelling pulmonary artery catheters. *JAMA* 233:891, 1975.

139. Myers ML, Austin TW, Sibbald WJ: Pulmonary artery catheter infections: a prospective study. *Ann Surg* 201:237, 1985.

140. Hanna R, Raad II: Diagnosis of catheter-related bloodstream infection. *Curr Infect Dis Rep* 7:413, 2005.

141. Chatzinikolaou I, Hanna R, Darouiche R, et al: Prospective study of the value of quantitative culture of organisms from blood collected through central venous catheters in differentiating between contamination and bloodstream infection. *J Clin Microbiol* 44:1834, 2006.

142. Weinstein RA, Stamm WE, Kramer L: Pressure monitoring devices: overlooked source of nosocomial infection. *JAMA* 236:936, 1976.

143. Singh SJ, Puri VK: Prevention of bacterial colonization of pulmonary artery catheters. *Infect Surg* 1984;853.

144. Heard SO, Davis RF, Sherertz RJ, et al: Influence of sterile protective sleeves on the sterility of pulmonary artery catheters. *Crit Care Med* 15:499, 1987.

145. Cobb DK, High KP, Sawyer RG, et al: A controlled trial of scheduled replacement of central venous and pulmonary artery catheters. *N Engl J Med* 327:1062, 1992.

146. Berry AJ, Geer RT, Marshall BE: Alteration of pulmonary blood flow by pulmonary artery occluded pressure measurement. *Anesthesiology* 51:164, 1979.

147. Schluger J, Green J, Giustra FX, et al: Complication with use of flow-directed catheter. *Am J Cardiol* 32:125, 1973.

148. Isner JM, Horton J, Ronan JAS: Systolic click from a Swan-Ganz catheter: phonoechocardiographic depiction of the underlying mechanism. *Am J Cardiol* 42:1046, 1979.

149. Lawson D, Kushkins LG: A complication of multipurpose pacing pulmonary artery catheterization via the external jugular vein approach [letter]. *Anesthesiology* 62:377, 1985.

150. McLellan BA, Jerman MR, French WJ, et al: Inadvertent Swan-Ganz catheter placement in the left pericardiophrenic vein. *Cathet Cardiovasc Diagn* 16:173, 1989.

151. Allyn J, Lichtenstein A, Koski EG, et al: Inadvertent passage of a pulmonary artery catheter from the superior vena cava through the left atrium and left ventricle into the aorta. *Anesthesiology* 70:1019, 1989.

152. Lazzam C, Sanborn TA, Christian F: Ventricular entrapment of a Swan-Ganz catheter: a technique for nonsurgical removal. *J Am Coll Cardiol* 13:1422, 1989.

153. Ginosar Y, Sprung CL: The Swan-Ganz catheter: twenty-five years of monitoring. *Crit Care Clin* 12:771, 1996.

154. Wiedermann HP, Matthay MA, Matthay RA: Cardiovascular-pulmonary monitoring in the intensive care unit, 2. *Chest* 85:656, 1984.

155. Friese RS, Shafi S, Gentilello LM: Pulmonary artery catheter use is associated with reduced mortality in severely injured patients: a National Trauma Data Bank analysis of 53,312 patients. *Crit Care Med* 34:1597, 2006.

156. Effectiveness of a computer application in improving pulmonary artery waveform interpretation, Massachusetts General Hospital.http://clinicaltrials.gov/ct/show/NCT00138073.

Seth T. Dahlberg

CHAPTER **5**

Temporary Cardiac Pacing

Temporary cardiac pacing may be urgently required for the treatment of cardiac conduction and rhythm disturbances commonly seen in patients treated in the intensive care unit (ICU). Therefore, ICU personnel should be familiar with the indications and techniques for initiating and maintaining temporary cardiac pacing as well as the possible complications of this procedure. Recommendations for training in the performance of transvenous pacing have been published by a Task Force of the American College of Physicians, American Heart Association and American College of Cardiology [1]. Competence in the performance of transvenous pacing also requires the operator to have training in central venous access (see Chapter 2) and hemodynamic monitoring (see Chapter 4).

INDICATIONS FOR TEMPORARY CARDIAC PACING

As outlined in Table 5-1, temporary pacing is indicated in the diagnosis and management of a number of serious rhythm and conduction disturbances [2,3].

BRADYARRHYTHMIAS

The most common indication for temporary pacing in the ICU setting is a hemodynamically significant or symptomatic bradyarrhythmia such as sinus bradycardia or high-grade atrioventricular (AV) block.

Sinus bradycardia and AV block are commonly seen in patients with acute coronary syndromes, hyperkalemia, myxedema, or increased intracranial pressure. Infectious processes such as endocarditis or Lyme disease [4] may impair AV conduction. Bradyarrhythmias also result from treatment or intoxication with digitalis, antiarrhythmic, beta-blocker, or calcium channel blocker medications and may also result from exaggerated vasovagal reactions to ICU procedures such as suctioning of the tracheobronchial tree in the intubated patient. Bradycardia-dependent ventricular tachycardia may occur in association with ischemic heart disease.

TACHYARRHYTHMIAS

Temporary cardiac pacing has been used in both prevention and termination of supraventricular and ventricular tachyarrhythmias [5]. Atrial pacing is often effective in terminating atrial flutter and paroxysmal nodal supraventricular tachycardia [6]. Atrial pacing in the ICU setting is most frequently performed when temporary epicardial electrodes have been placed during cardiac surgery. A critical pacing rate (usually 125% to 135% of the flutter rate) and pacing duration (usually about 10 seconds)

are important in the successful conversion of atrial flutter to sinus rhythm [7,8]. This method is often effective in patients with classic atrial flutter; however, it is typically ineffective for atypical or type II atrial flutter (rate 400 beats per minute, P waves upright in the inferior leads).

In some clinical situations pacing termination of atrial flutter may be more attractive than synchronized cardioversion, which requires sedation with its attendant risks. Pacing termination is the treatment of choice for atrial flutter in patients with epicardial atrial wires in place after cardiac surgery. It may be preferred as the means to convert atrial flutter in patients on digoxin and those with sick sinus syndrome, as these groups often demonstrate prolonged sinus pauses after DC cardioversion [9].

Temporary pacing has proved lifesaving in preventing paroxysmal polymorphic ventricular tachycardia in patients with prolonged QT intervals (torsades de pointes), particularly when secondary to drugs. Temporary cardiac pacing is the treatment of choice to stabilize the patient while a type I antiarrhythmic agent exacerbating ventricular irritability is metabolized [10]. In this situation, the pacing rate is set to provide a mild tachycardia. The effectiveness of cardiac pacing probably relates to decreasing the dispersion of refractoriness of the ventricular myocardium (shortening the QT interval).

Temporary ventricular pacing is also frequently successful in terminating ventricular tachycardia [11]. If ventricular tachycardia must be terminated urgently, cardioversion is mandated. However, in less urgent situations, conversion of ventricular tachycardia via rapid ventricular pacing may be useful. The success of this technique depends on the setting in which ventricular tachycardia occurs as well as the type of pacing used (rapid overdrive pacing or programmed extrastimulation). Programmed stimulation techniques are usually effective in terminating ventricular tachycardia in a patient with remote myocardial infarction or in the absence of heart disease. This technique is less effective when ventricular tachycardia complicates acute myocardial infarction or cardiomyopathy. Rapid ventricular pacing is most successful in terminating ventricular tachycardia when the ventricle can be "captured" (asynchronous pacing for 5 to 10 beats at a rate of 50 beats per minute greater than that of the underlying tachycardia). Extreme caution is advised, as it may be accompanied by acceleration of ventricular tachycardias in more than 40% of patients; a cardiac defibrillator should be immediately available at the bedside.

DIAGNOSIS OF RAPID RHYTHMS

Temporary atrial pacing electrodes allow accurate diagnosis of tachyarrhythmias when the morphology of the P wave and its relation to the QRS complexes cannot be determined from the

TABLE 5-1. Indications for Acute (Temporary) Cardiac Pacing

Conduction disturbances
   Symptomatic persistent third-degree AV block with inferior
     myocardial infarction
   Third-degree AV block, new bifascicular block (e.g., right bundle
     branch block and left anterior hemiblock, left bundle branch
     block, first-degree AV block), or alternating left and right bundle
     branch block complicating acute anterior myocardial infarction
   Symptomatic idiopathic third-degree AV block, or high-degree AV
     block

Rate disturbances
   Hemodynamically significant or symptomatic sinus bradycardia
   Bradycardia-dependent ventricular tachycardia
   AV dissociation with inadequate cardiac output
   Polymorphic ventricular tachycardia with long QT interval (torsades
     de pointes)
   Recurrent ventricular tachycardia unresponsive to medical therapy

Av, atrioventricular.

surface electrocardiogram (ECG) [12,13]. A recording of the atrial electrogram is particularly helpful in a rapid, regular, narrow-complex tachycardia in which the differential diagnosis includes atrial flutter with rapid ventricular response, and AV nodal reentrant or other supraventricular tachycardia. This technique is also useful to distinguish wide-complex tachycardias in which the differential diagnosis includes supraventricular tachycardia with aberrant conduction, sinus tachycardia with bundle branch block, and ventricular tachycardia.

To record an atrial ECG, the limb leads are connected in the standard fashion and a precordial lead (usually V_1) is connected to the proximal electrode of the atrial pacing catheter or to an epicardial atrial electrode. A rhythm strip is run at a rapid paper speed, simultaneously demonstrating surface ECG limb leads as well as the atrial electrogram obtained via lead V_1. This rhythm strip should reveal the conduction pattern between atria and ventricles as antegrade, simultaneous, retrograde, or dissociated.

ACUTE MYOCARDIAL INFARCTION

Temporary pacing may be used therapeutically or prophylactically in acute myocardial infarction. Recommendations for temporary cardiac pacing have been provided by a Task Force of the American College of Cardiology and the American Heart Association (Table 5-2) [14]. Bradyarrhythmias unresponsive to medical treatment that result in hemodynamic compromise require urgent treatment. Patients with anterior infarction and bifascicular block or Mobitz type II second-degree AV block, while hemodynamically stable, may require a temporary pacemaker, as they are at risk for sudden development of complete heart block with an unstable escape rhythm.

Prophylactic temporary cardiac pacing has aroused considerable debate for the role it may play in complicated anterior wall myocardial infarction [15]. Thrombolytic therapy or percutaneous coronary intervention, when indicated, should take precedence over placement of prophylactic cardiac pacing, as prophylactic pacing has not been shown to improve mortality. Transthoracic (transcutaneous) cardiac pacing is safe and usu-

ally effective [16–19] and would be a reasonable alternative to prophylactic transvenous cardiac pacing, particularly soon after thrombolytic therapy has been administered.

When right ventricular involvement complicates inferior myocardial infarction, cardiac output may be very sensitive to ventricular preload. Because coordinated atrial transport may be required for maintenance of effective stroke volume, AV sequential pacing is frequently the pacing modality of choice in patients with right ventricular infarction [20,21].

EQUIPMENT AVAILABLE FOR TEMPORARY PACING

Several methods of temporary pacing are currently available for use in the ICU. Transvenous pacing of the right ventricle or right atrium with a pacing catheter or modified pulmonary artery catheter is the most widely used technique; intraesophageal, transcutaneous, and epicardial pacing are also available.

TRANSVENOUS PACING CATHETERS

Some of the many transvenous pacing catheters available for use in the critical care setting are illustrated in Figure 5-1. Pacing catheters range in size from 4 French (Fr) (1.2 mm) to 7 Fr (2.1 mm). In urgent situations, or where fluoroscopy is unavailable, a flow-directed flexible balloon-tipped catheter (Fig. 5-1, top) may be placed in the right ventricle using ECG guidance. After advancing the catheter into the right ventricle, the balloon can be deflated and the catheter tip advanced to the right ventricular apex. While the balloon-tipped catheter may avoid the need for fluoroscopy, placement may be ineffective in the setting of low blood flow during cardiac arrest or in the presence of severe tricuspid regurgitation. Stiff catheters (Fig. 5-1, middle) are easier to manipulate but require insertion under fluoroscopic guidance.

A flexible J-shaped catheter (Fig. 5-1, bottom), designed for temporary atrial pacing, is also available [22]. This lead is positioned by "hooking" it in the right atrial appendage under fluoroscopic guidance, providing stable contact with the atrial endocardium. Either the subclavian or internal jugular venous approach may be used.

A multilumen pulmonary artery catheter is available with a right ventricular lumen. Placement of a small (2.4 Fr) bipolar pacing lead through the right ventricular lumen allows intracardiac pressure monitoring and pacing through a single catheter [23]. Details on its use and insertion are described in Chapter 4.

ESOPHAGEAL ELECTRODE

An esophageal "pill" electrode allows atrial pacing and recording of atrial depolarizations without requiring central venous cannulation. As mentioned, detecting atrial depolarization aids in the diagnosis of tachyarrhythmias. Esophageal pacing has also been used to terminate supraventricular tachycardia and atrial flutter [24]. Because the electrode can be uncomfortable and may not give consistent, stable capture, the esophageal electrode is typically limited to short-term use for diagnosis of arrhythmias in pediatric patients.

TABLE 5-2. ACC/AHA Recommendations for Treatment of Atrioventricular and Intraventricular Conduction Disturbances During STEMI

Intraventricular Conduction	Normal		1st-Degree AV Block AMI		1st-Degree AV Block Non-AMI		Mobitz I 2nd-Degree AV Block AMI		Mobitz I 2nd-Degree AV Block Non-AMI		Mobitz II 2nd-Degree AV Block AMI		Mobitz II 2nd-Degree AV Block Non-AMI	
	Action	Class	Action	Class	Action	Class	Action	Class	Action	Class	Action	Class	Action	Class
Normal	OB	1	OB	1	OB	1	OB	2B	OB	2A	OB	3	OB	3
	A	3	A	3	A	3	A*	3	A	3	A	3	A	3
	TC	3	TC	2B	TC	2B	TC	1	TC	1	TC	1	TC	1
	TV	3	TV	3	TV	3	TV	3	TV	3	TV	2A	TV	2A
Old or New Fascicular Block (LAFB or LPFB)	OB	1	OB	2B	OB	2B	OB	2B	OB	2B	OB	3	OB	3
	A	3	A	3	A	3	A*	3	A	3	A	3	A	3
	TC	2B	TC	1	TC	2A	TC	1	TC	1	TC	1	TC	1
	TV	3	TV	3	TV	3	TV	3	TV	3	TV	2A	TV	2B
Old BBB	OB	1	OB	3	OB	3	OB	3	OB	3	OB	3	OB	3
	A	3	A	3	A	3	A*	3	A	3	A	3	A	3
	TC	2B	TC	1	TC	1	TC	1	TC	1	TC	1	TC	1
	TV	3	TV	2B	TV	2B	TV	2B	TV	2B	TV	2A	TV	2A
New BBB	OB	3	OB	3	OB	3	OB	3	OB	3	OB	3	OB	3
	A	3	A	3	A	3	A*	3	A	3	A	3	A	3
	TC	1	TC	1	TC	1	TC	1	TC	1	TC	2B	TC	2B
	TV	2B	TV	2A	TV	2A	TV	2A	TV	2A	TV	1	TV	1
Fascicular Block + RBBB	OB	3	OB	3	OB	3	OB	3	OB	3	OB	3	OB	3
	A	3	A	3	A	3	A*	3	A	3	A	3	A	3
	TC	1	TC	1	TC	1	TC	1	TC	1	TC	2B	TC	2B
	TV	2B	TV	2A	TV	2A	TV	2A	TV	2A	TV	1	TV	1
Alternating Left and Right BBB	OB	3	OB	3	OB	3	OB	3	OB	3	OB	3	OB	3
	A	3	A	3	A	3	A*	3	A	3	A	3	A	3
	TC	2B	TC	2B	TC	2B	TC	2B	TC	2B	TC	2B	TC	2B
	TV	1	TV	1	TV	1	TV	1	TV	1	TV	1	TV	1

This table is designed to summarize the atrioventricular (column headings) and intraventricular (row headings) conduction disturbances that may occur during acute anterior or nonanterior STEMI, the possible treatment options, and the indications for each possible therapeutic option.

A, atropine; AMI, anterior myocardial infarction; AV, atrioventricular; BBB, bundle-branch block; LAFB, left anterior fascicular block; LPFB, left posterior fascicular block; MI, myocardial infarction; non-AMI, nonanterior myocardial infarction; OB, observe; RBBB, right bundle-branch block; STEMI, ST elevation myocardial infarction; TC, transcutaneous pacing; TV, temporary transvenous pacing.

Action: There are four possible actions, or therapeutic options, listed and classified for each bradyarrhythmia or conduction problem:

1. Observe: continued ECG monitoring, no further action planned.

2. A, and A*: atropine administered at 0.6 to 1.0 mg IV every 5 min to up to 0.04 mg/kg. In general, because the increase in sinus rate with atropine is unpredictable, this is to be avoided unless there is symptomatic bradycardia that will likely respond to a vagolytic agent, such as sinus bradycardia or Mobitz I, as denoted by the asterisk, above.

3. TC: application of transcutaneous pads and standby transcutaneous pacing with no further progression to transvenous pacing imminently planned.

4. TV: temporary transvenous pacing. It is assumed, but not specified in the table, that at the discretion of the clinician, transcutaneous pads will be applied and standby transcutaneous pacing will be in effect as the patient is transferred to the fluoroscopy unit for temporary transvenous pacing.

Class: Each possible therapeutic option is further classified according to ACC/AHA criteria as Class 1: indicated, 2A: probably indicated, 2B: possibly indicated, and 3: not indicated.

Level of Evidence: This table was developed from published observational case reports and case series, published summaries, not meta-analyses, of these data; and expert opinion, largely from the prereperfusion era. There are no published randomized trials comparing different strategies of managing conduction disturbances after STEMI. Thus, the level of evidence for the recommendations in this table is C.

How to Use the Table: Example: 54-year-old man is admitted with an anterior STEMI and a narrow QRS on admission. On day 1, he develops a right bundle-branch block (RBBB), with a PR interval of 0.28 seconds.

1. RBBB is an intraventricular conduction disturbance, so look at row "New BBB."
2. Find the column for "First-Degree AV Block."
3. Find the "Action" and "Class" cells at the convergence.
4. Note that "Observe" and "Atropine" are class 3, not indicated; transcutaneous pacing (TC) is class 1. Temporary transvenous pacing (TV) is class 2B. Copyright 2004 American College of Cardiology Foundation. [From Antman EM, Anbe DT, Armstrong PW, et al.: ACC/AHA guidelines for the management of patients with ST-elevation myocardial infarction—executive summary. A report of the American College of Cardiology/American Heart Association Task Force on Practice Guidelines (Writing Committee to revise the 1999 guidelines for the management of patients with acute myocardial infarction). *J Am Coll Cardiol* 44:671–719, 2004, with permission.]

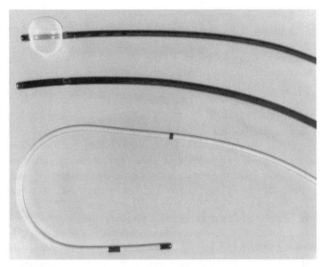

FIGURE 5-1. Cardiac pacing catheters. Several designs are available for temporary pacing in the critical care unit. **Top:** Balloon-tipped, flow-directed pacing wire. **Middle:** Standard 5 Fr pacing wire. **Bottom:** Atrial J-shaped wire.

TRANSCUTANEOUS EXTERNAL PACEMAKERS

Transcutaneous external pacemakers have external patch electrodes that deliver a higher current (up to 200 mA) and longer pulse duration (20–40 milliseconds) than transvenous pacemakers. External pacing can be implemented immediately and the risks of central venous access avoided. Some patients may require sedation for the discomfort of skeletal muscle stimulation from the high cutaneous current. Transcutaneous external pacemakers have been used to treat bradyasystolic cardiac arrest, symptomatic bradyarrhythmias, and overdrive pacing of tachyarrhythmias and prophylactically for conduction abnormalities during myocardial infarction. They may be particularly useful when transvenous pacing is unavailable, as in the prehospital setting, or relatively contraindicated, as during thrombolytic therapy for acute myocardial infarction [16–18,25–27). When continued pacing is needed, transvenous pacing is preferable.

EPICARDIAL PACING

The placement of epicardial electrodes requires open thoracotomy. These electrodes are routinely placed electively during cardiac surgical procedures for use during the postoperative period (12,13,28). Typically, both atrial and ventricular electrodes are placed for use in diagnosis of postoperative atrial arrhythmias and for AV pacing. Because ventricular capture is not always reliable, in patients with underlying asystole or an unstable escape rhythm, additional prophylactic transvenous pacing should be considered.

PULSE GENERATORS FOR TEMPORARY PACING

Newer temporary pulse generators are now capable of ventricular, atrial, and dual chamber sequential pacing with adjustable ventricular and atrial parameters that include pacing modes (synchronous or asynchronous), rates, current outputs (mA), sensing thresholds (mV), and AV pacing interval/delay (mil-

liseconds). Since these generators have atrial sensing/inhibiting capability, they are also set with an upper rate limit (to avoid rapid ventricular pacing while "tracking" an atrial tachycardia); in addition, an atrial pacing refractory period may be programmed (to avoid pacemaker-mediated/endless loop tachyarrhythmias).

Earlier models may be limited to sensing only ventricular depolarization. Without atrial sensing, if the intrinsic atrial rate exceeds the atrial pacing rate, the atrial pacing stimulus will fail to capture and AV sequential pacing will be lost with AV dissociation. Consequently, with these models, the pacing rate must be set continuously to exceed the intrinsic atrial rate to maintain AV sequential pacing.

CHOICE OF PACING MODE

A pacing mode must be selected when temporary cardiac pacing is initiated. Common modes for cardiac pacing are outlined in Table 5-3. The mode most likely to provide the greatest hemodynamic benefit should be selected. In patients with hemodynamic instability, establishing ventricular pacing is of paramount importance prior to attempts at AV sequential pacing.

Although ventricular pacing effectively counteracts bradycardia and is most frequently used in ICU patients, it cannot restore normal cardiac hemodynamics because it disrupts the synchronous relationship between atrial and ventricular contraction [29–31]. In patients with diseases characterized by noncompliant ventricles (ischemic heart disease, hypertrophic or congestive cardiomyopathy, aortic stenosis, and right ventricular infarction), the atrial contribution to ventricular stroke volume (the atrial "kick") may be quite substantial. In one study, loss of a properly timed atrial contraction in patients following inferior or anterior myocardial infarction was associated with a 25% decrease in systolic blood pressure and cardiac output [32].

Asynchronous contraction of the atria and ventricles (via random dissociation or retrograde ventriculoatrial conduction) results in increased left atrial pressure, reduced stroke volume and cardiac output, and intermittent mitral and tricuspid regurgitation.

In addition to the hemodynamic benefit of atrial or AV sequential pacing, the risk of atrial fibrillation or flutter may be reduced because of decreased atrial size and/or atrial pressure. This suggests that patients with intermittent atrial fibrillation may be better maintained in normal sinus rhythm with

TABLE 5-3. Common Pacemaker Modes for Temporary Cardiac Pacing

AOO	Atrial pacing: Pacing is asynchronous
AAI	Atrial pacing, atrial sensing: Pacing is on demand to provide a minimum programmed atrial rate
VOO	Ventricular pacing: Pacing is asynchronous
VVI	Ventricular pacing, ventricular sensing: Pacing is on demand to provide a minimum programmed ventricular rate
DVI	Dual-chamber pacing, ventricular sensing: Atrial pacing is asynchronous, ventricular pacing is on demand following a programmed AV delay
DDD	Dual-chamber pacing and sensing: Atrial and ventricular pacing is on demand to provide a minimum rate, ventricular pacing follows a programmed AV delay, and upper-rate pacing limit should be programmed

atrial or AV sequential pacing, rather than ventricular demand pacing.

PROCEDURE TO ESTABLISH TEMPORARY PACING

After achieving venous access, most often via the internal jugular or subclavian approach (see Chapter 2), the pacing catheter is advanced to the central venous circulation and then positioned in the right heart using fluoroscopic or ECG guidance [33,34]. To position the electrode using ECG guidance, the patient is connected to the limb leads of the ECG machine, and the distal (negative) electrode of the balloon-tipped pacing catheter is connected to lead V_1 with an alligator clip or a special adaptor supplied with the lead. Lead V_1 is then used to continuously monitor a unipolar intracardiac electrogram. The morphology of the recorded electrogram indicates the position of the catheter tip (Fig. 5-2). The balloon is inflated in the superior vena cava, and the catheter is advanced while observing the recorded intracardiac electrogram. When the tip of the catheter is in the right ventricle, the balloon is deflated and the catheter advanced to the right ventricular apex. The ST segment of the intracardiac electrogram is elevated due to a current of injury when the catheter tip contacts the ventricular endocardium.

After the tip of the pacing catheter is satisfactorily inserted in the right ventricular apex, the leads are connected to the ventricular output positions at the top of the pulse generator, with the pacemaker box in the off position. The pacemaker is then put on asynchronous mode and the ventricular rate set to exceed the patient's intrinsic ventricular rate by 10 to 20 beats

per minute. The threshold current for ventricular pacing is set at 5 to 10 mA. Then the pacemaker is switched on. Satisfactory ventricular pacing is evidenced by a wide QRS complex, with ST segment depression and T wave inversion immediately preceded by a pacemaker depolarization (spike). With pacing from the apex of the right ventricle, the paced rhythm usually demonstrates a pattern of left bundle branch block on the surface ECG [35].

Ventricular pacing is maintained as the output current for ventricular pacing is slowly reduced. The pacing threshold is defined as the lowest current at which consistent ventricular capture occurs. With the ventricular electrode appropriately positioned at or near the apex of the right ventricle, a pacing threshold of less than 0.5 to 1.0 mA should be achieved. If the output current for continuous ventricular pacing is consistently greater than 1 to 1.5 mA, the pacing threshold is too high. Possible causes of a high pacing threshold include relatively refractory endomyocardial tissue (fibrosis) or, most commonly, unsatisfactory positioning of the pacing electrode. The tip of the pacing electrode should be repositioned in the region of the ventricular apex until satisfactory ventricular capture at a current of less than 1.0 mA is consistently maintained. After the threshold current for ventricular pacing has been established at a satisfactory level, the ventricular output is set to exceed the threshold current at least threefold. This guarantees uninterrupted ventricular capture despite any modest increase in the pacing threshold.

The pacemaker is now in VOO mode. However, the pacing generator generally should be set in the VVI ("demand") mode, as this prevents pacemaker discharge soon after an intrinsic or spontaneous premature depolarization, while the heart lies in the electrically vulnerable period for induction of sustained ventricular arrhythmias [36]. To set the pacemaker in VVI mode, the pacing rate is set at 10 beats per minute less than the intrinsic rate and the sensitivity control is moved from asynchronous to the minimum sensitivity level. The sensitivity is gradually increased until pacing spikes appear. This level is the sensing threshold. The sensitivity is then set at a level slightly below the determined threshold and the pacing rate reset to the minimum desired ventricular rate.

If AV sequential pacing is desired, the atrial J-shaped pacing catheter should be advanced into the right atrium and rotated anteromedially to achieve a stable position in the right atrial appendage; positioning the atrial catheter usually requires fluoroscopy [34,37]. The leads are then connected to the atrial output of the pulse generator. The atrial current is set to 20 mA and the atrial pacing rate adjusted to at least 10 beats per minute greater than the intrinsic atrial rate. The AV interval is adjusted at 100 to 200 milliseconds (shorter intervals usually provide better hemodynamics), and the surface ECG is inspected for evidence of atrial pacing (electrode depolarization and capture of the atrium at the pacing rate).

The manifestation of atrial capture on ECG is atrial depolarization immediately following the atrial pacing spike. In patients with intact AV conduction, satisfactory atrial capture can be verified by shutting off the ventricular portion of the pacemaker and demonstrating AV synchrony during atrial pacing. As long as the atrial pacing rate continually exceeds the intrinsic sinus rate, the atrial P wave activity should track with the atrial pacing spike.

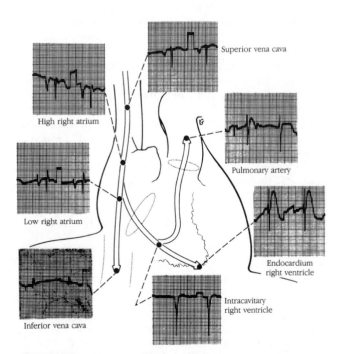

FIGURE 5-2.   Pattern of recorded electrogram at various locations in the venous circulation. [From Harthorne JW, McDermott J, Poulin FK: Cardiac pacing, in Johnson RA, Haber E, Austen WG (eds): *The Practice of Cardiology: The Medical and Surgical Cardiac Units at the Massachusetts General Hospital.* Boston: Little, Brown, 1980, with permission.]

The dual-chamber temporary pacemaker may not have atrial sensing capability. If not, the pacemaker will function in a DVI mode (see Table 5-3). Should the intrinsic atrial rate equal or exceed the atrial pacing rate, the atrial stimulus will fail to capture and AV sequential pacing will be lost. If the pacemaker has atrial sensing capability, the atrial sensing threshold should be determined and an appropriate level set. The pacer will then function in the DDD mode. The DDD mode is usually preferred, as it provides optimum cardiac hemodynamics through a range of intrinsic atrial rates. In this mode an upper-rate limit must be set to prevent rapid ventricular pacing in response to a paroxysmal supraventricular tachycardia.

COMPLICATIONS OF TEMPORARY PACING

Although temporary endocardial pacing can be accomplished from several alternate venous access sites, rational selection of the optimal route requires an understanding of the results and complications of each. Transvenous pacing in the ICU setting is most often performed via the internal jugular or subclavian approach.

Complications of temporary pacing from any venous access route include pericardial friction rub, arrhythmia, right ventricular perforation, cardiac tamponade, infection, arterial injury, diaphragmatic stimulation, phlebitis, and pneumothorax. Using predominantly the subclavian or internal jugular approaches, Donovan and Lee [38] reported a 7% rate of serious complications related to temporary cardiac pacing. The Mayo Clinic experience revealed that percutaneous cannulation of the right internal jugular vein provided the simplest, most direct route to the right-sided cardiac chambers [39].

Complications of internal jugular venous cannulation may include pneumothorax, carotid arterial injury, venous thrombosis, and pulmonary embolism (see Chapter 2) [40]. These risks are minimized by knowledge of anatomic landmarks, adherence to proven techniques, and use of a small-caliber needle to localize the vein before insertion of the large-caliber needle (for full discussion see Chapter 2). Full-dose systemic anticoagulation, thrombolytic therapy, and prior neck surgical procedures are relative contraindications to routine internal jugular vein cannulation [41].

Percutaneous subclavian venipuncture is also frequently used for insertion of temporary pacemakers [36,42]. When the operator has a good understanding of the subclavian anatomy, the latter procedure is relatively simple and safe (see Chapter 2). This approach should be avoided in patients with severe obstructive lung disease or a bleeding diathesis (including thrombolytic therapy), in whom the risk of pneumothorax or bleeding is increased.

Although insertion via direct cutdown of the brachial vein may be satisfactory for short-term pacing, percutaneous vascular access by the subclavian or internal jugular vein provides more stable long-term vascular access for temporary pacing (see Chapter 2). Insertion from the brachial vein reduces the risk of arterial injury, hematoma formation, and pneumothorax, but the motion of the patient's arm relative to the torso increases the risk of dislodgement of the pacing electrode from a stable ventricular or atrial position [39]. The risk of infection may also be increased with this approach. The brachial approach is still preferred for the patient receiving thrombolytic therapy or full-dose anticoagulation.

The femoral venous approach is used for electrophysiologic studies or during cardiac catheterization when the catheter is left in place for only a few hours. Although temporary cardiac pacing can be established through the percutaneous femoral approach, this approach is less desirable when long-term cardiac pacing is required, since there is a risk of deep venous thrombosis or infection around the catheter. In one study, venographic or autopsy evidence of deep venous thrombosis was present in 34% and pulmonary embolism in 50% of patients in whom a temporary pacing catheter had been inserted by the femoral venous approach [43]. A more recent study showed that a 75% incidence of venous thrombosis, documented by duplex ultrasound, was reduced to 12% by the use of intravenous heparin [44].

A 43% incidence of pacemaker malfunction (i.e., failure to sense or capture the R wave properly) and a 16.9% incidence of pacemaker-related complications were reported in 142 episodes of temporary pacemaker insertion by the brachial (61 cases) or femoral (81 cases) approach [45]. Austin et al. [41] reported pacemaker malfunction in 37% and complications in 20% of 100 patients requiring pacemaker insertion by the antecubital or femoral route. The Mayo Clinic's early experience with temporary cardiac pacing in the coronary care unit revealed a 17.9% incidence of malfunction of the temporary pacemaker and a 13.7% incidence of complications [45]. Over the 4-year interval from 1976 to 1980, as use of the antecubital route declined, so did the rate of complications (pacemaker malfunction, infection) when compared to the subclavian or internal jugular venous approaches.

REFERENCES

1. Francis GS, Williams SV, Achord JL, et al: Clinical competence in insertion of a temporary transvenous ventricular pacemaker: a statement for physicians from the ACP/ACC/AHA Task Force on Clinical Privileges in Cardiology. *Circulation* 89:1913, 1994.
2. Wiener I: Pacing techniques in the treatment of tachycardias. *Ann Intern Med* 93:326, 1980.
3. Silver MD, Goldschlager NG: Temporary transvenous cardiac pacing in the critical care setting. *Chest* 93:607, 1988.
4. McAlister HF, Klementowicz PT, Andrews C, et al: Lyme carditis: an important cause of reversible heart block. *Ann Intern Med* 110:339, 1989.
5. Wellens HJJ, Bar F, Gorges AP, et al: Electrical management of arrhythmias with emphasis on the tachycardia. *Am J Cardiol* 41:1025, 1978.
6. Wellens HJJ: Value and limitations of programmed electrical stimulation of the heart in the study and treatment of tachycardias. *Circulation* 57:845, 1978.
7. Wills JI, Jr., MacLean WAH, James TN, et al: Characterization of atrial flutter studies in man after open heart surgery using fixed atrial electrodes. *Circulation* 60:665, 1979.
8. Waldo AL, MacLean WAH, Karp RB, et al: Entrainment and interruption of atrial flutter with atrial pacing studies in man following open heart surgery. *Circulation* 56:737, 1977.
9. Das G, Anand K, Ankinfedu K, et al: Atrial pacing for cardioversion of atrial flutter in digitalized patients. *Am J Cardiol* 41:308, 1978.
10. Scarovsky S, Strasberg B, Lewin RF, et al: Polymorphous ventricular tachycardia—clinical features and treatment. *Am J Cardiol* 44:339, 1979.
11. Wellens HJJ, Schuilenburg RM, Durrer DL: Electrical stimulation of the heart in patients with ventricular tachycardia. *Circulation* 46:216, 1972.
12. Waldo AL, MacLean WAH, Cooper TB, et al: Use of temporarily placed epicardial atrial wire electrodes for the diagnosis and treatment of cardiac arrhythmias following open-heart surgery. *J Thorac Cardiovasc Surg* 76:500, 1978.
13. Waldo AL. *Cardiac Arrhythmias: Their Mechanisms, Diagnosis, and Management.* Philadelphia: JB Lippincott, 1987.
14. Antman EM, Anbe DT, Armstrong PW, et al: ACC/AHA guidelines for the management of patients with ST-elevation myocardial infarction—executive summary. A report of the American College of Cardiology/American Heart Association Task Force on Practice Guidelines (Writing Committee to revise the 1999 guidelines for the management of patients with acute myocardial infarction). *J Am Coll Cardiol* 44:671, 2004.
15. Lamas GA, Muller JE, Zoltan GT, et al: A simplified method to predict occurrence of complete heart block during acute myocardial infarction. *Am J Cardiol* 57:1213, 1986.

16. Falk RH, Ngai STA: External cardiac pacing: Influence of electrode placement on pacing threshold. *Crit Care Med* 14:931, 1986.

17. Hedges JR, Syverud SA, Dalsey WC, et al: Prehospital trial of emergency transcutaneous cardiac pacing. *Circulation* 76:1337, 1987.

18. Madsen JK, Meibom J, Videbak R, et al: Transcutaneous pacing: Experience with the Zoll noninvasive temporary pacemaker. *Am Heart J* 116:7, 1988.

19. Dunn DL, Gregory JJ: Noninvasive temporary pacing: Experience in a community hospital. *Heart Lung* 1:23, 1989.

20. Love JC, Haffajee CI, Gore JM, et al: Reversibility of hypotension and shock by atrial or atrioventricular sequential pacing in patients with right ventricular infarction. *Am Heart J* 108:5, 1984.

21. Topol EJ, Goldschlager N, Ports TA, et al: Hemodynamic benefit of atrial pacing in right ventricular myocardial infarction. *Ann Intern Med* 96:594, 1982.

22. Littleford PO, Curry RC, Jr., Schwartz KM, et al: Clinical evaluation of a new temporary atrial pacing catheter: results in 100 patients. *Am Heart J* 107:237, 1984.

23. Simoons ML, Demey HE, Bossaert LL, et al: The Paceport catheter: a new pacemaker system introduced through a Swan-Ganz catheter. *Cathet Cardiovasc Diagn* 15:66, 1988.

24. Benson DW: Transesophageal electrocardiography and cardiac pacing: the state of the art. *Circulation* 75:86, 1987.

25. Luck JC, Grubb BP, Artman SE, et al: Termination of sustained ventricular tachycardia by external noninvasive pacing. *Am J Cardiol* 61:574, 1988.

26. Kelly JS, Royster RL, Angert KC, et al: Efficacy of noninvasive transcutaneous cardiac pacing in patients undergoing cardiac surgery. *Anesthesiology* 70:747, 1989.

27. Blocka JJ: External transcutaneous pacemakers. *Ann Emerg Med* 18:1280, 1989.

28. Elmi F, Tullo NG, Khalighi K: Natural history and predictors of temporary epicardial pacemaker wire function in patients after open heart surgery. *Cardiology* 98:175, 2002.

29. Romero LR, Haffajee CI, Doherty P, et al: Comparison of ventricular function and volume with A-V sequential and ventricular pacing. *Chest* 80:346, 1981.

30. Knuse I, Arnman K, Conradson TB, et al: A comparison of the acute and long-term hemodynamic effects of ventricular inhibited and atrial synchronous ventricular inhibited pacing. *Circulation* 65:846, 1982.

31. Murphy P, Morton P, Murtaugh G, et al: Hemodynamic effects of different temporary pacing modes for the management of bradycardias complicating acute myocardial infarction. *Pacing Clin Electrophysiol* 15:391–396, 1992.

32. Chamberlain DA, Leinbach RC, Vassau CE, et al: Sequential atrioventricular pacing in heart block complicating acute myocardial infarction. *N Engl J Med* 282:577, 1970.

33. Bing OHL, McDowell JW, Hantman J, et al: Pacemaker placement by electrocardiographic monitoring. *N Engl J Med* 287:651, 1972.

34. Harthorne JW, McDermott J, Poulin FK: Cardiac pacing, in Johnson RA, Haber E, Austen WG (eds): *The Practice of Cardiology: The Medical and Surgical Cardiac Units at the Massachusetts General Hospital.* Boston: Little, Brown, 1980; p 219.

35. Morelli RL, Goldschlager N: Temporary transvenous pacing: resolving postinsertion problems. *J Crit Illness* 2:73, 1987.

36. Donovan KD: Cardiac pacing in intensive care. *Anaesth Intensive Care* 13:41, 1984.

37. Holmes DR Jr: Temporary cardiac pacing, in Furman S, Hayes DL, Holmes DR Jr (eds): *A Practice of Cardiac Pacing.* Mount Kisco, NY, Futura, 1989; p 209.

38. Donovan KD, Lee KY: Indications for and complications of temporary transvenous cardiac pacing. *Anaesth Intensive Care* 13:63, 1984.

39. Hynes JK, Holmes DR, Harrison CE: Five year experience with temporary pacemaker therapy in the coronary care unit. *Mayo Clin Proc* 58:122, 1983.

40. Chastre J, Cornud F, Bouchama A, et al: Thrombosis as a complication of pulmonary-artery catheterization via the internal jugular vein: prospective evaluation by phlebography. *N Engl J Med* 306:278, 1982.

41. Austin JL, Preis LK, Crampton RS, et al: Analysis of pacemaker malfunction and complications of temporary pacing in the coronary care unit. *Am J Cardiol* 49:301, 1982.

42. Linos DA, Mucha P, Jr., van Heerden JA: Subclavian vein: a golden route. *Mayo Clin Proc* 55:315, 1980.

43. Nolewajka AJ, Goddard MD, Brown TC: Temporary transvenous pacing and femoral vein thrombosis. *Circulation* 62:646, 1980.

44. Sanders P: Effect of anticoagulation on the occurrence of deep venous thrombosis associated with temporary transvenous femoral pacemakers. *Am J Cardiol* 88:798, 2001.

45. Lumia FJ, Rios JC: Temporary transvenous pacemaker therapy: An analysis of complications. *Chest* 64:604, 1973.

Naomi F. Botkin

CHAPTER **6**

Cardioversion and Defibrillation

The use of electric countershock to terminate arrhythmia was described over 200 years ago. Thanks to the pioneering work of Zoll et al. [1], Lown et al. [2], and Alexander et al. [3] in the second half of the twentieth century, the use of electric countershock gained widespread acceptance and became a staple in the treatment of cardiac arrhythmia. *Cardioversion* refers to the use of direct-current electric countershock to terminate arrhythmias other than ventricular fibrillation. In order to avoid triggering ventricular fibrillation, shocks are synchronized with the R wave. *Defibrillation*, on the other hand, refers to the termination of ventricular fibrillation with unsynchronized shocks. An understanding of both cardioversion and defibrillation is critical for intensive care unit personnel.

PHYSIOLOGY OF ARRHYTHMIA AND COUNTERSHOCK

Electric countershocks are capable of terminating arrhythmias that are due to reentry. Reentry refers to the phenomenon in which a wave of excitation travels repeatedly over a closed pathway or circuit of conduction tissue. In order for reentry to occur, there must be unidirectional block in one branch of the circuit. In addition, conduction down the unblocked pathway must be slow enough that the blocked pathway recovers excitability by the time the wave reaches the site of block in a retrograde fashion. Continuous electrical activation in such a circuit can lead to reentrant arrhythmias.

Most of the commonly encountered arrhythmias are due to a reentrant mechanism, including atrial fibrillation, atrial flutter, atrioventricular (AV) nodal reentrant tachycardia, most ventricular tachycardias, and ventricular fibrillation. Cardioversion and defibrillation terminate these arrhythmias by simultaneously depolarizing all excitable tissue, disrupting the process of reentry.

Arrhythmias due to disorders all of impulse formation (increased automaticity or triggered activity) do not respond to countershock. These include sinus tachycardia, focal atrial tachycardia, and some types of ventricular tachycardia. Table 6-1 categorizes arrhythmias by their responsiveness to electric countershock.

Insight into the effect of countershock on fibrillating myocardial cells has grown in the past few decades. Although it was initially thought that all ventricular activation fronts had to be terminated simultaneously to stop ventricular fibrillation [4], it is now believed that if the vast majority of myocardium is silenced, the remaining mass is insufficient to perpetuate the arrhythmia [5]. The effect of shock on fibrillating myocardium is complex and is dependent on multiple factors including energy,

shock waveform, and myocardial refractory state. It is known that electric countershock at low energy levels may fail to terminate ventricular fibrillation. Although subthreshold shocks may extinguish fibrillatory wavefronts, they will often reinitiate new wavefronts elsewhere in the ventricle, leading to the perpetuation of fibrillation [6]. Thus, it is necessary to deliver shocks above a particular threshold of energy for defibrillation to be successful. Furthermore, ventricular fibrillation can be triggered in patients not already in this rhythm if shocks are poorly timed. Synchronization of shocks with the R wave will minimize the risk.

INDICATIONS AND CONTRAINDICATIONS

Cardioversion and defibrillation are performed for a variety of reasons in the intensive care setting. In the case of hemodynamic instability due to tachyarrhythmia of nearly any variety, the urgent use of countershock is strongly indicated. One must be careful, however, not to mistake sinus tachycardia, which is commonly present in patients who are hypotensive for noncardiac reasons, for a shockable rhythm. The onset of congestive heart failure or angina in a patient with a tachyarrhythmia is also an indication for immediate countershock. In the absence of hemodynamic instability or significant symptoms, cardioversion is usually considered elective and the risks and benefits of the procedure must be carefully weighed.

Extreme caution should be exercised in patients with digitalis toxicity or electrolyte imbalance because of their increased risk of ventricular tachycardia or fibrillation after being shocked. Patients with severe conduction system disease may develop significant bradyarrhythmia after cardioversion. In addition, patients who have been in atrial fibrillation for a prolonged or indeterminate length of time are at risk for thromboembolism due to cardioversion; appropriate measures should be taken to minimize this risk (see below).

CLINICAL COMPETENCE

A clinical competence statement by the American College of Cardiology and American Heart Association outlines the cognitive and technical skills required for the successful and safe performance of elective external cardioversion (Table 6-2). A minimum of eight cardioversions should be supervised before a physician is considered competent to perform the procedure independently. In addition, a minimum of four procedures should be performed annually to maintain competence [7].

TABLE 6-1.   Classification of Tachyarrhythmias Based on Predicted Responses to Cardioversion/Defibrillation

Responsive (reentrant)
  Supraventricular arrhythmias
    Atrial fibrillation
    Atrial flutter
    Sinoatrial nodal reentrant tachycardia
    AV nodal reentrant tachycardia
    AV reciprocating tachycardia
  Ventricular arrhythmias
    Monomorphic ventricular tachycardia due to scar or bundle
      branch reentry
    Polymorphic ventricular tachycardia
    Ventricular flutter
    Ventricular fibrillation
Unresponsive (automatic)
  Supraventricular arrhythmias
    Sinus tachycardia
    Focal atrial tachycardias
    Junctional tachycardia
  Ventricular arrhythmias
    Idiopathic monomorphic ventricular tachycardia
    Accelerated idioventricular rhythm

METHODS

Patient Preparation

In the case of unconsciousness due to tachyarrhythmia, countershock must be performed urgently. In more elective settings, patient safety and comfort become paramount. As with any procedure, informed consent should be obtained. Patients

TABLE 6-2.   Cognitive and Technical Skills Necessary for Performing External Cardioversion

Physicians should have knowledge of the following:
  Electrophysiologic principles of cardioversion
  Indications for the procedure
  Anticoagulation management
  Proper use of antiarrhythmic therapy
  Use of sedation and the management of overdose
  Direct current cardioversion equipment, including the selection of
    appropriate energy and synchronization.
  Treatment of possible complications, including ACLS,
    defibrillation, and pacing
  Proper placement of paddles or pads
  Appropriate monitor display and recognition of arrhythmias
  Baseline 12-lead electrocardiogram reading, recognition of acute
    changes, drug toxicity, and contraindications
Physicians should have the following technical skills:
  Proper preparation of skin and electrode placement
  Achievement of artifactfree monitored strips and synchronization
    signal/marker
  Technically acceptable 12-lead electrocardiograms before and
    after DCCV
  Temporary pacing and defibrillation capabilities
  Ability to perform advanced cardiac life support, including proper
    airway management

From Tracy CM, Akhtar M, DiMarco JP, et al: American College of Cardiology/American Heart Association Clinical competence statement on invasive electrophysiology studies, catheter ablation, and cardioversion. *J Am Coll Cardiol* 36:1725–1736, 2000.

should refrain from eating and drinking for several hours in order to decrease the risk of aspiration. Constant heart rhythm monitoring should be used throughout the procedure and a 12-lead electrocardiogram should be obtained before and after the countershock.

Medications with rapid onset and short half-life are favored for achieving analgesia, sedation, and amnesia. The combination of a benzodiazepine, such as midazolam, and a narcotic, such as fentanyl, is a frequent choice in the absence of anesthesiology assistance. Propofol is often used when an anesthesiologist is present to assist with airway management and sedation. Existing hospital policies for monitoring during conscious sedation should be followed, including frequent assessment of blood pressure and pulse oximetry. Supplemental oxygen is delivered via nasal cannula, face mask, or—in the case of heavier sedation—AmbuBag. The goal of sedation should be minimal or no response to verbal stimulus. In such a state, a patient may cry out during the actual cardioversion but will nonetheless usually have no recollection of the procedure after recovery.

Shock Waveforms

Defibrillators that employ biphasic waveforms have largely replaced those utilizing monophasic waveforms. The chief advantage of biphasic waveforms is a lower defibrillation threshold, meaning shocks using biphasic waveforms require less energy to achieve defibrillation. It is thought that the first phase of the biphasic waveform stimulates the myocardium to defibrillate while the second phase lowers the defibrillation threshold, although the mechanism is not well understood [8]. Biphasic truncated exponential waveform and biphasic rectilinear waveform are both commercially available, with the former being more common. Randomized trials comparing the two types of waveforms in the cardioversion of atrial fibrillation have failed to show any significant difference in efficacy [9–11].

The efficacy of biphasic shocks in the termination of VF has been well established [12,13]. Furthermore, clinical studies of elective cardioversion have established the superiority of biphasic over monophasic waveform shocks [14,15]. For instance, one study demonstrated the equivalent efficacy of a 120 J to 200 J biphasic sequence with a 200 J to 360 J monophasic sequence [15]. Biphasic waveforms allow fewer shocks to be given and a lower total energy delivery [14]. Whether or not this translates into a significant clinical advantage remains to be demonstrated. However, there is evidence that biphasic shocks result in less dermal injury [14]. Although an animal model suggested better maintenance of cardiac function after biphasic shocks [16], human data on myocardial function are unavailable.

Electrodes

Until recently, hand-held paddles coated with conductive gel were the sole type of electrode used to deliver countershock. Self-adhesive pads have become more common in the past few years, although paddles are still used, especially in emergent cases. Limited data are available comparing the two modalities, but one study suggested the superiority of paddles over pads in cardioverting atrial fibrillation [17]. This phenomenon might be explained by the lower transthoracic impedance achieved with paddles [18]. Whichever modality is used, impedance can be minimized by avoiding positioning over breast tissue, by clipping body hair when it is excessive [19], and by delivering the shock during expiration [20].

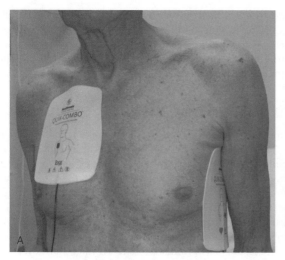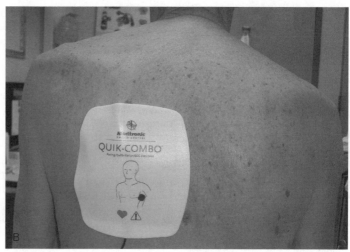

FIGURE 6-1. **A:** Self-adhesive defibrillator pads in the anterior and lateral positions. **B:** Self-adhesive defibrillator pad in the posterior position. When posterior positioning is used, the second pad is placed anteriorly.

The optimal anatomic placement of pads and paddles is controversial. Anterior-lateral and anterior-posterior placements are both acceptable (Fig. 6-1). The anterior paddle is placed on the right infraclavicular chest [21]. In anterior-lateral placement, the lateral paddle should be located lateral to the left breast and should have a longitudinal orientation, since this results in a lower transthoracic impedance than horizontal orientation [22]. When anterior-posterior positioning is used, the posterior pad is commonly located to the left of the spine at the level of the lower scapula, although some physicians favor placement to the right of, or directly over, the spine. There are data to suggest that anterior-posterior placement is more successful in the cardioversion of atrial fibrillation than anterior-lateral positioning when monophasic waveforms are used [23]. It is thought that anterior-posterior positioning directs more of the delivered energy to the atria than anterior-lateral placement. Since it has been shown that only 4% of the current flow from shock reaches the myocardium with the anterior-lateral position [24], any method that directs more energy to the atria should be beneficial. However, a study using defibrillators employing a biphasic waveform suggested pad position was not associated with cardioversion success [25].

TABLE 6-3. Checklist for Performing Cardioversion

Preparing the patient:
1. Ensure NPO status
2. Obtain informed consent
3. Apply self-adhesive pads (clip hair if needed)
4. Achieve adequate sedation
5. Monitor vital signs and cardiac rhythm throughout

Performing the cardioversion:
1. Select initial energy appropriate for specific device
2. Select the synchronization function
3. Confirm that arrhythmia is still present
4. Charge, clear, and deliver shock
5. If no change in rhythm, escalate energy as appropriate

NPO, nil per os.

Using the Defibrillator

External defibrillators are designed for easy operation. After the patient is adequately prepared and the electrodes are applied, attention may be turned to the device itself. If the QRS amplitude on the rhythm tracing is small and difficult to see, a different lead should be selected. If cardioversion—rather than defibrillation—is to be performed, the "synchronization" function should be selected. The appropriate initial energy is selected. Finally, the capacitor is charged, the area is cleared, and the shock is delivered. One should be aware that the synchronization function is automatically deselected after each shock in some devices, meaning that it must be manually reselected prior to any further shock delivery.

Table 6-3 provides a checklist for physicians involved in cardioversion. Table 6-4 gives recommendations for the initial energy selection for defibrillation and cardioversion of various arrhythmias. Recommendations specific to each device are available in the manufacturers' manuals and should be consulted by physicians unfamiliar with their particular device.

TREATMENT OF VENTRICULAR FIBRILLATION AND PULSELESS VENTRICULAR TACHYCARDIA

The algorithm for the treatment of pulseless ventricular tachycardia and ventricular fibrillation in the most recently published American Heart Association guidelines [21] contains some important changes from the previous guidelines. Rather than beginning with three "stacked" shocks, the guidelines

TABLE 6-4. Suggested Initial Energy for Cardioversion and Defibrillation

Rhythm	Monophasic	Biphasic
Ventricular fibrillation, pulseless ventricular tachycardia	360 J	120–200 J
Ventricular tachycardia with pulse	100 J	unknown
Atrial fibrillation	100–200 J	100–120 J
Atrial flutter	50–100 J	unknown

TABLE 6-5. Treatment of Ventricular Fibrillation and Pulseless Ventricular Tachycardia

Assess airway, breathing, and circulation
Assess rhythm
Deliver 1 shock
   Monophasic: 360 J
   Biphasic: use device specific energy; if unknown, 200 J
Resume compressions immediately and perform 5 cycles of CPR
Check rhythm—if still VT/VF, shock again
   Monophasic: 360 J
   Biphasic: same as first shock or higher dose
Resume compressions immediately and perform 5 cycles of CPR
Give a vasopressor during CPR, either before or after the second shock
   Epinephrine 1 mg IV/IO, repeat every 3–5 min, OR
   Vasopressin 40 U IV/IO may replace First or second dose of epinephrine
Check rhythm—if still VT/VF, shock again
Consider an antiarrhythmic before or after third shock:
   Amiodarone 300 mg IV/IO once, then consider additional 150 mg once OR
   Lidocaine 1 to 1.5 mg/kg first dose, then 0.5 to 0.75 mg/kg IV/IO, maximum 3 doses.

IO, intraosseous; IV, intravenous; VF, ventricular fibrillation; VT, ventricular tachycardia.

recommend only one shock followed by five cycles of cardiopulmonary resuscitation (CPR) before the rhythm is reassessed. This change was prompted by the observation that delivering three closely timed shocks involves a substantial interruption in CPR, which has been shown to be associated with a decreased chance of successful termination of ventricular fibrillation [26]. In the new algorithm, vasopressors (epinephrine or vasopressin) may be given before or after the second shock, and antiarrhythmics such as amiodarone and lidocaine may be considered before or after the third shock (Table 6-5). Both ventricular fibrillation and pulseless ventricular tachycardia are treated with unsynchronized, high-energy shocks of 360 J in the case of devices that use monophasic waveforms and 120 to 200 J with biphasic ones.

TREATMENT OF WIDE COMPLEX TACHYCARDIA WITH A PULSE

When a pulse is present, a regular, wide complex tachycardia may be either ventricular tachycardia or a supraventricular tachycardia with aberrant conduction. If signs of instability such as chest pressure, altered mental status, hypotension, or heart failure are present, urgent cardioversion is indicated. A starting energy of 100 J is recommended when a monophasic shock waveform is being used. The optimal initial energy with biphasic devices is unknown. The energy should be escalated with each successive shock, such as 100 J, 200 J, 300 J, and 360 J [21].

If the patient is stable, however, one might consider enlisting the assistance of an expert in distinguishing between ventricular and supraventricular arrhythmia. If this is not possible, it is safest to assume a ventricular etiology. Stable ventricular tachycardia may be treated initially with antiarrhythmic agents such as amiodarone. Elective cardioversion is usually performed.

Wide complex tachycardia that appears irregular is usually atrial fibrillation with aberrant conduction rather than ventricular tachycardia. Treatment should follow the recommendations for atrial fibrillation below, unless the Wolff-Parkinson-White Syndrome is suspected.

TREATMENT OF SUPRAVENTRICULAR TACHYCARDIA

The most common regular, narrow complex tachycardia is sinus tachycardia. Supraventricular tachycardia with a reentrant mechanism and atrial flutter are the next most common. Supraventricular tachycardia should be suspected when the arrhythmia starts suddenly, when it is more rapid than typical sinus tachycardia, and when P waves are absent or closely follow the QRS. Initial therapy involves vagal maneuvers and adenosine. If these fail, nondihydropyridine calcium channel antagonists or beta-blockers may terminate the arrhythmia. Cardioversion is indicated only rarely for clinical instability, usually in patients with underlying heart disease in whom the initial therapies fail.

TREATMENT OF ATRIAL FIBRILLATION AND FLUTTER

Rate Control

Although the majority of patients with atrial fibrillation and flutter remain hemodynamically stable, many develop bothersome symptoms such as palpitations, chest pressure, and, occasionally, pulmonary edema. Beta-blockers and nondihydropyridine calcium channel antagonists are used to slow the ventricular response rate by depressing AV nodal conduction. Many patients become asymptomatic or minimally symptomatic with adequate rate control, allowing the decision about cardioversion to be made electively.

Electrical Cardioversion

Cardioversion for atrial fibrillation or flutter is usually performed electively. The risk of thromboembolism dictates a thoughtful decision about treatment options. When cardioversion is performed, an appropriate initial starting dose is 100 to 200 J for monophasic waveform shock and 100 to 120 J for biphasic shock. Atrial flutter responds to lower energy, so a starting dose of 50 to 100 J is recommended with a monophasic waveform. The ideal starting energy for biphasic devices is unknown [21]. If atrial fibrillation or flutter fails to terminate, shock energy should be escalated.

Anticoagulation

Patients with atrial fibrillation or flutter may develop thrombus in the left atrial appendage or left atrial cavity, leading to thromboembolism during or after cardioversion. One study demonstrated a risk of pericardioversion thromboembolism of 5.3% in patients who were not anticoagulated and 0.8% in those who were [27].

There is general agreement that cardioversion of patients who have been in atrial fibrillation for less than 24 to 48 hours is very unlikely to cause thromboembolism. Current guidelines indicate that pericardioversion anticoagulation with heparin or low molecular weight heparin is optional in these patients [28]. Patients in whom the arrhythmia has been present for longer than 24 to 48 hours, or for an undetermined length of time, are felt to be at higher risk. When these patients do not require urgent cardioversion for reasons of symptomatology, there are two reasonable approaches.

In the first case, one may perform a transesophageal echocardiogram to assess for the presence of thrombus in the left atrial appendage [29,30]. If thrombus is not visualized, the patient is considered to be at low risk for thromboembolism, and cardioversion may be performed. Anticoagulation with warfarin to an international normalized ratio (INR) goal of 2.5 (range 2.0 to 3.0) is recommended for 4 weeks after cardioversion [7]. The reason for such a long period of anticoagulation after cardioversion is that the return of organized atrial mechanical activity can lag behind the restoration of normal sinus rhythm [31,32]. Unfractionated heparin should be administered until the INR is in the therapeutic range. Low molecular weight heparin has been demonstrated to be effective in preventing thromboembolism in small trials of atrial fibrillation patients undergoing cardioversion [33,34] but has not yet been incorporated into the guidelines.

The second approach is to defer cardioversion until the patient has been anticoagulated at a therapeutic level for at least 3 weeks. Cardioversion is then performed and the patient anticoagulated for a minimum of 4 weeks afterward [7].

Pharmacologic Cardioversion

Cardioversion can be achieved not only electrically but also pharmacologically. Pharmacologic cardioversion is used mainly for atrial fibrillation and flutter of relatively short duration. Although electrical cardioversion is quicker and has a higher probability of success, pharmacologic cardioversion does not require sedation. The risk of thromboembolism with pharmacologic cardioversion has not been well established but is thought to be similar to that of electric countershock because it is the return of sinus rhythm rather than the shock itself that is believed to precipitate thromboembolism.

Dofetilide, flecainide, ibutilide, propafenone, amiodarone, and quinidine have been demonstrated to have some degree of efficacy in restoring sinus rhythm [20]. Each of these medications has potential toxicities including malignant arrhythmias and hypotension. The risks and benefits should be carefully weighed when selecting a pharmacologic agent. Although beta-blockers and calcium channel antagonists are often believed to facilitate cardioversion, their efficacy has not been established in controlled trials.

Management of Resistant Atrial Fibrillation

Electrical cardioversion is unsuccessful in 10% to 30% of cases of atrial fibrillation [20] and up to 28% of cases of atrial flutter [35]. The duration of atrial fibrillation is inversely related to the probability of successful cardioversion.

When cardioversion fails, the operator's technique should be reviewed and modified. Electrode position may be altered, from anterior-posterior to anterior-lateral or vice versa. If paddles are being used, firmer pressure may be employed. If a device that delivers monophasic waveform shocks is being employed, it may be exchanged for one that delivers biphasic waveform shocks. Synchronized shocks from two separate defibrillators using electrical switches to coordinate the shocks may be performed [36]. An antiarrhythmic medication may be initiated prior to another attempt at cardioversion. Finally, transvenous cardioversion may be attempted (see below).

Although some patients fail to achieve sinus rhythm, many who are successfully cardioverted revert to atrial fibrillation within minutes, hours, or days. The administration of antiarrhythmic pharmacologic therapy decreases this possibility significantly [37]. However, given the adverse reactions associated with these medications, the necessity of maintaining sinus rhythm should be carefully considered. When atrial fibrillation is associated with substantial symptoms that are not alleviated by rate-controlling medications, antiarrhythmic therapy may be indicated. However, patients in whom the arrhythmia is well tolerated may be served as well by a strategy of rate control and anticoagulation [38].

Transvenous Cardioversion

Cardioversion using high-energy shocks delivered internally via a right atrial (RA) catheter and a backplate was described in 1988 [39]. This technique was demonstrated to be more efficacious than external cardioversion, especially in patients who are obese or who have chronic obstructive pulmonary disease [40]. Lower energy internal shock using an RA cathodal electrode and an anode in the coronary sinus or left pulmonary artery has also been described [41].

COMPLICATIONS

Burns

Countershock can cause first-degree burns and pain at the paddle or pad site. One study documented moderate to severe pain in nearly one quarter of patients undergoing cardioversion. Pain was directly related to total energy delivered and number of shocks [42]. Another study showed a lower rate of dermal injury with biphasic rather than monophasic shocks, probably due to the lower energy necessary with biphasic shocks [14]. The lowest effective energy should be used to minimize skin injury.

Thromboembolism

Cardioversion of atrial fibrillation and atrial flutter carries a risk of thromboembolism. One percent to 7% of patients in atrial fibrillation who undergo cardioversion without receiving anticoagulation may experience this complication [27,43]. The role of anticoagulation to diminish this risk is discussed above.

Arrhythmia

Bradyarrhythmias such as sinus arrest and sinus bradycardia are common immediately after countershock and are almost always short-lived. However, patients who have atrial fibrillation with a slow ventricular response in the absence of medications that slow AV conduction should be suspected of having conduction disease and are at higher risk for sustained bradyarrhythmia after cardioversion. The prophylactic placement of a transvenous or transcutaneous pacemaker may be considered in this situation [20].

Ventricular tachycardia and ventricular fibrillation can occasionally be precipitated by countershock, particularly in patients with digitalis toxicity or hypokalemia [44,45]. Elective cardioversion should therefore be avoided in patients with these conditions. If cardioversion or defibrillation must be performed urgently, one should anticipate the ventricular arrhythmias to be more refractory to shock than usual.

Myocardial Damage

Occasionally, one may see transient ST elevations on postcountershock electrocardiograms [46]. This is unlikely to signify myocardial injury. Although a study of cardioversion using higher-than-usual energy levels demonstrated an increase in creatine kinase-MB levels above that expected from skeletal muscle damage in 10% of patients, there was no elevation in troponin-T or -I seen [47]. This observation suggests that clinically significant myocardial damage from cardioversion or defibrillation is unlikely. Nonetheless, it has been suggested that any two consecutive shocks be delivered no less than one minute apart to minimize the chance of myocardial damage [48]. Of course, this recommendation applies only to nonemergent situations.

MISCELLANEOUS TOPICS

Patients with Implanted Pacemakers and Defibrillators

Patients with implanted pacemakers and defibrillators may undergo external cardioversion and defibrillation safely in most cases. However, one must be aware of the possibility that external energy delivery may alter the programming of the internal device. Furthermore, energy may be conducted down an internal lead, causing local myocardial injury and a resultant change in the pacing or defibrillation threshold [20]. The paddles or pads used for external electric countershock should never be placed over the internal device. In addition, interrogation of the device immediately after any external shock delivery is recommended.

Chest Thump

The use of a manual "thump" on the chest to successfully terminate ventricular tachycardia was described in several patients in 1970 [49]. The reason for its success is not well understood. Unfortunately, this technique may inadvertently trigger ventricular fibrillation if the blow happens to fall during the vulnerable period of the ventricle [50]. For this reason, chest thump is considered a therapy of last resort, administered only to a pulseless patient when a defibrillator is unavailable and unlikely to become available soon. It should not be administered when a pulse is present unless a defibrillator is immediately available.

Cardioversion and Defibrillation in Pregnancy

Cardioversion and defibrillation have been performed in all trimesters of pregnancy without obvious adverse fetal effects or premature labor [51,52]. It has been suggested that the fetal heart rhythm be monitored during cardioversion [53].

REFERENCES

1. Zoll PM, Linethal AJ, Gibson W, et al: Termination of ventricular fibrillation in man by externally applied countershock. N Eng J Med 25:727–732, 1956.
2. Lown B, Amarasingham R, Newman J: New method for terminating cardiac arrhythmias: Use of synchronized capacitor discharge. JAMA 182:548–555, 1962.
3. Alexander S, Kleiger R, Lown B: Use of external electric countershock in the treatment of ventricular tachycardia. JAMA 177:916–918, 1961.
4. Wiggers CJ: The mechanism and nature of ventricular defibrillation. Am Heart J 20:399–412, 1940.
5. Zipes DP, Fisher J, King RM, et al: Termination of ventricular fibrillation in dogs by depolarizing a critical amount of myocardium. Am J Cardiol 36:37–44, 1975.
6. Chen P-S, Shibata N, Dixon EG, et al: Comparison of the defibrillation threshold and the upper limit of vulnerability. Circulation 73:1022–1028, 1986.
7. Tracy CM, Akhtar M, DiMarco JP, et al: American College of Cardiology/American Heart Association clinical competence statement on invasive electrophysiology studies, catheter ablation, and cardioversion. J Am Coll Cardiol 36:1725–1736, 2000.
8. Ideker RE, Huang J, Walcott GP: Defibrillation waveforms, in Zipes DP, Jalife J (eds): Cardiac Electrophysiology From Cell to Bedside. 4th ed. Philadelphia, Saunders, Philadelphia, 2004; chap. 47, p 426–432.
9. Neal S, Ngarmukos T, Lessard D, et al: Comparison of the efficacy and safety of two biphasic defibrillator waveforms for the conversion of atrial fibrillation to sinus rhythm. Am J Cardiol 92:810–814, 2003.
10. Kim ML, Kim SG, Park DS, et al: Comparison of rectilinear biphasic waveform energy versus truncated exponential biphasic waveform energy for transthoracic cardioversion of atrial fibrillation. Am J Cardiol 94:1438–1440, 2004.
11. Alatawi F, Gurevitz O, White RD, et al: Prospective, randomized comparison of two biphasic waveforms for the efficacy and safety of transthoracic biphasic cardioversion or atrial fibrillation. Heart Rhythm 2:382–387, 2005.
12. Van Alem AP, Chapman FW, Lank P, et al: A prospective, randomised and blinded comparison of first shock success of monophasic and biphasic waveforms in out-of-hospital cardiac arrest. Resuscitation 58:17–24, 2003.
13. Schneider T, Martens, PR, Paschen H, et al: Multicenter, randomized, controlled trial of 150-J biphasic shocks compared with 200- to 360-J monophasic shocks in the resuscitation of out-of-hospital cardiac arrest victims. Circulation 101:1780–1787, 2000.
14. Page RL, Kerber RE, Russell JK, et al: Biphasic versus monophasic shock waveform for conversion of atrial fibrillation: the results of an international randomized, double-blind multicenter trial. J Am Coll Cardiol 39:1956–1963, 2002.
15. Scholten M, Szili-Torok T, Klootwijk P, et al: Comparison of monophasic and biphasic shocks for transthoracic cardioversion of atrial fibrillation. Heart 89:1032–1034, 2003.
16. Tang W, Weil MH, Sun S, et al: The effects of biphasic and conventional monophasic defibrillation on postresuscitation myocardial function. J Am Coll Cardiol 34:815–822, 1999.
17. Kirchhof P, Monnig G, Wasmer K, et al: A trial of self-adhesive patch electrodes and hand-held paddle electrodes for external cardioversion of atrial fibrillation. Eur Heart J 26:1292–1297, 2005.
18. Dodd TE, Deakin CD, Petley GW, et al: External defibrillation in the left lateral position—a comparison of manual paddles with self-adhesive pads. Resuscitation 63:283–286, 2004.
19. Sado DM, Deakin CD, Petley GW, et al: Comparison of the effects of removal of chest hair with not doing so before external defibrillation on transthoracic impedance. Am J Cardiol 93:98–100, 2004.
20. Fuster V, Ryden LE. Asinger RW, et al: ACC/AHA/ESC guidelines for the management of patients with atrial fibrillation. Eur Heart J 22:1852–1923, 2001.
21. American Heart Association Guidelines for Cardiopulmonary Resuscitation and Emergency Cardiovascular Care. Circulation 112[Suppl I]:1–211, 2005.
22. Deakin CD, Sado DM, Petley GW: Is the orientation of the apical defibrillation paddle of importance during manual external defibrillation? Resuscitation 56:25–34, 2003.
23. Kirchhof P, Eckardt L, Loh P, et al: Anterior-posterior versus anterior-lateral electrode positions for external cardioversion of atrial fibrillation: a randomised trial. Lancet 360:1275–1279, 2002.
24. Lerman BB, Deale OS: Relation between transcardiac and transthoracic current during defibrillation in humans. Circ Res 67:1420–1426, 1990.
25. Walsh SJ, McCarty D, McClelland AJ, et al: Impedance compensated biphasic waveforms for transthoracic cardioversion of atrial fibrillation: a multi-centre comparison of antero-apical and antero-posterior pad positions. Eur Heart J 26:1298–1302, 2005.
26. Eftestol T, Sunde K, Steen PA: Effects of interrupting precordial compressions on the calculated probability of defibrillation success during out-of-hospital cardiac arrest. Circulation 105:2270–2273, 2002.
27. Bjerkelund CJ, Orning OM: The efficacy of anticoagulant therapy in preventing embolism related to DC electrical conversion of atrial fibrillation. Am J Cardiol 23:208–216, 1969.
28. Singer DE, Albers GW, Dalen JE, et al: Antithrombotic therapy in atrial fibrillation: the Seventh ACCP Conference on Antithrombotic and Thrombolytic Therapy. Chest 126[Suppl 3]:429S–456S, 2004.
29. Klein AL, Grimm RA, Murray RD, et al: Use of transesophageal echocardiography to guide cardioversion in patients with atrial fibrillation. N Engl J Med 344:1411–1420, 2001.
30. Klein AL, Grimm RA, Jasper SE, et al: Efficacy of transesophageal echocardiography-guided cardioversion of patients with atrial fibrillation at six months: a randomized controlled trial. Am Heart J 151:380–389, 2006.
31. Manning WJ, Leeman DE, Gotch PJ, et al: Pulsed Doppler evaluation of atrial mechanical function after electrical cardioversion of atrial fibrillation. J Am Coll Cardiol 13:617–623, 1989.
32. O'Neill PG, Puleo PR, Bolli R, et al: Return of atrial mechanical function following electrical conversion of atrial dysrhythmias. Am Heart J 120:353–359, 1990.
33. Bechtold H, Gunzenhauser D, Sawitzki D, et al: Anticoagulation with the low-molecular-weight heparin dalteparin (Fragmin) in atrial fibrillation and TEE-guided cardioversion. Z Kardiol 92:532–539, 2003.
34. Yigit Z, Kucukoglu MS, Okcun B, et al: The safety of low-molecular weight heparins for the prevention of thromboembolic events after cardioversion of atrial fibrillation. Jpn Heart J 44:369–377, 2003.
35. Frithz G, Aberg H: Direct current conversion of atrial flutter. Acta Med Scand 187:271–274, 1970.
36. Saliba W, Juralti N, Chung MK, et al: Higher energy synchronized external direct current cardioversion for refractory atrial fibrillation. J Am Coll Cardiol 34:2031–2034, 1999.
37. Van Gelder IC, Crijns HJ, Tieleman RG, et al: Chronic atrial fibrillation. Success of serial cardioversion therapy and safety of oral anticoagulation. Arch Intern Med 156:2585–2592, 1996.

38. Wyse DG, Waldo AL, DiMarco JP, et al: A comparison of rate control and rhythm control in patients with atrial fibrillation. *N Engl J Med* 347:1825–1833, 2002.

39. Levy S, Lauribe P, Cointe R, et al: High energy transcatheter cardioversion of chronic atrial fibrillation. *J Am Coll Cardiol* 12:514–518, 1988.

40. Levy S, Lauribe P, Dolla E, et al: A randomized comparison of external and internal cardioversion of chronic atrial fibrillation. *Circulation* 86:1415–1420, 1992.

41. Levy S, Ricard P, Lau CP, et al: Multicenter low energy transvenous atrial defibrillation (XAD) trial results in different subsets of atrial fibrillation. *J Am Coll Cardiol* 29:750–756, 1997.

42. Ambler JJ, Sado DM, Zideman DA, et al: The incidence and severity of cutaneous burns following external DC cardioversion. *Resuscitation* 61:281–288, 2004.

43. Arnold AZ, Mick MJ, Mazurek RP, et al: Role of prophylactic anticoagulation for direct current cardioversion in patients with atrial fibrillation or atrial flutter. *J Am Coll Cardiol* 19:851–855, 1992.

44. Lown B, Kleiger R, Williams J: Cardioversion and digitalis drugs: changed threshold to electric shock in digitalized animals. *Circ Res* 17:519–531, 1965.

45. Aberg H, Cullhed I: Direct current countershock complications. *Acta Med Scand* 183:415–21, 1968.

46. Van Gelder IC, Crijns HJ, Van der LA, et al: Incidence and clinical significance of ST segment elevation after electrical cardioversion of atrial fibrillation and atrial flutter. *Am Heart J* 121:51–56, 1991.

47. Lund M, French JK, Johnson RN, et al: Serum troponins T and I after elective cardioversion. *Eur Heart J* 21:245–253, 2000.

48. Dahl CF, Ewy GA, Warner ED, et al: Myocardial necrosis from direct current countershock: effect of paddle electrode size and time interval between discharges. *Circulation* 50:956–961, 1974.

49. Pennington JE, Taylor J, Lown B: Chest thump for reverting ventricular tachycardia. *N Eng J Med* 283:1192–1195, 1970.

50. Yakaitis RW, Redding JS: Precordial thumping during cardiac resuscitation. *Crit Care Med* 1:22–26, 1973.

51. Vogel JH, Pryor K: Blound SG. Direct current defibrillation during pregnancy. *JAMA* 193:970–971, 1965.

52. Schroeder JS, Harrison DC: Repeated cardioversion during pregnancy. *Am J Cardiol* 27:445–446, 1971.

53. Meitus ML: Fetal electrocardiography and cardioversion with direct current countershock. *Dis Chest* 48:324–325, 1965.

CHAPTER **7**

Pericardiocentesis

Pericardiocentesis is a potentially life-saving procedure performed in the critical care setting. It is not carried out with sufficient frequency, however, to allow most physicians to master the procedure. This chapter reviews the indications for emergent and urgent pericardiocentesis, summarizes the pathobiology of pericardial effusions, and provides a step-by-step approach to pericardiocentesis, including management of patients following the procedure.

INDICATIONS FOR PERICARDIOCENTESIS

The initial management of patients with either a known or suspected pericardial effusion is largely determined by their overall clinical status. In the absence of hemodynamic instability or suspected purulent bacterial pericarditis, there is no need for emergent or urgent pericardiocentesis. It may, however, be performed for diagnostic purposes. A thorough noninvasive workup should be completed before consideration of an invasive diagnostic procedure [1]. Whenever possible, elective pericardiocentesis should be performed using echocardiographic guidance.

In contrast, the management of hemodynamically compromised patients requires emergent removal of pericardial fluid to restore adequate ventricular filling (preload) and hasten clinical stabilization. The exact method and timing of pericardiocentesis is ultimately dictated by the patient's overall degree of instability. Patients with hypotension unresponsive to fluid resuscitation and vasopressor support require immediate, often unguided (blind), pericardiocentesis. In this setting, there are no absolute contraindications to the procedure, and it should therefore be performed without delay at the patient's bedside.

Urgent pericardiocentesis is indicated for patients who are initially hypotensive but respond quickly to aggressive fluid resuscitation. The procedure should be performed within several hours of presentation while careful monitoring and hemodynamic support continue. As in elective circumstances, pericardiocentesis in these patients should be undertaken with appropriate visual guidance, the method of which depends on the physician's expertise and resources. The modalities used most commonly are echocardiography or computed tomography (CT).

Three additional points must be stressed regarding patients undergoing expedited pericardiocentesis. First, coagulation parameters—prothrombin time, partial thromboplastin time, and platelet count—should be checked and, when possible, quickly normalized prior to the procedure. An anti-Xa level is recommended for patients receiving low molecular weight heparin. Second, many critical care specialists and cardiologists advocate performance of all pericardiocentesis procedures in the catheterization laboratory with concomitant right heart pressure monitoring to document efficacy of the procedure and to exclude a constrictive element of pericardial disease [2]. The authors support this approach; however, excessive delays must be avoided. Finally, efforts to ensure a cooperative and stationary patient during the procedure greatly facilitate the performance, safety, and success of pericardiocentesis.

The clinical presentation of hemodynamically significant pericardial effusions varies widely among patients. A comprehensive understanding requires knowledge of normal pericardial anatomy and physiology.

ANATOMY

The pericardium is a membranous structure with two layers separated by a small potential space. The visceral pericardium is closely but loosely adherent to the epicardial surface. It is a monolayer of mesothelial cells and attaches to the epicardium by a loose collection of small blood vessels, lymphatics, and connective tissue. The parietal pericardium is a fibrous structure that defines the outer membrane. Its inner surface is also composed of a monolayer of mesothelial cells. The remainder of the parietal pericardium consists of a dense network of connective tissue that is relatively nondistendible; therefore, it defines the dimensions and shape of the pericardium [3].

Further anatomic definition of the pericardium is derived from multiple attachments of the parietal pericardium in the thorax. Superiorly, the fibrous parietal pericardium attaches to the ascending aorta just below the arch. The inferior portion adheres strongly to the fibrous center of the diaphragm on which it rests. Anteriorly, the outer membrane is anchored to the sternum and costal cartilages by ligaments, as well as by a less-organized collection of connective tissue. The posterior margin of the parietal pericardium abuts the esophagus and pleural sacs; here, the visceral pericardium is absent and the parietal pericardium attaches directly to the epicardium at the borders of the entrance of the inferior and superior vena cavae and pulmonary veins [4]. Beyond providing stability, these multiple attachments also limit the inherent elasticity and distensibility of the pericardium.

This complex anatomic arrangement provides an anchor for the contracting myocardium and results in a small space between the visceral and parietal layers (pericardial space). The pericardial space or sac usually contains a small volume (15 to 50 mL) of clear, serous fluid that is chemically similar to a plasma ultrafiltrate [5,6]. The mechanism responsible for the production of pericardial fluid is not well understood. A homeostasis usually exists between new production of pericardial fluid and its drainage into the venous circulation via lymphatics.

The major determinant of when and how pericardial effusions come to clinical attention is directly related to the speed at which they develop. Effusions that collect rapidly (over minutes to hours) may cause hemodynamic compromise with volumes of 250 mL or less. These effusions are usually located posteriorly and are often difficult to detect without echocardiography or other imaging modalities such as multislice CT or cardiac magnetic resonance imaging (MRI). In contrast, effusions developing slowly (over days to weeks) allow for hypertrophy and distention (stretch) of the fibrous parietal membrane. Volumes of 2,000 mL or greater may accumulate without significant hemodynamic compromise. These patients may present with symptoms owing to compression of adjacent thoracic structures, such as cough, dyspnea, dysphagia, or early satiety. Three other clinical conditions promote hemodynamic compromise, even in the absence of large pericardial effusions: intravascular hypovolemia, impaired ventricular systolic function, and ventricular hypertrophy with decreased elasticity of the myocardium (diastolic dysfunction).

PROCEDURE

Since the first blind or closed pericardiocentesis performed in 1840 [7], several different approaches have been described [8]. These approaches have varied considerably, particularly in the needle apparatus entry site. Marfan [9] described the subcostal approach in 1911, which then became the standard approach for unguided pericardiocentesis.

The advent of clinically applicable ultrasonography has opened a new chapter in diagnostic and therapeutic approaches to pericardial disease, allowing clinicians to quantitate and localize pericardial effusions quickly and noninvasively [10,11]. Work by Callahan et al. [12,13] at the Mayo Clinic established the efficacy and safety of two-dimensional echocardiography to guide pericardiocentesis. This has resulted in two major trends in clinical practice: First, two-dimensional echocardiography is commonly used to guide pericardiocentesis. Second, approaches other than the traditional subxiphoid method have been investigated owing to the ability to clearly define the anatomy (location and volume) of each patient's effusion [8,12,13]. Typically, a four-chamber view of the heart is obtained by positioning the transducer at the apex. After insertion of the pericardiocentesis needle (described later), appropriate positioning within the pericardial space can be confirmed by injecting 5 mL of agitated saline (contrast). Echocardiography can also be used to reposition the needle safely if fluid return is suboptimal. Standard fluoroscopy can be used to confirm needle and catheter positioning within the pericardial space.

Formulas for quantitating the amount of pericardial fluid by echocardiographic or fluoroscopic means have not been established. As a rule, however, an effusion of moderate size (at least 250 mL) is required for percutaneous pericardiocentesis.

Regardless of whether echocardiography or another guidance method is used, the subxiphoid approach remains the standard of practice. The materials required for bedside pericardiocentesis are listed in Table 7-1 (Fig. 7-1). Table 7-2 (Fig. 7-2) lists the materials required for simultaneous placement of an intrapericardial drainage catheter. The materials are available in prepackaged kits or individually. I do not have a preference; the key to success is immediate availability of the necessary materials.

TABLE 7-1. Materials for Percutaneous Pericardiocentesis

Site preparation
    Antiseptic
    Gauze
    Sterile drapes and towels
    Sterile gloves, masks, gowns, caps
    5-mL or 10-mL syringe with 25-gauge needle
    1% lidocaine (without epinephrine)
    Code cart
    Atropine (1-mg dose vial)
Procedure
    No. 11 blade
    20-mL syringe with 10 mL of 1% lidocaine (without epinephrine)
    18-gauge, 8-cm, thin-walled needle with blunt tip
    Multiple 20- and 40-mL syringes
    Hemostat
    Sterile alligator clip
    Electrocardiogram machine
    Three red-top tubes
    Two purple-top (heparinized) tubes
    Culture bottles
Postprocedure
    Suture material
    Scissors
    Sterile gauze and bandage

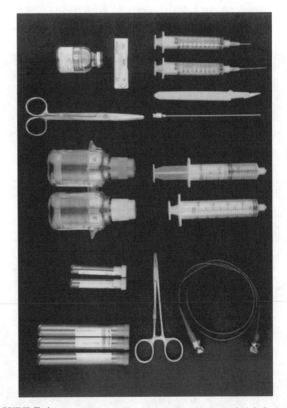

FIGURE 7-1. Materials required for pericardiocentesis (*clockwise from upper left*): 1% lidocaine solution, suture material, 10-mL syringe with 25-gauge needle, 10-mL syringe with 22-gauge needle, no. 11 blade, 18-gauge 8-cm thin-walled needle, 20-mL syringe, 30-mL syringe, alligator clip, hemostat, three red-top tubes, two purple-top tubes, culture bottles, scissors.

TABLE 7-2. Materials for Intrapericardial Catheter

Catheter placement
 Teflon-coated flexible J-curved guidewire
 6 Fr dilator
 8 Fr dilator
 8 Fr, 35-cm flexible pigtail catheter with multiple fenestrations
  (end and side holes)
Drainage system[a]
 Three-way stopcock
 Sterile IV tubing
 500-mL sterile collecting bag (or bottle)
 Sterile gauze and adhesive bag (or bottle)
 Suture material

[a]System described allows continuous drainage.

While the patient is being prepared for emergent or urgent pericardiocentesis, it is imperative that aggressive resuscitation measures are undertaken. Two large-bore peripheral intravenous lines should be placed for infusion of isotonic saline or colloid solutions. The use of inotropic agents and other vasoactive drugs (vasopressors) remains controversial [14–16], but when fluid resuscitation alone is inadequate, their use should be considered strongly.

The subxiphoid approach for pericardiocentesis is as follows:

1. Patient preparation. Assist the patient in assuming a comfortable supine position with the head of the bed elevated to approximately 45 degrees from the horizontal plane. It is

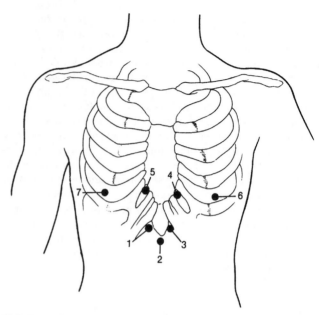

FIGURE 7-3. Selected locations for pericardiocentesis. In most cases, the subxiphoid approach (1 to 3) is preferred. [From Spodick DH: *Acute Pericarditis.* New York, Grune & Stratton, 1959, with permission.]

important for the patient to maintain this position during the procedure. Extremely dyspneic patients may need to be positioned fully upright, with a wedge if necessary. Elevation of the thorax allows free-flowing effusions to collect inferiorly and anteriorly, sites that are safest and easiest to access using the subxiphoid approach. The patient's bed should be placed at a comfortable height for the physician performing the procedure.

2. Needle entry site selection. Locate the patient's xiphoid process and the border of the left costal margin using inspection and careful palpation. The needle entry site should be 0.5 cm to the (patient's) left of the xiphoid process and 0.5 to 1.0 cm inferior to the costal margin (Fig. 7-3). It is essential that the surface anatomy be accurately defined before proceeding further. It is helpful to estimate (by palpation) the distance between the skin surface and the posterior margin of the bony thorax: This helps guide subsequent needle insertion. The usual distance is 1.0 to 2.5 cm, increasing with obesity or protuberance of the abdomen.

3. Site preparation. Strict sterile techniques must be maintained at all times in preparation of the needle entry site. Prepare a wide area in the subxiphoid region and lower thorax with a povidone-iodine solution and drape the field with sterile towels, leaving exposed the subxiphoid region. Raise a 1- to 2-cm subcutaneous wheal by infiltrating the needle entry site with 1% lidocaine solution (without epinephrine). Incise the skin with a no. 11 blade at the selected site after achieving adequate local anesthesia: This facilitates needle entry, which is at times difficult because of the absence of a bevel on the Teflon needle apparatus.

4. Insertion of the needle apparatus. Place the needle apparatus in the dominant hand (right-handed operators should stand to the patient's right and left-handed operators to the left) and insert it in the subxiphoid incision. The angle of

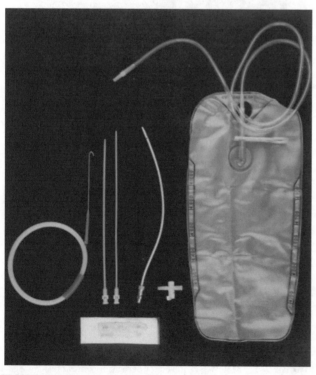

FIGURE 7-2. Materials required for intrapericardial catheter placement and drainage (*clockwise from lower left*): Teflon-coated flexible 0.035-inch J-curved guidewire, 8 Fr dilator, 6.3 Fr dilator, 8 Fr catheter with end and side holes (35-cm flexible pigtail catheter not shown), three-way stopcock, 500-mL sterile collecting bag and tubing, suture material.

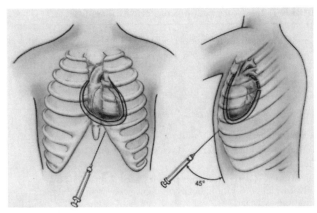

FIGURE 7-4. Insertion of the needle apparatus. After the subxiphoid region and lower thorax are prepared and adequate local anesthesia is given, the pericardiocentesis needle is inserted in the subxiphoid incision. The angle of entry (with the skin) should be approximately 45 degrees. The needle tip should be directed superiorly, toward the patient's left shoulder.

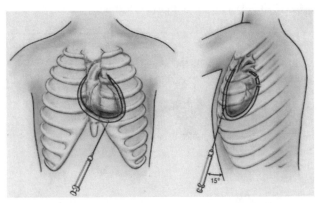

FIGURE 7-5. Needle direction. The needle tip should be reduced to 15 degrees once the posterior margin of the bony thorax has been passed. Needle advancement: The needle is advanced toward the left shoulder slowly while alternating between aspiration and injection. A "give" is felt, and fluid is aspirated when the pericardial space is entered.

entry (with the skin) should be approximately 45 degrees. Direct the needle tip superiorly, aiming for the patient's left shoulder. Continue to advance the needle posteriorly while alternating between aspiration and injection of lidocaine, until the tip has passed just beyond the posterior border of the bony thorax (Fig. 7-4). The posterior border usually lies within 2.5 cm of the skin surface. If the needle tip contacts the bony thorax, inject lidocaine after aspirating to clear the needle tip and anesthetize the periosteum. Then, walk the needle behind the posterior (costal) margin.

5. Needle direction. Reduce the angle of contact between the needle and skin to 15 degrees once the tip has passed the posterior margin of the bony thorax: This will be the angle of approach to the pericardium; the needle tip, however, should still be directed toward the patient's left shoulder. A 15-degree angle is used regardless of the height of the patient's thorax (whether at 45 degrees or sitting upright) (Fig. 7-5).

6. Needle advancement. Advance the needle slowly while alternating between aspiration of the syringe and injection of 1% lidocaine solution. If electrocardiographic guidance is used, apply the sterile alligator clip to the needle hub, being certain not to occlude the needle's lumen. Obtain a baseline lead V tracing and monitor a continuous tracing for the presence of ST-segment elevation or premature ventricular contractions (evidence of epicardial contact) as the needle is advanced. Advance the needle along this extrapleural path until either:

   a. A "give" is felt, and fluid is aspirated from the pericardial space (usually 6.0 to 7.5 cm from the skin) (Fig. 7-6). Some patients may experience a vasovagal response at this point and require atropine intravenously to increase their blood pressure and heart rate.

   b. ST-segment elevation or premature ventricular contractions are observed on the electrocardiographic lead V tracing when the needle tip contacts the epicardium. If ST-segment elevation or premature ventricular complexes occur, immediately (and carefully) withdraw the

needle toward the skin surface while aspirating. Avoid any lateral motion, which could damage the epicardial vessels. Completely withdraw the needle if no fluid is obtained during the initial repositioning.

The patient's hemodynamic status should improve promptly with removal of sufficient fluid. Successful relief of tamponade is supported by (a) a fall of intrapericardial pressure to levels between −3 and +3 mm Hg, (b) a fall in right atrial pressure and a separation between right and left ventricular diastolic pressures, (c) augmentation of cardiac output, (d) increased

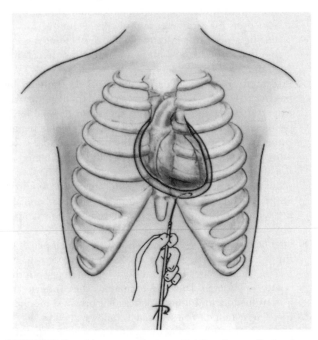

FIGURE 7-6. Placement technique. Holding the needle in place, a Teflon-coated, 0.035-in. guidewire is advanced into the pericardial space. The needle is then removed. After a series of skin dilations, an 8 Fr, 35-cm flexible pigtail catheter is placed over the guidewire into the pericardial space. Passage of dilators and the pigtail catheter is facilitated by a gentle clockwise/counterclockwise motion.

TABLE 7-3.   Diagnostic Studies Performed
on Pericardial Fluid

Hematocrit
White blood cell count with differential
Glucose
Protein
Gram's stain
Routine aerobic and anaerobic cultures
Smear and culture for acid-fast bacilli
Cytology
Cholesterol, triglyceride
Amylase
Lactate dehydrogenase
Special cultures (viral, parasite, fungal)
Antinuclear antibody
Rheumatoid factor
Total complement, C3

systemic blood pressure, and (e) reduced pulsus paradoxus to physiologic levels (10 mm Hg or less). An improvement may be observed after removal of the first 50
to 100 mL of fluid. If the right atrial pressure remains
elevated after fluid removal, an effusive-constrictive process should be considered. The diagnostic studies performed on pericardial fluid are outlined in Table 7-
3. Several options exist for continued drainage of the
pericardial space. The simplest approach is to use large-
volume syringes and aspirate the fluid by hand. This
approach is not always practical (i.e., in large-volume
effusions), however, and manipulation of the needle
apparatus may cause myocardial trauma. Alternatively,
some pericardiocentesis kits include materials and instructions for a catheter-over-needle technique for inserting a pericardial drain. Finally, the Seldinger technique may be used to place an indwelling pericardial
drain.

7. Placement technique. Create a track for the catheter by
passing a 6 French (Fr) dilator over a firmly held guidewire.
After removing the dilator, use the same technique to
pass an 8 Fr dilator. Then advance an 8 Fr flexible pigtail
catheter over the guidewire into the pericardial space. Remove the guidewire. Passage of the dilators is facilitated by
use of a torquing (clockwise/counterclockwise) motion. A
wider incision at the base of the guidewire may be required
to pass the dilators. Proper positioning of the catheter using radiography, fluoroscopy, or bedside echocardiography can be used to facilitate fluid drainage.

8. Drainage system [17–20]. Attach a three-way stopcock to
the intrapericardial catheter and close the system by attaching the stopcock to the sterile collecting bag with the
connecting tubing. The catheter may also be connected to
a transducer, allowing intrapericardial pressure monitoring. The system may be secured as follows:

   a. Suture the pigtail catheter to the skin, making sure the
   lumen is not compressed. Cover the entry site with a
   sterile gauze and dressing.

   b. Secure the drainage bag (or bottle) using tape at a
   level approximately 35 to 50 cm below the level of
   the heart. This system may be left in place for 48 to

TABLE 7-4.   Complications of Pericardiocentesis

Cardiac puncture with hemopericardium
Coronary artery laceration (hemopericardium or myocardial
  infarction)
Pneumothorax
Hemothorax
Arrhythmias
  Bradycardia
  Ventricular tachycardia/ventricular fibrillation
Trauma to abdominal organs (liver, gastrointestinal tract)
Hemorrhagic peritonitis
Cardiac arrest (predominantly pulseless electrical activity from
  myocardial perforation, but occasionally tachyarrhythmia or
  bradyarrhythmia) [a]
Transient biventricular dysfunction
Infection
Fistula formation
Pulmonary edema

---

[a]Incidence has varied from 0% to 5% in studies and was less common
in guided procedures, more common in "blind" procedures.
Permayer-Miulda G, Sagrista-Savleda J, Soler-Soler J: Primary acute peri-
cardial disease: a prospective study of 231 consecutive patients. *Am J
Cardiol* 56:623, 1985.
Wong B, Murphy J, Chang CJ, et al: The risk of pericardiocentesis. *Am
J Cardiol* 44:1110, 1979.
Krikorian JG, Hancock EW: Pericardiocentesis. *Am J Med* 65:808, 1978.

72 hours. Echocardiography or fluoroscopic guidance
may be used to reposition the pigtail catheter, facilitating complete drainage of existing pericardial fluid.

The catheter should be flushed manually every 4 to
6 hours using 10 to 15 cc of normal saline solution.

SHORT-TERM AND LONG-TERM MANAGEMENT

After pericardiocentesis, close monitoring is required to detect
evidence of recurrent tamponade and procedure-related complications. Table 7-4 lists the most common serious complications associated with pericardiocentesis [1,21,22]. Factors associated with an increased risk of complications include (a) small
effusion (less than 250 mL), (b) posterior effusion, (c) loculated effusion, (d) maximum anterior clear space (by echocardiography) less than 10 mm, and (e) unguided percutaneous

TABLE 7-5.   Major Surgical Options for the Management of
Pericardial Effusions

Procedure	Approach	Resection Margins
Pericardial window		
Subxiphoid	Subxiphoid	<9 cm^2 block
Pleural	Thoracotomy	<9 cm^2 block
Partial pericardiectomy	Thoracotomy	Right phrenic nerve; great vessels to diaphragmatic reflection
Complete pericardiectomy	Thoracotomy or sternotomy	Right phrenic nerve to left pulmonary vein: great vessels to midportion of diaphragmatic pericardium

TABLE 7-6.   Common Causes of Pericardial Effusion

Idiopathic

Malignancy (primary, metastatic; solid tumors, hematologic)

Uremia

Graft versus host disease

Extramedullary hematopoiesis

Postpericardiotomy syndrome

Connective tissue disease

Trauma
    Blunt
    Penetrating

Infection
    Viral (including HIV)
    Bacterial
    Fungal
    Tuberculosis

Aortic dissection

Complication of cardiac catheterization, percutaneous coronary intervention or pacemaker insertion

Myxedema

Postirradiation

---

approach. All patients undergoing pericardiocentesis should have a portable chest radiograph performed immediately after the procedure to exclude the presence of pneumothorax. In addition, a transthoracic two-dimensional echocardiogram should be obtained within several hours to evaluate the adequacy of pericardial drainage. Echocardiography can also be used to confirm drainage catheter placement.

Finally, careful technique is required to maintain the sterility of the pericardial catheter drainage system. With meticulous local care, the complication rate is exceptionally low, even when the catheter is left in place for 36 to 48 hours [12,18].

The long-term management of patients with significant pericardial fluid collections is beyond the scope of this chapter; however, the role of surgical intervention is reviewed briefly. The indications for surgical intervention are controversial and vary widely (Table 7-5) [2,23–28]. Several indications that have been established include: (a) pericardial disease with concomitant constrictive physiology, (b) known loculated or posteriorly located effusions not amenable to pericardiocentesis, (c) suspected purulent pericarditis, (d) effusions not successfully drained by pericardiocentesis, and (e) rapidly recurring effusions [2,29]. The etiology of the pericardial effusion (Table 7-6) and the patient's functional status are of central importance for determining the preferred treatment. Aggressive attempts at nonsurgical management of chronically debilitated patients or those with metastatic disease involving the pericardium may be appropriate [25,30,31]. Pericardial sclerosis with tetracycline, cisplatin or other agents has benefited carefully selected patients with malignant pericardial disease [30,32,33]. Patients with a guarded prognosis who fail aggressive medical therapy should be offered the least invasive procedure.

REFERENCES

1. Permayer-Miulda G, Sagrista-Savleda J, Soler-Soler J: Primary acute pericardial disease: a prospective study of 231 consecutive patients. *Am J Cardiol* 56:623, 1985.
2. Lovell BH, Braunwald E: Pericardial disease, in Braunwald E (ed). *Heart Disease: A Textbook of Cardiovascular Medicine*. Philadelphia, WB Saunders, 1988, p 1484.
3. Tandler J: Anatomie des Harsens. Jeng, Fischer, 1913. Quoted by Elias H, Boyd LJ: Notes on the anatomy, embryology and histology of the pericardium. *J NY Med Coll* 2:50, 1960.
4. Roberts WC, Spray TL: Pericardial heart disease: a study of its causes, consequences, and morphologic features, in Spodick D (ed): Pericardial Diseases. Philadelphia, FA Davis, 1976, p 17.
5. Shabatai R: Function of the pericardium, in Fowler NO (ed): *The Pericardium in Health and Disease*. Mount Kisco, NY, Futura, 1985, p 19.
6. Shabetai R. *The Pericardium*. New York, Grune & Stratton, 1981.
7. Schuh R: Erfahrungen uber de Paracentese der Brust und des Herz Beutels. *Med Jahrb Osterr Staates Wien* 33:388, 1841.
8. Tilkian AG, Daily EK: Pericardiocentesis and drainage, in Tilkian AG, Daily EK (eds): *Cardiovascular Procedures: Diagnostic Techniques and Therapeutic Approaches*. St. Louis, Mosby, 1986, p 231.
9. Marfan AB: Poncitian du pericarde par l espigahe. *Ann Med Chir Infarct* 15:529, 1911.
10. Tibbles CD, Porcaro W: Procedural applications of ultrasound. *Emerg Med Clin North Am* 22:797, 2004.
11. Rifkin RD, Mernoff DB: Noninvasive evaluation of pericardial effusion composition by computed tomography. *Am Heart J* 149:1120, 2005.
12. Callahan JA, Seward JB, Nishimura RA: 2-dimensional echocardiography-guided pericardiocentesis: experience in 117 consecutive patients. *Am J Cardiol* 55:476, 1985.
13. Callahan JA, Seward JB, Tajik AJ: Pericardiocentesis assisted by 2-dimensional echocardiography. *J Thorac Cardiovasc Surg* 85:877, 1983.
14. Callahan M: Pericardiocentesis in traumatic and non-traumatic cardiac tamponade. *Ann Emerg Med* 13:924, 1984.
15. Fowler NO, Guberman BA, Gueron M: Cardiac tamponade, in Eliot RS (ed): *Cardiac Emergencies*. 2nd ed. Mount Kisco, NY, Futura, 1982, p 415.
16. Seldinger S: Catheter replacement of the needle in percutaneous angiography. *Acta Radiol Diagn (Stockh)* 39:368, 1953.
17. Kapoor AS: Technique of pericardiocentesis and intrapericardial drainage, in Kapoor AS (ed): *International Cardiology*. New York, Springer-Verlag, 1989, p 146.
18. Kopecky SL, Callahan JA, Tajik AJ, et al: Percutaneous pericardial catheter drainage: report of 42 consecutive cases. *Am J Cardiol* 58:633, 1986.
19. Massumi RA, Rios JC, Ewy GA: Technique for insertion of an indwelling pericardial catheter. *Br Heart J* 30:333, 1960.
20. Patel AK, Kogolcharoen PK, Nallasivan M, et al: Catheter drainage of the pericardium: practical method to maintain long-term patency. *Chest* 92:1018, 1987.
21. Wong B, Murphy J, Chang CJ, et al: The risk of pericardiocentesis. *Am J Cardiol* 44:1110, 1979.
22. Krikorian JG, Hancock EW: Pericardiocentesis. *Am J Med* 65:808, 1978.
23. Piehler JM, Pluth JR, Schaff HV, et al: Surgical management of effusive pericardial disease: influence of extent of pericardial resection on clinical cause. *J Thorac Cardiovasc Surg* 90:506, 1985.
24. Little AG, Kremser PC, Wade JL, et al: Operation for diagnosis and treatment of pericardial effusions. *Surgery* 96:738, 1984.
25. Palatianos GM, Thuer RJ, Karser GA: Comparison of effectiveness and safety of operations on the pericardium. *Chest* 88:30, 1985.
26. Little AG, Fergusen MK: Pericardioscopy as adjunct to pericardial window. *Chest* 89:53, 1986.
27. Prager RL, Wilson CH, Border WH Jr: The subxiphoid approach to pericardial disease. *Ann Thorac Surg* 34:6, 1982.
28. Spodick DH: Pericardial windows are suboptimal. *Am J Cardiol* 51:607, 1983.
29. Rub RH, Moelleering RC: Clinical microbiologic and therapeutic aspects of purulent pericarditis. *Am J Med* 59:68, 1975.
30. Shepherd FA, Morgan C, Evans WK, et al: Medical management of malignant pericardial effusion by tetracycline sclerosis. *Am J Cardiol* 60:1161, 1987.
31. Morm JE, Hallonby D, Gonda A, et al: Management of uremia pericarditis: a report of 11 patients with cardiac tamponade and a review of the literature. *Ann Thorac Surg* 22:588, 1976.
32. Reitknecht F, Regal AM, Antkowiak JG, et al: Management of cardiac tamponade in patients with malignancy. *J Surg Oncol* 30:19, 1985.
33. Maisch B, Ristic AD, Pankuweit S, et al: Neoplastic pericardial effusion. Efficacy and safety of intrapericardial treatment with cisplatin. *Eur Heart J* 23:1625, 2002.

Robert A. Lancey

CHAPTER **8**

Chest Tube Insertion and Care

Chest tube insertion (tube thoracostomy) involves placement of a sterile tube into the pleural space to evacuate air or fluid into a closed collection system to restore negative intrathoracic pressure, promote lung expansion, and prevent potentially lethal levels of pressure from developing in the thorax. Although it is not as complex as many surgical procedures, serious and potentially life-threatening complications may result if chest tube insertion is performed without proper preparation or instruction. Insertion and care of chest tubes are common issues not only in the intensive care unit but throughout the hospital and have become a required component of the training for Advanced Trauma Life Support [1].

PLEURAL ANATOMY AND PHYSIOLOGY

Because the primary goal of chest tube placement is drainage of the pleural space, a basic knowledge of its anatomy and physiology is useful. The lung fills all but 10 cc of the pleural space in the normal physiologic state. This space is a closed, serous sac surrounded by two separate layers of mesothelial cells (the parietal and visceral pleurae), which are contiguous at the pulmonary hilum and the inferior pulmonary ligament. Normally, there is a negative intrapleural pressure of –2 to –5 cm water.

The parietal pleura is subdivided into four anatomic sections: the costal pleura (lining the ribs, costal cartilages, and intercostal spaces), the cervical pleura (on the most superior aspect of the pleural space), the mediastinal pleura (covering the medial aspect of the pleural space), and the diaphragmatic pleura. The visceral pleura completely covers and is adherent to the pulmonary parenchyma, extending into the interlobar fissures to varying degrees. The pleural layers are in close apposition and under normal physiologic conditions allow free expansion of the lung in a lubricated environment. In some areas, potential spaces exist where parietal pleural surfaces are in contact during expiration, most notably in the costodiaphragmatic and costomediastinal sinuses [2].

Drainage of the pleural space is necessary when the normal physiologic processes are disrupted. Violation of the visceral pleura allows accumulation of air (pneumothorax) and possibly blood (hemothorax) in the pleural space. Disruption of the parietal pleura may also result in a hemothorax if an underlying vascular structure is disrupted or a pneumothorax if the defect communicates to the environment.

Derangements of normal fluid dynamics in the pleural space may result in the accumulation of clinically significant effusions. Fluid is secreted into and reabsorbed from the pleural space by the parietal pleura, the latter process through stomas that drain into the lymphatic system and ultimately through the mediastinal, intercostal, phrenic, and substernal lymph nodes. Although up to 500 mL per day may enter the pleural space, normally less than 3 mL fluid is present at any given time [3]. This normal equilibrium may be disrupted by increased fluid entry into the space due to alterations in hydrostatic pressures (e.g., congestive heart failure) or oncotic pressures or by changes in the parietal pleura itself (e.g., inflammatory diseases). A derangement in lymphatic drainage, as with lymphatic obstruction by malignancy, may also result in excess fluid accumulation.

CHEST TUBE PLACEMENT

INDICATIONS

The indications for closed intercostal drainage encompass a variety of disease processes in the hospital setting (Table 8-1). The procedure may be performed to palliate a chronic disease process (e.g., drainage of malignant pleural effusions) or to relieve an acute, life-threatening process (e.g., decompression of a tension pneumothorax). Chest tubes also may provide a vehicle for pharmacologic interventions, as when used with antibiotic therapy for treatment of an empyema or to instill sclerosing agents to prevent recurrence of malignant effusions.

Pneumothorax

Accumulation of air in the pleural space is the most common indication for chest tube placement. Symptoms include tachypnea, dyspnea, and pleuritic pain, although some patients (in particular, those with a small spontaneous pneumothorax) may be asymptomatic. Physical findings include diminished breath sounds and hyperresonance to percussion on the affected side.

Diagnosis is often confirmed by chest radiography, demonstrating a thin opaque line beyond which exists a hyperlucent area without lung markings. Although the size of a pneumothorax may be estimated, this is at best a rough approximation of a three-dimensional space based on a two-dimensional view. Inspiratory and expiratory films may be helpful in equivocal situations, as may a lateral decubitus film with the suspected side up. Detection of an anterior pneumothorax in blunt trauma may be especially difficult and yet may be easily detected by chest computed tomographic (CT) scanning [4].

The decision to insert a chest tube for a pneumothorax is based on the patient's overall clinical status and may be aided by serial chest radiographs. Tube decompression is indicated in those who are symptomatic, who have a large or expanding pneumothorax, or who are being mechanically ventilated (the latter of whom may present acutely with deteriorating oxygenation and an increase in airway pressures, necessitating immediate decompression).

TABLE 8-1. Indications for Chest Tube Insertion

Pneumothorax
   Spontaneous
   Traumatic
   Necrotizing pneumonia
   Interstitial fibrosis
   Malignancy
      Primary
      Metastatic
   Bullous emphysema
   Pulmonary infarction
   Iatrogenic
      Central line placement
      Positive-pressure ventilation
      Thoracentesis
Hemothorax
   Traumatic
      Blunt
      Penetrating
   Iatrogenic
   Malignancy
      Primary
      Metastatic
   Infectious
   Pulmonary arteriovenous malformation
   Spontaneous pneumothorax
   Blood dyscrasias
   Ruptured thoracic aortic aneurysm
Empyema
   Parapneumonic
   Posttraumatic
   Postoperative
   Septic emboli
   Intraabdominal infection
Chylothorax
   Traumatic
      Blunt
      Penetrating
      Surgical
   Congenital
   Malignancy
   Miscellaneous
      Filariasis
      Tuberculosis
      Subclavian vein obstruction
Pleural effusion
   Transudate
   Exudate
      Malignancy
      Postoperative
      Iatrogenic
      Immunologic
      Inflammatory

A spontaneous pneumothorax occurs most commonly in tall, slender, young males secondary to rupture of apical alveoli and subsequent formation of subpleural blebs, which then rupture into the pleural space. An associated hemothorax from torn adhesions may occur in up to 5% of cases [5]. The risk of a recurrent ipsilateral spontaneous pneumothorax is as high as 50%, and the risk of a third episode is 60% to 80% [6].

A small, stable, asymptomatic pneumothorax can be followed with serial chest radiographs. Reexpansion occurs at the rate of approximately 1.25% of lung volume per day [7]. Definitive operative intervention beyond tube thoracostomy may include resection of apical blebs, pleurodesis, and/or pleurectomy via open thoracotomy or thoracoscopy. These procedures are often reserved for those with a persistent air leak or with recurrent spontaneous pneumothoraces.

Pneumothorax in trauma patients is often accompanied by bleeding (hemopneumothorax) and almost invariably requires tube decompression, especially if mechanical ventilation is planned, to avoid a life-threatening tension pneumothorax. Persistent leaking of air into the pleural space with no route of escape will ultimately collapse the affected lung, flatten the diaphragm, and eventually produce contralateral shift of the mediastinum. Compression of the contralateral lung and compromise of venous return result in progressive hypoxemia and hypotension. Emergency decompression with a 14- or 16-gauge catheter in the midclavicular line of the second intercostal space may be lifesaving while preparations for chest tube insertion are being made. In a hypotensive trauma patient, such pleural space decompression may be required before radiographic diagnosis of tension pneumothorax is confirmed.

Additional potential sources of pneumothorax are bullous disease, malignancies (particularly soft tissue sarcoma metastases), and necrotizing pneumonia. Iatrogenic causes include thoracentesis and central venous catheter insertion. The incidence of pneumothorax associated with attempts at subclavian vein access has been reported to be as high as 6%, and although the incidence is lower with an internal jugular approach, pneumothorax still may result (as the lung apices rise above the clavicles) [8]. Patients on mechanical ventilation, especially with elevated levels of positive end-expiratory pressure, are also at risk. In this setting, a tension pneumothorax may rapidly develop and require emergency measures as described above. Although prophylactic insertion of bilateral pleural tubes has been reported for patients on extremely high levels of positive end-expiratory pressure (greater than 40 cm H_2O), no controlled study has yet documented its benefit [9].

Hemothorax

Accumulation of blood in the pleural space can be classified as spontaneous, iatrogenic, or traumatic. Attempted thoracentesis or tube placement may result in injury to the intercostal or internal mammary arteries or to the pulmonary parenchyma. Up to a third of patients with traumatic rib fractures may have an accompanying pneumothorax or hemothorax [10]. Pulmonary parenchymal bleeding from chest trauma is often self-limited due to the low pressure of the pulmonary vascular system. However, systemic sources (intercostal, internal mammary or subclavian arteries, aorta, or heart) may persist and become life threatening.

Indications for open thoracotomy in the setting of traumatic hemothorax include initial blood loss greater than 1,500 mL or continued blood loss exceeding 500 mL over the first hour, 200 mL per hour after 2 to 4 hours, or 100 mL per hour after 6 to 8 hours, or in an unstable patient who does not respond to volume resuscitation [11–13]. Placement of large-bore [36 to 40 French (Fr)] drainage tubes encourages evacuation of blood and helps determine the need for immediate thoracotomy. Although some have advocated clamping the tube in the face of significant intrathoracic hemorrhage, this practice should be discouraged, as it fails to prevent hypotension and instead hinders ventilation [14].

Incomplete drainage of a traumatic hemothorax due to poor tube positioning or tube "thrombosis" may result in a chronic fibrothorax. Subsequent significant reduction of pulmonary reserve may occur as a result of restricted lung expansion. Early, aggressive evacuation of a retained hemothorax (via thoracoscopy or open thoracotomy) encourages full reexpansion and prevents empyema formation [15,16] in those who are able to tolerate the procedure. If the patient's condition mandates nonoperative management, a waiting period of several weeks allows an organized "peel" to form, facilitating its removal (decortication).

Spontaneous pneumothoraces may result from necrotizing pulmonary infections, pulmonary arteriovenous malformations, pulmonary infarctions, primary and metastatic malignancies of the lung and pleura, and tearing of adhesions between the visceral and parietal pleurae.

Empyema

Empyemas are pyogenic infections of the pleural space that may result from numerous clinical conditions, including necrotizing pneumonia, septic pulmonary emboli, spread of intraabdominal infections, or inadequate drainage of a traumatic hemothorax. Pyothorax as a complication of pneumonia is less common now than in the preantibiotic era, with the common organisms now being *Staphylococcus aureus* and anaerobic and Gram-negative microbes.

Definitive management includes evacuation of the collection and antibiotic therapy. Chest tube drainage is indicated for pleural collections with any of the following characteristics: pH less than 7.0, glucose less than 40 mg per dL, lactate dehydrogenase greater than 1,000 IU per L, frank purulence, or culture-positive specimens [17]. Large-bore drainage tubes (36 to 40 Fr) are used, and success is evidenced by resolving fever and leukocytosis, improving clinical status, and eventual resolution of drainage. The tube can then be removed slowly over several days, allowing a fibrous tract to form. If no improvement is seen, rib resection and open drainage may be indicated. Chronic empyema may require decortication or, in more debilitated patients, open flap drainage (Eloesser procedure). Fibrinolytic enzymes (urokinase or streptokinase) can also be instilled through the tube to facilitate drainage of persistent purulent collections or for hemothorax or malignant effusions [18–20].

Chylothorax

A collection of lymphatic fluid in the pleural space is termed *chylothorax*. Due to the immunologic properties of lymph, the collection is almost always sterile. As much as 1,500 mL per day may accumulate and may result in hemodynamic compromise or adverse metabolic sequelae as a result of loss of protein, fat, and fat-soluble vitamins. The diagnosis is confirmed by a fluid triglyceride level greater than 110 mg per dL or a cholesterol-triglyceride ratio of less than 1 [21,22].

Primary causes of chylothorax include trauma, surgery, malignancy, and congenital abnormalities. Surgical procedures most often implicated are those involving mobilization of the distal aortic arch and isthmus (e.g., repair of aortic coarctation, ligation of a patent ductus arteriosus, or repair of vascular rings) and esophageal resections [23]. Its appearance in the pleural space may be delayed for 7 to 10 days if there are postoperative dietary restrictions; the fluid may also collect in the posterior mediastinum before rupturing into the pleural space (often on the right side) [22]. Traumatic causes include crush or blast injuries, those that cause sudden hyperextension of the spine or neck, or even a bout of violent vomiting or coughing.

In the absence of trauma, malignancy must always be suspected. Leak occurs secondary to direct invasion of the thoracic duct or from obstruction by external compression or tumor emboli. Lymphosarcoma, lymphoma, and primary lung carcinomas are those most frequently implicated [22].

Treatment involves tube drainage along with aggressive maintenance of volume and nutrition. With hyperalimentation and intestinal rest (to limit flow through the thoracic duct), approximately 50% will resolve without surgery [24]. Although no consensus exists as to the optimal time to intervene surgically, a minimum of 2 weeks of observation is usually appropriate unless the patient is already malnourished [25,26]. Open thoracotomy may be necessary to ligate the duct and close the fistula.

Pleural Effusion

Management of a pleural effusion often begins with thoracentesis to identify the collection as either a transudative or exudative process. Treatment of *transudative* pleural effusions is aimed at controlling the underlying cause (e.g., congestive heart failure, nephrotic syndrome, cirrhosis). Tube thoracostomy is rarely indicated. *Exudative* effusions, however, often require tube drainage. Decubitus chest films before drainage are useful in determining whether the fluid is free flowing or loculated. If loculated, localization of the collection for proper tube placement may require use of ultrasound or CT scanning.

Malignancies (most commonly of the lung, breast, or lymph system) are a common cause of exudative effusions. Recurrence of effusion following thoracentesis may be as high as 97% in a month, with most recurring within 1 to 3 days [27]. Chest tube insertion serves not only to relieve symptoms and allow lung expansion but also to allow instillation of sclerosing agents that facilitate adherence of visceral to parietal surfaces and to obliterate potential spaces and prevent future fluid accumulation. Tube drainage alone without sclerosis may result in a recurrence rate as high as 100% within a month [27]. Chemical pleurodesis should be undertaken once apposition of pleural surfaces is complete and can be performed using any of a number of agents, including bleomycin, doxycycline, and talc [28–30].

CONTRAINDICATIONS

The most apparent contraindication to chest tube insertion seems obvious—lack of a pneumothorax or of a fluid collection in the pleural space—yet this distinction is not always clear. What may appear at first to be a pneumothorax may instead be a rib edge or a skinfold, the medial border of the scapula, or even the tract of a recently removed chest tube. A large bulla may also be mistaken for a pneumothorax, a circumstance in which attempted pleural tube placement may result in significant morbidity. An expiratory chest film, which highlights the pulmonary parenchyma by increasing its density, or a decubitus view with the suspected side up may help confirm the diagnosis, as may CT scanning. Likewise, an apparent pleural effusion may be a lung abscess or consolidated pulmonary parenchyma (e.g., pneumonia, atelectasis, etc.). Again, CT scanning or ultrasonography may prove helpful in delineating the pathology before tube placement.

History of a process that would promote pleural symphysis (such as a sclerosing procedure, pleurodesis, pleurectomy, or previous thoracotomy on the affected side) should raise caution and prompt evaluation with CT scanning to help identify the exact area of pathology and to direct tube placement away from areas where the lung is adherent to the chest wall. In a postpneumonectomy patient, the pleural tube should be placed above the original incision, as the diaphragm frequently rises to this height.

The possibility of herniation of abdominal contents through the diaphragm in patients with severe blunt abdominal trauma or stab wounds in the vicinity of the diaphragm requires more extensive evaluation before tube placement. In addition, coagulopathies should be corrected before tube insertion in a nonemergency setting.

TECHNIQUE

Chest tube insertion requires knowledge not only of the anatomy of the chest wall and intrathoracic and intraabdominal structures but also of general aseptic technique. The procedure should be performed or supervised only by experienced personnel, because the complications of an improperly placed tube may have immediate life-threatening results. Before tube placement, the patient must be evaluated thoroughly by physical examination and chest films to avoid insertion of the tube into a bulla or lung abscess, into the abdomen, or even into the wrong side. Particular care must be taken before and during the procedure to avoid intubation of the pulmonary parenchyma.

The necessary equipment is listed in Table 8-2. Sterile technique is mandatory whether the procedure is performed in the operating room, intensive care unit, emergency room, or on the ward. Detailed informed consent is obtained and contributes to reducing patient anxiety during the procedure. Careful titration of parenteral narcotics or benzodiazepines as well as careful and generous administration of local anesthetic agents provide for a relatively painless procedure. Standard, large-bore drainage tubes are made from either Silastic or rubber. Silastic tubes are either right angled or straight, have multiple drainage holes, and contain a radiopaque stripe with a gap to mark the most proximal drainage hole. They are available in sizes ranging from 6 to 40 Fr, with size selection dependent on the patient population

TABLE 8-2.   Chest Tube Insertion Equipment

Chlorhexidine or povidone-iodine solution
Sterile towels and drapes
Sterile sponges
1% lidocaine without epinephrine (40 mL)
10-mL syringe
18-, 21-, and 25-gauge needles
2 Kelly clamps
Mayo scissors
Standard tissue forceps
Towel forceps
Needle holder
0-Silk suture with cutting needle
Scalpel handle and no. 10 blade
Chest tubes (24, 28, 32, and 36 French)
Chest tube drainage system (filled appropriately)
Petrolatum gauze
2-in. adhesive tape
Sterile gowns and gloves, masks, caps

(6 to 24 Fr for infants and children) and the collection being drained (24 to 28 Fr for air, 32 to 36 Fr for pleural effusions, and 36 to 40 Fr for blood or pus). Recently, these have undergone technical changes to make them soft and more flexible. Smaller-caliber, Silastic types have been increasingly employed for chest drainage, particularly after open-heart surgery, to decrease pain and encourage earlier ambulation [31].

Before performing the procedure, it is important to review the steps to be taken and to ensure that all necessary equipment is available. Patient comfort and safety are paramount.

1. With the patient supine and the head of the bed adjusted for comfort, the involved side is elevated slightly with the ipsilateral arm brought up over the head (Fig. 8-1). Supplemental oxygen is administered as needed.

2. The tube is usually inserted through the fourth or fifth intercostal space in the anterior axillary line. An alternative entry site (for decompression of a pneumothorax) is the second intercostal space in the midclavicular line, but for cosmetic reasons and to avoid the thick pectoral muscles, the former site is preferable in adults.

3. Under sterile conditions, the area is prepared with 2% chlorhexidine in 70% isopropyl alcohol, and after allowing it to dry, is draped to include the nipple, which serves as a landmark. A 2- to 3-cm area is infiltrated with 1% lidocaine to raise a wheal two finger breadths below the intercostal space to be penetrated. (This allows for a subcutaneous tunnel to develop, through which the tube will travel, and discourages air entry into the chest following removal of the tube.)

4. A 2-cm transverse incision is made at the wheal, and additional lidocaine is administered to infiltrate the tissues through which the tube will pass, including a generous area in the intercostal space (especially the periosteum of the ribs above and below the targeted interspace). Care should be taken to anesthetize the parietal pleura fully, as it (unlike the visceral pleura) contains pain fibers. Each injection of lidocaine should be preceded by aspiration of the syringe to prevent injection into the intercostal vessels. Up to 30 to 40 mL lidocaine may be needed to achieve adequate local anesthesia (see Fig. 8-1).

5. To confirm the location of air or fluid, a thoracentesis is then performed at the proposed site of tube insertion. If air or fluid is not aspirated, the anatomy should be reassessed and chest radiographs and CT scans reexamined before proceeding.

6. A short tunnel is created to the chosen intercostal space, using Kelly clamps. After the intercostal muscles are bluntly divided, the closed clamp is carefully inserted through the parietal pleura, hugging the superior portion of the lower rib to prevent injury to the intercostal bundle of the rib above. The clamp is placed to a depth of less than 1 cm to prevent injury to the intrathoracic structures and is spread open approximately 2 cm (Fig. 8-2).

7. A finger is inserted into the pleural space to explore the anatomy and confirm proper location and lack of pleural symphysis. Only easily disrupted adhesions should be broken. Bluntly dissecting strong adhesions may tear the lung and initiate potentially troublesome bleeding from the systemic circulation.

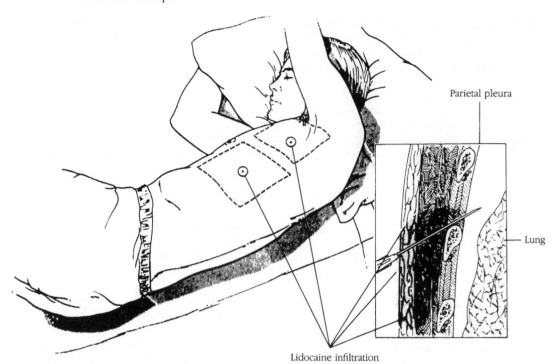

Parietal pleura

Lung

Lidocaine infiltration

FIGURE 8-1.   Proper patient positioning for chest tube insertion. Note that the involved side is slightly elevated, and the arm is flexed over the head. Lidocaine infiltrates progressively through the tissue.

8. The chest tube is inserted into the pleural space and positioned apically for a pneumothorax and dependently for fluid removal. All holes must be confirmed to be within the pleural space. The use of undue pressure or force to insert the tube should be avoided (Fig. 8-3).

9. The location of the tube should be confirmed by observing flow of air (seen as condensation within the tube) or fluid from the tube. It is then sutured to the skin securely to prevent slippage (Fig. 8-4). A horizontal mattress suture can be used to allow the hole to be tied closed when the tube is removed. An occlusive petrolatum gauze dressing is applied, and the tube is connected to a drainage apparatus and securely taped to the dressing and to the patient. All connections between the patient and the drainage apparatus must also be tight and securely taped.

COMPLICATIONS

Chest tube insertion may be accompanied by significant complications. In one series, insertion and management of pleural tubes in patients with blunt chest trauma carried a 9% incidence of complications [32]. Insertion alone is usually accompanied by a 1% to 2% incidence of complications even when performed by experienced personnel [32,33] (Table 8-3).

Unintentional placement of the tube through intercostal vessels or into the lung, heart, liver, or spleen can result in considerable morbidity and possible mortality [33,34]. Malposition of tubes within the pleural space may potentially limit effectiveness. Baldt et al. [34] found that nearly one of four chest tubes placed in a trauma setting was not positioned correctly, with 75% of these not functioning properly. Although adequate knowledge

of the anatomy in general and of the pathologic process in particular should prevent such occurrences, the most common mistake is placing the tube too low [35]. Reexpansion pulmonary edema on the affected side in the setting of a large, chronic, pleural effusion may be avoided by incremental removal of the fluid, limiting initial removal to no more than 1 L over the first 30 minutes. Factors that contribute to this process include an inelastic lung and negative-pressure drainage [36,37].

A residual pneumothorax may follow removal of the tube as a result of a persistent air leak, entry of air through the tube site during or after removal, or restricted expansion of the lung. These conditions may be differentiated based on serial chest films, as a persistent leak results in an increasing pneumothorax and requires replacement of the tube. A small, stable pneumothorax can be treated by sealing the wound securely and continued observation. If the pneumothorax is large or symptomatic, tube decompression is indicated.

Rarely, secondary infection of the pleural space may occur after chest tube insertion, resulting in an empyema. This is most common following treatment for a traumatic hemothorax. Numerous studies have examined the utility of prophylactic antibiotics for tube thoracostomy. Although it is generally accepted that antibiotics are of no benefit for decompression of a spontaneous pneumothorax [38], several investigations, including a meta-analysis of six randomized studies, suggested benefit of prophylactic antibiotic regimens directed against *Staphylococcus aureus* in patients undergoing tube thoracostomy in a trauma setting [39–41]. However, the Society of Thoracic Surgeons Workforce on Evidence-Based Medicine found no scientific evidence that the use of prophylactic antibiotics enhanced protection against infectious complications, and concluded that this practice should not be followed [42].

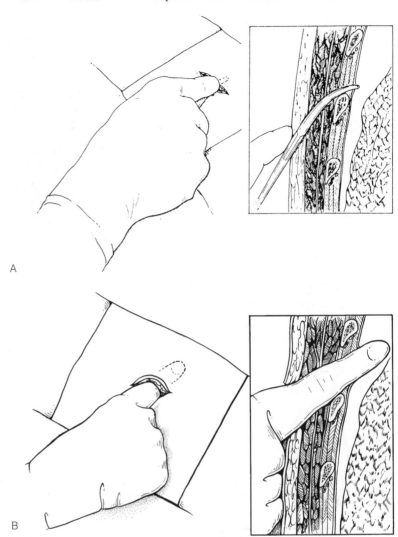

FIGURE 8-2.   **A:** The clamp penetrates the intercostal muscle. **B:** The index finger is gently inserted to explore the immediate area around the incision. No instruments are inserted into the pleural space at this time.

Because of their size and stiffness, chest tubes may limit ambulation and deep breathing. Pain associated with their presence as well as with their removal has come under scrutiny with efforts to encourage early ambulation and discharge [43,44], particularly following cardiac surgery [45]. They have also been found to impair pulmonary function, especially when placed through an intercostal space [46]. The use of small caliber, less rigid, Silastic drains has been found to be as safe and efficacious as the more rigid, conventional chest tubes [47,48], and they allow both more mobility and earlier discharge when used in open-heart surgery patients [49].

CHEST TUBE MANAGEMENT AND CARE

While a chest tube is in place, the tube and drainage system must be checked daily for adequate functioning. Most institutions use a three-chambered system that contains a calibrated collection trap for fluid, an underwater seal unit to allow escape of air while maintaining negative pleural pressure, and a suction regulator. Suction is routinely established at 15 to 20 cm water, controlled by the height of the column in the suction regulator unit, and maintained as long as an air leak is present. The drainage system is examined daily to ensure that appropriate levels are maintained in the underwater seal and suction regulator chambers. If suction is desired, bubbling should be noted in the suction regulator unit. Connections between the chest tube and the drainage system should be tightly fitted and securely taped. For continuous drainage, the chest tube and the tubing to the drainage system should remain free of kinks, should not be left in a dependent position, and should never be clamped. The tube can be milked and gently stripped, although with caution, as this may generate negative pressures of up to 1,500 mm Hg and can injure adjacent tissues [50]. Irrigation of the tube is discouraged. Dressing changes should be performed every 2 or 3 days and as needed. Adequate pain control is mandatory to encourage coughing and ambulation, to facilitate lung reexpansion.

Serial chest films are obtained routinely to evaluate the progress of drainage and to ensure that the most proximal drainage hole has not migrated from the pleural space (a situation that may result in pneumothorax or subcutaneous emphysema). If this occurs and the pathologic process is not corrected, replacement of the tube is usually indicated, especially if subcutaneous emphysema is developing. A tube should never

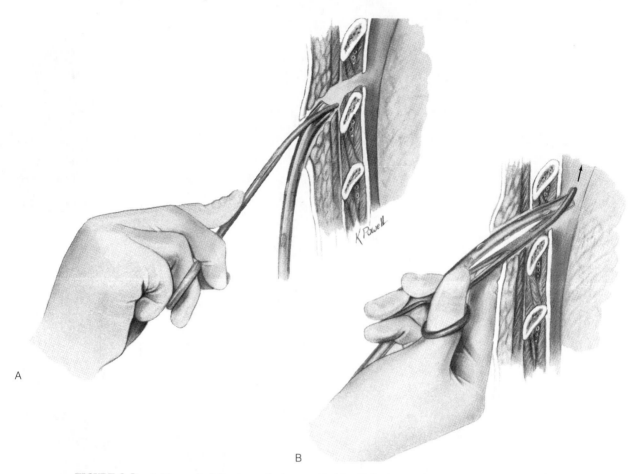

FIGURE 8-3. **A:** The end of the chest tube is grasped with a Kelly clamp and guided with a finger through the chest incision. **B:** The clamp is rotated 180 degrees to direct the tube toward the apex.

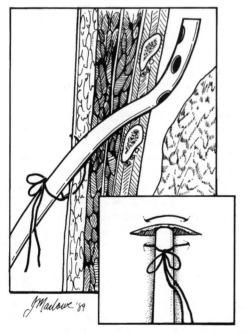

FIGURE 8-4. The tube is securely sutured to the skin with a 1-0 or 2-0 silk suture. This suture is left long, wrapped around the tube, and secured with tape. To seal the tunnel, the suture is tied when the tube is pulled out.

be readvanced into the pleural space, and if a tube is to be replaced it should always be at a different site rather than through the same hole. If a pneumothorax persists, increasing the suction level may be beneficial, but an additional tube may be required if no improvement results. Proper positioning may also be confirmed by chest CT scanning [51].

CHEST TUBE REMOVAL

Indications for removal of chest tubes include resolution of the pneumothorax or fluid accumulation in the pleural space, or both. For a pneumothorax, the drainage system is left on suction

TABLE 8-3. Complications of Chest Tube Insertion

Unintentional tube placement into vital structures
  (lung, liver, spleen, etc.)
Bleeding
Reexpansion pulmonary edema
Residual pneumothorax
Residual hemothorax
Empyema

until the air leak stops. If an air leak persists, brief clamping of the chest tube can be performed to confirm that the leak is from the patient and not the system. If, after several days, an air leak persists, placement of an additional tube may be indicated. When the leak has ceased for more than 24 to 48 hours (or if no fluctuation is seen in the underwater seal chamber), the drainage system is placed on water seal by disconnecting the wall suction, followed by a chest film several hours later. If no pneumothorax is present and no air leak appears in the system with coughing, deep breathing, and reestablishment of suction, the tube can be removed. For fluid collections, the tube can be removed when drainage is minimal, unless sclerotherapy is planned.

Tube removal is often preceded by oral or parenteral analgesia at an appropriate time interval [52]. The suture holding the tube to the skin is cut. As the patient takes deep breaths, the tube is removed and the hole simultaneously covered with an occlusive petrolatum gauze dressing at peak inspiration (at which point only positive pressure can be generated in the pleural space, minimizing the possibility of drawing air in). A chest radiograph is performed immediately to check for a pneumothorax and is repeated 24 hours later to rule out reaccumulation of air or fluid.

RELATED SYSTEMS

Percutaneous aspiration of the pleural space to relieve a pneumothorax with no active air leak has been reported. Although successful in up to 75% of cases of needle-induced or traumatic pneumothoraces, the success rate is less for those with a spontaneous pneumothorax [53,54]. Small-bore catheters placed via Seldinger technique or using a trocar have been successful for treatment of spontaneous and iatrogenic pneumothoraces [55–57].

Heimlich valves (one-way flutter valves that allow egress of air from pleural tubes or catheters) have also gained more use by facilitating ambulation and outpatient care for those with persistent air leaks [58,59].

REFERENCES

1. *Advanced Trauma Life Support Instructor Manual.* Chicago, American College of Surgeons, 1989, p 105.
2. DeMeester TR, Lafontaine E: The pleura, in Sabiston DC, Spencer FC (eds): *Surgery of the Chest.* Philadelphia, WB Saunders, 1990, p 444.
3. Sahn SA: Benign and malignant pleural effusions, in Shields TW (ed): *General Thoracic Surgery.* Philadelphia, Lea & Febiger, 1989, p 613.
4. Collins JA, Samra GS: Failure of chest x-rays to diagnose pneumothoraces after blunt trauma. *Anaesthesia* 53:69, 1998.
5. Deslauriers J, LeBlanc P, McClish A: Bullous and bleb diseases of the lung, in Shields TW (ed): *General Thoracic Surgery.* Philadelphia, Lea & Febiger, 1989, p 727.
6. Gobbel WG, Rhea WG, Nelson IA, et al: Spontaneous pneumothorax. *J Thorac Cardiovasc Surg* 46:331, 1963.
7. Kircher LT Jr, Swartzel RL: Spontaneous pneumothorax and its treatment. *JAMA* 155:24, 1954.
8. Bernard RW, Stahl WM: Subclavian vein catheterization: a prospective study, I. Non-infectious complications. *Ann Surg* 173:184, 1971.
9. Hayes DF, Lucas CE: Bilateral tube thoracostomy to preclude tension pneumothorax in patients with acute respiratory insufficiency. *Am Surg* 42:330, 1976.
10. Ziegler DW, Agarwal NN: The morbidity and mortality of rib fractures. *J Trauma* 37:975, 1994.
11. Sandrasagra FA: Management of penetrating stab wounds of the chest: assessment of the indications for early operation. *Thorax* 33:474, 1978.
12. McNamara JJ, Messersmith JK, Dunn RA, et al: Thoracic injuries in combat casualties in Vietnam. *Ann Thorac Surg* 10:389, 1970.
13. Boyd AD: Pneumothorax and hemothorax, in Hood RM, Boyd AD, Culliford AT (eds): *Thoracic Trauma.* Philadelphia, WB Saunders, 1989, p 133.
14. Ali J, Qi W: Effectiveness of chest tube clamping in massive hemothorax. *J Trauma* 38:59, 1995.
15. Collins MP, Shuck JM, Wachtel TL, et al: Early decortication after thoracic trauma. *Arch Surg* 113:440, 1978.
16. Meyer DM, Jessen ME, Wait MA, et al: Early evaluation of traumatic retained hemothoraces using thoracoscopy: a prospective, randomized trial. *Ann Thorac Surg* 64:1396, 1997.
17. Miller JI Jr: Infections of the pleura, in Shields TW (ed): *General Thoracic Surgery.* Philadelphia, Lea & Febiger, 1989, p 633.
18. Bouros D, Schiza S, Patsourakis G, et al: Intrapleural streptokinase versus urokinase in the treatment of complicated parapneumonic effusions: a prospective double-blind study. *Am J Respir Crit Care Med* 155:291, 1997.
19. Roupie E, Bouabdallah K, Delclaux C, et al: Intrapleural administration of streptokinase in complicated purulent pleural effusion: a CT-guided strategy. *Intensive Care Med* 22:1351, 1996.
20. Robinson LA, Moulton AL, Fleming WH, et al: Intrapleural fibrinolytic treatment of multiloculated thoracic empyemas. *Ann Thorac Surg* 57:803, 1994.
21. Staats RA, Ellefson RD, Budahn LL, et al: The lipoprotein profile of chylous and unchylous pleural effusions. *Mayo Clin Proc* 55:700, 1980.
22. Miller JI Jr: Chylothorax and anatomy of the thoracic duct, in Shields TW (ed): *General Thoracic Surgery.* Philadelphia, Lea & Febiger, 1989, p 625.
23. Bessone LN, Ferguson TB, Burford TH: Chylothorax. *Ann Thorac Surg* 12:527, 1971.
24. Ross JK: A review of the surgery of the thoracic duct. *Thorax* 16:12, 1961.
25. Williams KR, Burford TH: The management of chylothorax. *Ann Surg* 160:131, 1964.
26. Selle JG, Snyder WA, Schreiber JT: Chylothorax. *Ann Surg* 177:245, 1977.
27. Anderson CB, Philpott GW, Ferguson TB: The treatment of malignant pleural effusions. *Cancer* 33:916, 1974.
28. Hausheer FH, Yarbro JW: Diagnosis and treatment of malignant pleural effusions. *Semin Oncol* 12:54, 1985.
29. Milanez RC, Vargas FS, Filomeno LB, et al: Intrapleural talc for the treatment of malignant pleural effusions secondary to breast cancer. *Cancer* 75:2688, 1995.
30. Heffner JE, Standerfer RJ, Torstveit J, et al: Clinical efficacy of doxycycline for pleurodesis. *Chest* 105:1743, 1994.
31. Daly RC, Mucha P, Pairolero PC, et al: The risk of percutaneous chest tube thoracostomy for blunt thoracic trauma. *Ann Emerg Med* 14:865, 1985.
32. Terzi A, Feil B, Bonadamin C, et al: The use of flexible spiral drains after non-cardiac thoracic surgery: a clinical study. *Eur J Cardiovasc Surg* 27:134, 2005.
33. Millikan JS, Moore EE, Steiner E, et al: Complications of tube thoracostomy for acute trauma. *Am J Surg* 140:738, 1980.
34. Baldt MM, Bankier AA, Germann PS, et al: Complications after emergency tube thoracostomy: assessment with CT. *Radiology* 195:539, 1995.
35. Griffith JR, Roberts M: Do junior doctors know where to insert chest drains safely? *Postgrad Med J* 81:456, 2005.
36. Trapnell DH, Thurston JGB: Unilateral pulmonary edema after pleural aspiration. *Lancet* 1:1367, 1970.
37. Janocik SE, Roy TM, Killeen TR: Re-expansion pulmonary edema: a preventable complication. *J Ky Med Assoc* 91:143, 1993.
38. Neugebauer MK, Fosburg RG, Trummer MJ: Routine antibiotic therapy following pleural space intubation: a reappraisal. *J Thorac Cardiovasc Surg* 61:882, 1971.
39. Evans JT, Green JD, Carlin PE, et al: Meta-analysis of antibiotics in tube thoracostomy. *Am Surg* 61:215, 1995.
40. Stone HH, Symbas PN, Hooper CA: Cefamandole for prophylaxis against infection in closed tube thoracostomy. *J Trauma* 21:975, 1981.
41. Nichols RL, Smith JW, Muzik AC, et al: Preventive antibiotic usage in traumatic thoracic injuries requiring closed tube thoracostomy. *Chest* 106:1493, 1994.
42. Edwards FH, Engelman RM, Houck P, et al: The Society of Thoracic Surgeons Practice Guideline Series: antibiotic prophylaxis in cardiac surgery, Part I. Duration. *Ann Thorac Surg* 81:397, 2006.
43. Gift AG, Bolgiano CS, Cunningham J: Sensations during chest tube removal. *Heart Lung* 20:131, 1991.
44. Carson MM, Barton DM, Morrison CC, et al: Managing pain during mediastinal chest tube removal. *Heart Lung* 23:500, 1994.
45. Kinney MR, Kirchhoff KT, Puntillo KA: Chest tube removal practices in critical care units in the United States. *Am J Crit Care* 4:419, 1995.
46. Hagl C, Harringer W, Gohrbandt B, et al: Site of pleural drain insertion and early postoperative pulmonary function following coronary artery bypass grafting with internal mammary artery. *Chest* 115:757, 1999.
47. Lancey RA, Gaca C, Vander Salm TJ: The use of smaller, more flexible chest drains following open heart surgery. *Chest* 119:19, 2001.
48. Ishikura H, Kimura F: The use of flexible silastic drains after chest surgery: novel thoracic drainage. *Ann Thorac Surg* 81:231, 2006.
49. Frankel TL, Hill PC, Stamou SB, et al: Silastic drains versus conventional chest tubes after coronary artery bypass. *Chest* 124:108, 2003.
50. Landolfo K, Smith P: Postoperative care in cardiac surgery, in Sabiston DC, Spencer FC (eds): *Surgery of the Chest.* 6th ed. Philadelphia, WB Saunders, 1996, p 230.
51. Cameron EW, Mirvis SE, Shanmuganathan K, et al: Computed tomography of malpositioned thoracostomy drains: a pictorial essay. *Clin Radiol* 52:187, 1997.
52. Puntillo KA: Effects of intrapleural bupivacaine on pleural chest tube removal pain: a randomized controlled trial. *Am J Crit Care* 5:102, 1996.

53. Delius RE, Obeid FN, Horst HM, et al: Catheter aspiration for simple pneumothorax. *Arch Surg* 124:883, 1989.

54. Andrevit P, Djedaini K, Teboul JL, et al: Spontaneous pneumothorax: comparison of thoracic drainage vs. immediate or delayed needle aspiration. *Chest* 108:335, 1995.

55. Conces DJ, Tarver RD, Gray WC, et al: Treatment of pneumothoraces utilizing small caliber chest tubes. *Chest* 94:55, 1988.

56. Peters J, Kubitschek KR: Clinical evaluation of a percutaneous pneumothorax catheter. *Chest* 86:714, 1984.

57. Minami H, Saka H, Senda K, et al: Small caliber catheter drainage for spontaneous pneumothorax. *Am J Med Sci* 304:345, 1992.

58. McKenna RJ Jr, Fischel RJ, Brenner M, et al: Use of the Heimlich valve to shorten hospital stay after lung reduction surgery for emphysema. *Ann Thorac Surg* 61:1115, 1996.

59. Ponn RB, Silverman HJ, Federico JA: Outpatient chest tube management. *Ann Thorac Surg* 64:1437, 1997.

Stephen J. Krinzman
Richard S. Irwin

CHAPTER **9**

Bronchoscopy

Since its commercial introduction for clinical use in 1968, flexible bronchoscopy has had a dramatic impact on the approach and management of patients with a wide variety of respiratory problems [1]. The procedure revolutionized the practice of clinical chest medicine. It offers a variety of features and capabilities that have fostered its widespread use: (a) it is easily performed, (b) it is associated with few complications [2], (c) it is much more comfortable [3] and safer [4] for the patient than rigid bronchoscopy, (d) it exposes a far greater proportion of the tracheobronchial tree (especially the upper lobes) to direct visualization than does rigid bronchoscopy [5], (e) it does not require general anesthesia or the use of an operating room [3], and (f) it may be performed at the bedside [3]. For all of these reasons, flexible bronchoscopy has largely replaced rigid bronchoscopy as the procedure of choice for most endoscopic evaluations of the airway. On the other hand, rigid bronchoscopy may be the procedure of choice [1,6] for (a) brisk hemoptysis (200 mL per 24 hours), (b) extraction of foreign bodies, (c) endobronchial resection of granulation tissue that might occur after traumatic and/or prolonged intubation, (d) biopsy of vascular tumors (e.g., bronchial carcinoid) in which brisk and excessive bleeding can be controlled by packing, (e) endoscopic laser surgery, and (f) dilation of tracheobronchial strictures and placement of airway stents.

DIAGNOSTIC INDICATIONS

GENERAL CONSIDERATIONS

Because flexible bronchoscopy can be performed easily even in intubated patients, the same general indications apply to critically ill patients on ventilators and to noncritically ill patients; however, only the indications most commonly encountered in critically ill patients are discussed here.

COMMON INDICATIONS

Hemoptysis

Hemoptysis is one of the most common clinical problems for which bronchoscopy is indicated [7,8]. Whether the patient complains of blood streaking or massive hemoptysis (expectoration of greater than 600 mL in 48 hours) [9], bronchoscopy should be considered to localize the site of bleeding and to diagnose the cause. Localization of the site of bleeding is crucial if definitive therapy such as surgery becomes necessary, and it is also useful to guide angiographic procedures. Bronchoscopy

performed within 48 hours of the time that bleeding stops is more likely to localize the site of bleeding (34% to 91%) compared with delayed bronchoscopy (11% to 52%) [10]. Bronchoscopy is more likely to identify a bleeding source in patients with moderate or severe hemoptysis [11]. Clinical judgment must dictate whether and when bronchoscopy is indicated. For instance, it is not indicated in patients with obvious pulmonary embolism with infarction. Whenever patients have an endotracheal or tracheostomy tube in place, hemoptysis should always be evaluated, because it may indicate potentially life-threatening tracheal damage. Unless the bleeding is massive, a flexible bronchoscope, rather than a rigid bronchoscope, is the instrument of choice for evaluating hemoptysis.

Diffuse Parenchymal Disease

In patients with diffuse pulmonary disease, the clinical setting influences the choice of procedure. When diffuse pulmonary infiltrates suggest sarcoidosis, carcinomatosis, or eosinophilic pneumonia, transbronchoscopic lung forceps biopsy should be considered initially because it has an extremely high yield in these situations. Transbronchial lung biopsy has a low yield for the definitive diagnosis of inorganic pneumoconiosis and pulmonary vasculitides [12]; when these disorders are suspected, surgical lung biopsy is the procedure of choice. In the case of pulmonary fibrosis and acute interstitial pneumonitis, transbronchial biopsy does not provide adequate tissue for a specific histologic diagnosis, although by excluding infection the procedure may provide sufficient information to guide therapy.

When an infectious process is suspected, the diagnostic yield depends on the organism and the immune status of the patient. In immunocompetent patients, bronchoalveolar lavage (BAL) has a sensitivity of 87% for detecting respiratory pathogens [13], and a negative BAL quantitative culture has a specificity of 96% in predicting sterile lung parenchyma. In bone marrow transplant recipients with pulmonary complications, BAL is diagnostic in 31% to 66% of patients [14]. BAL has a relatively poor sensitivity for detecting fungal infections in this population (40%) [15]. Transbronchial biopsy adds little additional information with respect to infectious processes, with a yield of less than 10% in bone marrow recipients [15–17]. Although noninfectious causes of pulmonary infiltrates may be identified by transbronchial biopsy, findings are nonspecific in the great majority of cases and must be weighed against a major complication rate of 7% [16]. In AIDS patients, the sensitivity of lavage or transbronchial lung biopsy for identifying all opportunistic organisms can be as high as 87% [18,19]. Transbronchial biopsy adds significantly to the diagnostic yield in AIDS patients and may be the sole means of making a diagnoses in up to 24% of patients, including diagnoses of *Pneumocystis jiroveci, Cryptococcus neoformans, Mycobacterium tuberculosis,* and nonspecific interstitial pneumonitis [20]. Lavage alone may have a sensitivity of up to 97% for the diagnosis of *P. jiroveci* pneumonia [21]. However, because induced sputum samples can also be positive for *P. jiroveci* in up to 79% of cases [21], induced expectorated sputum, when available, should be evaluated first for this organism before resorting to bronchoscopy.

Acute Inhalation Injury

In patients exposed to smoke inhalation, flexible nasopharyngoscopy, laryngoscopy, and bronchoscopy are indicated to identify the anatomic level and severity of injury [22,23]. Prophylactic intubation should be considered if considerable upper airway mucosal injury is noted early; acute respiratory failure is more likely in patients with mucosal changes seen at segmental or lower levels [24]. Upper airway obstruction is a life-threatening problem that usually develops during the initial 24 hours after inhalation injury. It correlates significantly with increased size of cutaneous burns, burns of the face and neck, and rapid intravenous fluid administration [25].

Blunt Chest Trauma

Flexible bronchoscopy has a high yield in the evaluation of patients after major chest trauma. Patients may present with atelectasis, pulmonary contusion, hemothorax, pneumothorax, pneumomediastinum, or hemoptysis. Prompt bronchoscopic evaluation of such patients has a diagnostic yield of 53%; findings may include tracheal or bronchial laceration or transection (14%), aspirated material (6%), supraglottic tear with glottic obstruction (2%), mucus plugging (15%), and distal hemorrhage (13%) [26]. Many of these diagnoses may not be clinically evident and require surgical intervention.

Postresectional Surgery

Flexible bronchoscopy can identify a disrupted suture line causing bleeding and pneumothorax [27] following surgery and an exposed endobronchial suture causing cough [28].

Assessment of Intubation Damage

When a nasotracheal or orotracheal tube of the proper size is in place, the balloon can be routinely deflated and the tube withdrawn over the bronchoscope to look for subglottic damage. The tube is withdrawn up through the vocal cords and over the flexible bronchoscope and glottic and supraglottic damage sought. This technique may by useful after reintubation for stridor, or when deflation of the endotracheal tube cuff does not produce a significant air leak, suggesting the potential for life threatening upper airway obstruction when extubation takes place. In patients on long-term ventilatory assistance with cuffed tracheostomy tubes, flexible bronchoscopy can help differentiate aspiration from tracheoesophageal fistula. With the bronchoscope in the distal trachea, the patient is asked to swallow a dilute solution of methylene blue. The absence of methylene blue in the trachea and its presence leaking around and out of the tracheostomy stoma provide accurate evidence of a swallowing abnormality and the absence of a tracheoesophageal fistula.

Diagnosing Ventilator-Associated Pneumonia

Clinicians' ability to determine the probability of ventilator-associated pneumonia (VAP) is very limited, with a sensitivity of only 50% and a specificity of 58% [29]. Quantitative cultures obtained via bronchoscopy may thus play an important role in the diagnostic strategy. Quantitative cultures of BAL fluid and protected specimen brush (PSB), with thresholds of 10^4 colony forming units (cfu)/mL and 10^3 cfu/mL respectively, are most commonly employed prior to the initiation of antimicrobial therapy. Cultures of bronchial washings do not add to the diagnostic yield of quantitative BAL culture alone [30]. For a brief description of how to perform BAL and obtain PSB cultures, see the Procedure Section below.

For BAL, an evidence-based analysis of 23 prior investigations yields a sensitivity of 73% and a specificity of 82%, indicating that BAL cultures fail to diagnose VAP in almost one fourth of all cases [31]. A similar analysis of PSB cultures indicates a very wide range of results, with a sensitivity of 33% to greater than 95% and a median of 67%, and a specificity of 50% to 100% with a median of 95% [32,33]. PSB is thus more specific than it is sensitive, and negative results may not be sufficient to exclude the presence of VAP [34]. Blind protected telescoping catheter specimens perform similarly to bronchoscopically directed PSB cultures [35,36]. It is critical to note that colony counts change very quickly with antibiotic therapy. Within 12 hours of starting antibiotic therapy, 50% of all significant bacterial species initially identified in significant numbers had colony counts reduced to below the "pathogenic" threshold level. After 48 hours of therapy, only 14% of isolates are still present above threshold values [37]. It is therefore essential to obtain quantitative cultures before starting or changing antibiotics.

Despite the greater accuracy of quantitative bronchoscopic cultures, prospective randomized trials of early invasive diagnostic strategies employing bronchoscopy and quantitative lower respiratory tract cultures for VAP have not demonstrated significant advantages in mortality or other major clinical endpoints [38]. Recent evidence-based consensus guidelines for the management of VAP recommend obtaining quantitative or semiquantitative lower respiratory tract cultures when VAP is suspected, with subsequent management based on culture results and clinical response to therapy [39]. Further investigations will be required to clarify the role of quantitative cultures in management protocols.

THERAPEUTIC INDICATIONS

ATELECTASIS

Although atelectasis may be due to mucus plugging, bronchoscopy should be performed in patients who do not improve after chest physiotherapy to rule out endobronchial obstruction by carcinoma, foreign body, mucoid impaction, or clot. When atelectasis occurs in critically ill patients who had a normal chest film on admission, mucus plugging is the most likely cause [40]. Bronchoscopy has a success rate of up to 89% in cases of lobar atelectasis, but only produced clinical improvement in 44% of patients when performed for retained secretions [41]. One randomized trial found no advantage of bronchoscopy over a very aggressive regimen of frequent chest physiotherapy, recruitment maneuvers, saline nebulization, and postural drainage [42]. Occasionally, the direct instillation of acetylcysteine (Mucomyst) through the bronchoscope may be necessary to liquefy the thick, tenacious inspissated mucus [43]. Because acetylcysteine may induce bronchospasm in asthmatics, these patients must be pre-treated with a bronchodilator.

FOREIGN BODIES

Although the rigid bronchoscope is considered by many to be the instrument of choice for removing foreign bodies, devices with which to grasp objects are available for use with the flexible bronchoscope [44].

ENDOTRACHEAL INTUBATION

In patients with ankylosing spondylitis and other mechanical problems of the neck, the flexible bronchoscope may be used as an obturator for endotracheal intubation [27]. The bronchoscope with an endotracheal tube passed over it can be passed transnasally (after proper local anesthesia) through the vocal cords into the trachea. Then the tube can be passed over the scope. This same technique can be used in patients with tetanus complicated by trismus and in patients with acute supraglottitis [45]. In the latter two instances, the procedure should preferably be done in the operating room with an anesthesiologist and otolaryngologist present.

HEMOPTYSIS

On rare occasions where brisk bleeding threatens asphyxiation, endobronchial tamponade may stabilize the patient before definitive therapy is performed [46]. With the use of the flexible bronchoscope, usually passed through a rigid bronchoscope or endotracheal tube, a Fogarty catheter with balloon is passed into the bleeding lobar orifice. When the balloon is inflated and wedged tightly, the patient may be transferred to surgery or angiography for bronchial arteriography and bronchial artery embolization [47–49]. Hemostasis may also be achieved by utilizing flexible bronchoscopy to apply oxidized regenerated cellulose mesh to the bleeding site [50].

CENTRAL OBSTRUCTING AIRWAY LESIONS

Some patients with cancer and others with benign lesions that obstruct the larynx, trachea, and major bronchi can be treated by electrocautery, laser photoresection, cryotherapy, or phototherapy [51,52] through the bronchoscope. Flexible bronchoscopy can also be used to place catheters that facilitate endobronchial delivery of radiation (brachytherapy). Metal or silicone endobronchial stents can be placed bronchoscopically to relieve stenosis of large airways [53].

CLOSURE OF BRONCHOPLEURAL FISTULA

Bronchopleural fistula (BPF) is an acquired pathway between the bronchial tree and pleural space. After placement of a chest tube, drainage of the pleural space, and stabilization of the patient (e.g., infection, cardiovascular and respiratory systems), bronchoscopy can be used to visualize a proximal BPF or localize a distal BPF; it can also be used in attempts to close the BPF [54,55]. Although the published experience on bronchoscopically sealing BPFs is limited, a number of case reports have

suggested that a variety of materials, injected through the bronchoscope, may successfully seal BPFs [56,57]. These materials have included doxycycline and tetracycline followed by autologous blood instillation to form an obstructive blood clot, lead fishing weights or shot, tissue adhesive, fibrin glue, absorbable gelatin sponge, angiographic occlusion coils, silver nitrate, and balloon occlusion.

COMPLICATIONS

When performed by a trained specialist, *routine* flexible bronchoscopy is extremely safe. Mortality should not exceed 0.1% [2], and overall complications should not exceed 8.1% [2]. The rare deaths have been due to excessive premedication or topical anesthesia, respiratory arrest from hemorrhage, laryngospasm, or bronchospasm, and cardiac arrest from acute myocardial infarction [58,59]. Nonfatal complications occurring within 24 hours of the procedure include fever (1.2% to 24%) [2,60,61], pneumonia (0.6% to 6%) [2,60], vasovagal reactions (2.4%) [2], laryngospasm and bronchospasm (0.1% to 0.4%) [2,58], cardiac arrhythmias (0.9% to 4%) [2,62], pneumothorax (4% after transbronchial biopsy) [64], anesthesia-related problems (0.1%) [2,58], and aphonia (0.1%) [2]. Fever may occur in up to 24% of patients after bronchoscopy and appears to be cytokine mediated and uncommonly indicative of a true infection or bacteremia [61]. Transient bacteremias often occur (15.4% to 33%) after rigid bronchoscopy [63,64], probably due to trauma to the teeth and airways. Most investigations have found that the incidence of bacteremia after transoral flexible bronchoscopy is much lower (0.7%) [65]. Guidelines published by the American Heart Association recommend endocarditis prophylaxis for rigid but not for flexible bronchoscopy, except in high-risk cardiac patients such as those with prosthetic valves, where prophylaxis should be considered [66].

Although routine bronchoscopy is extremely safe, critically ill patients appear to be at higher risk of complications. Asthmatics are prone to develop laryngospasm and bronchospasm. Bone marrow transplant recipients are more likely to develop major bleeding during bronchoscopy (0% to 6%) [17,67], particularly if protected specimen brush or transbronchial lung biopsy is performed (7.7% versus 1.5% for BAL alone) [67]. Patients with uremia are at increased risk of bleeding [68]. One investigation found that aspirin use did not increase bleeding risk after transbronchial biopsy [69]. In critically ill, mechanically ventilated patents, bronchoscopy causes a transient decrease in Pao_2 (partial arterial oxygen pressure) of approximately 25% [70], and transbronchial lung biopsy is more likely to result in pneumothorax (7% to 23%) [71,72], particularly in patients with acute respiratory distress syndrome (ARDS) (up to 36%) [73]. Patients with ARDS also have more pronounced declines in oxygenation, with a mean decrease of more than 50% in the Pao_2 [70].

CONTRAINDICATIONS

Bronchoscopy should not be performed (a) unless an experienced bronchoscopist is available; (b) when the patient will not or cannot cooperate; (c) when adequate oxygenation cannot be maintained during the procedure; (d) in unstable cardiac patients [74–76]; and (e) in untreated symptomatic asthmatics [77]. The impact of coagulation parameters and antiplatelet agents on bleeding risk during transbronchial biopsy remains controversial [69,78]. In patients with recent cardiac ischemia, the major complication rate is low (3% to 5%) and is similar to that of other critically ill populations [79,80]. Although patients with stable carbon dioxide retention can safely undergo bronchoscopy with a flexible instrument [81], premedication, sedation during the procedure, and supplemental oxygen must be used with caution.

Consideration of bronchoscopy in neurologic and neurosurgical patients requires attention to the effects of bronchoscopy on intracranial pressure (ICP) and cerebral perfusion pressure (CPP). In patients with head trauma, bronchoscopy causes the ICP to increase by at least 50% in 88% of patients, and by at least 100% in 69% of patients, despite the use of deep sedation and paralysis [82]. Because mean arterial pressure tends to rise in parallel with ICP, there is often no change in CPP. No significant neurologic complications have been noted in patients with severe head trauma [82,83] or with space-occupying intracranial lesions with computed tomographic evidence of elevated ICP [84]. Bronchoscopy in such patients should be accompanied by deep sedation, paralysis, and medications for cerebral protection (thiopental, lidocaine). Cerebral hemodynamics should be continuously monitored to ensure that intracranial pressures and CPP are within acceptable levels. Caution is warranted in patients with markedly elevated baseline ICP or with borderline CPP.

PROCEDURE

AIRWAY AND INTUBATION

In nonintubated patients, flexible bronchoscopy can be performed by the transnasal route or transoral route with a bite block [1]. In intubated and mechanically ventilated patients, the flexible bronchoscope can be passed into the tube through a swivel adapter with a rubber diaphragm that will prevent loss of the delivered respiratory gases [85]. To prevent dramatic increases in airway resistance and an unacceptable loss of tidal volumes, the lumen of the endotracheal tube should be at least 2 mm larger than the outer diameter of the bronchoscope [86,87]. Thus, flexible bronchoscopy with an average adult-sized instrument (outside diameter of scope 4.8 to 5.9 mm) can be performed in a ventilated patient if there is an endotracheal tube in place that is 8 mm or larger in internal diameter. If the endotracheal tube is smaller, a pediatric bronchoscope (outside diameter 3.5 mm) or intubation endoscope (outside diameter 3.8 mm) must be used.

PREMEDICATION

Topical anesthesia may be achieved by hand-nebulized lidocaine and lidocaine jelly as a lubricant [1], and by instilling approximately 3 mL of 1% or 2% lidocaine at the main carina and, if needed, into the lower airways. Lidocaine is absorbed through the mucous membranes, producing peak serum concentrations that are nearly as high as when the equivalent dose is administered intravenously, although toxicity is rare if the total dose does not exceed 6 to 7 mg/kg. In patients with hepatic or cardiac insufficiency, lidocaine clearance is reduced, and the dose should be decreased to a maximum of 4 to 5 mg/kg [88]. Administering nebulized lidocaine prior to the procedure sub-

stantially increases the total lidocaine dose without improving cough or patient comfort [89]. Conscious sedation with incremental doses of midazolam, titrated to produce light sleep, produces amnesia in greater than 95% of patients, but adequate sedation may require a total of greater than 20 mg in some subjects [90]. Cough suppression is more effective when narcotics are added to benzodiazepine premedication regimens [90]. Premedication with intravenous atropine has not been found to reduce secretions, decrease coughing, or prevent bradycardia [91,92].

MECHANICAL VENTILATION

Maintaining adequate oxygenation and ventilation while preventing breath-stacking and positive end expiratory pressure (auto-PEEP) may be challenging when insertion of the bronchoscope reduces the effective lumen of the endotracheal tube by more than 50%. PEEP caused by standard scopes and tubes will approach 20 cm H_2O with the potential for barotrauma [86]. PEEP, if already being delivered, must be discontinued before inserting the scope [86]. The inspired oxygen concentration must be temporarily increased to 100% prior to starting the procedure [86]. With the help of a respiratory care practitioner, expired volumes should be constantly measured to ensure that they are adequate (tidal volumes usually have to be increased 40% to 50%) [88]. Meeting these ventilatory goals may require increasing the high pressure limit in volume cycled ventilation to near its maximal value, allowing the ventilator to generate the force needed to overcome the added resistance caused by the bronchoscope. Although this increases the measured peak airway pressure, the alveolar pressure is not likely to change significantly because the lung is protected by the resistance of the bronchoscope [93]. Alternatively, decreasing the inspiratory flow rate in an attempt to decrease measured peak pressures may paradoxically increase alveolar pressures by decreasing expiratory time and thus increasing auto-PEEP. Suctioning should be kept to a minimum and for short periods of time, because suctioning will decrease the tidal volumes being delivered [86].

QUANTITATIVE CULTURES

BAL is performed by advancing the bronchoscope until the tip wedges tightly in a distal bronchus from the area of greatest clinical interest. If the disease process is diffuse, perform the procedure in the right middle lobe because this is the area from which the best returns are most consistently obtained. Three aliquots of saline, typically 35 to 50 mL, are then instilled and withdrawn; in some protocols, the first aliquot is discarded to prevent contamination with more proximal secretions. A total instilled volume of 100 mL with at least 5% to 10% retrieved constitutes an adequate specimen [94]. PSB may be performed through a bronchoscope by advancing the plugged catheter assembly until it projects from the bronchoscope. When the area of interest is reached (e.g., purulent secretions can be seen), the distal plug is ejected, and the brush is then fully advanced beyond the protective sheath. After the specimen is obtained, the brush is pulled back into the sheath, and only then is the catheter assembly removed from the bronchoscope. Blinded plugged telescoping catheter (BPTC) specimens are obtained by advancing the catheter 30 to 40 cm into the airways through the endotracheal tube until resistance is met. The catheter is then withdrawn a few centimeters, and the inner catheter is advanced 2 to 3 cm beyond the tip of the outer sheath, extruding the plug. Three brief aspirations are then applied to the inner catheter, the catheter is withdrawn several centimeters into the outer sheath, and the assembly is then removed. The distal end is cut with sterile scissors distal to the inner catheter, the inner catheter is advanced, and 1 mL of sterile saline is flushed through the catheter and collected for culture [95].

REFERENCES

1. Sackner MA: Bronchofiberscopy. *Am Rev Respir Dis* 111:62, 1975.
2. Pereira W Jr, Kovnat DM, Snider GL: A prospective cooperative study of complications following flexible fiberoptic bronchoscopy. *Chest* 73:813, 1978.
3. Rath GS, Schaff JT, Snider GL: Flexible fiberoptic bronchoscopy: techniques and review of 100 bronchoscopies. *Chest* 63:689, 1973.
4. Lukomsky GI, Ovchinnikov AA, Bilal A: Complications of bronchoscopy: comparison of rigid bronchoscopy under general anesthesia and flexible fiberoptic bronchoscopy under topical anesthesia. *Chest* 79:316, 1981.
5. Kovnat DM, Rath GS, Anderson WM, et al: Maximal extent of visualization of bronchial tree by flexible fiberoptic bronchoscopy. *Am Rev Respir Dis* 110:88, 1974.
6. Prakash UBS, Stuffs SE: The bronchoscopy survey: some reflections. *Chest* 100:1660, 1991.
7. Khan MA, Whitcomb ME, Snider GL: Flexible fiberoptic bronchoscopy. *Am J Med* 61:151, 1976.
8. Selecky PA: Evaluation of hemoptysis through the bronchoscope. *Chest* 73[Suppl]:741, 1978.
9. Crocco JA, Rooney JJ, Fankushen DS, et al: Massive hemoptysis. *Arch Intern Med* 121:495, 1968.
10. Dweik RA, Stoller JK: Role of bronchoscopy in massive hemoptysis. *Clin Chest Med* 20:89–105, 1999.
11. Hirshberg B, Biran I, Glazer M, et al: Hemoptysis: etiology, evaluation, and outcome in a tertiary referral hospital. *Chest* 112:440–444, 1997.
12. Schnabel A, Holl-Ulrich K, Dahloff K, et al: Efficacy of transbronchial biopsy in pulmonary vasculitides. *Eur Respir J* 10:2738–2743, 1997.
13. Kirtland SH, Corley DE, Winterbauer RH, et al: The diagnosis of ventilator-associated pneumonia: a comparison of histologic, microbiologic, and clinical criteria. *Chest* 112:445, 1997.
14. Gruson D, Hilbert H, Valentino R, et al: Utility of fiberoptic bronchoscopy in neutropenic patients admitted to the intensive care unit with pulmonary infiltrates. *Crit Care Med* 28:2224, 2000.
15. Jain O, Sunder S, Mile Y, et al: Role of flexible bronchoscopy in immunocompromised patients with lung infiltrates. *Chest* 125:712, 2004.
16. Patel N, Lee P, Kim J, et al: The influence of diagnostic bronchoscopy on clinical outcomes comparing adult autologous and allogeneic bone marrow transplant recipients. *Chest* 127:1388, 2005.
17. White P, Bonacum JT, Miller CB: Utility of fiberoptic bronchoscopy in bone marrow transplant patients. *Bone Marrow Transplant* 20:681, 1997.
18. Emanuel D, Peppard J, Stover D, et al: Rapid immunodiagnosis of cytomegalovirus pneumonia by bronchoalveolar lavage using human and murine monoclonal antibodies. *Ann Intern Med* 104:476, 1986.
19. Broaddus C, Dake MD, Stulbarg MS, et al: Bronchoalveolar lavage and transbronchial biopsy for the diagnosis of pulmonary infections in the acquired immunodeficiency syndrome. *Ann Intern Med* 102:747, 1985.
20. Raoof S, Rosen MJ, Khan FA: Role of bronchoscopy in AIDS. *Clin Chest Med* 20:63, 1999.
21. Hopewell PC: *Pneumocystis carinii* pneumonia: diagnosis. *J Infect Dis* 157:1115, 1988.
22. Wanner A, Cutchavaree A: Early recognition of upper airway obstruction following smoke inhalation. *Am Rev Respir Dis* 108:1421, 1973.
23. Hunt JL, Agree RN, Pruitt BA Jr: Fiberoptic bronchoscopy in acute inhalation injury. *J Trauma* 15:641, 1975.
24. Brandstetter RD: Flexible fiberoptic bronchoscopy in the intensive care unit. *Intensive Care Med* 4:248, 1989.
25. Haponik EF, Meyers DA, Munster AM, et al: Acute upper airway injury in burn patients: serial changes of flow-volume curves and nasopharyngoscopy. *Am Rev Respir Dis* 135:360, 1987.
26. Hara KS, Prakash UBS: Fiberoptic bronchoscopy in the evaluation of acute chest and upper airway trauma. *Chest* 96:627, 1989.
27. Landa JF: Indications for bronchoscopy. *Chest* 73[Suppl]:686, 1978.
28. Albertini RE: Cough caused by exposed endobronchial sutures. *Ann Intern Med* 94:205, 1981.
29. Fartoukh M, Maitre B, Honore S, et al: Diagnosing pneumonia during mechanical ventilation: the clinical infection score revisited. *Am J Respir Crit Care Med* 168:173, 2003.
30. Pinckard JK, Kollef M, Dunne WM: Culturing bronchial washings obtained during bronchoscopy fails to add diagnostic utility to culturing the bronchoalveolar lavage fluid alone. *Diagn Microbiol Infect Dis* 43:99, 2002.
31. Torres A, El-Ebiary M: Bronchoscopic BAL in the diagnosis of ventilator-associated pneumonia. *Chest* 117:198, 2000.
32. Baughman RP: Protected-specimen brush technique in the diagnosis of ventilator associated pneumonia. *Chest* 117:203S, 2000.
33. Grossman RF, Fein A: Evidence-based assessment of diagnostic tests for ventilator associated pneumonia. *Chest* 117:177S, 2000.
34. Kirtland SH, Corley DE, Winterbauer RH, et al: The diagnosis of ventilator associated pneumonia: a comparison of histologic, microbiologic, and clinical criteria. *Chest* 112:445, 1997.
35. Brun-Bruisson C, Fartoukh M, Lechapt E, et al: Contribution of blinded protected quantitative specimens to the diagnostic and therapeutic management of ventilator-associated pneumonia. *Chest* 128:533, 2005.
36. Wood AY, Davit AJ, Ciraulo DL, et al: A prospective assessment of diagnostic efficacy of blind protected bronchial brushings compared to bronchoscope assisted lavage, bronchoscope-directed brushings, and blind endotracheal aspirates in ventilator assisted pneumonia. *J Trauma* 55:825, 2003.
37. Prats E, Dorca J, Pujol M, et al: Effects of antibiotics on protected specimen brush sampling in ventilator associated pneumonia. *Eur Respir J* 19:944, 2002.
38. Shorr AF, Sherner JH, Jackson WL, et al: Invasive approaches to the diagnosis of ventilator-associated pneumonia: a meta-analysis. *Crit Care Med* 33:46, 2005.
39. American Thoracic Society: Guidelines for the management of adults with hospital acquired, ventilator-associated, and healthcare-associated pneumonia. *Am J Respir Crit Care Med* 171:388, 2005.
40. Mahajan VK, Catron PW, Huber GL: The value of fiberoptic bronchoscopy in the management of pulmonary collapse. *Chest* 73:817, 1978.
41. Kreider ME, Lipson DA: Bronchoscopy for atelectasis in the ICU: a case report and review of the literature. *Chest* 124:344, 2003.
42. Marini JJ, Pierson DJ, Hudson LD: Acute lobar atelectasis: a prospective comparison of fiberoptic bronchoscopy and respiratory therapy. *Am Rev Respir Dis* 119:971, 1979.
43. Lieberman J: The appropriate use of mucolytic agents. *Am J Med* 49:1, 1970.
44. Cunanan OS: The flexible fiberoptic bronchoscope in foreign body removal: experience in 300 cases. *Chest* 73:725, 1978.
45. Giudice JC, Komansky HJ: Acute epiglottitis: the use of a fiberoptic bronchoscope in diagnosis and therapy. *Chest* 75:211, 1979.
46. Saw EC, Gottlieb LS, Yokoyama T, et al: Flexible fiberoptic bronchoscopy and endobronchial tamponade in the management of massive hemoptysis. *Chest* 70:589, 1976.
47. Bredin CP, Richardson PR, King TKC: Treatment of massive hemoptysis by combined occlusion of pulmonary and bronchial arteries. *Am Rev Respir Dis* 117:969, 1978.
48. Remy J, Arnaud A, Fardou H, et al: Treatment of hemoptysis by embolization of bronchial arteries. *Radiology* 122:33, 1977.
49. White RI, Kaufman SL, Barth KH: Therapeutic embolization with detachable silicone balloons: early clinical experience. *JAMA* 241:1257, 1979.
50. Valipour A, Kreuzer A, Koller H, et al: Bronchoscopy-guided topical hemostatic tamponade therapy for the management of life threatening hemoptysis. *Chest* 127:2113, 2005.
51. Seijo LM, Sterman DH: Interventional pulmonology. *N Engl J Med* 344:740, 2001.
52. Beamis J: Interventional pulmonology techniques for treating malignant large airway obstruction: an update. *Current Opin Pulm Med* 11:292, 2005.
53. Prakash UBS: Advances in bronchoscopic procedures. *Chest* 116:1404, 1999.
54. Powner DJ, Bierman MI: Thoracic and extrathoracic bronchial fistulas. *Chest* 100:480, 1991.
55. Baumann MH, Sahn SA: Medical management and therapy of bronchopleural fistulas in the mechanically ventilated patient. *Chest* 97:721, 1990.
56. Salmon CJ, Ponn RB, Westcott JL: Endobronchial vascular occlusion coils for control of a large parenchymal bronchopleural fistula. *Chest* 98:233, 1990.
57. Martin WR, Siefkin AD, Allen R: Closure of a bronchopleural fistula with bronchoscopic instillation of tetracycline. *Chest* 99:1040, 1991.
58. Credle WF, Smiddy JF, Elliott RC: Complications of fiberoptic bronchoscopy. *Am Rev Respir Dis* 109:67, 1974.
59. Suratt PM, Smiddy JF, Gruber B: Deaths and complications associated with fiberoptic bronchoscopy. *Chest* 69:747, 1976.
60. Pereira W, Kovnat DM, Khan MA, et al: Fever and pneumonia after flexible fiberoptic bronchoscopy. *Am Rev Respir Dis* 112:59, 1975.
61. Krause A, Hohberg B, Heine F, et al: Cytokines derived from alveolar macrophages induce fever after bronchoscopy and bronchoalveolar lavage. *Am J Resp Crit Care Med* 155:1793, 1997.
62. Stubbs SE, Brutinel WM: Complications of bronchoscopy, in Prakash USB (ed): *Bronchoscopy*, New York, Lippincott Williams & Wilkins, 1994; p 357.
63. Burman SO: Bronchoscopy and bacteremia. *J Thorac Cardiovasc Surg* 40:635, 1960.
64. Everett ED, Hirschmann JV: Transient bacteremia and endocarditis prophylaxis: a review. *Medicine* 56:61, 1977.
65. Yigla M, Oren I, Solomonov A, et al: Incidence of bacteraemia following fiberoptic bronchoscopy. *Eur Resp J* 14:789, 1999.
66. Dajani AS, Taubert KA, Wilson W, et al: Prevention of bacterial endocarditis: recommendations of the American Heart Association. *JAMA* 277:1794, 1997.
67. Dunagan DP, Baker AM, Hurd DD: Bronchoscopic evaluation of pulmonary infiltrates following bone marrow transplantation. *Chest* 111:135, 1997.
68. Zavala DC: Pulmonary hemorrhage in fiberoptic transbronchial biopsy. *Chest* 70:584, 1976.
69. Herth FJ, Becker HD, Ernst A: Aspirin does not increase bleeding complications after transbronchial biopsy. *Chest* 122:1461, 2002.
70. Trouillet JL, Guiguet M, Gibert C, et al: Fiberoptic bronchoscopy in ventilated patients: evaluation of cardiopulmonary risk under midazolam sedation. *Chest* 97:927, 1990.
71. Pincus PS, Kallenbach JM, Hurwitz MD, et al: Transbronchial biopsy during mechanical ventilation. *Crit Care Med* 15:1136, 1987.
72. O'Brien JD, Ettinger NA, Shevlin D: Safety and yield of transbronchial biopsy in mechanically ventilated patients. *Crit Care Med* 25:440, 1997.
73. Bulpa PA, Dive AM, Mertens L, et al: Combined bronchoalveolar lavage and transbronchial lung biopsy: safety and yield in ventilated patients. *Eur Respir J* 21:489, 2003.
74. Shrader DL, Lakshminarayan S: The effect of fiberoptic bronchoscopy on cardiac rhythm. *Chest* 73:821, 1978.
75. Lundgren R, Haggmark S, Reiz S: Hemodynamic effects of flexible fiberoptic bronchoscopy performed under topical anesthesia. *Chest* 82:295, 1982.

76. Luck JC, Messeder OH, Rubenstein MJ, et al: Arrhythmias from fiberoptic bronchoscopy. *Chest* 74:139, 1978.

77. Sahn SA, Scoggin C: Fiberoptic bronchoscopy in bronchial asthma: a word of caution. *Chest* 69:39, 1976.

78. Chinsky K: Bleeding risk and bronchoscopy: in search of the evidence in evidence-based medicine. *Chest* 127:1875, 2005.

79. Dweik RA, Mehta AC, Meeker DP, et al: Analysis of the safety of bronchoscopy after recent acute myocardial infarction. *Chest* 110:825, 1996.

80. Dunagan DP, Burke HL, Aquino SL, et al: Fiberoptic bronchoscopy in coronary care unit patients: indications, safety and clinical implications. *Chest* 114:1660, 1998.

81. Salisbury BG, Metzger LF, Altose MD, et al: Effect of fiberoptic bronchoscopy on respiratory performance in patients with chronic airways obstruction. *Thorax* 30:441, 1975.

82. Kerwin AJ, Croce MA, Timmons SD, et al: Effects of fiberoptic bronchoscopy on intracranial pressure in patients with brain injury; a prospective clinical study. *J Trauma* 48:878, 2000.

83. Peerless JR, Snow N, Likavec MJ, et al: The effect of fiberoptic bronchoscopy on cerebral hemodynamics in patients with severe head injury. *Chest* 108:962, 1995.

84. Bajwa MK, Henein S, Kamholz SL: Fiberoptic bronchoscopy in the presence of space-occupying intracranial lesions. *Chest* 104:101, 1993.

85. Reichert WW, Hall WJ, Hyde RW: A simple disposable device for performing fiberoptic bronchoscopy on patients requiring continuous artificial ventilation. *Am Rev Respir Dis* 109:394, 1974.

86. Lindholm C-E, Ollman B, Snyder JV, et al: Cardiorespiratory effects of flexible fiberoptic bronchoscopy in critically ill patients. *Chest* 74:362, 1978.

87. Lawson RW, Peters JI, Shelledy DC: Effects of fiberoptic bronchoscopy during mechanical ventilation in a lung model. *Chest* 118:824, 2000.

88. Milman N, Laub M, Munch EP, et al: Serum concentrations of lignocaine and its metabolite monoethylglycinexylidide during fiberoptic bronchoscopy in local anesthesia. *Respir Med* 92:40, 1998.

89. Stolz D, Chhajed PN, Leuppi J, et al: Nebulized lidocaine for flexible bronchoscopy: a randomized, double-blind, placebo-controlled trial. *Chest* 128:1756, 2005.

90. Williams TJ, Bowie PE: Midazolam sedation to produce complete amnesia for bronchoscopy: 2 years' experience at a district hospital. *Respir Med* 93:361, 1999.

91. Cowl CT, Prakash UBS, Kruger BR: The role of anticholinergics in bronchoscopy: a randomized clinical trial. *Chest* 118:188, 2000.

92. Williams T, Brooks T, Ward C: The role of atropine premedication in fiberoptic bronchoscopy using intravenous midazolam sedation. *Chest* 113:113, 1998.

93. Lawson RW, Peters JI, Shelledy DC: Effects of fiberoptic bronchoscopy during mechanical ventilation in a lung model. *Chest* 118:824, 2000.

94. Meyer, KC: The role of bronchoalveolar lavage in interstitial lung disease. *Clin Chest Med* 25:637, 2004.

95. Pham LH, Brun-Buisson C, Legrand P, et al: Diagnosis of nosocomial pneumonia in mechanically ventilated patients: comparison of a plugged telescoping catheter with a protected specimen brush. *Am Rev Resp Dis* 143:1055, 1991.

Mark M. Wilson
Richard S. Irwin

CHAPTER **10**

Thoracentesis

Thoracentesis is an invasive procedure that involves the introduction of a needle, cannula, or trocar into the pleural space to remove accumulated fluid or air. Although a few prospective studies have critically evaluated the clinical value and complications associated with it [1–3], most studies concerning thoracentesis have dealt with the interpretation of the pleural fluid analyses [4,5].

INDICATIONS

Although history (cough, dyspnea, or pleuritic chest pain) and physical findings (dullness to percussion, decreased breath sounds, and decreased vocal fremitus) suggest that an effusion is present, chest radiography or ultrasonic examination is essential to confirm the clinical suspicion. Thoracentesis can be performed for diagnostic or therapeutic reasons. When done for diagnostic reasons, the procedure should be performed whenever possible before any treatment has been given to avoid confusion in interpretation [6]. Analysis of pleural fluid has been shown to yield clinically useful information in more than 90% of cases [3]. The four most common diagnoses for symptomatic and asymptomatic pleural effusions are malignancy, congestive heart failure, parapneumonia, and postoperative sympathetic effusions [7]. A diagnostic algorithm for evaluation of a pleural effusion of unknown etiology is presented in Figure 10-1. In patients whose pleural effusion remains undiagnosed after thoracentesis and closed pleural biopsy, thoracoscopy should be considered for visualization of the pleura and directed biopsy. Thoracoscopy has provided a positive diagnosis in more than 80% of patients with recurrent pleural effusions that are not diagnosed by repeated thoracentesis, pleural biopsy, or bronchoscopy [8].

Therapeutic thoracentesis is indicated to remove fluid or air that is causing cardiopulmonary embarrassment or for relief of severe symptoms. Definitive drainage of the pleural space with a thoracostomy tube must be done for a tension pneumothorax and should be considered for pneumothorax that is slowly enlarging or the instillation of a sclerosing agent after drainage of a recurrent malignant pleural effusion [9].

CONTRAINDICATIONS

Absolute contraindications to performing a thoracentesis are an uncooperative patient, the inability to identify the top of the rib clearly under the percutaneous puncture site, a lack of expertise in performing the procedure, and the presence of a coagulation abnormality that cannot be corrected. Relative con-

traindications to a thoracentesis include entry into an area where known bullous lung disease exists, a patient on positive end expiratory pressure, and a patient who has only one "functioning" lung (the other having been surgically removed or that has severe disease limiting its gas exchange function). In these settings, it may be safer to perform the thoracentesis under ultrasonic guidance.

COMPLICATIONS

A number of prospective studies have documented that complications associated with the procedure are not infrequent [1,2,10]. The overall complication rate has been reported to be as high as 50% to 78% and can be further categorized as major (15% to 19%) or minor (31% to 63%) [2,3]. Complication rates appear to be indirectly related to experience level of the operator; the more experienced, the fewer the complications [11]. Although death due to the procedure is infrequently reported, complications may be life threatening [1].

Major complications include pneumothorax, hemopneumothorax, hemorrhage, hypotension, and reexpansion pulmonary edema. The reported incidence of pneumothorax varies between 3% and 30% [1–3,11–14], with up to one third to one half of those with demonstrated pneumothoraces requiring subsequent intervention. Various investigators have reported associations between pneumothorax and underlying lung disease (chronic obstructive pulmonary disease, prior thoracic radiation, prior thoracic surgery, lung cancer) [10,12,13,15], needle size and technique [3,15], number of passes required to obtain a sample [12,15], aspiration of air during the procedure [12], operator experience [1,3,10,11], use of a vacuum bottle [13], size of the effusion [2,15], and mechanical ventilation versus spontaneously breathing patients [16]. Some of the above-mentioned studies report directly contradictory findings compared to other similar studies. This is most apparent in the reported association between pneumothorax and therapeutic thoracentesis [3,10,15], which was not supported by subsequent large prospective trials [13,14]. The most likely explanation for this discrepancy in the literature concerning the presumed increased risk for pneumothorax for therapeutic over diagnostic procedures is the generally lower level of operator experience in the first group. Small sample sizes also limit the generalization of reported findings to allow for the delineation of a clear risk profile for the development of a pneumothorax due to thoracentesis. The presence of baseline lung disease, low level of operator experience with the procedure, and the use of positive-pressure mechanical ventilation appear for now to be the best-established

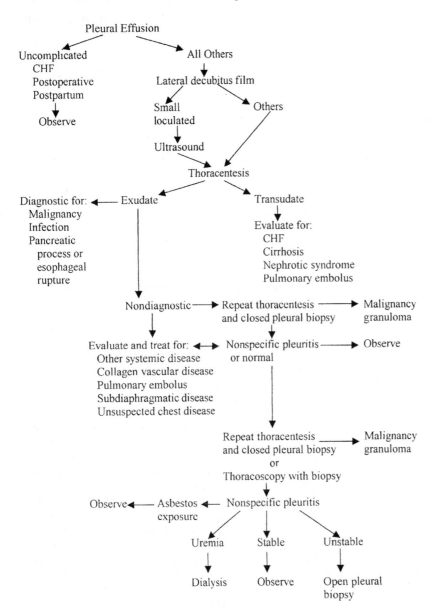

Pleural Effusion

Uncomplicated
CHF
Postoperative
Postpartum

All Others

Lateral decubitus film

Observe

Small
loculated

Others

Ultrasound

Thoracentesis

Diagnostic for: ◄── Exudate
Malignancy
Infection
Pancreatic
    process or
    esophageal
    rupture

Transudate

Evaluate for:
CHF
Cirrhosis
Nephrotic syndrome
Pulmonary embolus

Nondiagnostic ──► Repeat thoracentesis ──► Malignancy
                  and closed pleural biopsy   granuloma

Evaluate and treat for: ◄──► Nonspecific pleuritis ──► Observe
Other systemic disease   or normal
Collagen vascular disease
Pulmonary embolus
Subdiaphragmatic disease
Unsuspected chest disease

Repeat thoracentesis ────── Malignancy
and closed pleural biopsy   granuloma
        or
Thoracoscopy with biopsy

Observe ◄── Asbestos ◄── Nonspecific pleuritis
            exposure

Uremia   Stable   Unstable

Dialysis   Observe   Open pleural
                            biopsy

FIGURE 10-1.   Diagnostic algorithm for evaluation of pleural effusion. CHF, congestive heart failure. [From Smyrnios NA, Jederlinic PJ, Irwin RS: Pleural effusion in an asymptomatic patient. Spectrum and frequency of causes and management considerations. *Chest* 97:192, 1990, with permission.]

risk factors in the literature. Further research involving more patients is needed.

Although pneumothorax is most commonly due to laceration of lung parenchyma, room air may enter the pleural space if the thoracentesis needle is open to room air when a spontaneously breathing patient takes a deep breath (intrapleural pressure is subatmospheric). The pneumothorax may be small and asymptomatic, resolving spontaneously, or large and associated with respiratory compromise, requiring chest tube drainage. Hemorrhage can occur from laceration of an intercostal artery or inadvertent puncture of the liver or spleen, even if coagulation studies are normal. The risk of intercostal artery laceration is greatest in the elderly because of increased tortuosity of their vessels [17]. This last complication is potentially lethal, and open thoracotomy may be required to control the bleeding.

Hypotension may occur during the procedure (as part of a vasovagal reaction or tension pneumothorax) or hours after the procedure (most likely due to reaccumulation of fluid into the pleural space or the pulmonary parenchyma from the intravas-

cular space). Hypotension in the latter settings responds to volume expansion; it can usually be prevented by limiting pleural fluid drainage to 1 L or less. Other major complications are rare and include implantation of tumor along the needle tract of a previously performed thoracentesis [18], venous and cerebral air embolism (so-called pleural shock) [19,20], and inadvertent placement of a sheared off catheter into the pleural space [1].

Minor complications include dry tap or insufficient fluid, pain, subcutaneous hematoma or seroma, anxiety, dyspnea, and cough [2]. Reported rates for these minor complications range from 16% to 63% and depend on the method used to perform the procedure, with higher rates associated with the catheter-through-needle technique [2,3]. Dry tap and insufficient fluid are technical problems and expose the patient to increased risk of morbidity because of the need to perform a repeat thoracentesis. Under these circumstances, it is recommended that the procedure be repeated under direct sonographic guidance. Pain may originate from parietal pleural nerve endings from inadequate local anesthesia, inadvertent scraping of rib periosteum, or piercing an intercostal nerve during a misdirected needle thrust.

PROCEDURES

GENERAL CONSIDERATIONS

The most common techniques for performing thoracentesis are catheter-over-needle, needle only, and needle under direct sonographic guidance. The catheter-through-needle technique has been used much less frequently over the past decade.

TECHNIQUE FOR DIAGNOSTIC (NEEDLE-ONLY OR CATHETER-OVER-NEEDLE) REMOVAL OF FREELY FLOWING FLUID

The technique for diagnostic removal of freely flowing fluid is:

1. Obtain a lateral decubitus chest radiograph to confirm a free-flowing pleural effusion.
2. Describe the procedure to the patient and obtain written informed consent. Operators should be thoroughly familiar with the procedure they will be performing and should receive appropriate supervision from an experienced operator before performing thoracentesis on their own.
3. With the patient sitting, arms at sides, mark the inferior tip of the scapula on the side to be tapped. This approximates the eighth intercostal space and should be the lowest interspace punctured, unless it has been previously determined by sonography that a lower interspace can be safely entered or chest radiographs and sonography show the diaphragm to be higher than the eighth intercostal space.
4. Position the patient sitting at the edge of the bed, comfortably leaning forward over a pillow-draped, height-adjusted, bedside table (Fig. 10-2). The patient's arms should be crossed in front to elevate and spread the scapulae. An assistant should stand in front of the patient to prevent any unexpected movements.
5. Percuss the patient's posterior chest to determine the highest point of the effusion. The interspace below this point should be entered in the posterior axillary line, unless it is below the eighth intercostal space. Gently mark the superior aspect of the rib in the chosen interspace with your fingernail. (The inferior portion of each rib contains an intercostal artery and should be avoided.)
6. Cleanse the area with 2% chlorhexidine in 70% isopropyl alcohol and allow it to dry. Using sterile technique, drape the area surrounding the puncture site.
7. Anesthetize the superficial skin with 2% lidocaine using a 25-gauge needle. Change to an 18- to 22-gauge needle, 2 inches long, and generously anesthetize the deeper soft tissues, aiming for the top of the rib. Always aspirate through the syringe as the needle is advanced and before instilling lidocaine to ensure that the needle is not in a vessel or the pleural space. Carefully aspirate through the syringe as the pleura is approached (the rib is 1 to 2 cm thick). Fluid enters the syringe on reaching the pleural space. The patient may experience discomfort as the needle penetrates the well-innervated parietal pleura. Be careful not to instill anesthetic into the pleural space; it is

bactericidal for most organisms, including *Mycobacterium tuberculosis*. Place a gloved finger at the point on the needle where it exits the skin (to estimate the required depth of insertion) and remove the needle.
8. Attach a three-way stopcock to a 20-gauge, 1.5-inch needle and to a 50-mL syringe. The valve on the stopcock should be open to the needle to allow aspiration of fluid during needle insertion.
9. Insert the 20-gauge needle (or the catheter-over-needle apparatus) into the anesthetized tract with the bevel of the needle down and always aspirate through the syringe as the needle/catheter-over-needle is slowly advanced. When pleural fluid is obtained using the needle-only technique, stabilize the needle by attaching a clamp to the needle where it exits the skin to prevent further advancement of the needle into the pleural space. Once pleural fluid is obtained with the catheter-over-needle technique, direct the needle-catheter apparatus downward to ensure that the catheter descends to the most dependent area of the pleural space. Advance the catheter forward in a single smooth motion as the inner needle is simultaneously pulled back out of the chest.
10. Once pleural fluid can easily be obtained, fill a heparinized blood gas syringe from the side port of the three-way stopcock. Express all air bubbles from the sample, cap it, and place it in a bag containing iced slush for immediate transport to the laboratory.
11. Fill the 50-mL syringe and transfer its contents into the appropriate collection tubes and containers. Always maintain a closed system during the procedure to prevent room air from entering the pleural space. For most diagnostic studies, 50 mL should be ample fluid [21]. Always ensure that the three-way stopcock has the valve closed toward the patient when changing syringes.
12. When the thoracentesis is completed, remove the needle (or catheter) from the patient's chest. Apply pressure to the wound for several minutes, and then apply a sterile bandage.
13. Obtain a postprocedure upright end-expiratory chest radiograph if a pneumothorax is suspected [22].
14. Immediately after the procedure, draw venous blood for total protein and lactate dehydrogenase (LDH) determinations. These studies are necessary to interpret pleural fluid values (see the section Interpretation of Pleural Fluid Analysis).

TECHNIQUE FOR THERAPEUTIC REMOVAL OF FREELY FLOWING FLUID

To perform the technique for therapeutic removal of freely flowing fluid, steps 1 to 7 should be followed as described previously. Removal of more than 100 mL pleural fluid generally involves placement of a catheter into the pleural space to minimize the risk of pneumothorax from a needle during this longer procedure. Commercially available kits generally use a catheter-over-needle system, although catheter-through-needle systems are still available in some locations. Each kit should have a specific set of instructions for performing this procedure. Operators should be thoroughly familiar with the recommended procedure for the catheter system that they will be using and should

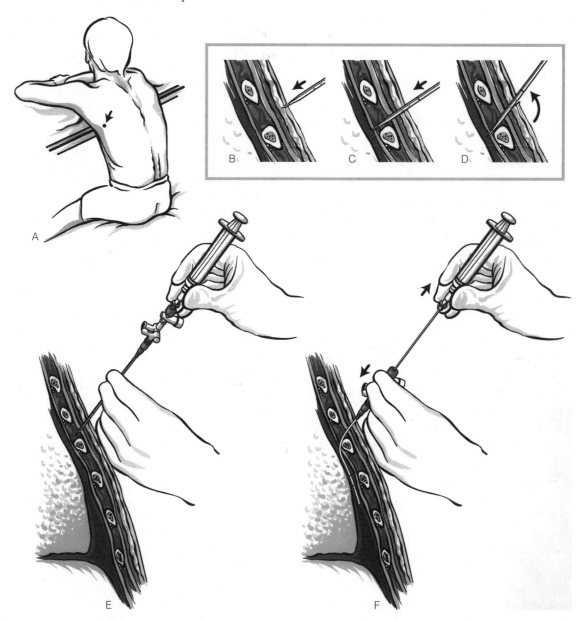

FIGURE 10-2. Catheter-over-needle technique for thoracentesis of freely flowing pleural field. **A:** The patient is comfortably positioned, sitting up and leaning forward over a pillow-draped, height-adjusted, bedside table. The arms are crossed in front of the patient to elevate and spread the scapulae. The preferred entry site is along the posterior axillary line. **B:** The catheter apparatus is gently advanced through the skin and across the upper surface of the rib. The needle is advanced several millimeters at a time while continuously aspirating through the syringe. **C:** As soon as the parietal pleura has been punctured, fluid will appear in the syringe. **D:** Before the catheter is advanced any farther, the apparatus is directed downward. **E,F:** In rapid sequence, the catheter is advanced fully to the chest wall and the needle withdrawn from the apparatus. The one-way valve in the apparatus maintains a closed system until the operator manually changes the position of the stopcock to allow drainage of the pleural fluid.

receive appropriate supervision from an experienced operator before performing thoracentesis on their own.

TECHNIQUE FOR THORACENTESIS BY DIRECTED GUIDANCE

When performing the technique for thoracentesis, a dynamic (real-time) sonographic scanner or computed tomography may be useful for the removal of freely flowing fluid (especially when present in small quantities) or in removal of loculated fluid [23]. They are first used to document the pleural effusion fluid level and the depth of needle insertion necessary to enter the pleural space and will ideally minimize the risk for pneumothorax. The protocol is similar to that described for the needle-only technique, but the needle can be inserted under direct guidance after localization of the effusion. The use of a catheter is optional in this setting.

TECHNIQUE FOR REMOVAL OF FREELY MOVING PNEUMOTHORAX

The technique for removal of freely moving pneumothorax is:

1. Follow the same catheter-over-needle protocol described for removing freely moving fluid, but position the patient supine with the head of the bed elevated 30 to 45 degrees.

2. Prepare the second or third intercostal space in the anterior midclavicular line (this avoids hitting the more medial internal mammary artery) for the needle and catheter insertion.

3. Have the bevel of the needle facing up and direct the needle upward so that the catheter can be guided toward the superior aspect of the hemithorax.

4. Air can be actively withdrawn by syringe or pushed out when intrapleural pressure is supraatmospheric (e.g., during a cough), as long as the catheter is intermittently open to the atmosphere. In the latter setting, air can leave but not reenter if the catheter is attached to a one-way check-valve apparatus (Heimlich valve) or if it is put to underwater seal.

5. When local anesthesia and skin cleansing are not possible because a tension pneumothorax is life threatening, perform the procedure without them. If a tension pneumothorax is known to be present and a chest tube is not readily available, quickly insert a 14-gauge needle into the second anterior intercostal space. If a tension pneumothorax is suspected and a 14-gauge needle and 16-gauge catheter are handy, place the catheter according to the above technique to avoid puncturing the lung. If a tension pneumothorax is present, air escapes under pressure. When the situation has stabilized and the tension pneumothorax has been diagnosed, leave the needle or catheter in place until a sterile chest tube can be inserted.

INTERPRETATION OF PLEURAL FLUID ANALYSIS

To determine the etiology of a pleural effusion, a number of tests on pleural fluid are helpful. A two-stage laboratory approach to the evaluation of pleural effusion should be used [24]. The initial determination should be to classify the effusion as a transudate or an exudate using the criteria discussed below. Additional studies can then be ordered to help establish a final diagnosis for the etiology of the pleural effusion, especially in the setting of an exudate.

TRANSUDATES VERSUS EXUDATES

A transudate is biochemically defined by meeting all of the following criteria: pleural fluid–serum total protein ratio of less than 0.5, pleural fluid–serum LDH ratio of less than 0.6, and absolute pleural fluid LDH of less than 200 IU [25], or less than two thirds the normal serum level. The former diagnostic criteria of pleural fluid specific gravity of less than 1.015 or total protein of less than 3.0 g/dL are no longer used.

TABLE 10-1.   Causes of Pleural Effusions

ETIOLOGIES OF EFFUSIONS THAT ARE VIRTUALLY ALWAYS TRANSUDATES

Congestive heart failure	Cirrhosis
Nephrotic syndrome	Atelectasis
Hypoalbuminemia	Peritoneal dialysis
Urinothorax	Constrictive pericarditis
Trapped lung	Superior vena caval obstruction

ETIOLOGIES OF EFFUSIONS THAT ARE TYPICALLY EXUDATES

Infections
Parapneumonic
Tuberculous pleurisy
Parasites (amebiasis, paragonimiasis, echinococcosis)
Fungal disease
Atypical pneumonias (virus, *Mycoplasma*, Q fever, *Legionella*)
Nocardia, Actinomyces
Subphrenic abscess
Hepatic abscess
Splenic abscess
Hepatitis
Spontaneous esophageal rupture

Noninfectious Inflammations
Pancreatitis
Benign asbestos pleural effusion
Pulmonary embolism
Radiation therapy
Uremic pleurisy
Sarcoidosis
Postcardiac injury syndrome
Hemothorax
Acute respiratory distress syndrome

Malignancies
Carcinoma
Lymphoma
Mesothelioma
Leukemia
Chylothorax

Chronically Increased Negative Intrapleural Pressure
Atelectasis
Trapped lung
Cholesterol effusion

Iatrogenic
Drug-induced (nitrofurantoin, methotrexate
Esophageal perforation
Esophageal sclerotherapy
Central venous catheter misplacement or migration
Enteral feeding tube in space

Connective Tissue Disease
Lupus pleuritis
Hepatic abscess
Rheumatoid pleurisy
Mixed connective tissue disease
Churg-Strauss syndrome
Wegener's granulomatosis
Familial Mediterranean fever

Endocrine Disorders
Hypothyroidism
Ovarian hyperstimulation syndrome

Lymphatic Disorders
Malignancy
Yellow nail syndrome
Lymphangioleiomyomatosis

Movement of Fluid from Abdomen to Pleural Space
Pancreatitis
Pancreatic pseudocyst
Meigs' syndrome
Carcinoma
Chylous ascites

Adapted from Sahn SA: The pleura. *Am Rev Respir Dis* 138:184, 1988.

An exudate is present when any of the foregoing criteria for transudates are not met. If a transudate is present, generally no further tests on pleural fluid are indicated [24] (Table 10-1). The one exception to this is the transudative pleural effusion due to urinothorax. Unless it is suspected and a pH and creatinine level from the pleural fluid is measured and compared to serum levels, this etiology may be missed. An acidotic transudate is characteristic of a urinothorax, and elevated pleural fluid creatinine confirms the diagnosis. If an exudate is present, further laboratory evaluation is warranted (Fig. 10-1). If subsequent testing does not narrow the differential diagnosis, a percutaneous pleural biopsy should be considered [7,26]. Thoracoscopy-guided pleural biopsy should be considered in patients with pleural effusion of unknown etiology despite the above-listed evaluation [8].

SELECTED TESTS THAT ARE POTENTIALLY HELPFUL TO ESTABLISH ETIOLOGY FOR A PLEURAL EFFUSION

pH

Pleural fluid pH determinations may have diagnostic and therapeutic implications [27–29]. For instance, the differential diagnosis associated with a pleural fluid pH of less than 7.2 is consistent with systemic acidemia, bacterially infected effusion (empyema), malignant effusion, rheumatoid or lupus effusion, tuberculous effusion, ruptured esophagus, noninfected parapneumonic effusion that needs drainage, and urinothorax. Pleural effusions with a pH of less than 7.2 are potentially sclerotic and require consideration for chest tube drainage to aid resolution [30,31].

Amylase

A pleural fluid amylase level that is twice the normal serum level or with an absolute value of greater than 160 Somogyi units may be seen in patients with acute and chronic pancreatitis, pancreatic pseudocyst that has dissected or ruptured into the pleural space, primary and metastatic cancer, and esophageal rupture.

Glucose

A low pleural fluid glucose value is defined as less than 50% of the normal serum value. In this situation, the differential diagnosis includes rheumatoid and lupus effusion, bacterial empyema, malignancy, tuberculosis, and esophageal rupture [4,31].

Triglyceride and Cholesterol

Chylous pleural effusions are biochemically defined by a triglyceride level greater than 110 mg/dL and the presence of chylomicrons on a pleural fluid lipoprotein electrophoresis [32]. The usual appearance of a chylous effusion is milky, but an effusion with elevated triglycerides may also appear serous. The measurement of a triglyceride level is therefore important. Chylous effusions occur when the thoracic duct has been disrupted somewhere along its course. The most common causes are trauma and malignancy (e.g., lymphoma) [32]. A pseudochylous effusion appears grossly milky because of an elevated cholesterol level, but the triglyceride level is normal. Chronic effusions, especially those associated with rheumatoid and tuberculous pleuritis, are characteristically pseudochylous [32].

Cell Counts and Differential

Although pleural fluid white blood cell count and differential are never diagnostic of any disease, it would be distinctly unusual for an effusion other than one associated with bacterial pneumonia to have a white blood cell count exceeding 50,000 per mm^3 [33]. In an exudative pleural effusion of acute origin, polymorphonuclear leukocytes predominate early, whereas mononuclear cells predominate in chronic exudative effusions. Although pleural fluid lymphocytosis is nonspecific, severe lymphocytosis (greater than 80% of cells) is suggestive of tuberculosis or malignancy. Finally, pleural fluid eosinophilia is nonspecific.

A red blood cell count of 5,000 to 10,000 cells per mm^3 must be present for fluid to appear pinkish. Grossly bloody effusions containing more than 100,000 red blood cells per mm^3 are most consistent with trauma, malignancy, or pulmonary infarction [33]. To distinguish a traumatic thoracentesis from a preexisting

hemothorax, several observations are helpful [4]. First, because a preexisting hemothorax has been defibrinated, it does not form a clot on standing. Second, a hemothorax is suggested when a pleural fluid hematocrit value is 50% or more of the serum hematocrit value.

Cultures and Stains

To maximize the yield from pleural fluid cultures, anaerobic and aerobic cultures should be obtained. If the sample of pleural fluid sent for culture is transported in an oxygen-free atmosphere (a capped glass syringe with all bubbles squirted out is all that is necessary), the microbiology laboratory can perform all necessary anaerobic, aerobic, fungal, and mycobacterial cultures and smears. Because acid-fast stains may be positive in up to 20% of tuberculous effusions [4], they should always be performed in addition to Gram's-stained smears. By submitting pleural biopsy pieces to pathology and microbiology laboratories, it is possible to diagnose up to 90% of tuberculous effusions percutaneously [25].

Cytology

Malignancies can produce pleural effusions by implantation of malignant cells on the pleura or impairment of lymphatic drainage secondary to tumor obstruction. The tumors that most commonly cause pleural effusions are lung, breast, and lymphoma. Pleural fluid cytology should be performed for an exudative effusion of unknown etiology, using at least 100 to 200 mL fluid. If initial cytology results are negative and strong clinical suspicion exists, additional samples of fluid can increase the chance of a positive result. In patients who are ultimately shown to have a malignancy as an etiology of their effusion, 59% have positive cytology on a single sample, 65% on the second sample, and 70% on the third sample [34]. The addition of a pleural biopsy increases the positive results to 81% [35]. In addition to malignancy, cytologic examination can definitively diagnose rheumatoid pleuritis [36]. The pathognomonic picture consists of slender, elongated macrophages and giant, round, multinucleated macrophages, accompanied by amorphous granular background material.

REFERENCES

1. Seneff MG, Corwin RW, Gold LH, et al: Complications associated with thoracentesis. *Chest* 89:97, 1986.
2. Collins TR, Sahn SA: Thoracentesis: clinical value, complications, technical problems, and patient experience. *Chest* 91:817, 1987.
3. Grogan D, Irwin RS, Channick R, et al: Complications associated with thoracentesis: a prospective randomized study comparing three different methods. *Arch Intern Med* 150:873, 1990.
4. Sahn SA: The differential diagnosis of pleural effusions. *West J Med* 137:99, 1982.
5. Heffner JE, Brown LK, Barbieri CA: Diagnostic value of tests that discriminate between exudative and transudative pleural effusions. *Chest* 111:970, 1997.
6. Romero-Candeira S, Fernandez C, Martin C, et al: Influence of diuretics on the concentration of proteins and other components of pleural transudates in patients with heart failure. *Am J Med* 110:681, 2001.
7. Smyrnios NA, Jederlinic PJ, Irwin RS: Pleural effusion in an asymptomatic patient. Spectrum and frequency of causes and management considerations. *Chest* 97:192, 1990.
8. Kendall SWH, Bryan AJ, Large SR, et al: Pleural effusions: is thoracoscopy a reliable investigation? A retrospective review. *Respir Med* 86:437, 1992.
9. Walker-Renard PB, Vaughan LM, Sahn SA: Chemical pleurodesis for malignant pleural effusions. *Ann Intern Med* 120:56, 1994.
10. Branstetter RD, Karetsky M, Rastogi R, et al: Pneumothorax after thoracentesis in chronic obstructive pulmonary disease. *Heart Lung* 23:67, 1994.
11. Bartter T, Mayo PD, Pratter MR, et al: Lower risk and higher yield for thoracentesis when performed by experimental operators. *Chest* 103:1873, 1993.
12. Doyle JJ, Hnatiuk OW, Torrington KG, et al: Necessity of routine chest roentgenography after thoracentesis. *Ann Intern Med* 124:816, 1996.

13. Petersen WG, Zimmerman R: Limited utility of chest radiograph after thoracentesis. *Chest* 117:1038, 2000.

14. Colt HG, Brewer N, Barbur E: Evaluation of patient-related and procedure-related factors contributing to pneumothorax following thoracentesis. *Chest* 116:134, 1999.

15. Raptopoulos V, Davis LM, Lee G, et al: Factors affecting the development of pneumothorax associated with thoracentesis. *AJR Am J Roentgenol* 156:917, 1991.

16. Gervais DA, Petersein A, Lee MJ: US-guided thoracentesis requirement for postprocedure chest radiography in patients who receive mechanical ventilation versus patients who breathe spontaneously. *Radiology* 204:503, 1997.

17. Carney PA, Ravin CE: Intercostal artery laceration during thoracentesis. *Chest* 75:520, 1979.

18. Stewart BN, Block AJ: Subcutaneous implantation of cancer following thoracentesis. *Chest* 66:456, 1974.

19. Wilson MM, Curley FJ: Gas embolism (Pt I). Venous gas emboli. *J Intensive Care Med* 11:182, 1996.

20. Wilson MM, Curley FJ: Gas embolism (Pt II). Arterial gas embolism and decompression sickness. *J Intensive Care Med* 11:261, 1996.

21. Sallach SM, Sallach JA, Vasquez E, et al: Volume of pleural fluid required for diagnosis of pleural malignancy. *Chest* 122:1913, 2002.

22. Aleman C, Alegre J, Armadans L, et al: The value of chest roentgenography in the diagnosis of pneumothorax after thoracentesis. *Am J Med* 107:340, 1999.

23. Kearney SE, Davies CW, Davies RJ, et al: Computed tomography and ultrasound in parapneumonic effusions and empyema. *Clin Radiol* 55:542, 2000.

24. Peterman TA, Speicher CE: Evaluating pleural effusions: a two stage laboratory approach. *JAMA* 252:1051, 1984.

25. Light RW, MacGregor MI, Luchsinger PC, et al: Pleural effusions: the diagnostic separation of transudates and exudates. *Ann Intern Med* 77:507, 1972.

26. Maskell NV, Gleeson FJO, Davies R: Standard pleural biopsy versus CT-guided cutting-needle biopsy for diagnosis of malignant disease in pleural effusions: a randomized controlled trial. *Lancet* 361:1326, 2003.

27. Burrows CM, Mathews WC, Colt HG: Predicting survival in patients with recurrent symptomatic malignant pleural effusions: an assessment of the prognostic values of physiologic, morphologic, and quality of life measures of extent of disease. *Chest* 117:73, 2000.

28. Heffner JE, Nietert PJ, Barbieri C: Pleural fluid pH as a predictor of survival for patients with malignant pleural effusions. *Chest* 117:79, 2000.

29. Heffner JE, Nietert PJ, Barbieri C: Pleural fluid pH as a predictor of pleordesis failure: analysis of primary data. *Chest* 117:87, 2000.

30. Heffner JE, Heffner JN, Brown LK: Multilevel and continuous pleural fluid pH likelihood ratios for draining parapneumonic effusions. *Respiration* 72:351, 2005.

31. Jimenez Castro D, Diaz Nuevo G, Sueiro A, et al: Pleural fluid parameters identifying complicated parapneumonic effusions. *Respiration* 72:357, 2005.

32. Staats BA, Ellefson RD, Budahn LL, et al: The lipoprotein profile of chylous and nonchylous pleural effusions. *Mayo Clin Proc* 55:700, 1980.

33. Light RS, Erozan YS, Ball WC: Cells in pleural fluid. *Arch Intern Med* 132:854, 1973.

34. Hausheer FH, Yarbro IW: Diagnosis and treatment of malignant pleural effusion. *Semin Oncol* 12:54, 1985.

35. Winkelman M, Pfitzer P: Blind pleural biopsy in combination with cytology of pleural effusions. *Acta Cytol* 25:373, 1981.

36. Naylor B: The pathognomonic cytologic picture of rheumatoid pleuritis. *J Clin Cytol Cytopathol* 34:465, 1990.

Kimberly A. Robinson
Deborah H. Markowitz
Richard S. Irwin

CHAPTER **11**

Arterial Puncture for Blood Gas Analysis

Analysis of a sample of arterial blood for pH_a, partial arterial carbon dioxide pressure ($Paco_2$), partial arterial oxygen pressure (Pao_2), bicarbonate, and percentage oxyhemoglobin saturation is performed with an arterial blood gas (ABG) analysis. Because an ABG can be safely and easily obtained and furnishes rapid and accurate information on how well the lungs and kidneys are working [1–3], it is the single most useful laboratory test in managing patients with respiratory and metabolic disorders. One should not rely on oximetry alone to evaluate arterial oxygen saturation (Sao_2) fully. Given the shape of the oxyhemoglobin saturation curve, there must be a substantial fall in Pao_2 before Sao_2 is altered to any appreciable degree and it is not possible to predict the level of Pao_2 and $Paco_2$ reliably using physical signs such as cyanosis [4] and depth of breathing [5]. Additionally, a discrepancy between Sao_2 measured by pulse oximetry and that calculated by the ABG can aid in the diagnosis of carboxyhemoglobinemia and methemoglobinemia.

Unsuspected hypoxemia or hypercapnia (acidemia) can cause a constellation of central nervous system and cardiovascular signs and symptoms. The clinician should have a high index of suspicion that a respiratory or metabolic disorder, or both, is present in patients with these findings and is most appropriately evaluated by obtaining an ABG. Although acute hypercapnia to 70 mm Hg (pH 7.16) and hypoxemia to less than 30 mm Hg may lead to coma and circulatory collapse, chronic exposures permit adaptation with more subtle effects [6]. Thus, the ABG provides the most important way of making a diagnostic assessment regarding the nature and severity of a respiratory or metabolic disturbance and of following its course over time.

Normal range of values for pH_a is 7.35 to 7.45 and 35 to 45 mm Hg for $Paco_2$ [7]. For Pao_2, the accepted predictive regression equation in nonsmoking, upright, normal individuals aged 40 to 74 years is [8]: $Pao_2 = 108.75 - (0.39 \times \text{age in years})$.

DRAWING THE ARTERIAL BLOOD GAS SPECIMEN

PERCUTANEOUS ARTERIAL PUNCTURE

The conventional technique of sampling arterial blood using a glass syringe is described in detail, because it is the standard to which all other methods are compared. The pulsatile arterial vessel is easily palpated in most cases. If a large enough needle is used, entry is apparent as the syringe fills spontaneously by the pressurized arterial flow of blood, without the need for applying a vacuum or using a vacuum-sealed collecting tube. It is logical to preferentially enter arteries that have the best collateral circulation so that, if spasm or clotting occurs, the distal tissue is not deprived of perfusion. Logic also dictates that puncture of a site where the artery is superficial is preferable, because entry is easiest and pain is minimized. The radial artery best fulfills the above criteria; it is very superficial at the wrist, and the collateral circulation to the hand by the ulnar artery provides sufficient collateral blood flow in approximately 92% of normal adults in the event of total occlusion of the radial artery [9].

The absence of a report of total occlusion of the radial artery after puncture for ABG in an adult with normal hemostasis and the absence of significant peripheral vascular disease attests to the safety of the percutaneous arterial puncture. It also suggests that determining the adequacy of collateral flow to the superficial palmar arch by Allen's test [10], a modification of Allen's test [11] (see Chapter 3), or Doppler ultrasound [9] before puncture is not routinely necessary in those patients with normal hemostasis and the absence of significant peripheral vascular disease. If radial artery sites are not accessible, dorsalis pedis, posterior tibial, superficial temporal (in infants), brachial, and femoral arteries are alternatives (see Chapter 3).

CONTRAINDICATIONS

Brachial and especially femoral artery punctures are not advised in patients with abnormal hemostatic mechanisms, because adequate vessel tamponade may not be possible in that these vessels are not located superficially, risking greater chance of complications [12]. If frequent sampling of superficial arteries in the same situation becomes necessary, arterial cannulation is recommended (see Chapter 3). Moreover, any vessel that has been reconstructed surgically should not be punctured for fear of forming a pseudoaneurysm, compromising the integrity of an artificial graft site or seeding the foreign body that could become a nidus for infection. This should also include avoidance of a femoral arterial puncture on the same side as a transplanted kidney.

The conventional recommended radial artery technique is as follows:

1. Put on protective gloves and sit in a comfortable position facing the patient.
2. With the patient's palm up, slightly hyperextend the wrist and palpate the radial artery. Severe hyperextension may obliterate the pulse.
3. Cleanse the skin with an alcohol swab.
4. With a 25-gauge needle, inject enough 1% lidocaine intradermally to raise a small wheal at the point where the skin puncture is to be made. The local anesthetic makes subsequent needle puncture with a 22-gauge needle less painful and often painless [13]. If local anesthesia is not given, however, the potential pain and anxiety, if associated with breath holding, may cause substantial blood gas changes. Thirty-five seconds of breath holding in normal subjects has been associated with a fall in PaO_2 of 50 mm Hg and a pH of 0.07 and a rise in $PaCO_2$ of 10 mm Hg [14].
5. Attach a needle no smaller than 22 gauge to a glass syringe that can accept 5 mL blood.
6. Wet the needle and syringe with a sodium heparin solution (1,000 units per mL). Express all excess solution.
7. With the needle, enter the artery at an angle of approximately 30 degrees to the long axis of the vessel. This insertion angle minimizes the pain due to inadvertently scraping the periosteum below the artery.
8. As soon as the artery is entered, blood appears in the syringe. Allow the arterial pressure to fill the syringe with at least 3 mL blood [15]. Do not apply suction by pulling on the syringe plunger.
9. Immediately after obtaining the specimen, expel any tiny air bubbles to ensure that the specimen will be anaerobic; then cap the syringe.
10. Roll the blood sample between both palms for 5 to 15 seconds to mix the heparin and blood. Apply pressure to the puncture site for 5 minutes or longer, depending on the presence of a coagulopathy. If the arterial sample was obtained from the brachial artery, compress this vessel so that the radial pulse cannot be palpated.
11. Immerse the capped sample in a bag of ice and water (slush) and immediately transport it to the blood gas laboratory.
12. Write on the ABG slip the time of the drawing and the conditions under which it was drawn (e.g., fraction of inspired oxygen, ventilator settings, position of the patient).

Deviations from these recommended techniques may introduce the following errors:

1. The syringe material may influence the results of PaO_2 (16–18). The most accurate results have been consistently obtained using a glass syringe. If plastic is used, the following errors may occur: (a) falsely low PaO_2 values may be obtained because plastic allows oxygen to diffuse to the atmosphere from the sample whenever the PO_2 exceeds 221 mm Hg; (b) plastic syringes with high surface area to volume ratios (e.g., 1-mL tuberculin syringes) worsen gas permeability errors as compared to standard 3-mL syringes. For this reason, butterfly infusion kits with their long thin tubing should not be used [19]; (c) plastic syringes tenaciously retain air bubbles, and extra effort is necessary to remove them [17]; (d) plastic impedes smooth movement of the plunger, which could have an impact on the clinician's confidence that arterial rather than venous blood has been sampled.
2. If suction is applied for plunger assistance, gas bubbles may be pulled out of the solution. If they are expelled, measured PaO_2 and $PaCO_2$ tensions may be falsely lowered [20].
3. Although liquid heparin is a weak acid, plasma pH is not altered because it is well buffered by hemoglobin. Mixing liquid heparin with blood dilutes dissolved gasses, shifting their concentration to that of heparin (PO_2 approximately 150 mm Hg, PCO_2 less than 0.3 mm Hg at sea level and room temperature). The degree of alteration depends on the amount of heparin relative to blood and the hemoglobin concentration [20–22]. The dilution error is no greater than 4% if a glass syringe and 22-gauge needle are only wetted with approximately 0.2 mL heparin and 3 to 5 mL blood collected. Any less heparin risks a clotted and unusable sample. Dilutional errors are avoided with the use of crystalline heparin, but this preparation is difficult to mix, which risks clotting of the specimen.
4. If an ABG specimen is not analyzed within 1 minute of being drawn or not immediately cooled to 2°C, the PO_2 and pH fall and PCO_2 rises because of cellular respiration and consumption of oxygen by leukocytes, platelets, and reticulocytes [23]. This is of particular concern in patients with leukemia (leukocytes greater than 40×10^9 per L) or thrombocytosis ($1,000 \times 10^9$ per L) [24].
5. Inadvertent sampling of a vein normally causes a falsely low PaO_2. A venous PO_2 greater than 50 mm Hg can be obtained if the sampling area is warmed. The PO_2 of "arterialized" venous blood can approximate PaO_2 when blood flow is greatly increased by warming, compromising the time for peripheral oxygen extraction.

COMPLICATIONS

Using the conventional radial artery technique described above, complications are unusual. They include a rare vasovagal episode, local pain, and limited hematomas, occurring no more than 0.58% of the time [1–3]. An expanding aneurysm of the radial artery and reflex sympathetic dystrophy [25] have been reported even more rarely after frequent punctures [26].

MEASUREMENTS FROM THE ARTERIAL BLOOD GAS SPECIMEN

Although pH, PCO_2, PO_2, bicarbonate, and SaO_2 are all usually reported, it is important to understand that the bicarbonate and SaO_2 are calculated, not directly measured. Although the calculated bicarbonate value is as reliable as the measured pH and PCO_2 values, given their immutable relationship through the Henderson-Hasselbalch equation, the calculated SaO_2 is often inaccurate because of the many variables that cannot be corrected for (e.g., 2,3-diphosphoglycerate, binding characteristics of hemoglobin).

The patient in the intensive care unit often requires serial ABG measurements to follow the progression of critical illness and guide therapy accordingly. Although it is understandable to interpret fluctuations in the ABG data as a sign of the patient's condition worsening or improving, depending on the trend, it is also important to appreciate that modest fluctuations may be due to deviations in the collection of the ABG specimen. Therefore, routine monitoring of ABGs without an associated change in patient status may not be warranted and may lead to an unproductive, lengthy, and expensive search for the cause.

When electrolytes and other blood values are measured from the unused portion of an ABG sample, clinicians should be aware of the following: Traditional liquid and crystalline heparins for ABG sampling are sodium-heparin salts, which artificially increase plasma sodium concentrations. Calcium and potassium bind to the negatively charged heparins, spuriously lowering their values. Lithium or electrolyte-balanced heparin is now available that contains physiologic concentrations of sodium and potassium, which should be used whenever sodium, potassium, ionized magnesium, ionized calcium, chloride, glucose, and lactate are measured in an ABG specimen [27–29]. Although lithium or balanced heparin minimizes the errors in electrolyte concentrations, dilutional error may still exist if excessive amounts are used for anticoagulation.

By convention, ABG specimens are analyzed at 37°C. Although no studies have demonstrated that correction for the patient's temperature is clinically necessary, blood gases drawn at temperatures greater than 39°C should probably be corrected for temperature [30]. Because the solubility of oxygen and carbon dioxide increases as blood is cooled to 37°C, the hyperthermic patient is more acidotic and less hypoxemic than uncorrected values indicate. Therefore, for each 1°C that the patient's temperature is greater than 37°C, Pao_2 should be increased 7.2%, $Paco_2$ increased 4.4%, and pH decreased 0.015. It is not necessary to correct the $Paco_2$ and pH in the hypothermic patient [31], because acid-base changes in vivo parallel the changes of blood in vitro. However, Pao_2 values must be corrected for temperature lest significant hypoxemia be overlooked. The Pao_2 at 37°C is decreased by 7.2% for each degree that the patient's temperature is less than 37°C.

It should also be noted that transport of an ABG specimen to the lab via a pneumatic tube system can result in alterations in Pao_2 secondary to contamination with room air. This effect is presumed to be due to pressure changes within the pneumatic tube system because the use of pressure tight transport containers obliterates the effect [32]. If a pneumatic tube system is to be used, one must be sure that all air bubbles are carefully expelled from the ABG specimen and that a pressure tight container is used. Otherwise, it may be best to hand-carry samples to the lab [32–34].

PHYSICIAN RESPONSIBILITY

Even when the ABG values of pH, Pco_2, Po_2, and bicarbonate appear consistently reliable, the clinician should periodically check the accuracy of the blood gas samples because the bicarbonate is calculated, not directly measured. Aliquots of arterial blood can be sent simultaneously for ABG analysis and to the chemistry laboratory for a total (T) CO_2 content. Accuracy of the blood gas laboratory's values can be checked using Henderson's simple mathematical equation, which is a re-

TABLE 11-1.   Relation between [H$^+$] and pH over a Normal Range of pH Values^a

pH	[H$^+$] (nM/L)
7.36	44
7.37	43
7.38	42
7.39	41
7.40	40
—	—
7.41	39
7.42	38
7.43	37
7.44	36

^{a}Note that pH 7.40 corresponds to hydrogen ion concentration of 40 nM/L and that, over the small range shown, each deviation in pH of 0.01 units corresponds to opposite deviation in [H$^+$] of 1 nM/L. For pH values between 7.28 and 7.45, [H$^+$] calculated empirically in this fashion agrees with the actual value obtained by means of logarithms to the nearest nM/L (nearest 0.01 pH unit). However, in the extremes of pH values, below pH 7.28 and above pH 7.45, the estimated [H$^+$] is always lower than the actual value, with the discrepancy reaching 11% at pH 7.10 and 5% at pH 7.50.
Modified from Kassirer J, Bleich H: Rapid estimation of plasma carbon dioxide tension from pH and total carbon dioxide content. *N Engl J Med* 171:1067, 1965.

arrangement of the Henderson-Hasselbalch equation [35]: [H$^+$] = 25 × $Paco_2$/Hco_3^-. [H$^+$] is solved by using the pH measured in the blood gas laboratory (Table 11-1). Measured arterial Tco_2 should be close to the calculated bicarbonate value. Venous Tco_2 should not be used in this exercise because it is often and normally up to 5 mEq/L greater than arterial Tco_2.

ALTERNATIVES

Although little progress has been made in noninvasive pH measurement, there have been four important areas of technologic development: oximetry, transcutaneous Po_2 and Pco_2 gas measurements, expired Pco_2, and indwelling intravascular electrode systems.

Many situations may arise whereby arterial blood samples are not available. For example, severe peripheral vascular disease makes radial arterial puncture difficult, or the patient refuses arterial blood sampling or cannulation. In general, in the absence of circulatory failure or limb ischemia, central and peripheral venous blood may substitute for arterial when monitoring acid-base and ventilatory status. In hemodynamically stable patients, pH_a is, on average, 0.03 units higher than central venous pH (pH_{cv}), and $Paco_2$ is lower than central venous carbon dioxide ($P_{cv}co_2$) by 5 mm Hg [36], and changes in each are tightly correlated [37]. Regression analysis reveals pH_a = (1.027 × pH_{cv}) − 0.156 and $Paco_2$ = (0.754 × $P_{cv}co_2$) + 2.75. In shock, the accentuated discrepancy may be due to increased carbon dioxide generated by the buffering of acids in conditions characterized by increased lactic acid production.

It must be made clear that, in the absence of warming a sampling area to collect "arterialized" venous blood, an arterial sample is still necessary for evaluation of accurate oxygenation status for precise measurements of Po_2 and alveolar-arterial oxygen gradient determination. Once the oxygenation and acid-base status have been identified, pulse oximetry can be used to follow trends in Sao_2 in stable or improving patients because serial ABGs are costly and risk vessel injury with repeated arterial punctures.

POINT OF CARE TESTING

Blood gas analysis is now routinely performed at the bedside with point of care testing (POCT) devices. Advantages of POCT include convenience and rapid turnaround time, theoretically improving the quality of patient care. With regards to pH, Po_2, and Pco_2, several studies have verified a high correlation between POCT results and conventional analysis methods [38,39].

REFERENCES

1. Fleming W, Bowen J: Complications of arterial puncture. *Milit Med* 139:307, 1974.
2. Petty T, Bigelow B, Levine B: The simplicity and safety of arterial puncture. *JAMA* 195:181, 1966.
3. Sackner M, Avery W, Sokolowski J: Arterial punctures by nurses. *Chest* 59:97, 1971.
4. Comoroe J, Botelho S: The unreliability of cyanosis in the recognition of arterial anoxemia. *Am J Med Sci* 214:1, 1947.
5. Mithoefer J, Bossman O, Thibeault D, et al: The clinical estimation of alveolar ventilation. *Am Rev Respir Dis* 98:868, 1968.
6. Weiss E, Faling L, Mintz S, et al: Acute respiratory failure in chronic obstructive pulmonary disease I. Pathophysiology. *Disease-a-Month* 1, October 1969.
7. Raffin T: Indications for arterial blood gas analysis. *Ann Intern Med* 105:390, 1986.
8. Cerveri I, Zoia M, Fanfulla F, et al: Reference values of arterial oxygen tension in the middle-aged and elderly. *Am J Respir Crit Care* 152:934, 1995.
9. Felix WJ, Sigel B, Popky G: Doppler ultrasound in the diagnosis of peripheral vascular disease. *Semin Roentgenol* 4:315, 1975.
10. Allen E: Thromboangiitis obliterans: methods of diagnosis of chronic occlusive arterial lesions distal to the wrist, with illustrative cases. *Am J Med Sci* 178:237, 1929.
11. Bedford R: Radial arterial function following percutaneous cannulation with 18- and 20-gauge catheters. *Anesthesiology* 47:37, 1977.
12. Macon WI, Futrell J: Median-nerve neuropathy after percutaneous puncture of the brachial artery in patients receiving anticoagulants. *N Engl J Med* 288:1396, 1973.
13. Giner J, Casan P, Belda J, et al: Pain during arterial puncture. *Chest* 110:1143, 1996.
14. Sasse S, Berry R, Nguyen T: Arterial blood gas changes during breath-holding from functional residual capacity. *Chest* 110:958, 1996.
15. Bloom S, Canzanello V, Strom J, et al: Spurious assessment of acid-base status due to dilutional effect of heparin. *Am J Med* 79:528, 1985.
16. Janis K, Gletcher G: Oxygen tension measurements in small samples: sampling errors. *Am Rev Respir Dis* 106:914, 1972.
17. Winkler J, Huntington C, Wells D, et al: Influence of syringe material on arterial blood gas determinations. *Chest* 66:518, 1974.
18. Ansel G, Douce F: Effects of syringe material and needle size on the minimum plunger-displacement pressure of arterial blood gas syringes. *Respir Care* 27:147, 1982.
19. Thelin O, Karanth S, Pourcyrous M, et al: Overestimation of neonatal Po_2 by collection of arterial blood gas values with the butterfly infusion set. *J Perinatol* 13:65, 1993.
20. Adams A, Morgan-Hughes J, Sykes M: pH and blood gas analysis: methods of measurement and sources of error using electrode systems. *Anaesthesia* 22:575, 1967.
21. Bloom S, Canzanello V, Strom J, et al: Spurious assessment of acid-base status due to dilutional effect of heparin. *Am J Med* 79:528, 1985.
22. Hansen J, Simmons D: A systematic error in the determination of blood Pco_2. *Am Rev Respir Dis* 115:1061, 1977.
23. Eldridge F, Fretwell L: Change in oxygen tension of shed blood at various temperatures. *J Appl Physiol* 20:790, 1965.
24. Schmidt C, Mullert-Plathe O: Stability of Po_2, Pco_2 and pH in heparinized whole blood samples: influence of storage temperature with regard to leukocyte count and syringe material. *Eur J Clin Chem Clin Biochem* 30:767, 1992.
25. Criscuolo C, Nepper G, Buchalter S: Reflex sympathetic dystrophy following arterial blood gas sampling in the intensive care unit. *Chest* 108:578, 1995.
26. Mathieu A, Dalton B, Fischer J, et al: Expanding aneurysm of the radial artery after frequent puncture. *Anesthesiology* 38:401, 1973.
27. Burnett R, Covington A, Fogh-Anderson N: Approved IFCC recommendations on whole blood sampling, transport and storage for simultaneous determination of pH, blood gases and electrolytes. *Eur J Clin Chem Clin Biochem* 33:247, 1995.
28. Lyon M, Bremner D, Laha T, et al: Specific heparin preparations interfere with the simultaneous measurement of ionized magnesium and ionized calcium. *Clin Biochem* 28:79, 1995.
29. Toffaletti J, Thompson T: Effects of blended lithium-zinc heparin on ionized calcium and general clinical chemistry tests. *Clin Chem* 41:328, 1995.
30. Curley F, Irwin R: Disorders of temperature control, I. hyperthermia. *J Intensive Care Med* 1:5, 1986.
31. Curley F, Irwin R: Disorders of temperature control, III. hypothermia. *J Intensive Care Med* 1:270, 1986.
32. Collinson PO, John CM, Gaze DC, Ferrigan LF, Cramp DG: Changes in blood gas samples produced by a pneumatic tube system. *J Clin Pathol* 55(2):105, 2002.
33. Astles JR, Lubarsky D, Loun B, et al: Pneumatic transport exacerbates interference of room air contamination in blood gas samples. *Arch Pathol Lab Med* 120(7):642, 1996.
34. Lu JY, Kao JT, Chien TI, et al: Effects of air bubbles and tube transportation on blood oxygen tension in arterial blood gas analysis. *J Formos Med Assoc* 102(4):246, 2003.
35. Kassirer J, Bleich H: Rapid estimation of plasma carbon dioxide tension from pH and total carbon dioxide content. *N Engl J Med* 272:1067, 1965.
36. Adrogue H, Rashad M, Gorin A, et al: Assessing acid-base status in circulatory failure; differences between arterial and central venous blood. *N Engl J Med* 320:1312, 1989.
37. Philips B, Peretz D: A comparison of central venous and arterial blood gas values in the critically ill. *Ann Intern Med* 70:745, 1969.
38. Sediame S, Zerah-Lancner F, d'Ortho MP, et al: Accuracy of the i-STAT bedside blood gas analyser. *Eur Respir J* 14(1):214, 1999.
39. Kampelmacher MJ, van Kesteren RG, Winckers EK: Instrumental variability of respiratory blood gases among different blood gas analysers in different laboratories. *Eur Respir J* 10(6):1341, 1997.

Scott E. Kopec
Ciaran J. McNamee

CHAPTER **12**

Tracheostomy

The terms *tracheotomy* and *tracheostomy* are interchangeable. Derived from the Greek words *tracheia arteria* (rough artery) and *tome* (incision), *tracheotomy* refers to the operation that opens the trachea, while *tracheostomy* results in the formation of a tracheostoma, or the opening itself. Although tracheostomy is referred to intermittently from the first century BC [1–3], it was not performed regularly until the 1800s when used by Trousseau and Bretonneau in the management of diphtheria. In the early 1900s, Chevalier Jackson [4], describing refinements to the operation, warned against tracheostomy involving the cricothyroid membrane or first tracheal ring because of the risk of injury to the cricoid cartilage and subsequent subglottic stenosis. During this period, the procedure was used to treat difficult cases of respiratory paralysis from poliomyelitis. Largely because of improvements in tubes and advances in clinical care, endotracheal intubation has become the treatment of choice for short-term airway management [3,5].

Although tracheostomy is occasionally required in critically ill and injured patients who cannot be intubated for various reasons (e.g., cervical spine injury, upper airway obstruction, laryngeal injury, anatomical considerations), the most common use of this procedure today is to provide long-term access to the airway in patients who are dependent on mechanical ventilation. With improvements in critical care medicine over the past 30 years, more patients are surviving initial episodes of acute respiratory failure, trauma, and extensive surgeries and are requiring prolonged periods of mechanical ventilation. It is now common practice to expeditiously convert these patients from translaryngeal intubation to tracheostomy. Tracheostomy is becoming a very common procedure in the intensive care unit (ICU). The prevalence of tracheostomies in ICU patients is at least 10% [6].

In this chapter we will review the indications, contraindications, complications, and techniques associated with tracheostomy. We will also discuss the timing of converting an orally intubated patient to tracheostomy.

INDICATIONS

The indications for tracheostomy can be divided into three general categories: to bypass obstruction of the upper airway, to provide an avenue for tracheal toilet and removal of retained secretions, and to provide a means for ventilatory support. These indications are summarized in Table 12-1 [7–13].

Anticipated prolonged ventilatory support, especially patients receiving mechanical ventilation via translaryngeal intubation, is the most common indication for placing a tracheostomy in the

ICU. There are several advantages and disadvantages of both translaryngeal intubation and tracheostomy in patients requiring prolonged ventilator support, and these are summarized in Table 12-2 [14–16]. Most authors feel that when the procedure is performed by a skilled surgical group, the potential benefits of tracheostomy over translaryngeal intubation for most patients justifies the application despite its potential risks. However, there are no detailed clinical trials consistently confirming the advantages of tracheostomy in patients requiring prolonged mechanical ventilation.

CONTRAINDICATIONS

There are no absolute contraindications to tracheostomy. Certain conditions, however, warrant special attention before anesthesia and surgery. In patients undergoing conversion from translaryngeal intubation to a tracheostomy for prolonged ventilatory support, the procedure should be viewed as an elective or semielective procedure. Therefore, the patient should be as medically stable as possible, and all attempts should be made to correct existing coagulopathies, including uremia. For obvious reasons, emergent tracheostomies for upper airway obstruction may need to be preformed when the patient is unstable or has a coagulopathy.

TIMING OF TRACHEOSTOMY

When to perform a tracheostomy on an intubated, critically ill patient has been very controversial. Recommendations range from performing a tracheostomy after just 3 days of translaryngeal intubation due to the risk of mucosal damage to the larynx and vocal cords [17], to more than 21 days based on reported high complication rates of open tracheostomies [18]. The reported low morbidity and mortality of bedside percutaneous tracheostomies confirm that it does not appear justified to avoid tracheostomy based solely on the risk of operative complications. The lower morbidity and mortality of the procedure shifts the risk-benefit ratio to more of a benefit in the majority of patients requiring prolonged ventilator support.

A more up-to-date approach regarding the timing of converting an intubated patient to a tracheostomy has been suggested by Heffner [14]. This recommendation takes into account the very low mortality and morbidity associated with placing a tracheostomy, plus the advantages and disadvantages of both translaryngeal intubation and tracheostomy. In summary, if a patient remains ventilator dependent after a week of translaryngeal intubation, a tracheostomy can be considered.

TABLE 12-1. Indications for Tracheostomy

Upper airway obstruction
    Laryngeal dysfunction: Vocal cord paralysis
    Trauma: Upper airway obstruction due to hemorrhage, edema, or
        crush injury; unstable mandibular fractures; injury to the larynx;
        cervical spine injuries
    Burns and corrosives: Hot smoke, caustic gases, corrosives
    Foreign bodies
    Congenital anomalies: Stenosis of the glottic or subglottic area
    Infections: Croup, epiglottitis, Ludwig's angina, deep neck space
        infections
    Neoplasms: Laryngeal cancer
    Postoperative: Surgeries of the base of the tongue and
        hypopharynx, rigid fixation of the mandibular
    Obstructive sleep apnea
Tracheal toilet
    Inability to clear secretions: Generalized weakness, altered mental
        status, excess secretions
    Neuromuscular disease
Ventilatory support: Prolonged or chronic

Kremer B, Botos-Kremer A, Eckel H, et al: Indications, complications, and surgical technique for pediatric tracheostomies. *J Pediatr Surg* 37:1556, 2002.
Bjure J: Tracheotomy: A satisfactory method in the treatment of acute epiglottis. A clinical and functional follow-up study. *Int J Pediatr Otorhinolaryngol* 3:37, 1981.
Hanline MH Jr: Tracheotomy in upper airway obstruction. *South Med J* 74:899, 1981.
Taicher S, Givol M, Peleg M, et al: Changing indications for tracheostomy in maxillofacial trauma. *J Oral Maxillofac Surg* 54:292, 1996.
Guilleminault C, Simmons FB, Motta J, et al: Obstructive sleep apnea syndrome and tracheostomy. *Arch Intern Med* 141:985, 1981.
Burwell C, Robin E, Whaley R, et al: Extreme obesity associated with alveolar hypoventilation. *Am J Med* 141:985, 1981.
Yung MW, Snowdon SL: Respiratory resistance of tracheostomy tubes. *Arch Otolaryngol* 110:591, 1984.

TABLE 12-2. Advantages and Disadvantages of Intubation and Tracheostomy [14–16]

Translaryngeal Intubation

Advantages	*Disadvantages*
Reliable airway during urgent intubation	Bacterial airway colonization
	Inadvertent extubation
Avoidance of surgical complications	Laryngeal injury
	Tracheal stenosis
	Purulent sinusitis (nasotracheal intubations)
	Patient discomfort

Tracheostomies

Advantages	*Disadvantages*
Avoids direct injury to the larynx	Complications (see Table 12-3)
Facilitates nursing care	Bacterial airway colonization
Enhances patient mobility	Cost
More secure airway	Surgical scar
Improved patient comfort	Tracheal and stomal stenosis
Permits speech	
Provides psychological benefit	
More rapid weaning from mechanical ventilation	
Better oral hygiene	
Decreased risk of nosocomal pneumonia	

Whether to perform the procedure or not should depend on the anticipated duration of ventilatory support and the benefits of a tracheostomy in that specific patient. If the patient appears to have minimal barriers to weaning, and appears likely to be successfully weaned and extubated within 7 days, tracheostomy should be avoided. In those patients whom it appears unlikely that they will successfully be weaned and extubated in 7 days, tracheostomy should be strongly considered. For those patients whose ability to wean and be extubated is unclear, the patient's status should be readdressed daily [14].

Some studies have suggested that early tracheostomy may be beneficial in some specific instances. Patients with blunt, multiple organ trauma have a shorter duration of mechanical ventilation, fewer episodes of nosocomial pneumonia [19], and a significant reduction in hospital costs [20] when the tracheostomy is performed within 1 week of their injuries. Similar benefits have been reported in patients with head trauma and poor Glasgow Coma Score [21–23], and patients with thermal injury [24], if a tracheostomy is performed within a week after the injury.

Several recent studies [25–27], coupled with a meta-analysis [28] sought to determine if performing an "early tracheostomy," that is, within 7 days of translaryngeal intubation, had any advantages over a "late tracheostomy" (greater than 7 days) in critically ill patients requiring mechanical ventilation. The meta-analysis combined five prospective studies and included 406 patients and suggested that early tracheostomy resulted in a decrease length of ICU stay by an average of 15.3 days, and a decrease in duration of mechanical ventilation by an average of 8.5 days [28]. Potential reasons for the decrease in duration of mechanical ventilation include easier weaning due to less dead space, less resistance, and less obstruction due to mucus plugging in patients with tracheostomies. There was no significant increase in hospital mortality or risk of hospital acquired pneumonia. However, there are obvious limitations to the meta-analysis. Currently there are three large randomized trials being performed in Europe addressing the timing of tracheostomy in critical ill patients on mechanical ventilation. Hopefully these studies, when concluded, can result in specific guidelines to the timing of tracheostomy.

PROCEDURES

EMERGENCY TRACHEOSTOMY

Emergency tracheostomy is a moderately difficult procedure requiring training and skill, experience, adequate assistance, time, lighting, and proper equipment and instrumentation. When time is short, the patient uncooperative, anatomy distorted, and the aforementioned requirements not met, tracheostomy can be very hazardous. Emergency tracheostomy comprises significant risks to nearby neurovascular structures, particularly in small children in whom the trachea is small and not well defined. The risk of complications from emergency tracheostomy is 2 to 5 times higher than for elective tracheostomy [29,30]. Nonetheless, there are occasional indications for emergency tracheostomy [31], including transected trachea, anterior neck trauma with crushed larynx [32], severe facial trauma, acute laryngeal obstruction or near impending obstruction, and pediatric (earlier than 12 years) patients requiring an emergency surgical airway in whom an cricothyrotomy is generally not advised. In emergency situations when there is inadequate time or personnel to perform an emergency tracheostomy, a cricothyrotomy may be a more efficient and expedient manner to provide an airway.

CRICOTHYROTOMY

Cricothyrotomy (cricothyroidotomy) was condemned in Jackson's [4] 1921 article on high tracheostomies because of excessive complications, particularly subglottic stenoses [33]. He emphasized the importance of the cricoid cartilage as an encircling support for the larynx and the trachea. However, a favorable report of 655 cricothyrotomies, with complication rates of only 6.1%, and no cases of subglottic stenoses [34], prompted reevaluation of cricothyrotomy for elective and emergency airway access. Further reports emphasized the advantages of cricothyrotomy over tracheostomy. These include technical simplicity, speed of performance, low complication rate [35–39], suitability as a bedside procedure, usefulness for isolation of the airway for median sternotomy [38,40], radical neck dissection [41], lack of need to hyperextend the neck, and formation of a smaller scar. Also, because cricothyrotomy results in less encroachment on the mediastinum, there is less chance of esophageal injury and virtually no chance of pneumothorax or tracheal arterial fistula [35]. Despite these considerations many authorities currently recommend cricothyrotomy should be used as an elective long-term method of airway access only in highly selective patients [33,35,41–43]. Use of cricothyrotomy in the emergency setting, particularly for managing trauma, is not controversial [44–46]. Emergency cricothyrotomy is useful because cricothyrotomy requires a small number of instruments and less training than tracheostomy and can be performed quickly as indicated as a means of controlling the airway in an emergency when oral or nasotracheal intubation is nonsuccessful or contraindicated. In emergency situations, translaryngeal intubations fail because of massive oral or nasal hemorrhage or regurgitation, structural deformities of the upper airway, muscle spasm and clenched teeth, and obstruction by foreign body through the upper airway [44]. Cricothyrotomy finds its greatest use in trauma management, axial or suspected cervical spine injury, alone or in combination with severe facial trauma, where nasotracheal and orotracheal intubation is both difficult and hazardous. Thus cricothyrotomy has an important role in emergency airway management [45].

Use and Contraindications

Cricothyrotomy should not be used to manage airway obstruction that occurred immediately after endotracheal extubation because the obstruction may be found below the larynx [4,35,45]; likewise, with primary laryngeal trauma or diseases such as tumor or an infection, cricothyrotomy may prove useless. It is contraindicated in infants and in children younger than 10 to 12 years, under all circumstances [45]. In this age group, percutaneous transtracheal ventilation may be a temporizing procedure until the tracheostomy can be performed.

Anatomy

The cricothyroid space is no larger than 7 to 9 mm in its vertical dimension, smaller than the outside diameter of most tracheostomy tubes (outside diameter 10.0 mm). The cricothyroid artery runs across the midline in the upper portion, and the membrane is vertically in the midline. The anterior superior edge of the thyroid cartilage is the laryngeal prominence. The cricothyroid membrane is approximately 2 to 3 cm below the laryngeal prominence and can be identified as an indentation immediately below the thyroid cartilage. The lower border of the cricothyroid membrane is the cricoid cartilage [38,39,43,46–48]. A description of the cricothyrotomy procedure is contained in standard surgical texts.

Complications

The report of incidents of short- and long-term complications of cricothyrotomy ranges from 6.1% [34] with procedures performed in an elective, well-controlled, carefully selected cases, to greater than 50% [44,46,49] for procedures performed under emergency or other suboptimal conditions. The incidence of subglottic stenosis after cricothyrotomy is 2% to 3% [33,35]. This major complication occurs at the tracheostomy or cricothyrotomy site but not at the cuff site [50]. Necrosis of cartilage due to iatrogenic injury to the cricoid cartilage or pressure from the tube on the cartilage may play a role [45]. Possible reasons that subglottic stenoses may occur more commonly with cricothyrotomy than with tracheostomy are as follows: the larynx is the narrowest part of the laryngotracheal airway; subglottic tissues, especially in children, are intolerant of contact; and division of the cricothyroid membrane and the cricoid cartilage destroy the only complete rings supporting the airway [3,33]. Furthermore, the range of tube sizes is limited due to the rigidity of the surrounding structures (cricoid and thyroid cartilage), and the curvature of the tracheostomy tube at this level may obstruct the airway due to potential posterior membrane impingement [51]. Prior laryngotracheal injury, as with prolonged translaryngeal intubation, is a major risk factor for the development of subglottic stenosis after cricothyrotomy [33,35].

The association of cricothyrotomy with these possible complications leads most authorities to consider replacing a cricothyrotomy within 48 to 72 hours with a standardized tracheostomy procedure. This is commonly done by an open surgical tracheostomy (OST), which occurs between the second and third tracheal ring as compared to a percutaneous dilational tracheostomy (PDT), which usually occurs between the cricoid cartilage and the first ring or the first and second ring [51].

TRACHEOSTOMY PROCEDURES IN THE INTENSIVE CARE UNIT

Tracheostomy is one of the most common surgical ICU procedures and it is commonly performed for weaning purposes and for airway protection for patients requiring prolonged ventilation. There are two major techniques for tracheostomy with various modifications that are described below. The different surgical tracheostomy techniques are well described in the references for this chapter and are briefly described below [52–54].

OPEN SURGICAL TRACHEOSTOMY

In OST the patient's neck is extended and the surgical field is exposed from the chin to several inches below the clavicle. This area is prepped and draped and prophylactic antibiotics are administered at the discretion of the surgeon. A vertical or horizontal incision may be used; however, a horizontal incision will provide a better cosmetic result. The platysma muscle is divided in line with the incision and the strap muscles are separated in the midline. The thyroid isthmus is then mobilized superiorly or is divided as needed to access the trachea. In the event of a low-lying cricoid cartilage, dissection on the anterior wall of the trachea helps to mobilize the trachea out of the mediastinum, and also the use of a cricoid hook will elevate the trachea to expose the second or third tracheal ring. Following identification of the second or third tracheal ring, a vertical tracheostomy is created or a tracheal flap (Bjork flap) is fashioned to create a fistulous tract by suturing the tracheal mucosal flap to the skin in the incision.

Variations on this technique include the use of retention sutures through the lateral aspect of the tracheal walls for retraction purposes during tracheostomy tube insertion and for expeditious reinsertion of a tracheostomy tube in the event of accidental tube decannulation [54,55].

PERCUTANEOUS DILATION TECHNIQUES

The PDT are divided into several techniques; however, all are alike in that they depend on the basic technique of guidewire placement through the anterior tracheal wall, followed by dilation over this guidewire to create a tracheal stoma. This is all accomplished with provision of adequate monitoring of O_2 saturations as well as adequate monitoring of cardiac rhythm and blood pressure. To achieve early successful tracheal cannulation within the operating room use end-tidal CO_2 monitoring via the fresh tracheostomy tube and in the ICU by capnography [56]. There are several different modifications from the original technique that was described by Ciaglia et al. [57] in 1988.

1. In the original technique, following the perforation of the first or second tracheal membrane, a tracheal stoma is created by the passage of several progressive larger dilators. The tracheostomy tube is carried into the stoma on an appropriately sized dilator once a sufficient stoma has been created.

2. A simple modification of this technique was first developed in 1989 by Schachner et al. [58] (Rapitrach instrument) (Fig. 12-1), which is a forceps device with a cutting edge on a cone that is introduced over the guidewire. Following tracheal penetration an adequate tract is created by pressure on the handles, which open the jaws of the cone to create a stoma. This instrument is not available in the US market because of posterior tracheal wall tears and lacerations of the balloon cuff of the new tracheostomy tube.

3. Griggs [59] in 1990 described a similar apparatus to the Rapitrach but with reduced tendency for tracheal or cuff lacerations. This device again accommodates a central guidewire in a tracheal spreader but lacks the sharp cutting edge. However, there is a potential with this instrument to damage contiguous structures or the posterior wall of the trachea.

4. In 1999, Ciaglia modified the original sequential dilating instrument to use only a single dilator covered with a hydrophilic membrane, which is progressively tapered to open the tracheal stoma with one smooth passage. The advantage of this technique in comparison to the original Ciaglia technique is the rapidity with which this can be performed and the prevention of the loss of tidal volume, which occurs with each progressive dilatation when the dilator is removed from the airway [60,61]. However, concern has been expressed about the potential for anterior cartilage fractures or posterior tracheal wall damage due to the excessive force used to make tracheal stoma formation with this technique.

5. The Perc Twist (Fig. 12-2) has been recently introduced, which consists of a screwlike dilator that follows the guidewire into the tracheal lumen and is designed to lift upward and thereby theoretically prevent posterior tracheal wall damage. However, studies have not clearly shown the value of the Perc Twist device in comparison to the single dilator technique [62].

6. A translaryngeal technique was described in 1997 by Fantoni and Ripamonti [63] and designed to reduce the incidence of posterior tracheal wall lacerations (Fig. 12-3). This technique is the only one where dilation of the stoma is in a retrograde passage from the inside of the trachea with all the force applied upward, thereby avoiding posterior wall trauma. However, it requires some experience and relies on the guidewire exiting through the mouth rather than passing distally into the airway (this early problem was resolved with modifications) [60,64,65]. The guide wire is then attached to a tapered end of a special tracheostomy tube and it is then pulled upward through the anterior tracheal wall, which theoretically limits damage to the posterior tracheal wall. Following the removal of the trocar, the tube is then rotated 180 degrees to point toward the carina. This technique appears to be a valid one, although it is operator dependent. Complications appear to be reduced with experience [60,65,66].

Both techniques (PDT) or (OST) can be performed in either the ICU or the operating room. Multiple analyses have been done with prospective studies as well as with case control studies [53,55,67]. There have been two meta-analyses comparing OST with PDT. Dulguerov et al. [68] reviewed 3,512 patients from 48 studies (1960–1996) and concluded that open surgical tracheostomy was more favorable than percutaneous dilational tracheostomy. However, Freeman et al. [69] reviewed the literature using only the best prospective controlled studies (1991–1999) and arrived at the conclusion that there is no difference between percutaneous tracheostomy and open surgical tracheostomy.

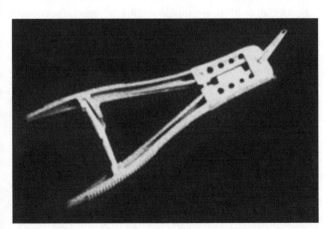

FIGURE 12-1.   Picture of the Rapitrach (Fresenius, Runcorn, Cheshire, UK). [From Lams E, Ravalia A: Percutaneous and surgical tracheostomy. *Hosp Med* 64:36–39, 2003, with permission.]

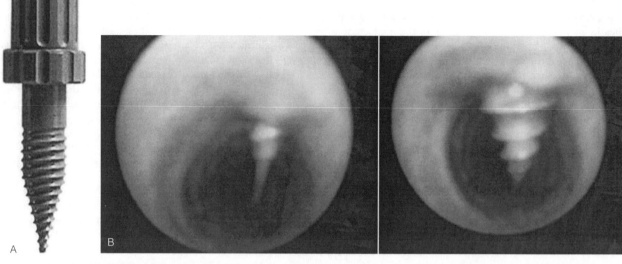

FIGURE 12-2. A picture of the Perc Twist dilating device (**A**), with pictures of the device within the trachea (**B**). [From Byhahn C, Wilke HJ, Halbig S, et al: Percutaneous tracheostomy: Ciaglia Blue Rhino versus the basic Ciaglia technique of percutaneous dilational tracheostomy. *Anaesth Analg* 91:882, 2000, with permission.]

Subsequent critiques of these papers indicate the inherent weakness of heterogeneous patient populations and the use of case series and nonrandomized studies in meta-analyses [70–72]. It is likely that experience and technical modifications allow both techniques to be performed in appropriate patients with the same degree of safety and efficiency (less than 1% procedure related mortality) [67].

Other factors have been used to justify the use of one procedure over the other such as cost efficiency [73,74], bleeding, infection, procedural time, and estimated time from the decision to proceed to successful completion of the procedure [67]. Each factor can be used to justify one procedure over another, but it is likely that institutional practice variations and operator experience are more important in the selection of one procedure over another. This is particularly relevant with respect to the target population where ICU daily expenses far outweigh the procedural costs of either technique [75], and the expected patient mortality can reach as high as 35% [76].

It is probably more important to judiciously use the institutional resources and the operator experience in providing the "best" tracheal technique for these compromised patients. It is possible that the target population may vary from one institution to another (cardiac versus trauma versus neurosurgical versus medical ICU patients), which may influence the decision to perform one technique over another.

Nonetheless, there are certain distinct advantages of PDT that can be outlined as follows: (a) easier access for timing of the procedure; (b) reduced operating room and manpower utilization; (c) less expense than OST (even if both procedures are performed in the ICU); (d) no requirement for transportation of critically ill patients to an operating room; (e) improved cosmetic result; (f) possibly reduced stomal infection and reduced tracheal secretions in the parastomal area due to the tight fitting of the stoma around the tracheostomy tube.

OST should be performed instead of PST in the following patients: (a) patients with more severe respiratory distress (FIO$_2$ greater than 0.60, positive end expiratory pressure greater than 10, complicated translaryngeal intubation or a nonpalpable cricoid cartilage or a cricoid cartilage less than 3 cm above the sternal notch [73]); (b) obese patients with abundant pretracheal subcutaneous fat; (c) patients with large goiters; (d) abnormal airways secondary to congenital acquired conditions; (e) the need for the constant attendance of a second physician to monitor ventilation or circulatory abnormalities; (f) abnormal bleeding diathesis that cannot be adequately corrected by coagulation factors [77].

Overall, candidates selected for tracheostomy are rarely concerned about the end cosmetic result given their ability to improve from the primary condition that led to the tracheostomy to begin with. Transportation issues in patients requiring a tracheostomy are usually of less concern considering that OST can be performed in the ICU. In addition, patients who are so compromised that they cannot be transported to the operating room should be considered poor candidates for a PDT.

Operator experience, the patient population, as well as the hospital environment and resources may be the most important critical factors with respect to procedure selection. Proponents performing both techniques support an efficiency and ease of PDT in good risk patients with a reduction in paratracheal infections and secretions as compared to OST. At the University of Massachusetts Medical Center, both techniques are used to cater to inherent differences between patients. PDT in the ICU is used for low risk patients; while poor risk patients undergo a hybrid procedure in the operating room or in the ICU. In this hybrid procedure, operative exposure of the appropriate tracheal ring is performed with a 3-cm cervical incision equal to the size required for a PDT. This incision allows the appropriate identification of the tracheal ring with mobilization of the isthmus of the thyroid or mobilization of the trachea out of the mediastinum for patients with a foreshortened neck. Thereafter, a small puncture is made on the anterior wall of the trachea and the guidewire of the Blue Rhinoceros tracheostomy dilator (Cook Critical Care, Bloomington, IN) is then inserted into the trachea. Following that, a tracheostoma is created with a

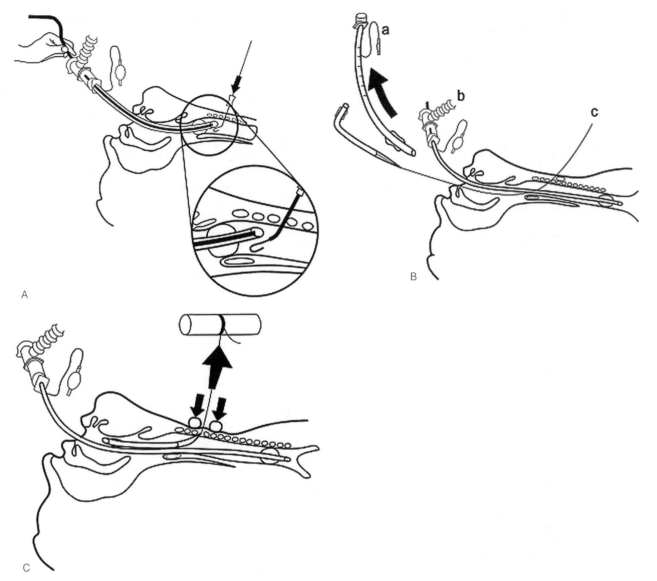

FIGURE 12-3. Sketches of the trocar-tracheostomy tube being pulled through the anterior tracheal wall, as initially described by Fantoni et al. [From Westphal K, Byhahn C, Rinne T, et al: Tracheostomy in cardiosurgical patients: surgical tracheostomy versus cialgia and fantoni methods. *Ann Thorac Surg* 68:486, 1999, with permission.]

single dilator technique followed by insertion of the appropriate tracheostomy tube as required. Bronchoscopy is used for preoperative as well as postoperative control of secretions as well as identification and verification that the tracheostoma is correctly placed. This technique is aimed at providing the safest approach to patient care; it uses the advantages of both OST and PDT techniques and can be performed in either the operating room or the ICU.

TUBES AND CANNULAS

Characteristics of a good tracheostomy tube are flexibility to accommodate varying patient anatomies, inert material, wide internal diameter, the smallest external diameter possible, a smooth surface to allow easy insertion and removal, and sufficient length to be secure once placed but not so long as to impinge the carina or other tracheal parts [78]. Until the late

1960s, when surgeons began to experiment with silicone and other synthetic materials, tracheostomy tubes and cannulas were made of metal. At present, almost all tracheostomy tubes are made of synthetic material. One disadvantage of a silicone tube over a metal one is the increased thickness of the tube wall, resulting in a larger outer diameter. Silicone tubes are available with or without a cuff. The cuff allows occlusion of the airway around the tube, which is necessary for positive-pressure ventilation. It may also minimize aspiration. In the past, cuffs were associated with a fairly high incidence of tracheal stenosis caused by ischemia and necrosis of the mucous membrane and subsequent cicatricial contracture at the cuff site [79,80]. High-volume, low-pressure cuffs diminish pressure on the wall of the trachea, thereby minimizing (but not eliminating) problems due to focal areas of pressure necrosis [81]. Cuff pressures should always be maintained at less than 30 cc H_2O, as higher pressures impair mucosal capillary blood flow leading to ischemic injury to the trachea [82]. Cuff pressures should be checked with a manometer daily in critically ill patients. Once the patient is weaned from mechanical ventilation, the cuff should be deflated, or consideration should be given to placing an uncuffed tracheostomy tube until the patient can be decannulated. If the only purpose of the tube is to secure the airway (sleep apnea) or to provide access for suctioning secretions, a tube without a cuff can be placed.

POSTOPERATIVE CARE

The care of a tracheostomy tube after surgery is important. Highlighted below are some specific issues that all intensivists need to know when caring for patients with tracheostomies.

WOUND AND DRESSING CARE

Daily examinations of the stoma are important in identifying infections or excoriations of the skin at the tracheostomy site [83]. In addition, keeping the wound clean and free of blood and secretions is very important, especially in the immediate post-tracheostomy period. Dressing changes should be preformed at least twice a day and when the dressings are soiled. Some authors recommend cleaning the stoma with 1:1 mixture of hydrogen peroxide and sterile saline [83]. When changing dressings and tapes, special care is needed to avoid accidental dislodging of the tracheostomy tube.

INNER CANNULAS

The inner cannulas should be used at all times in the ICU. They serve to extend the life of the tracheostomy tubes by preventing the buildup secretions within the tracheostomy. The inner cannulas can be easily removed and either cleaned or replaced with a sterile, disposable one. Disposable inner cannulas have the advantage of quick and efficient changing, a decrease in nursing time, decrease risk of cross-contamination, and guaranteed sterility [84]. The obturator should be kept at the bedside at all times in the event that reinsertion of the tracheostomy is necessary.

HUMIDIFICATION

One of the functions of the upper airway is to moisten and humidify inspired air. Since tracheostomies bypass the upper airway, it is vital to provide patients who have tracheostomies with warm, humidified air. Humidification of inspired gases will prevent complications in patients with tracheostomies. Failure to humidify the inspired gases can obstruct the tube by inspissated secretions, impair mucociliary clearance, and decrease cough [85,86].

SUCTIONING

Patients with tracheostomies frequently have increased amounts of airway secretions coupled with decreased ability to clear them effectively. Keeping the airways clear of excess secretions is important in decreasing the risk of lung infection and airway plugging [83]. Suctioning is frequently required in patients with poor or ineffective cough. Suction techniques should remove the maximal amount of secretions while causing the least

amount of airway trauma [87,88]. Routine suctioning, however, is not recommended [89].

TRACHEOSTOMY TUBE CHANGES

Tracheostomy tubes do not require routine changing. In general, the tube only needs to be changed under the following conditions: (a) there is a functional problem with it, such as an air leak in the balloon; (b) when the lumen is narrowed due to the buildup of dried secretions; (c) when switching to a new type of tube; or (d) when downsizing the tube prior to decannulation. Ideally, a tracheostomy tube should not be changed until 7 to 10 days after its initial placement. The reason for this is to allow the tracheal stoma and the tract to mature. Patients who have their tracheostomy tube changed before the tract is fully mature risk having the tube misplaced into the soft tissue of the neck. If the tracheostomy tube needs to be replaced before the tract has had time to mature, the tube should be changed over a guide, such as a suction catheter or tube changer [90,91].

ORAL FEEDING AND SWALLOWING DYSFUNCTION ASSOCIATED WITH TRACHEOSTOMIES

Great caution should be exercised before initiating oral feedings in patients with tracheostomy. Numerous studies have demonstrated that patients are at a significantly increased risk for aspiration when a tracheostomy is in place.

Physiologically, patients with tracheostomies are more likely to aspirate because the tracheostomy tube tethers the larynx, preventing its normal upward movement needed to assist in glottic closure and cricopharyngeal relaxation [92,93]. Tracheostomy tubes also disrupt normal swallowing by compressing the esophagus and interfering with deglutition [94], decreasing duration of vocal cord closure [95], and resulting in uncoordinated laryngeal closure [96]. In addition, prolonged orotracheal intubation can result in prolonged swallowing disorders even after the endotracheal tube is converted to a tracheostomy [97]. It is therefore not surprising that more than 65% of patients with tracheostomies aspirate when swallowing [98–100]. It is felt that 77% of the episodes are clinically silent [101,102].

Before attempting oral feedings in a patient with a tracheostomy, several objective criteria must be met. Obviously, the patient must be consistently alert, appropriate, and able to follow complex commands. The patient should also have adequate cough and swallowing reflexes, adequate oral motor strength, and a significant respiratory reserve [103]. These criteria are probably best assessed by a certified speech therapist. However, clinical assessment may only identify 34% of the patients at high risk for aspiration [104]. Augmenting the bedside swallowing evaluation by coloring feedings or measuring the glucose in tracheal secretions may not increase the sensitivity in detecting the risk of aspiration [105,106]. A video barium swallow may identify between 50% to 80% of patients with tracheostomies who are at a high risk to aspirate oral feeding [102,104]. A laryngoscopy to observe directly a patient's swallowing mechanics, coupled with a video barium swallow, may be more sensitive in predicting which patients are at risk for aspiration [104]. Scintigraphic studies may be the most sensitive test to determining which patients are aspirating [107], and it is much easier to perform than endoscopy. Plugging of the tracheostomy [107] or using a Passy-Muir valve [108] may reduce aspiration in patients with tracheostomies who are taking oral feedings, but this is not a universal finding [109].

Because of the high risk for aspiration and the difficulty assessing which patients are at high risk to aspirate, we do not institute oral feedings in our patients with tracheostomy in the ICU. We believe that the potential risks of a percutaneous endoscopically placed gastrostomy feeding tube is much less than the risk of aspiration of oral feedings and its complications (i.e., recurrent pneumonia, acute respiratory distress syndrome, and prolonged weaning). Typically we perform both procedures in the same setting to minimize the anesthesia load to the patient. We are, however, unaware of any prospective studies addressing the complications between these two methods of providing enteric nutritional support in patients with tracheostomies.

COMPLICATIONS

Tracheostomies, whether inserted by percutaneous dilatation or by the open surgical procedure, are associated with a variety of complications. These complications are best grouped by the time of occurrence after the placement and are divided into immediate, intermediate, and late complications (Table 12-3) [16]. The reported incidence of complications varies from as low as 4% [110] to as high as 65% [111], with reported mortality rates from 0.03% to 0.6% [68,112]. Complication rates appear to decrease with increasing experience of the physician performing the procedure [113]. Posttracheostomy mortality and morbidity is usually due to iatrogenic tracheal laceration [114], hemorrhage, tube dislodgment, infection, or obstruction. Neurosurgical patients have a higher posttracheostomy complication rate than other patients [115,116]. Tracheostomy is more hazardous in children than in adults and carries special risks in the very young, often related to the experience of the surgeon [117]. A comprehensive understanding of immediate, intermediate, and late complications of tracheostomy and their management is essential for the intensivist.

OBSTRUCTION

Obstruction of the tracheostomy tube is a potentially life-threatening complication. The tube may become plugged with clotted blood or inspissated secretions. In this case, the inner cannula should be removed immediately and the patient suctioned. Should that fail, it may be necessary to remove the outer cannula also, a decision that must take into consideration the reason the tube was placed and the length of time it has been in place. Obstruction may also be due to angulation of the distal end of the tube against the anterior or posterior tracheal wall. An undivided thyroid isthmus pressing against the angled tracheostomy tube can force the tip against the anterior tracheal wall, whereas a low superior transverse skin edge can force the tip of the tracheostomy tube against the posterior tracheal wall. An indication of this type of obstruction is an expiratory wheeze. Division of the thyroid isthmus and proper placement of transverse skin incisions prevent anterior or posterior tube angulation and obstruction [118].

TABLE 12-3.   Complications of Tracheostomies

Immediate Complications (0–24 hours)
  Tube displacement
  Arrhythmia
  Hypotension
  Hypoxia/hypercapnia
  Loss of airway control
  Pneumothorax
  Pneumomediastinum
  Acute surgical emphysema
  Major hemorrhage
  Bacteremia
  Esophageal injury (*uncommon*)
  Cardiorespiratory arrest (*uncommon*)
  Tracheo-laryngeal injury (*uncommon*)
  Crushed airway from dilational tracheostomy-*uncommon*
Intermediate Complications (from day 1 to day 7)
  Persistent bleeding
  Tube displacement
  Tube obstruction (mucus, blood)
  Major atelectasis
  Wound infection/cellulitis
Late Complications (>day 7)
  Tracheoinnominate artery fistula
  Tracheomalacia
  Tracheal stenosis
  Necrosis and loss of anterior tracheal cartilage
  Tracheoesophageal fistula
  Major aspiration
  Chronic speech and swallowing deficits
  Tracheocutaneous fistula

Conlan AA, Kopec SE: Tracheostomy in the ICU. *J Intensive Care Med* 15:1, 2000.
Angel LF, Simpson CB: Comparison of surgical and percutaneous dilational tracheostomy. *Clin Chest Med* 24:423, 2003.
Epstein SK: Late complications of tracheostomy. *Respir Care* 50:542, 2005.
Durbin CG: Early complications of tracheostomy. *Respir Care* 50:511, 2005.

TUBE DISPLACEMENT/DISLODGMENT

Dislodgment of a tracheostomy tube that has been in place for 2 weeks or longer is managed simply by replacing the tube. If it cannot be immediately replaced or if it is replaced and the patient cannot be ventilated (indicating that the tube is not in the trachea), orotracheal intubation should be performed. Immediate postoperative displacement can be fatal if the tube cannot be promptly replaced and the patient cannot be reintubated.

Dislodgment in the early postoperative period is usually caused by one of several technical problems. Failure to divide the thyroid isthmus may permit the intact isthmus to ride up against the tracheostomy tube and thus displace it [118]. Excessively low placement of the stoma (i.e., below the second and third rings) can occur when the thoracic trachea is brought into the neck by overextending the neck or by excessive traction on the trachea. When the normal anatomical relationships are restored, the trachea recedes below the suprasternal notch, causing the tube to be dislodged from the trachea [118,119]. The risk of dislodgment of the tracheostomy tube, a potentially lethal complication, can be minimized by (a) transection of the thyroid isthmus at surgery, if indicated; (b) proper placement of the stoma; (c) avoidance of excessive neck hyperextension and/or tracheal traction; (d) application of sufficiently tight tracheostomy tube retention tapes; and (e) suture of the tracheostomy tube flange to the skin in patients with short necks. Some surgeons apply retaining sutures to the trachea for use in the early postoperative period in case the tube becomes dislodged, allowing the trachea to be pulled into the wound for reintubation. Making a Bjork flap involves suturing the inferior edge of the trachea stoma to the skin, thus allowing a sure pathway for tube placement. Bjork flaps, however, tend to interfere with swallowing and promote aspiration [120]. Reintubation of a tracheostomy can be accomplished by using a smaller, beveled endotracheal tube and then applying a tracheostomy tube over the smaller tube, using the Seldinger technique [121]. Using a nasogastric tube as a guidewire has also been described [122].

If a tracheostomy becomes dislodged within 7 to 10 days of surgery, we recommend translaryngeal endotracheal intubation to establish a safe airway. The tracheostomy tube can then be replaced under less urgent conditions, with fiberoptic guidance if needed.

SUBCUTANEOUS EMPHYSEMA

Approximately 5% of patients develop subcutaneous emphysema after tracheostomy [121]. It is most likely to occur when dissection is extensive and/or the wound is closed tightly. Partial closure of the skin wound is appropriate, but the underlying tissues should be allowed to approximate naturally. Subcutaneous emphysema generally resolves over the 48 hours after tracheostomy, but when the wound is closed tightly and the patient is coughing or on positive-pressure ventilation, pneumomediastinum, pneumopericardium, and/or tension pneumothorax may occur [118].

PNEUMOTHORAX AND PNEUMOMEDIASTINUM

The cupola of the pleura extends well into the neck, especially in patients with emphysema; thus, the pleura can be damaged during tracheostomy. This complication is more common in the pediatric age group because the pleural dome extends more cephalad in children [1]. The incidence of pneumothorax after tracheostomy ranges from 0% to 5% [1,110,121]. Many surgeons routinely obtain a postoperative chest radiograph.

HEMORRHAGE

Minor postoperative fresh tracheostomy bleeding occurs in up to 37% of cases [1] and is probably the most common complication of this procedure. Postoperative coughing and straining can cause venous bleeding by dislodging a clot or ligature. Elevating the head of the bed, packing the wound, and/or using homeostatic materials usually controls minor bleeding. Major bleeding can occur in up to 5% of tracheotomies and is due to hemorrhage from the isthmus of the thyroid gland, loss of a ligature from one of the anterior jugular veins, or injury to the transverse jugular vein that crosses the midline just above the jugular notch [123]. Persistent bleeding may require a return to the operating room for management. Techniques to decrease the likelihood of early posttracheostomy hemorrhage include (a) use of a vertical incision; (b) careful dissection in the midline, with care to pick up each layer of tissue with instruments rather than simply spreading tissues apart; (c) liberal use of ligatures rather than electrocautery; and (d) careful division and suture ligation of the thyroid isthmus. Late hemorrhage after tracheostomy is usually due to bleeding granulation tissue or another relatively minor cause. However, in these late cases, a tracheoinnominate artery fistula needs to be ruled out.

TRACHEOINNOMINATE ARTERY FISTULA

At one point, it had been reported that 50% of all tracheostomy bleeding occurring more than 48 hours after the procedure was due to an often fatal complication of rupture of the innominate artery caused by erosion of the tracheostomy tube at its tip or cuff into the vessel [121]. However, since the advent of the low-pressure cuff, the incidence of this complication has decreased considerably and occurs less than 1% of the time [124].

Eighty-five percent of tracheal-innominate fistulas occur within the first month after tracheostomy [125], although it has been reported as late as 7 months after operation. Other sites of delayed exsanguinating posttracheostomy hemorrhage include the common carotid artery, superior and inferior thyroid arteries, aortic arch, and innominate vein [125]. Rupture and fistula formation are caused by erosion through the trachea into the artery due to excessive cuff pressure or by angulation of the tube tip against the anterior trachea. Infection and other factors that weaken local tissues, such as malnourishment and steroids, also seem to play a role [126]. The innominate artery rises to about the level of the sixth ring anterior to the trachea, and low placement of the stoma can also create close proximity of the tube tip or cuff to the innominate artery. Rarely, an anomaly of the innominate, occurring with an incidence of 1% to 2% [125], is responsible for this disastrous complication. Pulsation of the tracheostomy tube is an indication of potentially fatal positioning [125]. Initially, hemorrhage from a tracheal-innominate fistula is usually not exsanguinating. Herald bleeds must be investigated promptly using fiberoptic tracheoscopy. If a tracheal-innominate fistula seems probable (minimal tracheitis, anterior pulsating erosions), the patient should be taken to the operating room for evaluation. Definitive management involves resection of the artery [127]. The mortality rate approaches 100%, even with emergent surgical intervention [128]. Sudden exsanguinating hemorrhage may be managed by hyperinflation of the tracheostomy cuff tube or reintubation with an endotracheal tube through the stoma, attempting to place the cuff at the level of the fistula. A lower neck incision with blind digital compression on the artery may be part of a critical resuscitative effort [129]. If a tracheoinnominate artery fistula is suspected, the patient should be evaluated in the operating room, and preparations should be made for a possible sternotomy.

MISPLACEMENT OF TUBE

Misplacement of the tube error occurs at the time of surgery or when the tube is changed or replaced through a fresh stoma. If not recognized, associated mediastinal emphysema and tension pneumothorax can occur, along with alveolar hypoventilation. Injury to neurovascular structures, including the recurrent laryngeal nerve, is possible [119]. The patient must be orally intubated or the tracheostoma recannulated. Some advise placing retaining sutures in the trachea at the time of surgery. The availability of a tracheostomy set at the bedside after tracheostomy facilitates emergency reintubation.

STOMAL INFECTIONS

An 8% to 12% incidence of cellulitis or purulent exudate is reported with tracheostomy [1,121]. The risk of serious infection is less than 0.5% [110]. Attention to the details of good stoma care and early use of antibiotics are advised. However, prophylactic antibiotics are not recommended [130].

TRACHEOESOPHAGEAL FISTULA

Tracheoesophageal fistula caused by injury to the posterior tracheal wall and cervical esophagus occurs in less than 1% of patients, more commonly in the pediatric age group. Early postoperative fistula is a result of iatrogenic injury during the procedure [121,129]. The chances of creating a fistula can be minimized by entering the trachea initially with a horizontal incision between two tracheal rings (the second and third), thereby eliminating the initial cut into a hard cartilaginous ring [118]. A late tracheoesophageal fistula may be due to tracheal necrosis caused by tube movement or angulation, as in neck hyperflexion, or excessive cuff pressure [119,121,129]. A tracheoesophageal fistula should be suspected in patients with cuff leaks, abdominal distention, recurrent aspiration pneumonia, and reflux of gastric fluids through the tracheostomy site. It may be demonstrated on endoscopy and contrast studies. Tracheoesophageal fistulas require surgical repair. For patients who could not tolerate a major surgical procedure, placement of an esophageal and a tracheal stent may be used [131–133].

TRACHEAL STENOSIS

Some degree of tracheal stenosis is seen in 40% to 60% of patients with tracheostomies [112,134]. However, 3% to 12% of these stenoses are clinically significant enough to require intervention [135]. Stenosis most commonly occurs at the level of the stoma or just above the stoma but distal to the vocal cords [128]. The stenosis typically results from bacterial infection or chondritis of the anterior and lateral tracheal walls. Granulation tissue usually develops first. Ultimately the granulation tissue matures, becoming fibrous and covered with a layer of epithelium. The granulation tissue itself can also result in other complications, such as obstructing the airway at the level of the stoma, making changing the tracheostomy tube difficult and occluding tube fenestrations. Identified risk factors for developing tracheal stenosis include sepsis, stomal infections, hypotension, advanced age, male gender, corticosteroid use, excess motion of the tracheostomy tube, oversized tube, prolonged placement, elevated cuff pressures, and excessive excision of the anterior trachea cartilage [111,128,136]. Using properly sized tracheostomy tubes, inflating cuffs only when indicated, and maintaining intracuff pressures below 15 to 20 mm Hg may decrease the incidence of tracheal stenosis [137]. Tracheal stenosis, as well as other long-term complications, appears to be less with the percutaneous procedure [138–140].

Treatment options for granulation tissue include topical strategies (such as topical antibiotic or steroids, silver nitrate, and polyurethane form dressings), or surgical strategies (laser excision, electrocautery, and surgical removal) [128]. Treatment options for symptomatic tracheal stenosis include dilatation with a rigid bronchoscopy with coring, intralumen laser excision, or surgical resection with end-to-end tracheal anastomosis [111,141].

TRACHEOMALACIA

Tracheomalacia is a weakening of the tracheal wall resulting from ischemic injury to the trachea, followed by chondritis, then destruction, and necrosis of the tracheal cartilage [128]. Consequently, there is collapse of the affected portion of the trachea with expiration, resulting in airflow limitation, air trapping, and retention of airway secretions. Tracheomalacia may ultimately result in the patient's failing to wean from mechanical ventilation. A short-term therapeutic approach to tracheomalacia is to place a longer tracheostomy tube to bypass the area of malacia. Long-term treatment options include stenting, tracheal resection, or tracheoplasty [128].

DYSPHAGIA AND ASPIRATION

The major swallowing disorder associated with tracheostomy is aspiration. (See the section Oral Feeding and Swallowing Dysfunction.) Because of the high risk for aspiration, we do not recommend oral feeding in ICU patients with tracheostomies.

TRACHEOCUTANEOUS FISTULA

Although the tracheostoma generally closes rapidly after decannulation, a persistent fistula may occasionally remain, particularly when the tracheostomy tube is present for a prolonged period. If this complication occurs, the fistula tract can be excised and the wound closed primarily under local anesthesia [142].

CONCLUSION

Tracheostomy is one of the most common surgical procedures preformed in the ICU and is the airway of choice for patients requiring mechanical ventilation for more than 2 weeks. The exact timing for converting patients to tracheostomy is not entirely clear, so the physician must weight the risks and benefits of tracheostomy versus translaryngeal intubation and estimate the expected duration of mechanical ventilation for each individual patient. The physician performing the tracheostomy procedure needs to assess each patient to determine the best technique (whether it be performed bedside percutaneously or open in the operating room) for that specific patient. The patient's medical condition, the physician's experience with the various techniques, and the hospital's resources all need to be considered in determining the type of procedure performed.

REFERENCES

1. Goldstein SI, Breda SD, Schneider KL: Surgical complications of bedside tracheotomy in an otolaryngology residency program. *Laryngoscope* 97:1407, 1987.
2. Heffner JE, Miller KS, Sahn SA: Tracheostomy in the intensive care unit, 1: indication, techniques, management. *Chest* 90:269, 1986.
3. Goodall EW: The story of tracheotomy. *Br J Child Dis* 31:167, 1934.
4. Jackson C: High tracheotomy and other errors: the chief causes of chronic laryngeal stenosis. *Surg Gynecol Obstet* 32:392, 1921.
5. McClelland RMA: Tracheostomy: its management and alternatives. *Proc R Soc Med* 65:401, 1972.

6. Fischler L, Erhart S, Kleger GR, et al: Prevalence of tracheostomy in ICU patients. *Intensive Care Med* 26:1428, 2000.

7. Kremer B, Botos-Kremer A, Eckel H, et al: Indications, complications, and surgical technique for pediatric tracheostomies. *J Pediatr Surg* 37:1556, 2002.

8. Bjure J: Tracheotomy: A satisfactory method in the treatment of acute epiglottis. A clinical and functional follow-up study. *Int J Pediatr Otorhinolaryngol* 3:37, 1981.

9. Hanline MH Jr: Tracheotomy in upper airway obstruction. *South Med J* 74:899, 1981.

10. Taicher S, Givol M, Peleg M, et al: Changing indications for tracheostomy in maxillofacial trauma. *J Oral Maxillofac Surg* 54:292, 1996.

11. Guilleminault C, Simmons FB, Motta J, et al: Obstructive sleep apnea syndrome and tracheostomy. *Arch Intern Med* 141:985, 1981.

12. Burwell C, Robin E, Whaley R, et al: Extreme obesity associated with alveolar hypoventilation. *Am J Med* 141:985, 1981.

13. Yung MW, Snowdon SL: Respiratory resistance of tracheostomy tubes. *Arch Otolaryngol* 110:591, 1984.

14. Heffner JE: Tracheostomy application and timing. *Clin Chest Med* 24:389, 2003.

15. Durbin CG: Indications for and timing of tracheostomy. *Respir Care* 50:483, 2005.

16. Conlan AA, Kopec SE: Tracheostomy in the ICU. *J Intensive Care Med* 15:1, 2000.

17. Colice GL: Resolution of laryngeal injury following translaryngeal intubation. *Am Rev Respir Dis* 142(2 part 1):361, 1992.

18. Marsh HM, Gillespie DJ, Baumgartner AE: Timing of tracheostomy in the critically ill patient. *Chest* 96:190, 1989.

19. Lesnik I, Rappaport W, Fulginiti J, et al: The role of early tracheostomy in blunt, multiple organ trauma. *Am Surg* 58:346, 1992.

20. Armstrong PA, McCarthy MC, Peoples JB: Reduced use of resources by early tracheostomy in ventilator-dependent patients with blunt trauma. *Surgery* 124:763, 1998.

21. Teoh WH, Goh KY, Chan C: The role of early tracheostomy in critically ill neurosurgical patients. *Ann Acad Med Singapore* 30:234, 2001.

22. Koh WY, Lew TWK, Chin NM, et al: Tracheostomy in a neuro-intensive care setting: indications and timing. *Anaesth Intensive Care* 25:365, 1997.

23. D'Amelio LF, Hammond JS, Spain DA, et al: Tracheostomy and percutaneous endoscopic gastrostomy in the management of the head-injured patient. *Am Surg* 60:180, 1994.

24. Sellers BJ, Davis BL, Larkin PW, et al: Early predictors of prolonged ventilator dependence in thermally injured patients. *J Trauma* 43:899, 1997.

25. Rumbak MJ, Newton M, Truncale T, et al: A prospective, randomized study comparing early percutaneous dilational tracheostomy to prolonged translaryngeal intubation in critically ill medical patients. *Crit Care Med* 32:1689, 2004.

26. Blot F: A study of early tracheostomy in patients undergoing prolonged mechanical ventilation. *Rev Mal Respir* 20:411, 2003.

27. Dongelmans DA, Schultz MJ: Early or late tracheostomy. *Crit Care Med* 33:466, 2004.

28. Griffiths J, Barber VS, Morgan L, et al: Systematic review and meta-analysis of studies of the timing of tracheostomy in adult patients undergoing artificial ventilation. *BMJ* 330:1243, 2005.

29. Stock CM, Woodward CG, Shapiro BA, et al: Perioperative complications of elective tracheostomy in critically ill patients. *Crit Care Med* 14:861, 1986.

30. Skaggs JA, Cogbill CL: Tracheostomy: management, mortality, complications. *Am Surg* 35:393, 1969.

31. American College of Surgeons Committee on Trauma: *Advanced Trauma Life Support Course for Physicians, Instructor Manual.* Chicago, American College of Surgeons, 1985; p 159.

32. Kline SN: Maxillofacial trauma, in Kreis DJ, Gomez GA (eds): *Trauma Management.* Boston, Little, Brown, 1989.

33. Esses BA, Jafek BW: Cricothyroidotomy: a decade of experience in Denver. *Ann Otol Rhinol Laryngol* 96:519, 1987.

34. Brantigan CO, Grow JB: Cricothyroidotomy: elective use in respiratory problems requiring tracheotomy. *J Thorac Cardiovasc Surg* 71:72, 1976.

35. Cole RR, Aguilar EA: Cricothyroidotomy versus tracheotomy: an otolaryngologist's perspective. *Laryngoscope* 98:131, 1988.

36. Boyd AD, Romita MC, Conlan AA, et al: A clinical evaluation of cricothyroidotomy. *Surg Gynecol Obstet* 149:365, 1979.

37. Sise MJ, Shacksord SR, Cruickshank JC, et al: Cricothyroidotomy for long term tracheal access. *Ann Surg* 200:13, 1984.

38. O'Connor JV, Reddy K, Ergin MA, et al: Cricothyroidotomy for prolonged ventilatory support after cardiac operations. *Ann Thorac Surg* 39:353, 1985.

39. Lewis GA, Hopkinson RB, Matthews HR: Minitracheotomy: a report of its use in intensive therapy. *Anesthesia* 41:931, 1986.

40. Pierce WS, Tyers FO, Waldhausen JA: Effective isolation of a tracheostomy from a median sternotomy wound. *J Thorac Cardiovasc Surg* 66:841, 1973.

41. Morain WD: Cricothyroidotomy in head and neck surgery. *Plast Reconstr Surg* 65:424,1980.

42. Kuriloff DB, Setzen M, Portnoy W, et al: Laryngotracheal injury following cricothyroidotomy. *Laryngoscope* 99:125, 1989.

43. Hawkins ML, Shapiro MB, Cue JI, et al: Emergency cricothyrotomy: a reassessment. *Am Surg* 61:52, 1995.

44. Mace SE: Cricothyrotomy. *Emerg Med* 6:309, 1988.

45. Robinson RJS, Mulder DS : Airway control, in Mattox KL , Feliciano DV, Moore EE (eds): *Trauma.* New York, McGraw-Hill, 2000; p 171.

46. McGill J, Clinton JE, Ruiz E: Cricothyrotomy in the emergency department. *Ann Emerg Med* 11:361, 1982.

47. Terry RM, Cook P: Hemorrhage during minitracheotomy: reduction of risk by altered incision. *J Laryngol Otol* 103:207, 1989.

48. Cutler BS: Cricothyroidotomy for emergency airway, in Vander Salm TJ, Cutler BS, Wheeler HB (eds): *Atlas of Bedside Procedures.* Boston, Little, Brown, 1988; p 231.

49. Erlandson MJ, Clinton JE, Ruiz E, et al: Cricothyrotomy in the emergency department revisited. *J Emerg Med* 7:115, 1989.

50. Brantigan CO, Grow JB: Subglottic stenosis after cricothyroidotomy. *Surgery* 91:217, 1982.

51. Epstein SK: Anatomy and physiology of tracheostomy. *Respir Care* 50:476, 2005.

52. DeBoisblanc BP: Percutaneous dilational tracheostomy techniques. *Clin Chest Med* 24:399, 2003.

53. Lams E, Ravalia A: Percutaneous and surgical tracheostomy. *Hosp Med* 64:36, 2003.

54. Walts PA, Murthy SC, DeCamp MM: Techniques of surgical tracheostomy. *Clin Chest Med* 24:413, 2003.

55. Durbin CG: Technique for performing tracheostomy. *Respir Care* 50:488, 2005.

56. Mallick A, Venkatanath D, Elliot SC, et al: A prospective randomized controlled trial of capnography vs. bronchoscopy for Blue Rhino percutaneous tracheostomy. *Anaesthesia* 58:864, 2003.

57. Ciaglia P, Firsching R, Syniec C: Elective percutaneous dilatational tracheostomy: a new simple beside procedure. Preliminary report. *Chest* 87:715, 1985.

58. Schachner A, Ovil J, Sidi J, et al: Percutaneous tracheostomy: a new method. *Crit Care Med* 17:1052, 1989.

59. Griggs WM, Worthley LI, Gilligan JE, et al: A simple percutaneous tracheostomy technique. *Surg Gynecol Obstet* 170:543, 1990.

60. Byhahn C, Wilke HJ, Halbig S, et al: Percutaneous tracheostomy: Ciaglia Blue Rhino versus the basic Ciaglia technique of percutaneous dilational tracheostomy. *Anaesth Analg* 91:882, 2000.

61. Jeffery JL, Cheathan MML, Sagraves SG, et al: Percutaneous dilational tracheostomy: a comparison of single versus multiple dilator techniques. *Crit Care Med* 29:1251, 2001.

62. Byhahn C, Westphel K, Menninger D, et al: Single dilator percutaneous tracheostomy: a comparison of Percu twist and Ciaglia blue vinyl techniques. *Intensive Care Med* 28:1262, 2002.

63. Fantoni A, Ripamonti D: A non-derivative, non-surgical tracheostomy: the translaryngeal method. *Intensive Care Med* 23:386, 1997.

64. Westphal K, Byhahan C, Wilke AJ, et al: Percutaneous tracheostomy: a clinical comparison of dilational (Ciaglia) and translaryngeal (Fantoni) techniques. *Anesth Analg* 89:938, 1999.

65. Cantais E, Kaiser E, Le-Goff Y, et al: Percutaneous tracheostomy: prospective comparison of the translaryngeal technique versus the forceps-dilational technique in one hundred critically ill adults. *Crit Care Med* 30:815, 2002.

66. Antonelli M, Michetti V, DiPalma A, et al: Percutaneous translaryngeal versus surgical tracheostomy: a randomized trial with 1-year double blind follow-up. *Crit Care Med* 33:1015, 2005.

67. Angel LF, Simpson CB: Comparison of surgical and percutaneous dilational tracheostomy. *Clin Chest Med* 24:423, 2003.

68. Dulguerov P, Gysin C, Perneger TV, et al: Percutaneous or surgical tracheostomy: a meta-analysis. *Crit Care Med* 27:1617, 1999.

69. Freeman BD, Isabella K, Lin N, et al: A meta-analysis of prospective trials comparing percutaneous and surgical tracheostomy in critically ill patients. *Chest* 118:412, 2000.

70. Anderson JD, Rabinovici R, Frankel HL: Percutaneous dilational tracheostomy vs open tracheostomy. *Chest* 120:1423, 2001.

71. Heffner JE: Percutaneous dilational vs standard tracheostomy: a meta-analysis but not the final analysis. *Chest* 118:1236, 2000.

72. Susanto I: Comparing percutaneous tracheostomy with open surgical tracheostomy. *BMJ* 324:3, 2002.

73. Massick DD, Yao S, Powell DM, et al: Bedside tracheostomy in the intensive care unit: a perspective randomized trial comparing surgical tracheostomy with endoscopically guided percutaneous dilational tracheotomy. *Laryngoscope* 111:494, 2001.

74. McHenry CR, Raeburn CD, Lange RL, et al: Percutaneous tracheostomy: a cost-effective alternative to standard open tracheostomy. *Am Surg* 63:646, 1997.

75. Garland A: Improving the ICU: part 1. *Chest* 127:2151, 2005.

76. Combes A, Luyt CE, Trouillet JL, et al: Adverse effects on a referral intensive care unit's performance of accepting patients transferred from another intensive care unit. *Crit Care Med* 33:705, 2005.

77. Stocchetti N, Parma A, Lamperti M, et al: Neurophysiologic consequences of three tracheostomy techniques: a randomized study in neurosurgical patients. *Neurosurg Anesthesiol* 12:307, 2000.

78. Lewis RJ: Tracheostomies: indications, timing, and complications. *Clin Chest Med* 13:137, 1992.

79. Cooper JD, Grillo HC: The evolution of tracheal injury due to ventilatory assistance through cuffed tubes: a pathologic study. *Ann Surg* 169:334, 1969.

80. Stool SE, Campbell JR, Johnson DG: Tracheostomy in children: the use of plastic tubes. *J Pediatr Surg* 3:402, 1968.

81. Grillo HZ, Cooper JD, Geffin B, et al: A low pressured cuff for tracheostomy tubes to minimize tracheal inner injury. *J Thorac Cardiovasc Surg* 62:898, 1971.

82. Seegobin RD, van Hasselt GL: Endotracheal cuff pressure and tracheal mucosal blood flow, endoscopic study of effects of four large volume cuffs. *BMJ* 288:965, 1984.

83. Wright SE, van Dahn K: Long-term care of the tracheostomy patient. *Clin Chest Med* 24:473, 2003.

84. Crow S: Disposable tracheostomy inner cannula. *Infect Control* 7:285, 1986.

85. Forbes AR: Temperature, humidity and mucous flow in the intubated trachea. *Br J Anaesth* 46:29, 1974.

86. Chalon J, Patel C, Ali M, et al: Humidity and the anaesthetized patient. *Anesthiol* 50:195, 1979.

87. Shekelton M, Nield DM: Ineffective airway clearance related to artificial airway. *Nurs Clin North Am* 22:167, 1987.

88. Johnson KL, Kearney PA, Johnson SB, et al: Closed versus open endotracheal suctioning: costs and physiologic consequences. *Crit Care Med* 22:658, 1994.

89. Lewis RM: Airway clearance techniques for patients with artificial airways. *Respir Care* 47:808, 2002.

90. Gilsdorf, JR: Facilitated endotracheal and tracheostomy tube replacement. *Surg Gynecol Obstet* 159:587, 1984.

91. Young JS, Brady WJ, Kesser B, et al: A novel method for replacement of a dislodged tracheostomy tube: the nasogastric tube guidewire technique. *J Emerg Med* 14:205, 1996.

92. Bonanno PC: Swallowing dysfunction after tracheostomy. *Ann Surg* 174:29, 1971.

93. Shelly R: The post-insertion protocol for management of the Olympic tracheostomy button in neurosurgical patients. *J Neurosurg Nursing* 13:294, 1981.

94. Betts RH: Posttracheostomy aspiration. *N Engl J Med* 273:155, 1965.

95. Shaker R, Dodds WJ, Dantas EO: Coordination of deglutitive glottic closure with oropharyngeal swallowing. *Gastroenterol* 98:1478, 1990.

96. Buckwater JA, Sasaki CT: Effect of tracheostomy on laryngeal function. *Otolaryngol Clin North Am* 21:701, 1988.

97. Devita MA, Spierer-Rundback MS: Swallowing disorders in patients with prolonged intubation or tracheostomy tubes. *Crit Care Med* 18:1328, 1990.

98. Cameron JL, Reynolds J, Zuidema GD: Aspiration in patients with tracheostomies. *Surg Gynecol Obstet* 136:68, 1973.

99. Bone DK, Davis JL, Zuidema GD, et al: Aspiration pneumonia. *Ann Thorac Surg* 18:30, 1974.

100. Muz J, Mathog RH, Nelson R, et al: Aspiration in patients with head and neck cancer and tracheostomy. *Am J Otolaryngol* 10:282, 1989.

101. Panmunzio TG: Aspiration of oral feedings in patients with tracheostomies. *AACN Clin Issues. Advance Practice in Acute Critical Care* 7:560, 1996.

102. Elpern EH, Scott MG, Petro L, et al: Pulmonary aspiration in mechanically ventilated patients with tracheostomies. *Chest* 105:563, 1994.

103. Godwin JE, Heffner JE: Special critical care considerations in tracheostomy management. *Clin Chest Med* 12:573, 1991.

104. Tolep K, Getch CL, Criner GJ: Swallowing dysfunction in patients receiving prolonged mechanical ventilation. *Chest* 109:167, 1996.

105. Metheny NA, Clouse RE: Bedside methods for detecting aspiration in tube-fed patients. *Chest* 111:724, 1997.

106. Thompson-Henry S, Braddock B: The modified Evan's blue dye procedure fails to detect aspiration in the tracheostomized patient: five case reports. *Dysphagia* 10:172, 1995.

107. Muz J, Hamlet S, Mathog R, et al: Scintigraphic assessment of aspiration in head and neck cancer patients with tracheostomy. *Head Neck* 16:17, 1994.

108. Dettelbach MA, Gross RD, Mahlmann J, et al: Effect of the Passy-Muir valve on aspiration in patients with tracheostomy. *Head Neck* 17:297, 1995.

109. Leder SB, Tarro JM, Burell MI: Effect of occlusion of a tracheostomy tube on aspiration. *Dysphagia* 11:254, 1996.

110. Goldenberg D, Ari EG, Golz A, et al: Tracheostomy complications: a retrospective study of 1130 cases. *Otolaryngol Head Neck Surg* 123:495, 2000.

111. Sue RD, Susanto I: Long-term complications of artificial airways. *Clin Chest Med* 24:457, 2003.

112. Walz MK, Peitgen K, Thurauf N, et al: Percutaneous dilatational tracheostomy—early results and long-term outcome of 326 critically ill patients. *Intensive Care Med* 24:685, 1998.

113. Petros S, Engelmann L: Percutaneous dilatational tracheostomy in a medical ICU. *Intensive Care Med* 23:630, 1997.

114. Massard G, Rouge C, Dabbagh A, et al: Tracheobronchial lacerations after intubation and tracheostomy. *Ann Thorac Surg* 61:1483, 1996.

115. Dunham CM, LaMonica C: Prolonged tracheal intubation in the trauma patient. *J Trauma* 24:120, 1984.

116. Miller JD, Kapp JP: Complications of tracheostomies in neurosurgical patients. *Surg Neurol* 22:186, 1984.

117. Shinkwin CA, Gibbin KP: Tracheostomy in children. *J R Soc Med* 89:188, 1996.

118. Kirchner JA: Avoiding problems in tracheotomy. *Laryngoscope* 96:55, 1986.

119. Kenan PD: Complications associated with tracheotomy: prevention and treatment. *Otolaryngol Clin North Am* 12:807, 1979.

120. Malata CM, Foo IT, Simpson KH, et al: An audit of Bjork flap tracheostomies in head and neck plastic surgery. *Br J Oral Maxillofac Surg* 34:42, 1996.

121. Heffner JE, Miller KS, Sahn SA: Tracheostomy in the intensive care unit, 2: complications. *Chest* 90:430, 1986.

122. Young JS, Brady WJ, Kesser B, et al: A novel method for replacement of the dislodged tracheostomy tube: the nasogastric tube guidewire technique. *J Emerg Med* 14:205, 1996.

123. Muhammad JK, Major E, Wood A, et al: Percutaneous dilatational tracheostomy: hemorrhagic complications and the vascular anatomy of the anterior neck. *Internat J Oral Maxillofacial Surg*; 29:217, 2000.

124. Schaefer OP, Irwin RS: Tracheoarterial fistula: an unusual complication of tracheostomy. *J Intensive Care Med* 10:64, 1995.

125. Mamikunian C: Prevention of delayed hemorrhage after tracheotomy. *Ear Nose Throat J* 67:881, 1988.

126. Oshinsky AE, Rubin JS, Gwozdz CS: The anatomical basis for post-tracheotomy innominate artery rupture. *Laryngoscope* 98:1061, 1988.

127. Keceligil HT, Erk MK, Kolbakir F, et al: Tracheoinnominate artery fistula following tracheostomy. *Cardiovasc Surg* 3:509, 1995.

128. Epstein SK: Late complications of tracheostomy. *Respir Care* 50:542, 2005.

129. Thomas AN: The diagnosis and treatment of tracheoesophageal fistula caused by cuffed tracheal tubes. *J Thorac Cardiovasc Surg* 65:612, 1973.

130. Myers EN, Carrau RL: Early complications of tracheostomy. Incidence and management. *Clin Chest Med* 12:589, 1991.

131. Dartevelle P, Macchiarini P: Management of acquired tracheoesophageal fistula. *Chest Surg Clin North Am* 6:819, 1996.

132. Albes JM, Prokop M, Gebel M, et al: Bifurcate tracheal stent with foam cuff for tracheoesophageal fistula: utilization of reconstruction modes on spiral computer tomography. *Thorac Cardiovasc Surg* 42:367, 1994.

133. Wolf M, Yellin A, Talmi YP, et al: Acquired tracheoesophageal fistula in critically ill patients. *Ann Otol Rhinol Laryngol* 109(8 part 1):731, 2000.

134. Dollner R, Verch M, Schweiger P, et al: Laryngotracheoscopic findings in long-term follow-up after Griggs tracheostomy. *Chest* 122:206, 2002.

135. Streitz JM, Shapshay SM: Airway injury after tracheostomy and endotracheal intubation. *Surg Clin North Am* 71:1211, 1991.

136. Stauffer JL, Olsen DE, Petty TL: Complications and consequences of endotracheal intubation and tracheostomy: a prospective study of 150 critically ill adult patients. *Am J Med* 70:65, 1981.

137. Arola MK, Puhakka H, Makela P: Healing of lesions caused by cuffed tracheotomy tubes and their late sequelae: a follow-up study. *Acta Anaesthesiol Scand* 24:169, 1980.

138. Friedman Y, Franklin C: The technique of percutaneous tracheostomy: using serial dilation to secure an airway with minimal risk. *J Crit Illness* 8:289, 1993.

139. Crofts SL, Alzeer A, McGuire GP, et al: A comparison of percutaneous and operative tracheostomies in intensive care patients. *Can J Anaesth* 42:775, 1995.

140. Hill BB, Zweng TN, Manley RH, et al: Percutaneous dilational tracheostomy: report of 356 cases. *J Trauma* 41:38, 1996.

141. Zietek E, Matyja G, Kawczynski M: Stenosis of the larynx and trachea: diagnosis and treatment. *Otolaryngol Pol* 55:515, 2001.

142. Hughes M, Kirchner JA, Branson RJ: A skin-lined tube as a complication of tracheostomy. *Arch Otolaryngol* 94:568, 1971.

Alexander J. Eckardt
Wahid Wassef

CHAPTER **13**

Gastrointestinal Endoscopy

Gastrointestinal (GI) endoscopy has evolved into an essential diagnostic and therapeutic tool for the treatment of critically ill patients in the new millennium. The introduction of new endoscopic techniques and rapid improvements in our therapeutic armamentarium has led to major improvements in the management of patients in intensive care units (ICUs) worldwide. This chapter will review general aspects, current indications, contraindications, techniques, complications, and future directions of gastrointestinal endoscopy in the critically ill.

HISTORICAL ASPECTS

The introduction of the Lichtleiter (light conductor) by the German physician Phillip Bozzini [1] in 1804 marks the beginning of the modern era of endoscopy. This endoscope was the first to combine a light source with an optical system and a series of viewing tubes. The pioneering work of Rudolf Schindler led to the introduction of the semiflexible gastroscope. In 1941, Schindler founded the American Gastroscopic Club, now better known as the American Society of Gastrointestinal Endoscopy (ASGE) [2]. Basil Hirschowitz, from Ann Arbor University in Michigan, is recognized for the development of the first fiberoptic endoscope in the late 1950s [3]. Almost a decade later, Overholt [4] extended the use of the fiberoptic endoscope to examine the colon. Therapeutic endoscopy entered the field of gastroenterology in the 1970's. Wolff and Shinya's [5] introduction of snare-polypectomy marked the beginning of a new era in gastrointestinal endoscopy, namely the era of therapeutic endoscopy. Continuing technical advances over the past three decades have made therapeutic endoscopy an invaluable tool for the treatment of the critically ill.

ENDOSCOPES

Many of the basic principles of the Lichtleiter still hold true for modern endoscopes. Today's flexible endoscopes are composed of a control section, an insertion tube, and a connector section [6]. The control section is held in the operator's left hand. Wheels and buttons on the handle of the instrument control tip deflection (up/down, left/right), suction, and air and water insufflation (Fig. 13-1). The insertion tube is attached to the control section and varies in length, diameter, and stiffness characteristics. It contains one or two instrument channels, air- and water channels, and either a fiberoptic bundle or an electronic video system. The connector section has a light guide, an air pipe, and contacts for the processor/light source.

Standard front-viewing endoscopes used for diagnostic and therapeutic endoscopy are the esophagogastroduodenoscope (EGD), the colonoscope, and the push-enteroscope. They differ in diameter, length, and stiffness. Standard endoscopes are capable of visualizing the upper GI tract to the third or fourth portion of the duodenum, the colon, and terminal ileum. Enteroscopes can visualize parts of the jejunum. The side-viewing duodenoscope is predominantly used for endoscopic retrograde cholangio-pancreatography (ERCP), but can also be useful in the management of other duodenal lesions. ERCP uses fluoroscopy for imaging of the biliary tree. Contrast dye is injected through a catheter that is advanced through the operating channel into the bile duct or pancreatic duct. A sphinctertome is generally used to cut the sphincter of Oddi prior to stone extraction or other interventions (e.g., stenting, dilatation, etc.).

INDICATIONS

The indications for gastrointestinal endoscopy in the ICU are summarized in Table 13-1. Generally, endoscopy should only be performed if the results alter patient management. As outlined in Table 13-1, common indications for upper GI endoscopy in the ICU are upper GI bleeding, caustic or foreign body ingestion, and placement of feeding tubes. GI endoscopy in patients with clinically insignificant bleeding or chronic GI complaints should be postponed until their medical/surgical illnesses improve. Endoscopy would only be indicated in critically ill patients with occult blood loss, if anticoagulation or thrombolytic therapy is contemplated.

UPPER GASTROINTESTINAL ENDOSCOPY

Upper GI Bleeding

With an estimated 300,000 admissions annually, acute upper GI bleeding (UGIB) is one of the most common medical emergencies [7]. It is defined as the presence of melena, hematemesis, or blood in the nasogastric (NG) aspirate. Studies have shown improved outcomes of UGIBs in critically ill patients with hemodynamic instability or continuing transfusion requirements, if they are managed endoscopically [8,9]. The distinction between nonvariceal (peptic ulcer, esophagitis, Mallory-Weiss-tear, angiodysplasia, etc.) and variceal lesions (esophageal or gastric varices) is made endoscopically, allowing for targeted therapy [10,11]. Furthermore, endoscopic stigmata help to prognosticate risk of rebleeding in peptic ulcers, occasionally revealing lesions that require surgical or radiologic intervention [12].

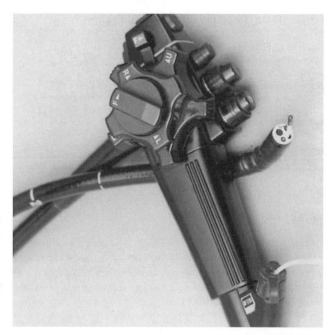

FIGURE 13-1. Video upper endoscope. Note the control knobs controlling tip deflection, buttons controlling suction and air and water insufflation, and the tip of the insertion tube with a heater probe catheter protruding through the operating channel.

Foreign Body Ingestion

Foreign body ingestions (FBI) occur commonly. They can be divided into two groups: food impactions and caustic ingestion. Food impactions constitute the majority of FBI. Although most will pass spontaneously, EGD should always be performed to look for the underlying cause of obstruction (strictures, rings, etc.). Endoscopic removal of the food bolus is necessary in 10% to 20% of cases, and 1% of patients will ultimately require surgery [13]. Although caustic ingestions only constitute a small number of FBI, they are frequently life-threatening, especially when they occur intentionally in adults. Endoscopy is safe and should be performed for prognostication and triage [14].

TABLE 13-1. Indications for Gastrointestinal (GI) Endoscopy

Upper GI Endoscopy
   Upper GI bleeding (variceal or nonvariceal)
   Caustic or foreign body ingestion
   Placement of feeding or drainage tubes
Endoscopic Retrograde Cholangiopancreatography
   Severe gallstone pancreatitis
   Severe cholangitis
   Bile leak
Lower GI Endoscopy
   Lower GI bleeding
   Decompression of nontoxic megacolon or sigmoid volvulus
   Unexplained diarrhea in the immunocompromised
     (graft versus host disease Cytomegalovirus infection, etc.)

Feeding Tubes

Enteral nutrition improves outcomes in critically ill patients and is preferred over parenteral nutrition in patients with a functional GI tract [15]. Although naso- or oroenteric feeding tubes may be used for short-term enteral nutrition, these tubes are felt to carry a higher risk of aspiration, displacement, and sinus infections than endoscopically placed percutaneous tubes. Percutaneous endoscopic gastrostomy (PEG), jejunal extension through a PEG (PEG-J), or direct endoscopic jejunostomy (D-PEJ) [16] are appropriate for many patients in the ICU. They are especially useful in patients with a reversible disease process, likely to require more than 4 weeks of artificial nutrition (e.g., neurologic injury, tracheostomy, neoplasms of the upper aerodigestive tract, etc.) [17]. PEG-J and D-PEJ tubes are appropriate for patients with severe gastroesophageal reflux, gastroparesis, or repeated feeding-related aspiration. Endoscopic gastrostomies or jejunostomies may also be indicated for decompression in patients with GI obstruction [18]. Although this is a technically simple procedure that can be performed at the bedside under conscious sedation, its risks and benefits should always be weighed carefully [19].

ENDOSCOPIC RETROGRADE CHOLANGIO-PANCREATOGRAPHY

The most common indication for urgent ERCP is complicated biliary obstruction from gallstones. Four randomized-controlled trials have studied the role of ERCP in acute gallstone pancreatitis, as summarized in a recent metaanalysis [20]. These and other studies showed that ERCP improves outcomes in the presence of cholangitis, progressive jaundice, or severe pancreatitis [21–23]. ERCP with sphincterotomy or stenting is also indicated for the diagnosis and treatment of postoperative (hepatobiliary surgery) or trauma-related bile leaks [24–27].

LOWER GASTROINTESTINAL ENDOSCOPY

Colonoscopy and flexible sigmoidoscopy are used much less frequently than upper endoscopy in the ICU. The main indications for urgent colonoscopy are lower GI bleeding, colonic pseudo-obstruction (Oglivie's syndrome), volvulus, and evaluation for infection (Cytomegalovirus [CMV], clostridium difficile) in the immuno-compromised, or graft versus host disease (GVHD) in the transplant patient [28,29].

Lower GI Bleeding

Acute lower GI bleeding (LGIB) is defined as bleeding from a source distal to the ligament of Treitz for less than 3 days and is predominantly a disease of the elderly [30]. Common causes are diverticular bleeding, ischemic colitis, and vascular abnormalities. However, as many as 11% of patients initially suspected to have a LGIB are ultimately found to have an UGIB [31]. Therefore, UGIB sources should always be considered first in patients with LGIB. Once an upper GI source has been excluded, colonoscopy should be performed. Although urgent colonoscopy within 24 to 48 hours has shown to decrease the length of hospital stay [32,33] and endoscopic intervention is often successful, 80% to 85% of LGIBs stop spontaneously [34]. If the bleeding is severe or a source cannot be identified at colonoscopy, a technetium (TC) 99m red blood cell scan with or without angiography should be considered [35,36].

Volvulus and Acute Colonic Pseudoobstruction

Acute colonic obstruction is considered a medical emergency. Imaging studies (abdominal plain films, computed tomography [CT] scan) are needed to differentiate "true" mechanical obstruction from acute colonic pseudoobstruction, because these entities are managed differently.

VOLVULUS. Colonic volvulus is the third most common cause of mechanical colonic obstruction in the western world, following neoplasms and diverticular disease [37]. It presents a "closed-loop obstruction" with risk for ischemia, perforation, and death. Decompressive endoscopy with minimal inflation of air resolves the acute obstruction in the majority of cases (81%) [38]. Despite a high recurrence rate (23% to 57%), colonoscopy is often considered the initial procedure of choice in the absence of intestinal ischemia [38,39].

ACUTE COLONIC PSEUDOOBSTRUCTION. Acute colonic pseudoobstruction (ACPO) is characterized by massive colonic dilatation without mechanical obstruction. It is a feared complication in critically ill patients with risk of spontaneous perforation and an estimated mortality rate of 50% [40]. A water-soluble contrast enema or CT should be performed to rule out mechanical obstruction if no air is visualized in the rectum on plain films. Initial management should include intravenous fluids (IVF), frequent repositioning, NG- and rectal tube placement, correction of metabolic imbalances, and discontinuation of medications known to slow intestinal transit [40,41]. Based on a double-blind, placebo-controlled, randomized trial, the parasympathomimetic agent neostigmine is now considered the treatment of choice if supportive measures fail [42]. This agent should only be given in the absence of contraindications and under close cardiorespiratory monitoring with atropine at the bedside. Endoscopic decompression is performed if the above measures fail. Recurrence rates range from 18% to 50% and may improve with placement of a decompression tube beyond the splenic flexure [43]. Percutaneous, endoscopic, or surgical cecostomy presents another alternative, but is rarely needed.

Diarrhea in the Immunocompromised

Diarrhea in the immunocompromised host may have considerable impact on morbidity and mortality. Endoscopy may aid in the diagnosis of infections (e.g., C. difficile or CMV) [44] and GVHD [29] and thus alter therapeutic management.

CONTRAINDICATIONS

Absolute and relative contraindications for endoscopic procedures are outlined in Table 13-2. Generally, endoscopy is contraindicated when the patient is unstable, when the risks of the procedure outweigh its benefit, when adequate patient cooperation or consent cannot be obtained, or when there is a suspected or known perforated viscus [45]. However, occasionally, there are exceptions to these rules. In these cases, resuscitation and endoscopic intervention would need to go on simultaneously.

TABLE 13-2.   Contraindications to Endoscopy

Absolute Contraindications
   Suspected or impending perforated viscus
   Risks to the patient outweigh benefits of the procedure
Relative Contraindications
   Adequate patient cooperation or consent cannot be obtained
   Hemodynamic instability or myocardial infarction
   Inadequate airway protection or hypoxemia
   Severe coagulopathy or thrombocytopenia
   Inflammatory changes with increased risk of perforation
     (e.g., diverticulitis or severe inflammatory bowel disease)

COMPLICATIONS

Although major complications of endoscopic procedures are infrequent, critically ill patients may be particularly sensitive to adverse outcomes due to multiple comorbidities. Complications can be divided into two groups: (a) general complications, and (b) specific complications (Table 13-3)

TECHNIQUES

Proper patient preparation is essential for safe and complete endoscopic examinations. Key elements of planning interventional endoscopic procedures include appropriate resuscitation, reversal of coagulopathies, determination of the need for adjunctive therapy (e.g., antibiotics, proton pump inhibitors, octreotide), and proper sedation as clinically indicated [46]. General aspects that apply to all endoscopic procedures will be discussed hereafter, followed by a specific description of endoscopic and adjunctive therapies.

GENERAL PATIENT PREPARATION

All patients presenting for GI endoscopy should have a history and physical examination, intravenous (IV) access, informed consent, and adequate preparation. Supplemental oxygen is used routinely with conscious sedation to prevent hypoxia, and vital signs are closely monitored in all patients [47].

TABLE 13-3.   Complications of Endoscopy

General Complications
   Complications of conscious sedation (cardiopulmonary,
    allergic, paradoxical reactions, etc.)
   Bleeding (e.g., treatment of lesions, sphincterotomy, etc)
   Perforation (caused by endoscope, accessories, or air insufflation)
   Aspiration
   Myocardial ischemia
Specific Complications (Examples)
   Endoscopic retrograde cholangio-pancreatography:
   Pancreatitis, cholangitis, etc.
   Percutaneous endoscopic gastrostomy:
   Tube occlusion, leakage, unintentional removal, skin infection, etc.
   Sclerotherapy: Ulceration, mediastinitis, etc.
   Stenting procedures: Stent migration

UPPER GASTROINTESTINAL ENDOSCOPY

Upper Gastrointestinal Bleeding

The most common indication for EGD is UGIB, which can be divided into variceal and nonvariceal hemorrhage. In either case, certain issues need to be addressed prior to endoscopy:

NEED FOR NASOGASTRIC TUBE LAVAGE. Nasogastric tube (NGT) lavage is the first step in diagnosing an UGIB source and has been shown to predict high-risk lesions in the presence of red blood [48]. In addition, it may aid in improving visualization at subsequent endoscopy. A negative NGT lavage does not rule out a duodenal bleeding source, because the pylorus may prevent reflux of blood into the stomach. Even the presence of a bilious aspirate does not completely rule out a high-risk lesion, because bleeding can be intermittent.

NEED FOR PROKINETICS. Large clots or residual blood may obscure visualization of the bleeding lesion during EGD. Successful treatment of an underlying lesion and accurate diagnosis strongly depends on good visualization. The use of the prokinetic agent erythromycin (250 mg in 50 mL of normal saline IV, 20 minutes prior to the procedure) has been shown to significantly improve visualization during EGD and to decrease the need for a "second-look" endoscopy [49,50]. Although metoclopramide may theoretically have a similar effect, this has not been studied extensively.

NEED FOR ENDOTRACHEAL INTUBATION. Uncooperative, confused, or hypoxemic patients may require endotracheal intubation with deep sedation or general anesthesia prior to the procedure. Although endotracheal intubation does not significantly alter the risk of acquired pneumonia or cardiovascular events [51], it generates controlled conditions during the procedure and may help prevent massive aspiration (especially in patients with variceal bleeding).

Nonvariceal Upper Gastrointestinal Bleeding

The treatment of a nonvariceal UGIB depends on the endoscopic findings [12]. Therefore, targeted irrigation should be performed to uncover and treat the underlying lesion, if an adherent clot is found. This approach may reduce the risk of rebleeding and need for surgical intervention, but does not affect the need for transfusions, length of hospitalization, or mortality [52]. Aggressive removal of clots (suction or guillotine technique) should only be performed by experienced endoscopists with surgical backup, since it carries the risk of reactivating a bleed. If active bleeding or a nonbleeding visible vessel is identified, endoscopic hemostatic techniques have been shown to be helpful.

Endoscopic methods for hemostasis include injection therapy, thermal therapies, and mechanical hemostasis with clips (Table 13-4). The combination of injection therapy with thermal coaptive therapy is superior to either alone [7,53,54]. Although no single solution for endoscopic injection therapy appears superior to another, an epinephrine-saline solution is usually injected in large volumes (13 to 20 mL) in four quadrants surrounding the lesion. Heater probe and multipolar-electrocoagulation instruments are subsequently applied with firm pressure to achieve optimal coaptation. Mechanical hemostasis, with hemoclips, has been recently added to our

TABLE 13-4. Endoscopic Methods for Hemostatis

Thermal Methods of Hemostasis
 Heater Probe
 Multipolar electrocoagulation (bicap)
 Neodymium yttrium-aluminium-garnet (YAG) laser
 Argon plasma coagulation
Injection Therapy for Hemostasis
 Distilled water or saline
 Epinephrine (adrenaline)
 Sclerosants (Cyanoacrylate, polidocanol, ethanol, ethanolamine
  oleate, sodium tetradecyl sulfate, sodium morrhuate)
 Thrombin, Fibrin-glue
Mechanical Methods
 Clips
 Band ligation
 Detachable loops

armamentarium. Evidence suggests that the use of clips may be especially useful in the treatment of critically ill patients [55,56]. However, clips may have limited efficacy in certain anatomic locations, such as the posterior duodenum, surgical margins, or the proximal stomach [57]. Argon plasma coagulation (APC) is a noncoaptive technique that provides current to tissues by means of ionized argon gas. This method is most commonly used in the treatment of arteriovenous malformations (AVMs). The YAG laser has fallen out of favor in the acute management of high-risk patients, because of its poor portability and associated high cost.

ADJUNCTIVE THERAPY. Whatever method of hemostasis is used, patients with nonvariceal UGIB need to be placed on antisecretory therapy with a proton pump inhibitor (PPI) following endoscopic hemostasis [8,53]. Both, oral and IV PPIs, have been shown to reduce rebleeding after endoscopic treatment of bleeding peptic ulcers with high-risk stigmata. High-dose IV PPI appears to decrease the need for surgery, while the effect on mortality remains controversial [58,59]. The optimal dosing of pantoprazole, the only IV PPI currently approved in the United States, has not been determined. Empirically, a dose of 40 mg IV twice a day is administered until the patient is switched to an oral PPI.

Variceal Upper Gastrointestinal Bleeding

In patients with variceal UGIB, endoscopic variceal ligation (EVL) has become the procedure of choice [60]. With this technique the varix is suctioned into a banding device attached to the tip of the endoscope, and a rubber band is then deployed at its base to obliterate the varix. In contrast, endoscopic sclerotherapy (EST) causes obliteration by injection of a sclerosing agent (e.g., sodium morrhuate) in or around the bleeding varix. A metaanalysis by Laine and Cook [61] suggested that EVL was superior to EST in all major outcomes (recurrent bleeding, local complications such as ulcers or strictures, time to variceal obliteration, and survival). However, EST is effective in controlling active bleeding in over 90% of cases and can be injected even with poor visualization during an active bleed.

Endoscopic methods (EST, EVL, injection of fibrin glue, etc.) have also been used for the treatment of bleeding gastric varices in small and mostly uncontrolled studies. However, these methods carry a considerable risk of rebleeding and mortality and patients with bleeding gastric varices generally require urgent placement of a transjugular intrahepatic portosystemic shunt (TIPS) [62].

ADJUNCTIVE THERAPY. If a variceal hemorrhage is suspected in patients with severe UGIB, with a clinical history or physical exam suggesting portal hypertension, adjunctive therapy should be initiated immediately in the absence of contraindications. Both somatostatin analogues (octreotide) or vasopressin and its analogues have been used intravenously to reduce portal pressures and prevent recurrent bleeding. A recent metaanalysis slightly favored octreotide over terlipressin/vasopressin in the control of esophageal variceal bleeding [63]. Octreotide is usually given as a onetime bolus of 50 to 100 mcg IV, followed by 25 to 50 mcg IV/hr for 3 to 5 days. In addition, prophylactic antibiotics should be given to patients with active variceal bleeding for the prevention of bacterial infections [64–66]. Recent data suggest that the use of prophylactic antibiotics after endoscopic treatment of a variceal bleed may also decrease the risk of rebleeding [67]. In contrast to nonvariceal hemorrhage, volume resuscitation should be performed judiciously, because bleeding appears to be directly related to portal pressures.

Enteric Feeding Tubes

The most widely used technique for the placement of enteric feeding tubes is the "pull-technique" [15]. This technique involves an initial EGD with visualization of the gastric mucosa. The light source of the endoscope is used for transillumination and can be visualized through the abdominal wall by the endoscopist in a darkened room. The endoscopist verifies the position by endoscopic visualization of the finger indentation that is applied from the outside. After sterile preparation of the skin a large bore (15-gauge) needle is advanced into the stomach under endoscopic visualization. A guidewire is passed through the needle into the stomach and pulled out through the mouth after grasping it with the endoscope. The feeding tube with a tapered tip and a rubber bumper at the proximal end is then attached to the wire and pulled through the skin after a small incision is made to allow easy passage.

A thin jejunal feeding tube can be fed through the PEG from the outside and advanced endoscopically into the jejunum to form a PEG-J. The D-PEJ technique is a modification of PEG placement. It is considerably more difficult to perform and therefore not widely used [15]. Tube feeds are usually started after reevaluating the patient within 24 hours.

LOWER GASTROINTESTINAL ENDOSCOPY

By definition, urgent colonoscopy is performed within 12 to 48 hours. In contrast to EGD, specific preparation is required to cleanse the colon. Rapid purge preparation is usually achieved by drinking 4 or more liters of polyethylene-glycol based solutions. Approximately one third of hospitalized patients require an NGT for this type of preparation [68]. Metoclopramide (10 mg IV × 1), administered prior to starting the preparation, may help to control nausea and promote gastric emptying [31]. Sigmoidoscopy or colonoscopy for volvulus or colonic decompression can be performed in the unprepared colon. The treatment options for LGIB are similar to the treatment of UGIB (see above) and should be based on the stigmata of bleeding that are identified.

ENDOSCOPIC RETROGRADE CHOLANGIO-PANCREATOGRAPHY

Detailed description of ERCP is beyond the scope of this chapter. Duodenoscopes used for ERCP are distinct from other endoscopes in that they are side-viewing and have an "elevator" that allows for adjustment of the direction of catheters as they exit the endoscope. There are a number of small diameter instruments that are used to cannulate the pancreaticobiliary tree and implant stents for drainage. Catheters, stents, and sphincterotomes are the basic accessories used for this procedure [69].

FUTURE DIRECTIONS

With the start of the new millennium rapid advances have been made in the development of new techniques, which are already starting to enter clinical practice [70]. Advances in endoscopic imaging by using special dyes, high-resolution optical coherence tomography, or narrow-band imaging allow for the diagnosis of even subtle mucosal abnormalities. Small bowel imaging has been revolutionized by the introduction of wireless video capsule endoscopy (VCE), which made endoscopic visualization of the entire small bowel possible. Double-balloon enteroscopy is a new exciting technique that will allow for therapeutic intervention, targeting lesions identified on VCE. These and other technical advances are likely to have a major impact on the future treatment of GI disorders in general and may evolve into valuable tools in management of the critically ill in particular.

REFERENCES

1. Bozzini P: Lichtleiter, eine Erfindung zur Anschauung innerer Teile und Krankheiten nebst der Abbildung von Dr. Bozzini, Arzt zu Frankfurt am Main. *J praktischen Arzneykunde Wundarzneykunst* 14:107–111, 1806.
2. Edmonson JM: The archives and instrument collection of the American Society for Gastrointestinal Endoscopy. *Gastrointest Endosc* 60:969–977, 2004.
3. Hirschowitz BI, Curtiss LE, Peter CW, et al: Demonstration of a new gastroscope, the "fiberscope." *Gastroenterology* 35:50–53, 1958.
4. Overholt BF: Clinical experience with the fiber sigmoidoscope. *Gastrointest Endosc* 15:27, 1968.
5. Wolff WI, Shinya H: Colonofiberoscopy. *JAMA* 217:1509–1512, 1971.
6. Bosco JJ, Barkun AN, Isenberg GA, et al: Gastrointestinal endoscopes. *Gastrointest Endosc* 58:822–30, 2003.
7. Wassef W: Upper gastrointestinal bleeding. *Curr Opin Gastroenterol* 20:538–545, 2004.
8. Adler DG, Leighton JA, Davila RE, et al: ASGE guideline: the role of endoscopy in acute non-variceal upper-GI hemorrhage. *Gastrointest Endosc* 60:497–504, 2004.
9. Chak A, Cooper GS, Lloyd LE, et al: Effectiveness of endoscopy in patients admitted to the intensive care unit with upper GI hemorrhage. *Gastrointest Endosc* 53:6–13, 2001.
10. Kupfer Y, Cappell MS, Tessler S: Acute gastrointestinal bleeding in the intensive care unit. The intensivist's perspective. *Gastroenterol Clin North Am* 29:275–307, 2000.
11. Beejay U, Wolfe MM: Acute gastrointestinal bleeding in the intensive care unit. The gastroenterologist's perspective. *Gastroenterol Clin North Am* 29:309–336, 2000.
12. Laine L, Peterson WL: Bleeding peptic ulcer. *N Engl J Med* 331:717–727, 1994.
13. Eisen GM, Baron TH, Dominitz JA, et al: Guideline for the management of ingested foreign bodies. *Gastrointest Endosc* 55:802–806, 2002.
14. Poley JW, Steyerberg EW, Kuipers EJ, et al: Ingestion of acid and alkaline agents: outcome and prognostic value of early upper endoscopy. *Gastrointest Endosc* 60:372–377, 2004.
15. Eisen GM, Baron TH, Dominitz JA, et al: Role of endoscopy in enteral feeding. *Gastrointest Endosc* 55:699–701, 2002.
16. Fan AC, Baron TH, Rumalla A: Comparison of direct percutaneous endoscopic jejunostomy and PEG with jejunal extension. *Gastrointest Endosc* 56:890–894, 2002.
17. DeLegge MH, McClave SA, DiSario JA, et al: Ethical and medicolegal aspects of PEG-tube placement and provision of artificial nutritional therapy. *Gastrointest Endosc* 62:952–959, 2005.
18. Herman LL, Hoskins WJ, Shike M: Percutaneous endoscopic gastrostomy for decompression of the stomach and small bowel. *Gastrointest Endosc* 38:314–318, 1992.
19. Hallenbeck J: Reevaluating PEG tube placement in advanced illnesses. *Gastrointest Endosc* 62:960–961, 2005.
20. Sharma VK, Howden CW: Metaanalysis of randomized controlled trials of endoscopic retrograde cholangiography and endoscopic sphincterotomy for the treatment of acute biliary pancreatitis. *Am J Gastroenterol* 94:3211–3214, 1999.

21. Fogel EL, Sherman S: Acute biliary pancreatitis: when should the endoscopist intervene? *Gastroenterology* 125:229–235, 2003.

22. Adler DG, Baron TH, Davila RE, et al: ASGE guideline: the role of ERCP in diseases of the biliary tract and the pancreas. *Gastrointest Endosc* 62:1–8, 2005.

23. Lai EC, Mok FP, Tan ES, et al: Endoscopic biliary drainage for severe acute cholangitis. *N Engl J Med* 326:1582–1586, 1992.

24. Bhattachrjya S, Puleston J, Davidson BR, et al: Outcome of early endoscopic biliary drainage in the management of bile leaks after hepatic resection. *Gastrointest Endosc* 57:526–530, 2003.

25. Kaffes AJ, Hourigan L, De Luca N, et al: Impact of endoscopic intervention in 100 patients with suspected postcholecystectomy bile leak. *Gastrointest Endosc* 61:269–275, 2005.

26. Sandha GS, Bourke MJ, Haber GB, et al: Endoscopic therapy of bile leak based on a new classification: results in 207 patients. *Gastrointest Endosc* 60:567–574, 2004.

27. Lubezky N, Konikoff FM, Rosin D, et al: Endoscopic sphincterotomy and temporary internal stenting for bile leaks following complex hepatic trauma. *Br J Surg* 93:78–81, 2006.

28. Southworth M, Taffet SL, Levien DH, et al: Colonoscopy in critically ill patients. What conditions call for it? *Postgrad Med* 88:159–163, 1990.

29. Oomori S, Takagi S, Kikuchi T, et al: Significance of colonoscopy in patients with intestinal graft-versus-host disease after hematopoietic stem cell transplantation. *Endoscopy* 37:346–350, 2005.

30. Davila RE, Rajan E, Adler DG, et al: ASGE guideline: the role of endoscopy in the patient with lower GI-bleeding. *Gastrointest Endosc* 62:656–660, 2005.

31. Jensen DM, Machicado GA: Diagnosis and treatment of severe hematochezia. The role of urgent colonoscopy after purge. *Gastroenterology* 95:1569–1574, 1988.

32. Strate LL, Syngal S: Timing of colonoscopy: impact on length of hospital stay in patients with acute lower GI bleeding. *Am J Gastroenterol* 98:317–322, 2003.

33. Schmulewitz N, Fisher DA, Rockey DC: Early colonoscopy for acute lower GI bleeding predicts shorter hospital stay: a retrospective study of experience in a single center. *Gastrointest Endosc* 58:841–846, 2003.

34. Farrell JJ, Friedman LS: Review article: the management of lower gastrointestinal bleeding. *Aliment Pharmacol Ther* 21:1281–1298, 2005.

35. Strate LL, Syngal S: Predictors of utilization of early colonoscopy vs. radiography for severe lower intestinal bleeding. *Gastrointest Endosc* 61:46–52, 2005.

36. Green BT, Rockey DC, Portwood G: Urgent colonoscopy for evaluation and management of acute lower gastrointestinal hemorrhage: a randomized controlled trial. *Am J Gastroenterol* 100:1–8, 2005.

37. Frizelle FA, Wolff BG: Colonic volvulus. *Adv Surg* 29:131–139, 1996.

38. Grossmann EM, Longo WE, Stratton MD, et al: Sigmoid volvulus in Department of Veterans Affairs Medical Centers. *Dis Colon Rectum* 43:414–418, 2000.

39. Martinez Ares D, Yanez Lopez J, Souto Ruzo J, et al: Indication and results of endoscopic management of sigmoid volvulus. *Rev Esp Enferm Dig* 95:544–548, 2003.

40. Saunders MD, Kimmey MB: Systematic review: acute colonic pseudo-obstruction. *Aliment Pharmacol Ther* 22:917–925, 2005.

41. Eisen GM, Baron TH, Dominitz JA, et al: Acute colonic pseudo-obstruction. *Gastrointest Endosc* 56:789–792, 2002.

42. Ponec RJ, Saunders MD, Kimmey MB: Neostigmine for the treatment of acute colonic pseudo-obstruction. *N Engl J Med* 341:137–141, 1999.

43. Geller A, Petersen BT, Gostout CJ: Endoscopic decompression for acute colonic pseudo-obstruction. *Gastrointest Endosc* 44:144–150, 1996.

44. Johal SS, Hammond J, Solomon K, et al: Clostridium difficile associated diarrhoea in hospitalized patients: onset in the community and hospital and role of flexible sigmoidoscopy. *Gut* 53:673–677, 2004.

45. American Society for Gastrointestinal Endoscopy: Appropriate use of gastrointestinal endoscopy. *Gastrointest Endosc* 52:831–837, 2000.

46. Wassef W, Rullan R: Interventional endoscopy. *Curr Opin Gastroenterol* 21:644–652, 2005.

47. Waring JP, Baron TH, Hirota WK, et al: Guidelines for conscious sedation and monitoring during gastrointestinal endoscopy. *Gastrointest Endosc* 58:317–322, 2003.

48. Aljebreen AM, Fallone CA, Barkun AN: Nasogastric aspirate predicts high-risk endoscopic lesions in patients with acute upper-GI bleeding. *Gastrointest Endosc* 59:172–178, 2004.

49. Coffin B, Pocard M, Panis Y, et al: Erythromycin improves the quality of EGD in patients with acute upper GI bleeding: a randomized controlled study. *Gastrointest Endosc* 56:174–179, 2002.

50. Frossard JL, Spahr L, Queneau PE, et al: Erythromycin intravenous bolus infusion in acute upper gastrointestinal bleeding: A randomized, controlled, double-blind trial. *Gastroenterology* 123:17–23, 2002.

51. Rudolph SJ, Landsverk BK, Freeman ML: Endotracheal intubation for airway protection during endoscopy for severe upper GI hemorrhage. *Gastrointest Endosc* 57:58–61, 2003.

52. Kahi CJ, Jensen DM, Sung JJY, et al: Endoscopic therapy versus medical therapy for bleeding peptic ulcer with adherent clot: a metaanalysis. *Gastroenterology* 129:855–862, 2005.

53. Barkun A, Bardou M, Marshall JK, et al: Consensus recommendations for managing patients with nonvariceal upper gastrointestinal bleeding. *Ann Intern Med* 139:843–857, 2003.

54. Chung SSC, Lau JYW, Sung JJY, et al: Randomised comparison between adrenaline injection alone and adrenaline injection plus heater probe treatment for actively bleeding ulcers. *BMJ* 314:1307–1311, 1997.

55. Ohta S, Yukioka T, Ohta S, et al: Hemostasis with hemoclipping for severe gastrointestinal bleeding in critically ill patients. *Am J Gastroenterol* 91:701–704, 1996.

56. Goto H, Ohta S, Yamaguchi Y, et al: Prospective evaluation of hemoclip application with injection of epinephrine in hypertonic saline solution for hemostasis in unstable patients with shock caused by upper GI bleeding. *Gastrointest Endosc* 56:78–82, 2002.

57. Lee YC, Wang HP, Yang CS, et al: Endoscopic hemostasis of a bleeding marginal ulcer: hemoclipping or dual therapy with epinephrine injection and heater probe thermocoagulation. *J Gastroenterol Hepatol* 17:1220–1225, 2002.

58. Bardou M, Toubouti Y, Benhaberou-Brun D, et al: Meta analysis: proton-pump inhibition in high-risk patients with acute peptic ulcer bleeding. *Aliment Pharmacol Ther* 21:677–686, 2005.

59. Leontiadis GI, Sharma VK, Howden CW: Systematic review and metaanalysis of proton pump inhibitor therapy in peptic ulcer bleeding. *BMJ* 330:568–570, 2005.

60. Qureshi W, Adler DG, Davila R, et al: ASGE guideline: the role of endoscopy in the management of variceal hemorrhage, updated July 2005. *Gastrointest Endosc* 62:651–655, 2005.

61. Laine L, Cook D: Endoscopic ligation compared with sclerotherapy for treatment of esophageal variceal bleeding: a metaanalysis. *Ann Intern Med* 123:280–287, 1995.

62. Sharara AI, Rockey DC: Gastroesophageal variceal bleed. *N Engl J Med* 345:669–681, 2001.

63. Corley DA, Cello JP, Akisson W, et al: Octreotide for acute esophageal variceal bleeding: a metaanalysis. *Gastroenterology* 120:946–954, 2001.

64. Runyon BA: Management of adult patients with ascites due to cirrhosis. *Hepatology* 39:1–16, 2004.

65. Hirota WK, Petersen K, Baron TH, et al: American Society for Gastrointestinal Endoscopy. Guidelines for antibiotic propylaxis for GI endoscopy. *Gastrointest Endosc* 58:475–482, 2003.

66. Pauwels A, Mostefa-Kara N, Debenes B, et al: Systemic antibiotic prophylaxis after gastrointestinal hemorrhage in cirrhotic patients with a high risk of infection. *Hepatology* 24:802–806, 1996.

67. Hou MC, Lin HC, Liu TT, et al: Antibiotic prophylaxis after endoscopic therapy prevents rebleeding in acute variceal hemorrhage: a randomized trial. *Hepatology* 39:746–753, 2004.

68. Elta GH: Technological review. Urgent colonoscopy for acute lower-GI bleeding. *Gastrointest Endosc* 59:402–408, 2004.

69. Brugge WR, Van Dam J: Pancreatic and biliary endoscopy. *N Engl J Med* 341:1808–1816, 1999.

70. Mallery S, Van Dam J: Endoscopic practice at the start of the new millennium. *Gastroenterology* 118:S129-S147, 2000.

CHAPTER **14**

Paracentesis and Diagnostic Peritoneal Lavage

ABDOMINAL PARACENTESIS

INDICATIONS

Abdominal paracentesis is a simple procedure that can be easily performed at the bedside in the intensive care unit and may provide important diagnostic information or therapy in critically ill patients with ascites. Diagnostic abdominal paracentesis is usually performed to determine the exact etiology of the accumulated ascites or to ascertain whether infection is present, as in spontaneous bacterial peritonitis [1]. It can also be used in any clinical situation in which the analysis of a sample of peritoneal fluid might be useful in ascertaining a diagnosis and guiding therapy. The evaluation of ascites should therefore include a diagnostic paracentesis with ascitic fluid analysis.

As a therapeutic intervention, abdominal paracentesis is usually performed to drain large volumes of abdominal ascites [2]. Ascites is the most common presentation of decompensated cirrhosis, and its development heralds a poor prognosis, with a 50% 2-year survival rate. Effective first-line therapy for ascites includes sodium restriction (2 g per day), use of diuretics, and large-volume paracentesis. Ideally, a combination of a loop diuretic and aldosterone antagonist is used. When tense or refractory ascites is present, large-volume paracentesis is safe and effective and has the advantage of producing immediate relief from ascites and its associated symptoms [3]. Ten percent of cirrhotic patients develop refractory ascites, which carries substantial morbidity and has a 1-year survival of less than 50%. A Cochrane Database Systematic Review compared transjugular intrahepatic portosystemic stent-shunts (TIPS) versus paracentesis standard treatment in patients with refractory ascites due to cirrhosis. TIPS removed ascites more effectively than paracentesis, and after 12 months, the beneficial effects of TIPS on ascites was still present. However, no differences in mortality, gastrointestinal bleeding, infection or sepsis, acute renal failure, and disseminated intravascular coagulation were identified, and hepatic encephalopathy occurred significantly more often in the TIPS group [4].

Therapeutic abdominal paracentesis can be palliative by diminishing abdominal pain from distention or improving pulmonary function by allowing better diaphragmatic excursion in patients who have ascites refractory to aggressive medical management [5]. Paracentesis is also used for percutaneous decompression of resuscitation-induced abdominal compartment syndrome related to the development of acute tense ascites [6,7].

TECHNIQUES

Before abdominal paracentesis is initiated, a catheter must be inserted to drain the urinary bladder, and correction of any underlying coagulopathy or thrombocytopenia should be considered. A consensus statement from the International Ascites Club states that "there are no data to support the correction of mild coagulopathy with blood products prior to therapeutic paracentesis, but caution is needed when severe thrombocytopenia is present" [3]. The practice guideline from the American Association for the Study of Liver Diseases states that routine correction of prolonged prothrombin time or thrombocytopenia is not required when experienced personnel perform paracentesis [8]. This has been confirmed in a study of 1,100 large-volume paracenteses in 628 patients [9]. But in critically ill patients, there is still uncertainty as to the optimal platelet count and prothrombin time for the safe conduct of paracentesis.

The patient must next be positioned correctly. If he or she is critically ill, the procedure is performed in the supine position. If the patient is clinically stable and abdominal paracentesis is being performed for therapeutic volume removal of ascites, the patient can be placed in the sitting position, leaning slightly forward, to increase the total volume of ascites removed.

The site for paracentesis on the anterior abdominal wall is then chosen (Fig. 14-1). The preferred site is in the lower abdomen, just lateral to the rectus abdominis muscle and inferior to the umbilicus. It is important to stay lateral to the rectus abdominis muscle to avoid injury to the inferior epigastric artery and vein. In patients with chronic cirrhosis and caput medusae (engorged anterior abdominal wall veins), these visible vascular structures must be avoided. Injury to these veins can cause significant bleeding because of underlying portal hypertension and may result in hemoperitoneum. The left lower quadrant of the abdominal wall is preferred over the right lower quadrant for abdominal paracentesis because critically ill patients often have cecal distention. The ideal site is therefore in the left lower quadrant of the abdomen, lateral to the rectus abdominis muscle in the midclavicular line and inferior to the umbilicus. It has also been determined that the left lower quadrant is significantly thinner and the depth of ascites greater compared with the infraumbilical midline position, confirming the left lower quadrant as the preferred location for paracentesis [10].

If the patient had previous abdominal surgery limited to the lower abdomen, it may be difficult to perform a paracentesis in the lower abdomen, and the upper abdomen may be chosen. The point of entry, however, remains lateral to the rectus

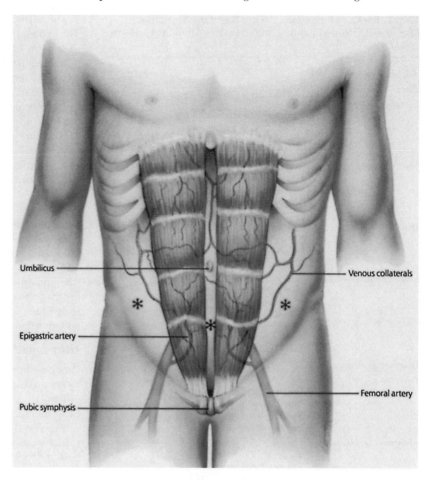

FIGURE 14-1.   Suggested sites for paracentesis.

abdominis muscle in the midclavicular line. If there is concern that the ascites is loculated because of previous abdominal surgery or peritonitis, abdominal paracentesis should be performed under ultrasound guidance to prevent iatrogenic complications.

Abdominal paracentesis can be performed by the needle technique, the catheter technique, or with ultrasound guidance. Diagnostic paracentesis usually requires 20 to 50 mL peritoneal fluid and is commonly performed using the needle technique. However, if large volumes of peritoneal fluid are required (i.e., for cytologic examination), the catheter technique is used because it is associated with a lower incidence of complications. Therapeutic paracentesis, as in the removal of large volumes of ascites, should always be performed with the catheter technique. Ultrasound guidance can be helpful in diagnostic paracentesis using the needle technique or in therapeutic paracentesis with large volume removal using the catheter technique.

Needle Technique

With the patient in the appropriate position and the access site for paracentesis determined, the patient's abdomen is prepared with 10% povidone-iodine solution and sterilely draped. If necessary, intravenous sedation is administered to prevent the patient from moving excessively during the procedure (see Chapter 20). Local anesthesia, using 1% or 2% lidocaine with 1:200,000 epinephrine is infiltrated into the site. A skin wheal is created with the local anesthetic, using a short 25- or 27-gauge needle. Then, using a 22-gauge, 1.5-inch needle, the local anesthetic is infiltrated into the subcutaneous tissues and anterior abdominal wall, with the needle perpendicular to the skin. Before the anterior abdominal wall and peritoneum are infiltrated, the skin is pulled taut inferiorly, allowing the peritoneal cavity to be entered at a different location than the skin entrance site, thereby decreasing the chance of ascitic leak. This is known as the *Z-track technique*. While tension is maintained inferiorly on the abdominal skin, the needle is advanced through the abdominal wall fascia and peritoneum, and local anesthetic is injected. Intermittent aspiration identifies when the peritoneal cavity is entered, with return of ascitic fluid into the syringe. The needle is held securely in this position with the left hand, and the right hand is used to withdraw approximately 20 to 50 mL ascitic fluid into the syringe for a diagnostic paracentesis.

Once adequate fluid is withdrawn, the needle and syringe are withdrawn from the anterior abdominal wall and the paracentesis site is covered with a sterile dressing. The needle is removed from the syringe, because it may be contaminated with skin organisms. A small amount of peritoneal fluid is sent in a sterile container for Gram's-stained smear and culture and sensitivity testing. The remainder of the fluid is sent for appropriate studies, which may include cytology, cell count and differential, protein, specific gravity, amylase, pH, lactate dehydrogenase, bilirubin, triglycerides, and albumin. A serum to ascites albumin gradient (SAAG) greater than 1.1 g per dL is indicative of

TABLE 14-1. Etiologies of Ascites Based on Normal or Diseased Peritoneum and Serum to Ascites Albumin Gradient (SAAG)

Normal Peritoneum

Portal Hypertension (SAAG > 1.1 g/dL)

Hepatic congestion

          Congestive heart failure
          Constrictive pericarditic
          Tricuspid insufficiency
          Budd-Chiari syndrome

Liver disease

          Cirrhosis
          Alcoholic hepatitis
          Fulminant hepatic failure
          Massive hepatic metastases

Hypoalbuminemia (SAAG < 1.1 g/dL)

          Nephrotic syndrome
          Protein-losing enteropathy
          Severe malnutrition with anasarca

Miscellaneous Conditions (SAAG < 1.1 g/dL)

          Chylous ascites
          Pancreatic ascites
          Bile ascites
          Nephrogenic ascites
          Urine ascites
          Ovarian disease

Diseased Peritoneum (SAAG < 1.1 g/dL)

Infections

          Bacterial peritonitis
          Tuberculous peritonitis
          Fungal peritonitis
          HIV-associated peritonitis

Malignant Conditions

          Peritoneal carcinomatosis
          Primary mesothelioma
          Pseudomyxoma peritonei
          Hepatocellular carcinoma

Other Rare Conditions

          Familial Mediterranean fever
          Vasculitis
          Granulomatous peritonitis
          Eosinophilic peritonitis

portal hypertension and cirrhosis (Table 14-1) [11]. Peritoneal fluid can be sent for smear and culture for acid-fast bacilli if tuberculous peritonitis is in the differential diagnosis.

Catheter Technique

The patient is placed in the proper position, and the anterior abdominal wall site for paracentesis is prepared and draped in the usual sterile fashion. Aseptic technique is used throughout the procedure. The site is anesthetized with local anesthetic as described for the needle technique. A 22-gauge, 1.5-inch needle attached to a 10-mL syringe is used to document the free return of peritoneal fluid into the syringe at the chosen site. This needle is removed from the peritoneal cavity and a catheter-over-needle assembly is used to gain access to the peritoneal cavity. If the anterior abdominal wall is thin, an 18- or 20-gauge angiocath can be used as the catheter-over-needle assembly. If the anterior abdominal wall is quite thick, as in obese patients, it may be necessary to use a long (5.25-inch) catheter-over-needle assembly (18- or 20-gauge) or a percutaneous single-lumen central venous catheter (18- or 20-gauge) and gain access to the peritoneal cavity using the Seldinger technique.

The peritoneal cavity is entered as for the needle technique. The catheter-over-needle assembly is inserted perpendicular to the anterior abdominal wall using the Z-track technique; once peritoneal fluid returns into the syringe barrel, the catheter is advanced over the needle, the needle is removed, and a 20- or 50-mL syringe is connected to the catheter. The tip of the catheter is now in the peritoneal cavity and can be left in place until the appropriate amount of peritoneal fluid is removed. This technique, rather than the needle technique, should be used when large volumes of peritoneal fluid must be removed, because complications (e.g., intestinal perforation) may occur if a needle is left in the peritoneal space for an extended period.

When the Seldinger technique is used in patients with a large anterior abdominal wall, access to the peritoneal cavity is initially gained with a needle or catheter-over-needle assembly. A guidewire is then inserted through the needle and an 18- or 20-gauge single-lumen central venous catheter threaded over the guidewire. It is very important to use the Z-track method for the catheter technique to prevent development of an ascitic leak, which may be difficult to control and may predispose the patient to peritoneal infection.

Ultrasound Guidance Technique

Patients who have had previous abdominal surgery or peritonitis are predisposed to abdominal adhesions, and it may be quite difficult to gain free access into the peritoneal cavity for diagnostic or therapeutic paracentesis. Ultrasound-guided paracentesis can be very helpful in this population by providing accurate localization of the peritoneal fluid collection and determining the best abdominal access site. This procedure can be performed using the needle or catheter technique as described above, depending on the volume of peritoneal fluid to be drained. Once the fluid collection is localized by the ultrasound probe, the abdomen is prepared and draped in the usual sterile fashion. A sterile sleeve can be placed over the ultrasound probe so that there is direct ultrasound visualization of the needle or catheter as it enters the peritoneal cavity. The needle or catheter is thus directed to the area to be drained, and the appropriate amount of peritoneal or ascitic fluid is removed. If continued drainage of a loculated peritoneal fluid collection is desired, the radiologist can place a chronic indwelling peritoneal catheter using a percutaneous guidewire technique (see Chapter 21).

The use of ultrasound guidance for drainage of loculated peritoneal fluid collections has markedly decreased the incidence of iatrogenic complications related to abdominal paracentesis. If the radiologist does not identify loculated ascites on the initial ultrasound evaluation and documents a large amount of peritoneal fluid that is free in the abdominal cavity, he or she can then indicate the best access site by marking the anterior abdominal wall with an indelible marker. The paracentesis can then be performed by the clinician and repeated whenever necessary. This study can be performed at the bedside in the intensive care unit with a portable ultrasound unit.

COMPLICATIONS

The most common complications related to abdominal paracentesis are bleeding and persistent ascitic leak. Because most patients in whom ascites have developed also have some component of chronic liver disease with associated coagulopathy and thrombocytopenia, it is very important to consider correction of any underlying coagulopathy before proceeding with abdominal paracentesis. In addition, it is very important to select an avascular access site on the anterior abdominal wall. The Z-track technique is very helpful in minimizing persistent ascitic leak and should always be used. Another complication associated with abdominal paracentesis is intestinal or urinary bladder perforation, with associated peritonitis and infection. Intestinal injury is more common when the needle technique is used. Because the needle is free in the peritoneal cavity, iatrogenic intestinal perforation may occur if the patient moves or if intraabdominal pressure increases with Valsalva maneuver or coughing. Urinary bladder injury is less common and underscores the importance of draining the urinary bladder with a catheter before the procedure. This injury is more common when the abdominal access site is in the suprapubic location; therefore, this access site is not recommended. Careful adherence to proper technique of paracentesis minimizes associated complications.

In patients who have large-volume chronic abdominal ascites, such as that secondary to hepatic cirrhosis or ovarian carcinoma, transient hypotension, and paracentesis-induced circulatory dysfunction (PICD) syndrome may develop during therapeutic abdominal paracentesis. PICD is characterized by hyponatremia, azotemia, and an increase in plasma renin activity. A significant inverse correlation between changes in plasma renin activity and systemic vascular resistance has been demonstrated in those patients following paracentesis, suggesting that peripheral arterial vasodilation may be responsible for this circulatory dysfunction. Evidence is accumulating that PICD is secondary to an accentuation of an already established arteriolar vasodilation with multiple etiologies, including the dynamics of paracentesis (the rate of ascitic fluid extraction), release of nitric oxide from the vascular endothelium, and mechanical modifications due to abdominal decompression [12].

PICD is associated with an increased mortality and may be prevented with the administration of plasma expanders. It is very important to obtain reliable peripheral or central venous access in these patients so that fluid resuscitation can be performed if transient hypotension develops during the procedure. A recent study randomized 72 patients to receive albumin or saline after total paracentesis [13]. The incidence of PICD was significantly higher in the saline group versus the albumin group (33.3% vs. 11.4%, $p = 0.03$). However, no significant differences were found when less than 6 L of ascitic fluid was evacuated (6.7% vs. 5.6%, $p = 0.9$). Significant increases in plasma renin activity were found 24 hours and 6 days after paracentesis when saline was used, whereas no changes were observed with albumin. Albumin was more effective than saline in the prevention of PICD, but is not required when less than 6 L of ascitic fluid is evacuated. Therefore, the administration of albumin intravenously (6 to 8 g/L of ascites removed) is recommended with large-volume paracentesis (>6L). There have been five randomized controlled trials comparing volume expansion with albumin with other plasma expanders including dextran, collagen-based colloids, and hydroxyethyl starch [14–18]. All studies have documented that synthetic plasma expanders were as effective as albumin at preventing the clinical complications of paracentesis, namely hyponatremia or renal impairment. However, only one study examined prevention of PICD (defined by an increased in plasma renin activity or aldosterone concentration), and de-

termined that albumin prevented this more effectively than synthetic plasma expanders [13].

Two randomized trials comparing terlipressin (a vasoconstrictor) versus albumin in PICD in cirrhosis documented that both terlipressin and albumin prevented paracentesis-induced renal impairment in these patients [19,20]. Terlipressin may be as effective as intravenous albumin in preventing PICD in patients with cirrhosis.

Large-volume ascites removal in such patients is only transiently therapeutic; the underlying chronic disease induces reaccumulation of the ascites. Percutaneous placement of a tunneled catheter is a viable and safe technique to consider in patients who have symptomatic malignant ascites that require frequent therapeutic paracentesis for relief of symptoms [21].

DIAGNOSTIC PERITONEAL LAVAGE

Before the introduction of diagnostic peritoneal lavage (DPL) by Root et al. [22] in 1965, nonoperative evaluation of the injured abdomen was limited to standard four-quadrant abdominal paracentesis. Abdominal paracentesis for evaluation of hemoperitoneum was associated with a high false-negative rate. This clinical suspicion was confirmed by Giacobine and Siler [23] in an experimental animal model of hemoperitoneum documenting that a 500-mL blood volume in the peritoneal cavity yielded a positive paracentesis rate of only 78%. The initial study by Root et al. [22] reported 100% accuracy in identification of hemoperitoneum using 1 L peritoneal lavage fluid. Many subsequent clinical studies confirmed these findings, with the largest series reported by Fischer et al. [24] in 1978. They reviewed 2,586 cases of DPL and reported a false-positive rate of 0.2%, false-negative rate of 1.2%, and overall accuracy of 98.5%. Since its introduction in 1965, DPL has been a cornerstone in the evaluation of hemoperitoneum due to blunt and penetrating abdominal injuries. However, it is nonspecific for determination of type or extent of organ injury.

Recent advances have led to the use of ultrasound (focused assessment with sonography in trauma [FAST]) and rapid helical computed tomography (CT) in the emergent evaluation of abdominal trauma and have significantly decreased the use of DPL in the evaluation of abdominal trauma to less than 1% [25–27].

INDICATIONS

The primary indication for DPL is evaluation of blunt abdominal trauma in patients with associated hypotension. If the patient is hemodynamically stable and can be transported safely, computed tomographic scan of the abdomen and pelvis is the diagnostic method of choice. If the patient is hemodynamically unstable or requires emergent surgical intervention for a craniotomy, thoracotomy, or vascular procedure, it is imperative to determine whether there is a coexisting intraperitoneal source of hemorrhage to prioritize treatment of life-threatening injuries. Ultrasound or DPL can be used to diagnose hemoperitoneum in patients with multisystem injury or those who require general anesthesia for treatment of associated traumatic injuries. Patients with associated thoracic or pelvic injuries should also have definitive evaluation for abdominal trauma, and DPL can be used in these individuals. DPL can also be used to evaluate for traumatic hollow viscus injury, and a cell count ratio (defined as the ratio between white blood cell and red blood cell count in the lavage fluid divided by the ratio of the same parameters in the peripheral blood) less than or equal to 1 had a specificity of 97% and sensitivity of 100% in over 300 DPLs [28].

DPL can also be used to evaluate penetrating abdominal trauma, however its role differs from that in blunt abdominal trauma [29]. A hemodynamically unstable patient with abdominal penetrating injury requires no further investigation and immediate laparotomy. Instead, the role of DPL in the *hemodynamically stable* patient with penetrating abdominal injury is to identify hemoperitoneum and hollow viscus or diaphragmatic injury. DPL has also been recommended as the initial diagnostic study in stable patients with penetrating trauma to the back and flank, defining a red blood cell count greater than 1,000 mm^3 as a positive test [30]. Implementation of this protocol decreased the total celiotomy rate from 100% to 24%, and the therapeutic celiotomy rate increased from 15% to 80%.

DPL may prove useful in evaluation for possible peritonitis or ruptured viscus in patients with an altered level of consciousness but no evidence of traumatic injury. DPL can be considered in critically ill patients with sepsis to determine whether intraabdominal infection is the underlying source. When DPL is used to evaluate intraabdominal infection, a white blood cell count greater than 500 cells per mm^3 of lavage fluid is considered positive. DPL can also serve a therapeutic role. It is very effective in rewarming patients with significant hypothermia. It may potentially be used therapeutically in pancreatitis, fecal peritonitis, and bile pancreatitis, but multiple clinical studies have not documented its efficacy in these cases.

DPL should not be performed in patients with clear signs of significant abdominal trauma and hemoperitoneum associated with hemodynamic instability. These patients should undergo emergent celiotomy. Pregnancy is a relative contraindication to DPL; it may be technically difficult to perform because of the gravid uterus and is associated with a higher risk of complications. Bedside ultrasound evaluation of the abdomen in the pregnant trauma patient is associated with least risk to the woman and to the fetus. An additional relative contraindication to DPL is multiple previous abdominal surgeries. These patients commonly have multiple abdominal adhesions, and it may be very difficult to gain access to the free peritoneal cavity. If DPL is indicated, it must be performed by the open technique to prevent iatrogenic complications such as intestinal injury.

TECHNIQUES

Three techniques can be used to perform DPL: the closed percutaneous technique, the semiclosed technique, and the open technique. The closed percutaneous technique, introduced by Lazarus and Nelson [31] in 1979, is easy to perform, can be done rapidly, is associated with a low complication rate, and is as accurate as the open technique. It should not be used in patients who have had previous abdominal surgery or a history of abdominal adhesions. The open technique entails the placement of the peritoneal lavage catheter into the peritoneal cavity under direct visualization. It is more time consuming than the closed percutaneous technique. The semiclosed technique requires a smaller incision than the open technique and uses a peritoneal lavage catheter with a metal stylet to gain entrance into the peritoneal cavity. It has become less popular as clinicians

have become more familiar and skilled with the Lazarus-Nelson closed technique.

The patient must be placed in the supine position for all three techniques. A catheter is placed into the urinary bladder and a nasogastric tube is inserted into the stomach to prevent iatrogenic bladder or gastric injury. The nasogastric tube is placed on continuous suction for gastric decompression. The skin of the anterior abdominal wall is prepared with 10% povidone-iodine solution and sterilely draped, leaving the periumbilical area exposed. Standard aseptic technique is used throughout the procedure. Local anesthesia with 1% or 2% lidocaine with 1:200,000 epinephrine is used as necessary throughout the procedure. The infraumbilical site is used unless there is clinical concern of possible pelvic fracture and retroperitoneal or pelvic hematoma, in which case the supraumbilical site is optimal.

Closed Percutaneous Technique

With the closed percutaneous technique (Fig. 14-2), local anesthesia is infiltrated inferior to the umbilicus and a 5-mm skin incision is made just at the inferior umbilical edge. An 18-gauge needle is inserted through this incision and into the peritoneal cavity, angled toward the pelvis at approximately a 45-degree angle with the skin. The penetration through the linea alba and then through the peritoneum is felt as two separate "pops." A J-tipped guidewire is passed through the needle and into the peritoneal cavity, again directing the wire toward the pelvis by maintaining the needle at a 45-degree angle to the skin. The 18-gauge needle is then removed and the peritoneal lavage catheter inserted over the guidewire into the peritoneal cavity, using a twisting motion and guided inferiorly toward the pelvis. The guidewire is then removed, and a 10-mL syringe is attached to the catheter for aspiration. If free blood returns from the peritoneal catheter before the syringe is attached, or if gross blood returns in the syringe barrel, hemoperitoneum has been documented; the catheter is removed, and the patient is transported quickly to the operating room for emergent celiotomy. If no gross blood returns on aspiration through the catheter, peritoneal lavage is performed using 1 L Ringer's lactate solution or normal saline that has been previously warmed to prevent hypothermia. The fluid is instilled into the peritoneal cavity through the peritoneal lavage catheter; afterward, the peritoneal fluid is allowed to drain out of the peritoneal cavity by gravity until the fluid return slows. A minimum of 250 mL lavage fluid is considered a representative sample of the peritoneal fluid [32]. A sample is sent to the laboratory for determination of red blood cell count, white blood cell count, amylase concentration, and presence of bile, bacteria, or particulate matter. When the lavage is completed, the catheter is removed and a sterile dressing applied over the site. Suture approximation of the skin edges is not necessary when the closed technique is used for DPL.

Semiclosed Technique

Local anesthetic is infiltrated in the area of the planned incision and a 2- to 3-cm vertical incision made in the infraumbilical or supraumbilical area. The incision is continued sharply down through the subcutaneous tissue and linea alba, and the peritoneum is then visualized. Forceps, hemostats, or Allis clamps are used to grasp the edges of the linea alba and elevate the fascial edges to prevent injury to underlying abdominal structures. The peritoneal lavage catheter with a metal inner stylet is inserted through the closed peritoneum into the peritoneal

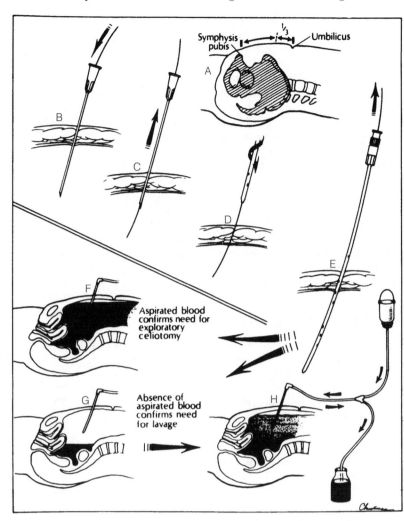

FIGURE 14-2. The closed percutaneous technique for diagnostic peritoneal lavage, using a Seldinger guidewire method.

cavity at a 45-degree angle to the anterior abdominal wall, directed toward the pelvis. When the catheter–metal stylet assembly is in the peritoneal cavity, the peritoneal lavage catheter is advanced into the pelvis and the metal stylet removed. A 10-mL syringe is attached to the catheter, and aspiration is conducted as previously described. When the lavage is completed, the fascia must be reapproximated with sutures, the skin closed, and a sterile dressing applied.

Open Technique

After the administration of appropriate local anesthetic, a vertical midline incision approximately 3 to 5 cm long is made. This incision is commonly made in the infraumbilical location, but in patients with presumed pelvic fractures or retroperitoneal hematomas or in pregnant patients, a supraumbilical location is preferred. The vertical midline incision is carried down through the skin, subcutaneous tissue, and linea alba under direct vision. The linea alba is grasped on either side using forceps, hemostats, or Allis clamps, and the fascia is elevated to prevent injury to the underlying abdominal structures. The peritoneum is identified, and a small vertical peritoneal incision is made to gain entrance into the peritoneal cavity. The peritoneal lavage catheter is then inserted into the peritoneal cavity under direct visualization and advanced inferiorly toward the pelvis. It is inserted without the

stylet or metal trocar. When in position, a 10-mL syringe is attached for aspiration. If aspiration of the peritoneal cavity is negative (i.e., no gross blood returns), peritoneal lavage is performed as described above. As in the semiclosed technique, the fascia and skin must be reapproximated to prevent dehiscence or evisceration, or both.

A prospective randomized study documented that the Lazarus-Nelson technique of closed percutaneous DPL can be performed faster than the open procedure [33]. The procedure times with the closed technique varied from 1 to 3 minutes, compared with 5 to 24 minutes for the open technique. In addition, it was documented that the closed percutaneous technique is as accurate as the open procedure and was associated with a lower incidence of wound infections and complications. The closed percutaneous technique, using the Seldinger technique, should therefore be used initially in all patients except those who have had previous abdominal surgery or in pregnant patients. This has been confirmed in a study of 2,501 DPLs performed over a 75-month period for blunt or penetrating abdominal trauma [34]. The majority (2,409, or 96%) were performed using the percutaneous or "closed" technique, and 92 (4%) were done open because of pelvic fractures, previous scars, or pregnancy. Open DPL was less sensitive than closed DPL in patients who sustained blunt trauma (90% vs. 95%) but slightly more sensitive in determining penetration (100% vs. 96%). Overall, there were few (21, or 0.8%) complications, and the overall sensitivity, specificity, and accuracy were 95%, 99%, and 98% respectively using a red blood cell count of 100,000 per mm^3 in blunt trauma and 10,000 per mm^3 in penetrating trauma as the positive threshold. A metaanalysis concluded that the closed DPL technique is comparable to the standard open DPL technique in terms of accuracy and major complications, with the advantage of reduced performance time with closed DPL, which is offset by increased technical difficulties and failures [35].

Cotter et al. [36] reported a modification of DPL that allows more rapid infusion and drainage of lavage fluid. This modification uses cystoscopy irrigation tubing for instillation and drainage of the peritoneal lavage fluid. The cystoscopy irrigation system dramatically reduced influx and efflux times, saving an average of 19 minutes per patient for the completion of peritoneal lavage. This modification can be applied to the closed percutaneous or open technique for DPL to decrease the procedure time in critically ill patients.

INTERPRETATION OF RESULTS

The current guidelines for interpretation of positive and negative results of DPL are listed in Table 14-2. A positive result can be estimated by the inability to read newsprint or typewritten print through the lavage fluid as it returns through clear plastic tubing. This test is not reliable, however, and a quantitative red blood cell (RBC) count in a sample of the peritoneal lavage fluid must be performed [37]. For patients with nonpenetrating abdominal trauma, a RBC count greater than 100,000 cells per mm^3 of lavage fluid is considered positive and requires emergent celiotomy. Fewer than 50,000 RBC per mm^3 is considered negative and RBC counts of 50,000 to 100,000 per mm^3 are considered indeterminate. The guidelines for patients with penetrating abdominal trauma are much less clear with clinical studies using a RBC count of greater than 1,000 or 10,000 cells per mm^3 to greater than 100,000 cells per mm^3 as the criterion for a positive DPL in patients with penetrating thoracic or abdominal trauma. The lower the threshold the more sensitive the test, but the higher the nontherapeutic laparotomy rate.

Determination of hollow viscus injury by DPL is much more difficult. A white blood cell count greater than 500 cells per mm^3 of lavage fluid or an amylase concentration greater than 175 units per dL of lavage fluid is usually considered positive. These studies, however, are not as accurate as the use of red blood cell count in the lavage fluid to determine the presence of hemoperitoneum. One study in patients with blunt abdominal trauma determined that the white blood cell count in lavage fluid has a positive predictive value of only 23% and probably should not be used as an indicator of a positive DPL [38]. Other studies analyzed alkaline phosphatase levels in DPL fluid to determine whether this assay is helpful in the diagnosis of hollow viscus injuries [39,40]. The results have been variable. One study of 545 patients who sustained blunt or penetrating abdominal injury determined that alkaline phosphatase levels greater than ten in the DPL effluent were predictive of hollow visceral injury with a specificity of 99.4% and a sensitivity of 93.3% [40]. Additional studies are required to confirm these results and establish the use of alkaline phosphatase levels as a positive indicator of significant intraabdominal injury. A prospective study used a diagnostic algorithm of initial abdominal ultrasound, followed by helical CT and subsequent DPL (if CT was suggestive of blunt bowel or mesenteric injury) using a cell count ratio (defined as the ratio between white blood cell and red blood cell count in the lavage fluid divided by the ratio of the same parameters in the peripheral blood) greater than or equal to 1 to determine need for laparotomy in patients with blunt abdominal injuries [41]. This proposed algorithm had a high accuracy (100%) while requiring the performance of DPL in only a few (2%) patients.

It must be stressed that DPL is not accurate for determination of retroperitoneal visceral injuries or diaphragmatic injuries [42]. The incidence of false-negative DPL results is approximately 30% in patients who sustained traumatic diaphragmatic rupture. In addition, DPL is insensitive in detecting subcapsular hematomas of the spleen or liver that are contained, with no evidence of hemoperitoneum. Although DPL is now used in the evaluation of nontraumatic intraabdominal pathology, the criteria for positive lavage in these patients have not yet been established. Additional clinical studies are needed.

COMPLICATIONS

Complications of DPL by the techniques described here include malposition of the lavage catheter, injury to the intraabdominal organs or vessels, iatrogenic hemoperitoneum, wound infection or dehiscence, evisceration, and possible unnecessary laparotomy. DPL is a very valuable technique, however, and if it is performed carefully, with attention to detail, these complications are minimized. In the largest series published to date, with

TABLE 14-2.   Interpretation of Diagnostic Peritoneal Lavage Results

Positive

Nonpenetrating Abdominal Trauma
  Immediate gross blood return via catheter
  Immediate return of intestinal contents or food particles
  Aspiration of 10 mL blood via catheter
  Return of lavage fluid via chest tube or urinary catheter
  Red blood cell (RBC) count >100,000/mm^3
  White blood cell (WBC) count >500/mm^3
  Cell count ratio (defined as the ratio between WBC and RBC
    count in the lavage fluid divided by the ratio of the same
    parameters in the peripheral blood) ≥1
  Amylase >175 U/100 mL

Penetrating Abdominal Trauma
  Immediate gross blood return via catheter
  Immediate return of intestinal contents or food particles
  Aspiration of 10 mL blood via catheter
  Return of lavage fluid via chest tube or Foley catheter
  RBC count used is variable, from >1,000/mm^3 to >100,000/mm^3
  WBC count >500/mm^3
  Amylase >175 U/100 mL

Negative

Nonpenetrating Abdominal Trauma
  RBC count <50,000/mm^3
  WBC count <100/mm^3
  Cell count ratio (defined as the ratio between WBC and RBC
    count in the lavage fluid divided by the ratio of the same
    parameters in the peripheral blood) <1
  Amylase <75 U/100 mL

Penetrating Abdominal Trauma
  RBC count used is variable, from <1,000/mm^3 to <50,000/mm^3
  WBC count <100/mm^3
  Amylase <75 U/100 mL

over 2,500 DPLs performed, the complications rate was 0.8% [34]. Wound infection, dehiscence, and evisceration are more common with the open technique; therefore, the closed percutaneous technique is recommended in all patients who do not have a contraindication to this technique. Knowledge of all techniques is necessary, however, because the choice of technique should be based on the individual patient's presentation.

REFERENCES

1. Caruntu FA, Benea L: Spontaneous bacterial peritonitis: pathogenesis, diagnosis and treatment. *J Gastrointestin Liver Dis* 15(1):51, 2006.
2. Garcia N, Sanyal AJ: Ascites. *Curr Treat Options Gastroenterol* 4:527, 2001.
3. Moore KP, Wong F, Gines P, et al: The management of ascites in cirrhosis: report on the consensus conference of the International Ascites Club. *Hepatology* 38(1):258, 2003.
4. Saab S, Nieto JM, Ly D, et al: TIPS versus paracentesis for cirrhotic patients with refractory ascites. *Cochrane Database Syst Rev* (3):CD4889, 2004.
5. Zervos EE, Rosemurgy AS: Management of medically refractory ascites. *Am J Surg* 181:256, 2001.
6. Parra MW, Al-Khayat H, Smith HG, et al: Paracentesis for resuscitation-induced abdominal compartment syndrome: an alternative to decompressive laparotomy in the burn patient. *J Trauma* 60(5):1119, 2006.
7. Latenser BA, Kowal-Vern A, Kimball D, et al: A pilot study comparing percutaneous decompression with decompressive laparotomy for acute abdominal compartment syndrome in thermal injury. *J Burn Care Rehabil* 23(3):190, 2002.
8. Runyon BA: Management of adult patients with ascites caused by cirrhosis. *Hepatology* 39: 841, 2004.
9. Grabau CM, Crago SF, Hoff LK, et al: Performance standards for therapeutic abdominal paracentesis. *Hepatology* 40:484, 2004.
10. Sakai H, Sheer TA, Mendler MH, et al: Choosing the location for non-image guided abdominal paracentesis. *Liver Int* 25(5):984, 2005.
11. Dittrich S, Yordi LM, DeMattos AA: The value of serum-ascites albumin gradient for the determination of portal hypertension in the diagnosis of ascites. *Hepatogastroenterology* 48:166, 2001.
12. Sola-Vera J, Such J: Understanding the mechanisms of paracentesis-induced circulatory dysfunction. *Eur J Gastroenterol Hepatol* 16(3):295, 2004.
13. Sola-Vera J, Minana J, Ricart E, et al: Randomized trial comparing albumin and saline in the prevention of paracentesis-induced dysfunction in cirrhotic patients with ascites. *Hepatology* 37(5):1147, 2003.
14. Gines A, Fernandez-Esparrach G, Monescillo A, et al: Randomized trial comparing albumin, dextran-70 and polygeline in cirrhotic patients with ascites treated by paracentesis. *Gastroenterology* 111:1002, 1996.
15. Altman C, Bernard B, Roulot D, et al: Randomized comparative multicenter study of hydroxyethyl starch versus albumin as a plasma expander in cirrhotic patients with tense ascites treated with paracentesis. *Eur J Gastroenterol Hepatol* 10:5, 1998.
16. Planas R, Gines P, Arroyo V, et al: Dextran-70 versus albumin as plasma expanders in cirrhotic patients with ascites treated with total paracentesis. Results of a randomized study. *Gastroenterology* 99:1736, 1990.
17. Salerno F, Badalamenti S, Lorenzano E, et al: Randomized comparative study of hemaccel vs. albumin infusion after total paracentesis in cirrhotic patients with refractory ascites. *Hepatology* 13:707, 1991.
18. Fassio E, Terg R, Landeira G, et al: Paracentesis with dextran 70 vs paracentesis with albumin in cirrhosis with tense ascites. Results of a randomized study. *J Hepatol* 14:310, 1992.
19. Singh V, Kumar R, Nain CK, et al: Terlipressin versus albumin in paracentesis-induced circulatory dysfunction in cirrhosis: a randomized study. *J Gastroenterl Hepatol* 21(1 Pt 2):303, 2006.
20. Moreau R, Asselah T, Condat B, et al: Comparison of the effect of terlipressin and albumin on arterial blood volume in patients with cirrhosis and tense ascites treated by paracentesis: a randomized pilot study. *Gut* 50(1):90, 2002.
21. Rosenberg SM: Palliation of malignant ascites. *Gastroenterol Clin North Am* 35(1):189, xi 2006.
22. Root H, Hauser C, McKinley C, et al: Diagnostic peritoneal lavage. *Surgery* 57:633, 1965.
23. Giacobine JW, Siler VE: Evaluation of diagnostic abdominal paracentesis with experimental and clinical studies. *Eur Gynecol Obstet* 110:676, 1960.
24. Fischer R, Beverlin B, Engrav L, et al: Diagnostic peritoneal lavage 14 years and 2586 patients later. *Am J Surg* 136:701, 1978.
25. Ollerton JE, Sugrue M, Balogh Z, et al: Prospective study to evaluate the influence of FAST on trauma patient management. *J Trauma* 60(4):785, 2006.
26. Kirkpatrick AW, Sirois M, Laupland KB, et al: Prospective evaluation of hand-held focused abdominal sonography for trauma (FAST) in blunt abdominal trauma. *Can J Surg* 48(6):453, 2005.
27. Fang JF, Wong YC, Lin BC, et al: Usefulness of multidetector computed tomography for the initial assessment of blunt abdominal trauma patients. *World J Surg* 30(2):176, 2006.
28. Fang JF, Chen RJ, Lin BC: Cell count ratio: New criterion of diagnostic peritoneal lavage for detection of hollow organ perforation. *J Trauma* 45(3):540, 1998.
29. Sriussadaporn S, Pak-art R, Pattaratiwanon M, et al: Clinical uses of diagnostic peritoneal lavage in stab wounds of the anterior abdomen: a prospective study. *Eur J Surg* 168(8–9): 490, 2002.
30. Boyle EM, Maier RV, Salazar JD, et al: Diagnosis of injuries after stab wounds to the back and flank. *J Trauma* 42:260, 1997.
31. Lazarus HM, Nelson JA: A technique for peritoneal lavage without risk or complication. *Surg Gynecol Obstet* 149:889, 1979.
32. Sweeney JF, Albrink MH, Bischof E, et al: Diagnostic peritoneal lavage: volume of lavage effluent needed for accurate determination of a negative lavage. *Injury* 25:659, 1994.
33. Howdieshell TR, Osler RM, Demarest GB: Open versus closed peritoneal lavage with particular attention to time, accuracy and cost. *Am J Emerg Med* 7:367, 1989.
34. Nagy KK, Roberts RR, Joseph KT, et al: Experience with over 2500 diagnostic peritoneal lavages. *Injury* 31:479, 2000.
35. Hodgson NF, Stewart TC, Girotti MJ: Open or closed diagnostic peritoneal lavage for abdominal trauma? A metaanalysis. *J Trauma* 48(6):1091, 2000.
36. Cotter CP, Hawkins ML, Kent RB, et al: Ultrarapid diagnostic peritoneal lavage. *J Trauma* 29:615, 1989.
37. Gow KW, Haley LP, Phang PT: Validity of visual inspection of diagnostic peritoneal lavage fluid. *Can J Surg* 39:114, 1996.
38. Soyka J, Martin M, Sloan E, et al: Diagnostic peritoneal lavage: is an isolated WBC count greater than or equal to 500/mm³ predictive of intra-abdominal trauma requiring celiotomy in blunt trauma patients? *J Trauma* 30:874, 1990.
39. Megison SM, Weigelt JA: The value of alkaline phosphatase in peritoneal lavage. *Ann Emerg Med* 19:5, 1990.
40. Jaffin JH, Ochsner G, Cole FJ, et al: Alkaline phosphatase levels in diagnostic peritoneal lavage as a predictor of hollow visceral injury. *J Trauma* 34:829, 1993.
41. Menegaux F, Tresallet C, Gosgnach M, et al: Diagnosis of bowel and mesenteric injuries in blunt abdominal trauma: A prospective study. *Am J Emerg Med* 24(1):19, 2006.
42. Fischer RP, Freeman T: The inadequacy of peritoneal lavage in diagnosing acute diaphragmatic rupture. *J Trauma* 16:538, 1976.

Marie T. Pavini
Juan Carlos Puyana

CHAPTER **15**

Gastroesophageal Balloon Tamponade for Acute Variceal Hemorrhage

Gastroesophageal variceal hemorrhage is an acute and catastrophic complication that occurs in one third to one half of patients with portal pressures greater than 12 mm Hg [1]. Because proximal gastric varices and varices in the distal 5 cm of the esophagus lie in the superficial lamina propria, they are more likely to bleed and more likely to respond to endoscopic treatment [2]. Variceal rupture is likely a factor of size, wall thickness, and portal pressure, and may be predicted by Child-Pugh class, red wale markings indicating epithelial thickness, and variceal size [1]. Whereas urgent endoscopy, sclerotherapy, and band ligations are considered first-line treatments, balloon tamponade remains a valuable intervention in the treatment of bleeding esophageal varices. Balloon tamponade is accomplished using a multilumen tube with esophageal and gastric cuffs that can be inflated to compress esophageal varices and gastric submucosal veins thereby providing hemostasis through tamponade.

HISTORICAL DEVELOPMENT

In 1930, Westphal described the use of an esophageal sound as a means of controlling variceal hemorrhage. In 1947, successful control of hemorrhage by balloon tamponade was achieved by attaching an inflatable latex bag to the end of a Miller-Abbot tube. In 1949, a two-balloon tube was described by Patton and Johnson. A triple-lumen tube with gastric and esophageal balloons (one lumen for gastric aspiration and the other two for balloon inflation) was described by Sengstaken and Blakemore in 1950. In 1953, Linton proposed a single gastric balloon tube with a suction lumen below the balloon as a diagnostic tool to differentiate between gastric and esophageal bleed and a larger balloon (800 mL) capable of compressing the submucosal veins in the cardia, thereby minimizing flow to the esophageal veins. An additional suction port above Linton's gastric balloon was introduced by Nachlas in 1955. The Minnesota tube was described in 1968 as a modification of the Sengstaken-Blakemore tube, incorporating the esophageal suction port, which will be described later.

ROLE OF BALLOON TAMPONADE IN THE MANAGEMENT OF BLEEDING ESOPHAGEAL VARICES

Treatment of portal hypertension to prevent variceal rupture includes primary and secondary prophylaxis. Primary prophylaxis consists of beta-blockers, band ligation, and endoscopic surveillance, and secondary prophylaxis includes nitrates, transjugular intrahepatic portosystemic shunt (TIPS), and surgical shunt [3]. Appropriate management of acute variceal bleeding involves multiple simultaneous and sequential modalities. A number of studies comparing the efficacy of balloon tamponade against sclerotherapy have shown that the incidence and severity of complications and success in controlling bleeding favor the use of sclerotherapy or band ligation as the first line of treatment [4,5]. The decision to use other therapeutic alternatives depends on the response to the initial therapy, the severity of the hemorrhage, and the patient's underlying condition.

Splanchnic vasoconstrictors such as octreotide, terlipressin (the only agent shown to decrease mortality), or vasopressin (with nitrates to reduce cardiac side effects) decrease portal blood flow and pressure and should be administered as soon as possible [6–8]. In fact, Pourriat et al. [9] advocate administration of octreotide by emergency medical personnel before patient transfer to the hospital. Recombinant activated factor VII has been reported to achieve hemostasis in bleeding esophageal varices unresponsive to standard treatment and may also be considered [10]. Emergent therapeutic endoscopy in conjunction with pharmacotherapy is more effective than pharmacotherapy alone and is also performed as soon as possible. Band ligation has a lower rate of rebleeding and complications when compared with sclerotherapy and should be performed preferentially, provided visualization is adequate to ligate varices successfully [3,11]. Tissue adhesives such as polidocanol and cyanoacrylate delivered through an endoscope are being used and studied outside the United States.

Balloon tamponade is performed to control massive variceal hemorrhage with the hope that band ligation or sclerotherapy and secondary prophylaxis will then be possible (Fig. 15-1). If bleeding continues beyond these measures, then TIPS [12] is

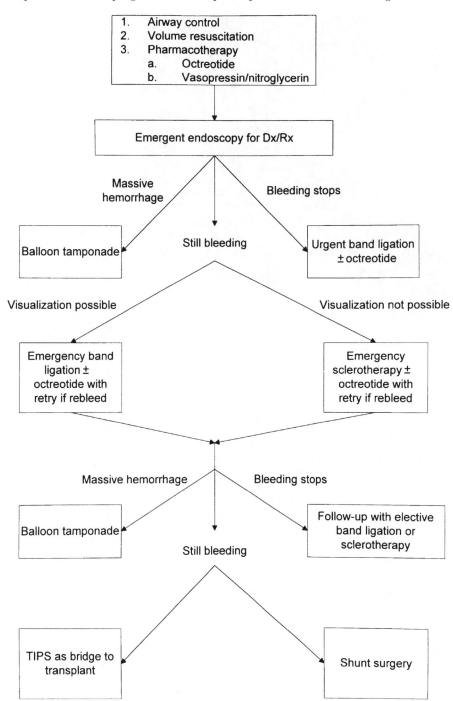

FIGURE 15-1. Management of esophageal variceal hemorrhage. Dx, diagnosis; Rx, therapy; TIPS, transjugular intrahepatic portosystemic shunt.

considered. Shunt surgery [13] may be considered if TIPS is contraindicated. Other alternatives include percutaneous transhepatic embolization, emergent esophageal transection with stapling [14], esophagogastric devascularization with esophageal transection and splenectomy, and hepatic transplantation. If gastric varices are noted, therapeutic options include endoscopic administration of the tissue adhesive cyanoacrylate, TIPS, balloon-occluded retrograde transvenous obliteration [15], balloon-occluded endoscopic injection therapy [16], and

devascularization with splenectomy, shunt surgery, and liver transplantation.

INDICATIONS AND CONTRAINDICATIONS

A Sengstaken-Blakemore or Minnesota tube is indicated in patients with a diagnosis of esophageal variceal hemorrhage in which neither band ligation nor sclerotherapy is technically possible, readily available, or has failed [17]. If at all possible,

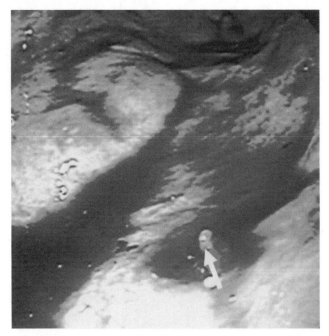

FIGURE 15-2. Esophageal varices as seen by endoscopy. The white nipple (*arrow*) indicates a recent platelet plug. (Courtesy of Dale Janik, MD.)

making an adequate anatomic diagnosis is critical before any of these balloon tubes are inserted. Severe upper gastrointestinal bleeding attributed to esophageal varices in patients with clinical evidence of chronic liver disease results from other causes in up to 40% of cases. The observation of a white nipple sign (platelet plug) is indicative of a recent variceal bleed (Fig. 15-2). The tube is contraindicated in patients with recent esophageal surgery or esophageal stricture [18]. Some authors do not recommend balloon tamponade when a hiatal hernia is present, but there are reports of successful hemorrhage control in some of these patients [19].

TECHNICAL AND PRACTICAL CONSIDERATIONS

AIRWAY CONTROL

Endotracheal intubation (see Chapter 1) is imperative in patients with hemodynamic compromise, encephalopathy, or both. The incidence of aspiration pneumonia is directly related to the presence of encephalopathy or impaired mental status [20]. Suctioning of pulmonary secretions and blood that accumulates in the hypopharynx is facilitated in patients who have been intubated. Sedatives and analgesics are more readily administered in intubated patients and may be required often because balloon tamponade is poorly tolerated in most patients. The incidence of pulmonary complications is significantly lower when endotracheal intubation is routinely used [21].

HYPOVOLEMIA, SHOCK, AND COAGULOPATHY

Adequate intravenous access should be obtained with large-bore venous catheters and fluid resuscitation should be undertaken with crystalloids and colloids. A central venous catheter or pulmonary artery catheter may be required to monitor intravascular

filling pressures, especially in patients with severe cirrhosis, advanced age, or underlying cardiac and pulmonary disease. The hematocrit should be maintained above 28%, and coagulopathy should be treated with fresh-frozen plasma and platelets. Four to six units of packed red cells should always be available in case of severe recurrent bleeding, which commonly occurs in these patients.

CLOTS AND GASTRIC DECOMPRESSION

Placement of an Ewald tube and aggressive lavage and suctioning of the stomach and duodenum facilitates endoscopy, diminishes the risk of aspiration, and may help control hemorrhage from causes other than esophageal varices. It should be removed prior to balloon tamponade.

INFECTION AND ULCERATION

Mortality is increased if infection is present in bleeding cirrhotic patients. The rate of early rebleeding is also increased in the presence of infection [22]. Prophylactic antibiotic use reduces the incidence of early rebleeding and increases survival [23]. Intravenous proton pump inhibitors are more efficacious than histamine 2 receptor antagonists in maintaining gastric pH at a goal of 7. Ulcers can form from sclerotherapy or from direct cuff pressure during balloon tamponade. Shaheen et al. [24] found that the postbanding ulcers in patients receiving a proton pump inhibitor were 2 times smaller than those in patients who had not received a proton pump inhibitor.

TUBES, PORTS, AND BALLOONS

Several studies have published combined experience with tubes such as the Linton and Nachlas tube [25,26]. The techniques described here are limited to the use of the Minnesota (Fig. 15-3) and Sengstaken-Blakemore (Fig. 15-4) tubes. All lumens should be patent, and the balloons inflated and checked for leaks. The baseline compliance of the gastric balloon should be tested by placing 100-mL aliquots of air, ensuring that the manometer attached (using a Y connector) does not increase by more than 15 mm Hg with each aliquot. Final pressure at maximum recommended inflation is recorded [27]. Both balloons are then completely deflated using suction, and clamped with rubber hemostats or plugged before lubrication. Although the Minnesota tube enjoys a fourth lumen that allows suctioning above the esophageal balloon[20], the Sengstaken-Blakemore tube must have a 14 to 18 French nasogastric tube secured a few centimeters proximal to the esophageal balloon to be used for esophageal decompression. The nasogastric tube should be used even if the esophageal balloon is not inflated because inflation of the gastric balloon precludes proper drainage of esophageal secretions [28].

INSERTION AND PLACEMENT OF THE TUBE

The head of the bed should be elevated to reduce the risk of aspiration. The tube should be generously lubricated with lidocaine jelly. It can be inserted through the nose or mouth, but the nasal route is not recommended in patients with coagulopathy. The tube is passed into the stomach. Auscultation in the epigastrium while air is injected through the gastric lumen verifies

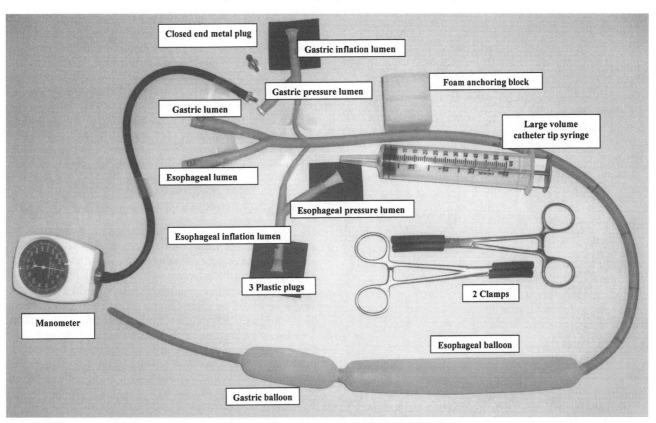

FIGURE 15-3.   Minnesota tube.

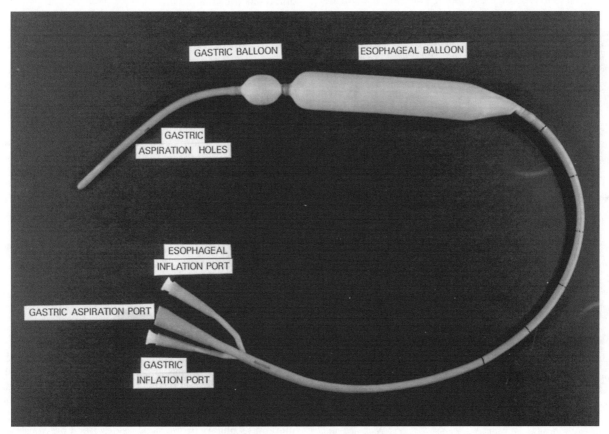

FIGURE 15-4.   Sengstaken-Blakemore tube.

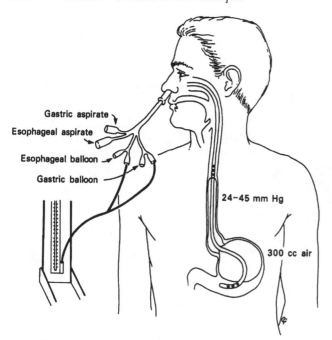

FIGURE 15-5.   Proper positioning of the Minnesota tube.

the position of the tube, but the position of the gastric balloon must be confirmed radiologically at this time. The gastric balloon is inflated with no more than 80 mL of air, and a (portable) radiograph is obtained that includes the upper abdomen and lower chest (Figs. 15-5 and 15-6). When it is documented that the gastric balloon is below the diaphragm, it should be further

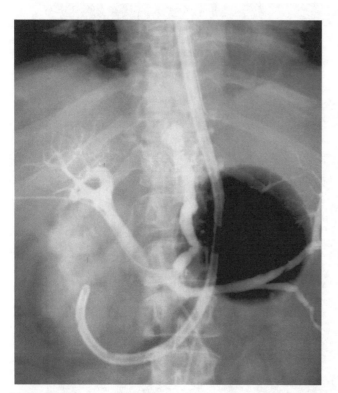

FIGURE 15-6.   Radiograph showing correct position of the tube; the gastric balloon is seen below the diaphragm. Note the Salem sump above the gastric balloon and adjacent to the tube. (Courtesy of Ashley Davidoff, MD.)

inflated with air, slowly, to a volume of 250 to 300 mL. The gastric balloon of the Minnesota tube can be inflated to 450 mL. Tube balloon inlets should be clamped with rubber-shod hemostats after insufflation. Hemorrhage is frequently controlled with insufflation of the gastric balloon alone without applying traction, but in patients with torrential hemorrhage, it is necessary to apply traction (vide infra). If the bleeding continues, the esophageal balloon should be inflated to a pressure of approximately 45 mm Hg (bedside manometer). This pressure should be monitored and maintained. Some authors inflate the esophageal balloon in all patients immediately after insertion [26].

FIXATION AND TRACTION TECHNIQUES

Fixation and traction on the tube depend on the route of insertion. When the nasal route is used, traction should not be applied against the nostril because this can easily cause skin and cartilage necrosis. When traction is required, the tube should be attached to a cord that is passed over a pulley in a bed with an overhead orthopaedic frame and aligned directly as it comes out of the nose to avoid contact with the nostril. This system allows maintenance of traction with a known weight (500 to 1,500 g) that is easily measured and constant. When the tube is inserted through the mouth, traction is better applied by placing a football helmet on the patient and attaching the tube to the face mask of the helmet after a similar weight is applied for tension. Pressure sores can occur in the head and forehead when the helmet does not fit properly or when it is used for a prolonged period. Several authors recommend overhead traction for oral and nasal insertion [29].

MAINTENANCE AND MONITORING

Tautness and inflation should be checked an hour after insertion, allowing for only transient fluctuations of as much as 30 mm Hg with respirations and esophageal spasm. Sedation or a pressure decrease may be necessary if elevated pressures persist. Soft restraints should also be in use. The tube is left in place a minimum of 24 hours with gastric balloon tamponade maintained continuously for up to 48 hours. The esophageal balloon should be deflated for 5 minutes every 6 hours to help prevent mucosal ischemia and esophageal necrosis. Radiographic assurance of correct placement should be obtained every 24 hours and when dislodgement is suspected (Fig. 15-7). A pair of scissors should be left at the bedside in case rapid decompression becomes necessary as balloon migration can acutely obstruct the airway or rupture the esophagus.

REMOVAL OF THE TUBE

Once hemorrhage is controlled, the esophageal balloon is deflated first; the gastric balloon is left inflated for an additional 24 to 48 hours. If there is no evidence of bleeding, the gastric balloon is deflated, and the tube is left in place 24 hours longer. If bleeding recurs, the balloon is reinflated. The tube is removed if no further bleeding occurs. Because rebleeding can occur in up to two thirds of patients within 3 months without therapy, secondary prophylaxis, as described previously should be started [3].

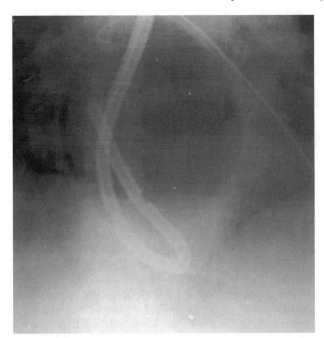

FIGURE 15-7. Chest radiograph showing distal segment of the tube coiled in the chest and the gastric balloon inflated above the diaphragm in the esophagus. (Courtesy of Ashley Davidoff, MD.)

COMPLICATIONS

Rebleeding when the cuff(s) is deflated should be anticipated. The highest risk of rebleeding is in the first few days after balloon deflation. By 6 weeks, the risk of rebleeding returns to premorbid risk level. Independent predictors of mortality in patients undergoing balloon tamponade described by Lee et al. [30] include blood transfusion greater than 10 units, coagulopathy, presence of shock, Glasgow Coma Score, and total volume of sclerosing agent (ethanolamine).

Aspiration pneumonia is the most common complication of balloon tamponade. The severity and fatality rate is related to the presence of impaired mental status and encephalopathy in patients with poor control of the airway. The incidence ranges from 0% to 12%. Acute laryngeal obstruction and tracheal rupture are the most severe of all complications and the worst examples of tube migration. Migration of the tube occurs when the gastric balloon is not inflated properly after adequate positioning in the stomach or when excessive traction (greater than 1.5 kg) is used, causing migration cephalad to the esophagus or hypopharynx. Mucosal ulceration of the gastroesophageal junction is common and is directly related to prolonged traction time (greater than 36 hours). Perforation of the esophagus is reported as a result of misplacing the gastric balloon above the diaphragm (Fig. 15-6). It is imperative that the position be confirmed radiologically immediately after passing the tube and before the gastric balloon is inflated with more than 80 mL of air as rupture of the esophagus carries a high mortality rate, especially in patients with severe hemorrhage who already have serious physiologic impairment. The incidence of complications that are a direct cause of death ranges from 0% to 20%. Unusual complications, such as impaction, result from obstruction of the balloon ports making it impossible to deflate the balloon. Occasionally, surgery is required to remove the tube. Other complications include necrosis of the nostrils and nasopharyngeal bleeding.

Acknowledgments

The authors thank Claire LaForce for her help collecting references and Nancy Meszaros, RN, BSN, for her help with figures and pictures. Ms. LaForce and Ms. Meszaros are both from Rutland Regional Medical Center, Rutland, VT. For their help with photography, thanks also to Charles F. Foltz and Susan A. Bright, Medical Media Service, West Roxbury Veterans Administration Medical Center, West Roxbury, MA.

REFERENCES

1. Rikkers LF: Surgical complications of cirrhosis and portal hypertension, in Townsend CM, Beauchamp RD, Evers BM, et al (eds): *Sabiston's Textbook of Surgery.* 17th ed. Philadelphia, WB Saunders, 2004; p 1175.
2. Tsokos M, Turk EE: Esophageal variceal hemorrhage presenting as sudden death in outpatients. *Arch Pathol Lab Med* 126:1197, 2002.
3. Zaman A, Chalasani N: Bleeding caused by portal hypertension. *Gastroenterol Clin North Am* 34:623, 2005.
4. Idezuki Y, Sanjo K, Bandai Y, et al: Current strategy for esophageal varices in Japan. *Am J Surg* 160:98, 1990.
5. Cipolletta L, Bianco MA, Rotondano G, et al: Emergency endoscopic ligation of actively bleeding gastric varices with a detachable snare. *Gastrointest Endosc* 47:400, 1998.
6. Sandford NL, Kerlin P: Current management of oesophageal varices. *Aust N Z Med J* 25:528, 1995.
7. Stein C, Korula J: Variceal bleeding: what are the options? *Postgrad Med* 98:143, 1995.
8. Erstad B: Octreotide for acute variceal bleeding. *Ann Pharmacother* 35:618, 2001.
9. Pourriat JL, Leyacher S, Letoumelin P, et al: Early administration of terlipressin plus glyceryl trinitate to control active upper gastrointestinal bleeding in cirrhotic patients *Lancet* 346:865, 1995.
10. Romero-Castro R, Jimenez-Saenz M, Pellicer-Bautista F, et al: Recombinant-activated factor VII as hemostatic therapy in eight cases of severe hemorrhage from esophageal varices. *Clin Gastroenterol Hepatol* 2:78, 2004.
11. Avgerinos A, Armonis A, Manolakpoulos S, et al: Endoscopic sclerotherapy versus variceal ligation in the long-term management of patients with cirrhosis after variceal bleeding: a prospective randomized study. *J Hepatol* 26:1034, 1997.
12. Banares R, Casado M, Rodriquez-Laiz JM, et al: Urgent transjugular intrahepatic portosystemic shunt for control of acute variceal bleeding. *Am J Gastroenterol* 93:75, 1998.
13. Lewis JJ, Basson MD, Modlin IM: Surgical therapy of acute esophageal variceal hemorrhage. *Dig Dis Sci* 10[Suppl 1]:46, 1992.
14. Mathur SK, Shah SR, Soonawala ZF, et al: Transabdominal extensive oesophagastric devascularization with gastro-oesophageal stapling in the management of acute variceal bleeding. *Br J Surg* 84:413, 1997.
15. Kitamoto M, Imamura M, Kamada K et al: Balloon-occluded retrograde transvenous obliteration of gastric fundal varices with hemorrhage. *AJR Am J Roentgenol* 178:1167, 2002.
16. Shiba M, Higuchi K, Nakamura K, et al: Efficacy and safety of balloon-occluded endoscopic injection sclerotherapy as a prophylactic treatment for high-risk gastric fundal varices: a prospective, randomized, comparative clinical trial. *Gastrointest Endosc* 56:522, 2002.
17. Burnett DA, Rikkers LF: Nonoperative emergency treatment of variceal hemorrhage. *Surg Clin North Am* 70:291, 1990.
18. McCormick PA, Burroughs AK, McIntyre N: How to insert a Sengstaken-Blakemore tube. *Br J Hosp Med* 43:274, 1990.
19. Minocha A, Richards RJ: Sengstaken-Blakemore tube for control of massive bleeding from gastric varices in hiatal hernia. *J Clin Gastroenterol* 14:36, 1992.
20. Pasquale MD, Cerra FB: Sengstaken-Blakemore tube placement. *Crit Care Clin* 8:743, 1992.
21. Cello JP, Crass RA, Grendell JH, et al: Management of the patient with hemorrhaging esophageal varices. *JAMA* 256:1480, 1986.
22. Papatheodoridis GV, Patch D, Webster JM, et al: Infection and hemostasis in decompensated cirrhosis: a prospective study using thromboelastography. *Hepatology* 29:1085, 1999.
23. Pohl J, Pollmann K, Sauer P, et al: Antibiotic prophylaxis after variceal hemorrhage reduces incidence of early rebleeding. *Hepatogastroenterology* 51(56):541, 2004.
24. Shaheen NJ, Stuart E, Schmitz S, et al: Pantoprazole reduces the size of postbanding ulcers after variceal band ligation: a randomized control trial. *Hepatology* 41:588, 2005.
25. Teres J, Cecilia A, Bordas JM, et al: Esophageal tamponade for bleeding varices: controlled trial between the Sengstaken-Blakemore tube and the Linton-Nachlas tube. *Gastroenterology* 75:566, 1978.
26. Panes J, Teres J, Bosch J, et al: Efficacy of balloon tamponade in treatment of bleeding gastric and esophageal varices: results in 151 consecutive episodes. *Dig Dis Sci* 33:454, 1998.
27. Panacek EA: Balloon tamponade of esophageal varices, in Roberts JR, Hedges JR (eds): *Clinical Procedures in Emergency Medicine.* 4th ed. Philadelphia, Saunders, 2004; p 817.
28. Boyce HW: Modification of the Sengstaken-Blackmore balloon tube. *Nord Hyg Tidskr* 267:195, 1962.
29. Hunt PS, Korman MG, Hansky J, et al: An 8-year prospective experience with balloon tamponade in emergency control of bleeding esophageal varices. *Dig Dis Sci* 27:413, 1982.
30. Lee H, Hawker FH, Selby W, et al: Intensive care treatment of patients with bleeding esophageal varices: results, predictors of mortality, and predictors of the adult respiratory distress syndrome. *Crit Care Med* 20:1555, 1992.

Lena M. Napolitano

CHAPTER **16**

Endoscopic Placement of Feeding Tubes

INDICATIONS FOR ENTERAL FEEDING

Nutritional support is an essential component of intensive care medicine. It has become increasingly evident that nutritional support administered via the enteral route is far superior to total parenteral nutrition [1–10]. The Canadian Clinical Practice Guidelines for Nutrition Support in Critically Ill Adults [1], the European Society for Clinical Nutrition and Metabolism (ESPEN) Guidelines on Enteral Nutrition for Intensive Care [2], and the Practice Management Guidelines for Nutritional Support of the Trauma Patient [3] all strongly recommend that enteral nutrition be used in preference to parenteral nutrition. An evidence-based consensus statement on the management of critically ill patients with severe acute pancreatitis also recommended that enteral nutrition be used in preference to parenteral nutrition [11]. A more recent systematic review also concluded that patients with severe acute pancreatitis should begin enteral nutrition early because such therapy modulates the stress response, promotes more rapid resolution of the disease process, and results in better outcome [12].

Although there are absolute or relative contraindications to enteral feeding in selected cases, most critically ill patients can receive some or all of their nutritional requirements via the gastrointestinal tract. Even when some component of nutritional support must be provided intravenously, feeding via the gut is desirable.

Provision of nutrition through the enteral route aids in prevention of gastrointestinal mucosal atrophy, thereby maintaining the integrity of the gastrointestinal mucosal barrier. Derangements in the barrier function of the gastrointestinal tract may permit the systemic absorption of gut-derived microbes and microbial products (bacterial translocation), which has been implicated as important in the pathophysiology of syndromes of sepsis and multiple organ system failure [13–15]. Other advantages of enteral nutrition are preservation of immunologic gut function and normal gut flora, improved use of nutrients, and reduced cost. Some studies suggest that clinical outcome is improved and infectious complications are decreased in patients who receive enteral nutrition compared with parenteral nutrition [16–18]. Additional clinical studies suggest that immune-enhancing enteral diets (immunonutrition) containing specialty nutrients (e.g., arginine, glutamine, nucleotides, and omega-3 fatty acids) may also reduce septic complications [19–23] but are not associated with an overall mortality advantage.

Several developments, including new techniques for placement of feeding tubes, availability of smaller caliber, minimally reactive tubes, and an increasing range of enteral formulas, have expanded the ability to provide enteral nutritional support to critically ill patients. Enteral feeding at a site proximal to the pylorus may be absolutely or relatively contraindicated in patients with increased risk of pulmonary aspiration, but feeding more distally (particularly distal to the ligament of Treitz) decreases the likelihood of aspiration. Other relative or absolute contraindications to enteral feeding include fistulas, intestinal obstruction, upper gastrointestinal hemorrhage, and severe inflammatory bowel disease. Enteral feeding is not recommended in patients with severe malabsorption or early in the course of severe short-gut syndrome.

ACCESS TO THE GASTROINTESTINAL TRACT

After deciding to provide enteral nutrition, the clinician must decide whether to deliver the formula into the stomach, duodenum, or jejunum, and determine the optimal method for accessing the site, based on the function of the patient's gastrointestinal tract, duration of enteral nutritional support required, and risk of pulmonary aspiration. Gastric feeding provides the most normal route for enteral nutrition, but it is commonly poorly tolerated in the critically ill patient because of gastric dysmotility with delayed emptying [24]. Enteral nutrition infusion into the duodenum or jejunum may decrease the incidence of aspiration because of the protection afforded by a competent pyloric sphincter; however, the risk of aspiration is not completely eliminated by feeding distal to the pylorus [25–27]. Infusion into the jejunum is associated with the lowest risk of pulmonary aspiration. An advantage of this site of administration is that enteral feeding can be initiated early in the postoperative period, because postoperative ileus primarily affects the colon and stomach and only rarely involves the small intestine. However, the early use of postpyloric feeding instead of gastric feeding in critically ill adult patients with no evidence of impaired gastric emptying was not associated with significant clinical benefits [28].

TECHNIQUES

Enteral feeding tubes can be placed via the transnasal, transoral, or percutaneous transgastric or transjejunal routes. If these procedures are contraindicated or unsuccessful, the tube may be placed by endoscopy, using endoscopic and laparoscopic technique, or surgically via a laparotomy [29,30].

NASOENTERIC ROUTE

Nasoenteric tubes are the most commonly used means of providing enteral nutritional support in critically ill patients. This route is preferred for short-term to intermediate-term enteral support when eventual resumption of oral feeding is anticipated. It is possible to infuse enteral formulas into the stomach using a conventional 16 or 18 French (Fr) polyvinyl chloride nasogastric tube, but patients are usually much more comfortable if a small-diameter silicone or polyurethane feeding tube is used. Nasoenteric tubes vary in luminal diameter (6 to 14 Fr) and length, depending on the desired location of the distal orifice: Stomach, 30 to 36 inches; duodenum, 43 inches; jejunum, at least 48 inches. Some tubes have tungsten-weighted tips designed to facilitate passage into the duodenum via normal peristalsis; others have a stylet. Most are radiopaque. Newer tubes permit gastric decompression while delivering formula into the jejunum.

Nasoenteric feeding tubes should be placed with the patient in a semi-Fowler's or sitting position. The tip of the tube should be lubricated, placed in the patient's nose, and advanced to the posterior pharynx. If the patient is alert and can follow instructions, the patient should be permitted to sip water as the tube is slowly advanced into the stomach. To avoid unintentional airway placement and serious complications, position of the tube should be ascertained after it has been inserted to 30 cm. Acceptable means of documenting intraesophageal location of the tube include a chest radiograph or lack of CO_2 detection through the lumen of the tube by capnography or colorimetry. If the tube is in the airway, CO_2 will be detected and the tube must be removed. Proper final placement of the tube in the stomach must be confirmed by chest or upper abdominal radiograph before tube feeding is begun. The following methods to assess final tube placement are unreliable and do not assess tube misdirection into the lower respiratory tract: Auscultation over the left upper quadrant with air insufflation through the tube, assessment of pH with gastric content aspiration, and easy passage of the tube to its full length with the absence of gagging and coughing [31,32]. The tube should be securely taped to the nose, forehead, or cheek without tension.

Delayed gastric emptying has been confirmed in critically ill patients and may contribute to gastric feeding intolerance. One study randomized 80 critically ill patients to gastric feeding with erythromycin (200 mg intravenously [IV] every 8 hours as a prokinetic agent) or through a transpyloric feeding tube, and identified that the two were equivalent in achieving goal caloric requirements [33]. Spontaneous transpyloric passage of enteral feeding tubes in critically ill patients is commonly unsuccessful secondary to the preponderance of gastric atony. The addition of a tungsten weight to the end of enteral feeding tubes and the development of wire or metal stylets in enteral feeding tubes are aimed at improving the success rate for spontaneous transpyloric passage. Once the tube is documented to be in the stomach, various bedside techniques, including air insufflation, pH-assisted, magnet-guided [34], and spontaneous passage with or without motility agents may help to facilitate transpyloric feeding tube passage.

Intravenous metoclopramide and erythromycin have been recommended as prokinetic agents. But a Cochrane Database Systematic review concluded that doses of 10 or 20 mg of intravenous metoclopramide were equally ineffective in facilitating transpyloric feeding tube placement [35]. No matter which techniques are used to facilitate transpyloric passage of enteral feeding tubes, these tubes must be inserted by skilled practitioners using defined techniques [36,37].

If the tube does not pass into the duodenum on the first attempt, placement can be attempted under endoscopic assistance or fluoroscopic guidance. Endoscopic placement of nasoenteral feeding tubes is easily accomplished in the critically ill patient and can be performed at the bedside using portable equipment [38–42]. Transnasal or transoral endoscopy can be used for placement of nasoenteral feeding tubes in critically ill patients [42]. The patient is sedated appropriately (see Chapter 20), and topical anesthetic is applied to the posterior pharynx with lidocaine or benzocaine spray. A nasoenteric feeding tube 43 to 48 inches long with an inner wire stylet is passed transnasally into the stomach. The endoscope is inserted and advanced through the esophagus into the gastric lumen. An endoscopy forceps is passed through the biopsy channel of the endoscope and used to grasp the tip of the enteral feeding tube. The endoscope, along with the enteral feeding tube, is advanced distally into the duodenum as far as possible (Fig. 16-1).

The endoscopy forceps and feeding tube remain in position in the distal duodenum as the endoscope is withdrawn back into the gastric lumen. The endoscopy forceps are opened, the feeding tube released, and the endoscopy forceps withdrawn carefully back into the stomach. On first pass, the feeding tube is usually lodged in the second portion of the duodenum. The portion of the feeding tube that is redundant in the stomach is advanced slowly into the duodenum using the endoscopy forceps to achieve a final position distal to the ligament of Treitz (Fig. 16-2). An abdominal radiograph is obtained at the completion of the procedure to document the final position of the nasoenteral feeding tube. Endoscopic placement of postpyloric enteral feeding tubes is highly successful, eliminates the risk of transporting the patient to the radiology department for fluoroscopic placement, and allows prompt achievement of nutritional goals because enteral feeding can be initiated immediately after the procedure.

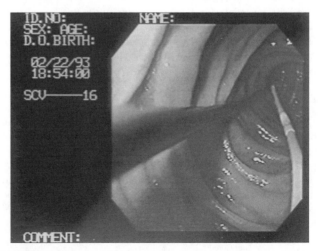

FIGURE 16-1. Endoscopic placement of nasoenteral feeding tube. Endoscopy forceps and gastroscope advance the feeding tube in the duodenum.

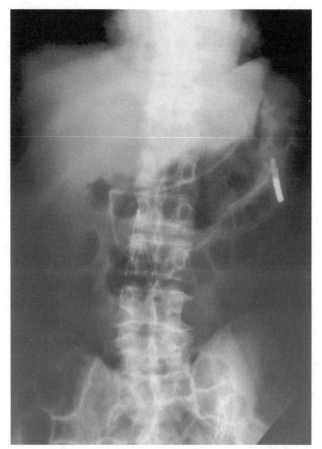

FIGURE 16-2. Abdominal radiograph documenting the optimal position of an endoscopically placed nasoenteral feeding tube, past the ligament of Treitz.

The recent development of ultrathin endoscopes (outer diameter 5.1 to 5.9 mm vs. 9.8 mm in standard gastroscope) has enabled nasoenteric feeding tube placement via transnasal endoscopy using an over-the-wire technique. A recent study documented a 90% success rate with endoscopic procedure duration of approximately 13 minutes, shorter than fluoroscopic procedure duration, and without the need for additional sedation [43]. Unsedated transnasal ultrathin endoscopy can also be used for feeding tube or percutaneous endoscopic gastrostomy (PEG) placement in patients who are unable to undergo transoral endoscopy, i.e. those that have partial or complete occlusion of the mouth [44].

PERCUTANEOUS ROUTE

Percutaneous endoscopic gastrostomy tube placement, introduced by Ponsky et al. [45] in 1990, has become the procedure of choice for patients requiring prolonged enteral nutritional support. The PEG tubes range in size from 20 to 28 Fr. PEG rapidly replaced open gastrostomy as the method of choice for enteral nutrition. Unlike surgical gastrostomy, PEG does not require general anesthesia and laparotomy and eliminates the discomfort associated with chronic nasoenteric tubes. This procedure can be considered in patients who have normal gastric emptying and low risk for pulmonary aspiration, and can be performed in the operating room, an endoscopy unit, or at the bedside in the intensive care unit with portable endoscopy equipment.

PEG should not be performed in patients with near or total obstruction of the pharynx or esophagus, in the presence of coagulopathy, or when transillumination is inadequate. Relative contraindications are ascites, gastric cancer, and gastric ulcer. Previous abdominal surgery is not a contraindication. The original method for PEG was the pull technique; more recent modifications are the push and introducer techniques.

Pull Technique

The pull technique is performed with the patient in the supine position. The abdomen is prepared and draped. The posterior pharynx is anesthetized with a topical spray or solution (e.g., benzocaine spray or viscous lidocaine), and IV sedation (e.g., 1 to 2 mg of midazolam) (see Chapter 20) is administered. A prophylactic antibiotic, usually a first-generation cephalosporin, is administered before the procedure. The fiberoptic gastroscope is inserted into the stomach, which is then insufflated with air. The lights are dimmed, and the assistant applies digital pressure to the anterior abdominal wall in the left subcostal area approximately 2 cm below the costal margin, looking for the brightest transillumination (light reflex). The endoscopist should be able to clearly identify the indentation in the stomach created by the assistant's digital pressure on the anterior abdominal wall (digital reflex); otherwise, another site should be chosen.

When the correct spot has been identified, the assistant anesthetizes the anterior abdominal wall. The endoscopist then introduces a polypectomy snare through the endoscope. A small incision is made in the skin, and the assistant introduces a large-bore catheter-needle stylet assembly into the stomach and through the snare. The snare is then tightened securely around the catheter. The inner stylet is removed, and a looped insertion wire is introduced through the catheter and into the stomach. The cannula is slowly withdrawn so the snare grasps the wire. The gastroscope is then pulled out of the patient's mouth with the wire firmly grasped by the snare. The end of the transgastric wire exiting the patient's mouth is then tied to a prepared gastrostomy tube. The assistant pulls on the end of the wire exiting from the abdominal wall while the endoscopist guides the lubricated gastrostomy tube into the posterior pharynx and the esophagus. With continued traction, the gastrostomy tube is pulled into the stomach so that it exits on the anterior abdominal wall. The gastroscope is reinserted into the stomach to confirm adequate placement of the gastrostomy tube against the gastric mucosa and to document that no bleeding has occurred. The intraluminal portion of the tube should contact the mucosa, but excessive tension on the tube should be avoided because this can lead to ischemic necrosis of the gastric wall. The tube is secured to the abdominal wall using sutures. Feedings may be initiated immediately after the procedure or 24 hours later.

Push Technique

The push technique method is similar to that of the pull technique. The gastroscope is inserted and a point on the anterior abdominal wall localized, as for the pull technique. Rather than introducing a looped insertion wire, however, a straight guidewire is snared and brought out through the patient's mouth by withdrawing the endoscope and snare together. A commercially developed gastrostomy tube (Sachs-Vine) with a tapered end is then passed in an aboral direction over the wire, which is held taut. The tube is grasped and pulled out the rest of the way. The gastroscope is reinserted to check the position and tension on the tube.

Introducer Technique

The introducer technique method uses a peel-away introducer technique originally developed for the placement of cardiac pacemakers and central venous catheters. The gastroscope is inserted into the stomach, and an appropriate position for placement of the tube is identified. After infiltration of the skin with local anesthetic, a 16-gauge or 18-gauge needle is introduced into the stomach. A J-tipped guidewire is inserted through the needle into the stomach and the needle is withdrawn. Using a twisting motion, a 16 Fr introducer with a peel-away sheath is passed over the guidewire into the gastric lumen [46,47]. The guidewire and introducer are removed, leaving in place the sheath that allows placement of a 14 Fr Foley catheter. The sheath is peeled away after the balloon is inflated with 10 mL of normal saline.

Percutaneous Endoscopic Gastrostomy/Jejunostomy

If postpyloric feeding is desired (especially in patients at high risk for pulmonary aspiration), a PEG/jejunostomy may be performed. The tube allows simultaneous gastric decompression and duodenal/jejunal enteral feeding [48]. A second, smaller feeding tube can be attached and passed through the gastrostomy tube and advanced endoscopically into the duodenum or jejunum. When the PEG is in position, a guidewire is passed through it and grasped using endoscopy forceps. The guidewire and endoscope are passed into the duodenum as distally as possible. The jejunal tube is then passed over the guidewire through the PEG into the distal duodenum and advanced into the jejunum, and the endoscope is withdrawn. An alternative method is to grasp a suture at the tip of the feeding tube or the distal tip of the tube itself and pass the tube into the duodenum using forceps advanced through the biopsy channel of the endoscope. This obviates the need to pass the gastroscope into the duodenum, which may result in dislodgment of the tube when the endoscope is withdrawn.

Direct Percutaneous Endoscopic Jejunostomy

Jejunostomy tubes can be placed endoscopically by means of a PEG with jejunal extension (PEG-J) or by direct percutaneous jejunostomy (PEJ) [49,50]. Because the size of the jejunal extension of the PEG-J tube is significantly smaller than the size of the direct PEJ, some have suggested that the PEJ provides more stable jejunal access for those who require long-term jejunal feeding. Unfortunately, a low success rate (68%) and a high adverse event rate (22.5%) has been documented in the largest series to date [51].

FLUOROSCOPIC TECHNIQUE

Percutaneous gastrostomy and gastrojejunostomy can also be performed using fluoroscopy [52,53]. The stomach is insufflated with air using a nasogastric tube or a skinny needle if the patient is obstructed proximally. Once the stomach is distended and position is checked again with fluoroscopy, the stomach is punctured with an 18-gauge needle. A heavy-duty wire is passed and the tract is dilated to 7 Fr. A gastrostomy tube may then be inserted into the stomach. An angiographic catheter is introduced and manipulated through the pylorus. The percutaneous tract is then further dilated, and the gastrojejunostomy tube is advanced as far as possible.

COMPLICATIONS

The most common complication after percutaneous placement of enteral feeding tubes is infection, usually involving the cutaneous exit site and surrounding tissue [54]. Gastrointestinal hemorrhage has been reported but is usually due to excessive tension on the tube, leading to necrosis of the stomach wall. Gastrocolic fistulas, which develop if the colon is interposed between the anterior abdominal wall and stomach when the needle is introduced, have been reported. Adequate transillumination aids in avoiding this complication. Separation of the stomach from the anterior abdominal wall can occur, resulting in peritonitis when enteral feeding is initiated. In most instances, this complication is caused by excessive tension on the gastrostomy tube. Another potential complication is pneumoperitoneum, secondary to air escaping after puncture of the stomach during the procedure, and is usually clinically insignificant. If the patient develops fever and abdominal tenderness, a gastrografin study should be obtained to exclude the presence of a leak.

All percutaneous gastrostomy and jejunostomy procedures described here have been established as safe and effective. The method is selected based on the endoscopist's experience and training and the patient's nutritional needs.

SURGICAL PROCEDURES

Since the advent of PEG, surgical placement of enteral feeding tubes is usually performed as a concomitant procedure as the last phase of a laparotomy performed for another indication. Occasionally, an operation solely for tube placement is performed in patients requiring permanent tube feedings when a percutaneous approach is contraindicated or unsuccessful. In these cases, the laparoscopic approach to enteral access should be considered [55]. Laparoscopic gastrostomy was introduced in 2000, 10 years after the PEG. Patients who are not candidates for PEG, due to head and neck cancer, esophageal obstruction, large hiatal hernia, gastric volvulus, or overlying intestine or liver, should be considered for laparoscopic gastrostomy or jejunostomy.

GASTROSTOMY

Gastrostomy is a simple procedure when performed as part of another intraabdominal operation. It should be considered when prolonged enteral nutritional support is anticipated after surgery.

Complications are quite common after surgical gastrostomy. This may reflect the poor nutritional status and associated medical problems in many patients who undergo this procedure. Potential complications include wound infection, dehiscence, gastrostomy disruption, internal or external leakage, gastric hemorrhage, and tube migration.

NEEDLE-CATHETER JEJUNOSTOMY

The needle-catheter jejunostomy procedure consists of the insertion of a small (5 Fr) polyethylene catheter into the small intestine at the time of laparotomy for another indication. Kits containing the necessary equipment for the procedure are available from commercial suppliers. A needle is used to create a submucosal tunnel from the serosa to the mucosa on the antimesenteric border of the jejunum. A catheter is inserted through the needle, and then the needle is removed. The catheter is brought out through the anterior abdominal wall, and the limb of jejunum is secured to the anterior abdominal wall with sutures. The tube can be used for feeding immediately after the operation. The potential complications are similar to those associated with gastrostomy, but patients may have a higher incidence of diarrhea. Occlusion of the needle-catheter jejunostomy is common because of its small luminal diameter, and elemental nutritional formulas are preferentially used.

TRANSGASTRIC JEJUNOSTOMY

Critically ill patients who undergo laparotomy commonly require gastric decompression and a surgically placed tube for enteral nutritional support. Routine placement of separate gastrostomy and jejunostomy tubes is common in this patient population and achieves the objective of chronic gastric decompression and early initiation of enteral nutritional support through the jejunostomy. Technical advances in surgically placed enteral feeding tubes led to the development of transgastric jejunostomy [56] and duodenostomy tubes, which allow simultaneous decompression of the stomach and distal feeding into the duodenum or jejunum. The advantage of these tubes is that only one enterotomy into the stomach is needed, eliminating the possible complications associated with open jejunostomy tube placement. In addition, only one tube is necessary for gastric decompression and jejunal feeding, eliminating the potential complications of two separate tubes for this purpose. The transgastric jejunostomy tube is placed surgically in the same manner as a gastrostomy tube, and the distal portion of the tube is advanced manually through the pylorus into the duodenum, with its final tip resting as far distally as possible in the duodenum or jejunum (Fig. 16-3). The transgastric jejunostomy tube is preferred to transgastric duodenostomy tubes because it is associated with less reflux of feedings into the stomach and a decreased risk of aspiration pneumonia. Surgical placement of transgastric jejunostomy tubes at the time of laparotomy is rec-

ommended for patients who will likely require prolonged gastric decompression and enteral feeding.

DELIVERING THE TUBE-FEEDING FORMULA

The enteral formula can be delivered by intermittent bolus feeding, gravity infusion, or continuous pump infusion.

In the intermittent bolus method, the patient receives 300 to 400 mL of formula every 4 to 6 hours. The bolus is usually delivered with the aid of a catheter-tipped, large-volume (60-mL) syringe. The main advantage of bolus feeding is simplicity. This approach is often used for patients requiring prolonged supplemental enteral nutritional support after discharge from the hospital. Bolus feeding can be associated with serious side effects, however. Bolus enteral feeding into the stomach can cause gastric distention, nausea, cramping, and aspiration. The intermittent bolus method should not be used when feeding into the duodenum or jejunum because boluses of formula can cause distention, cramping, and diarrhea.

Gravity-infusion systems allow the formula to drip continuously during 16 to 24 hours or intermittently during 20 to 30 minutes, 4 to 6 times per day. This method requires constant monitoring because the flow rate can be extremely irregular. The main advantages of this approach are simplicity, low cost, and close simulation of a normal feeding pattern.

Continuous pump infusion is the preferred method for the delivery of enteral nutrition in the critically ill patient. A peristaltic pump can be used to provide a continuous infusion of formula at a precisely controlled flow rate, which decreases problems with distention and diarrhea. Gastric residuals tend to be smaller with continuous pump-fed infusions, and the risk of aspiration may be decreased. In adult burn and trauma patients, continuous feedings are associated with less stool frequency and shorter time to achieve nutritional goals [57,58].

MEDICATIONS

When medications are administered via an enteric feeding tube, it is important to be certain the drugs are compatible with each other and with the enteral formula. In general, medications should be delivered separately rather than as a combined bolus. For medications that are better absorbed in an empty stomach, tube feedings should be suspended for 30 to 60 minutes before administration.

Medications should be administered in an elixir formulation via enteral feeding tubes whenever possible to prevent occlusion of the tube. Enteral tubes should always be flushed with 20 mL of saline after medications are administered. To use an enteral feeding tube to administer medications dispensed in tablet form, often the pills must be crushed and delivered as slurry mixed with water. This is inappropriate for some medications, however, such as those absorbed sublingually or formulated as a sustained-released tablet or capsule.

COMPLICATIONS

Enteral tube placement is associated with few complications if practitioners adhere to appropriate protocols and pay close attention to the details of the procedures.

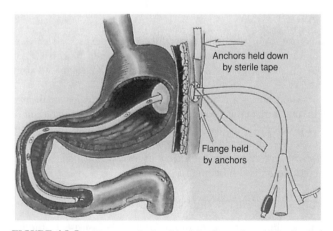

FIGURE 16-3.   Transgastric duodenal feeding tube, which allows simultaneous gastric decompression and duodenal feeding, can be placed percutaneously (with endoscopic or fluoroscopic assistance) or surgically.

NASOPULMONARY INTUBATION

Passage of an enteral feeding tube into the tracheobronchial tree most commonly occurs in patients with diminished cough or gag reflexes due to obtundation, altered mental status, or other causes such as the presence of endotracheal intubation [59]. The presence of a tracheostomy or endotracheal tube does not guarantee proper placement. A chest (or upper abdominal) radiograph should always be obtained before initiating tube feedings with a new tube to ensure that the tube is properly positioned. Endotracheal or transpulmonary placement of a feeding tube can be associated with pneumothorax, hydrothorax, pneumonia, pulmonary hemorrhage, abscess formation, or death. A chest radiograph or a means of detecting CO_2 through the tube after it has been inserted 30 cm should be obtained to prevent inadvertent placement of small-bore feeding tubes into the lungs.

ASPIRATION

Pulmonary aspiration is a serious and potentially fatal complication of enteral nutritional support [60]. The incidence of this complication is variable and depends on the patient population studied. The two most common bedside tests for detecting aspiration in tube-fed patients include adding dye to the formula and observing for its appearance in tracheobronchial secretions, and using glucose oxidase reagent strips to test tracheobronchial secretions for glucose-containing enteral formula [61]. No large prospective clinical trials have validated the use and safety of bedside monitors for aspiration, and their use should be abandoned. Nonrecumbent positioning is an evidence-based method for aspiration prevention that needs to be initiated in all patients receiving enteral nutrition.

Major risk factors for aspiration include obtundation or altered mental status, absence of cough or gag reflexes, delayed gastric emptying, gastroesophageal reflux, and feeding in the supine position. The risk of pulmonary aspiration is minimized when the enteral feeding tube is positioned in the jejunum past the ligament of Treitz.

GASTROINTESTINAL INTOLERANCE

Delayed gastric emptying is sometimes improved by administering the prokinetic agents metoclopramide (10 to 20 mg IV) or erythromycin (200 mg IV). Dumping syndrome (i.e., diarrhea, distention, and abdominal cramping) can limit the use of enteral feeding. Dumping may be caused by delivering a hyperosmotic load into the small intestine.

Diarrhea in critically ill patients should not be attributed to intolerance of enteral feeding until other causes are excluded. Other possible etiologies for diarrhea include medications (e.g., magnesium-containing antacids, quinidine), alterations in gut microflora due to prolonged antibiotic therapy, antibiotic-associated colitis, ischemic colitis, viral or bacterial enteric infection, electrolyte abnormalities, and excessive delivery of bile salts into the colon. Diarrhea can also be a manifestation of intestinal malabsorption because of enzyme deficiencies or villous atrophy [62].

Even if diarrhea is caused by enteral feeding, it can be controlled in nearly 50% of cases by instituting a continuous infusion of formula (if bolus feedings are used), slowing the rate of infusion, changing the formula, adding fiber to the enteral formula, or adding antidiarrheal agents (e.g., tincture of opium).

METABOLIC COMPLICATIONS

Prerenal azotemia and hypernatremia can develop in patients fed with hyperosmolar solutions. The administration of free water, either added to the formula or as separate boluses to replace obligatory losses, can avert this situation. Deficiencies of essential fatty acids and fat-soluble vitamins can develop after prolonged support with enteral solutions that contain minimal amounts of fat. Periodic enteral supplementation with linoleic acid or IV supplementation with emulsified fat can prevent this [63]. The amount of linoleic acid necessary to prevent chemical and clinical fatty acid deficiency has been estimated to be 2.5 to 20.0 g per day.

BACTERIAL CONTAMINATION

Bacterial contamination of enteral solutions [64–66] occurs when commercial packages are opened and mixed with other substances, and more commonly occurs with hospital-formulated and powdered feeds that require preparation compared to commercially prepared, ready-to-feed enteral formulas supplied in cans. The risk of contamination also depends on the duration of feeding. Contaminated formula may also play a significant role in the etiology of diarrhea in patients receiving enteral nutrition.

OCCLUDED FEEDING TUBES

Precipitation of certain proteins when exposed to an acid pH may be an important factor leading to the solidifying of formulas. Most premixed intact protein formulas solidify when acidified to a pH less than 5. To prevent occlusion of feeding tubes, the tube should be flushed with saline before and after checking residuals. Small-caliber nasoenteric feeding tubes should be flushed with 20 mL of saline every 4 to 6 hours to prevent tube occlusion, even when enteral feedings are administered by continuous infusion.

Medications are a frequent cause of clogging. When administering medications enterally, liquid elixirs should be used, if available, because even tiny particles of crushed tablets can occlude the distal orifice of small-caliber feeding tubes. If tablets are used, it is important to crush them to a fine powder and solubilize them in liquid before administration. In addition, tubes should be flushed with saline before and after the administration of any medications.

Several maneuvers are useful for clearing a clogged feeding tube. The tube can be irrigated with warm saline, a carbonated liquid, cranberry juice, or a pancreatic enzyme solution (e.g., Viokase). Commonly, a mixture of lipase, amylase, and protease (Pancrease) dissolved in sodium bicarbonate solution (for enzyme activation) is instilled into the tube with a syringe and the tube clamped for approximately 30 minutes to allow enzymatic degradation of precipitated enteral feedings. The tube is then vigorously flushed with saline. The pancreatic enzyme solution was successful in restoring tube patency in 96% of cases where formula clotting was the likely cause of occlusion and use of cola or water had failed [67,68]. Prevention of tube clogging with flushes and pancreatic enzyme are therefore the methods of choice in maintenance of chronic enteral feeding tubes.

REFERENCES

1. Heyland DK, Dhaliwal R, Drover JW, et al: Canadian clinical practice guidelines for nutrition support in mechanically ventilated, critically ill adult patients. *JPEN J Parenter Enteral Nutr* 27(5):355, 2003.
2. Kreymann KG, Berger MM, Duetz NEP, et al: ESPEN guidelines on enteral nutrition: intensive care. *Clin Nutr* 25(2):210, 2006.
3. Jacobs DG, Jacobs DO, Kudsk KA, et al: Practice management guidelines for nutritional support of the trauma patient. *J Trauma* 57:660, 2004.
4. Gramlich L, Kichian K, Pinlla J, et al: Does enteral nutrition compared to parenteral nutrition result in better outcomes in critically ill adult patients? A systematic review of the literature. *Nutrition* 20(10):843, 2004.
5. Heyland DK, Dhaliwal R, Day A, et al: Validation of the Canadian clinical practice guidelines for nutrition support in mechanically ventilated, critically ill adult patients: results of a prospective observational study. *Crit Care Med* 32(11):2260, 2004.
6. Dhaliwal R, Jurewitch B, Harrietha D, et al: Combination enteral and parenteral nutrition in critically ill patients: harmful or beneficial? A systematic review of the evidence. *Intensive Care Med* 30(8):1666, 2004.
7. Mackenzie SL, Zygun DA, Whitmore BL, et al: Implementation of a nutrition support protocol increases the proportion of mechanically ventilated patients reaching enteral nutrition targets in the adult intensive care unit. *JPEN J Parenter Enteral Nutr* 29(2):74, 2005.
8. Napolitano LM, Bochicchio G: Enteral feeding in the critically ill. *Curr Opin Crit Care* 6:1, 2000.
9. Marik PE, Zaloga GP: Early enteral nutrition in acutely ill patients: a systematic review. *Crit Care Med* 29(12):2264, 2001.
10. Zaloga GP: Parenteral and enteral nutrition in adult inpatients with functioning gastrointestinal tracts: assessment of outcomes. *Lancet* 367(9516):1101, 2006.
11. Nathens AB, Curtis JR, Beale RJ 2004; et al. Management of the critically ill patient with severe acute pancreatitis. *Crit Care Med* 32:2524.
12. McClave SA, Chang WK, et al: Nutrition support in acute pancreatitis: a systematic review of the literature. *JPEN J Parenter Enteral Nutr* 30(2):143, 2006.
13. Napolitano LM, Baker CC: Bacterial translocation: fact or fancy? *Adv Trauma Crit Care* 7: 79, 1992.
14. Alverdy JC, Aoys E, Moss G: Total parenteral nutrition promotes bacterial translocation from the gut. *Surgery* 104:185, 1988.
15. Li J, Kudsk KA, Gocinski B, et al: Effects of parenteral and enteral nutrition on gut-associated lymphoid tissue. *J Trauma* 39:44, 1995.
16. Moore FA, Moore EE, Jones TN, et al: TEN versus TPN following major abdominal trauma—reduced septic morbidity. *J Trauma* 29:916, 1989.
17. Moore FA, Feliciano DV, Andrassy RJ, et al: Early enteral feeding, compared with parenteral, reduces postoperative septic complications: the results of a meta-analysis: *Ann Surg* 216:172, 1992.
18. Kudsk KA, Croce MA, Fabian TC, et al: Enteral vs. parenteral feeding: effects on septic morbidity following blunt and penetrating abdominal trauma. *Ann Surg* 215:503, 1992.
19. Beale RJ, Bryg DJ, Bihari DJ: Immunonutrition in the critically ill: a systematic review of clinical outcome. *Crit Care Med* 27:2799, 1999.
20. Heys SD, Walker LG, Smith I, et al: Enteral nutritional supplementation with key nutrients in patients with critical illness and cancer: a meta-analysis of randomized controlled clinical trials. *Ann Surg* 299:467, 1999.
21. Heyland DK, Novak F, Drover JW, et al: Should immunonutrition become routine in critically ill patients? A systematic review of the evidence. *JAMA* 286:944, 2001.
22. Montejo JC, Zarazaga A, Lopez-Martinez J, et al: Immunonutrition in the intensive care unit: a systematic review and consensus statement. *Clin Nutr* 22(3):221, 2003.
23. Schulman AS, Willcutts KF, Claridge JA, et al: Does the addition of glutamine to enteral feeds affect patient mortality? *Crit Care Med* 33(11):2501, 2005.
24. Ritz MA, Fraser R, Edwards N, et al: Delayed gastric emptying in ventilated critically ill patients: measurement by 13 C-octanoic acid breath test. *Crit Care Med* 29:1744, 2001.
25. McClave SA, DeMeo MT, DeLegge MH, et al: North American Summit on aspiration in the critically ill patient: consensus statement. *JPEN J Parenter Enteral Nutr* 26[6 Suppl]:S80, 2002.
26. Esparza J, Boivin MA, Hartshorne MF, et al: Equal aspiration rates in gastrically and transpylorically fed critically ill patients. *Intensive Care Med* 27:660, 2001.
27. Marik PE, Zaloga GP: Gastric versus post-pyloric feeding: a systematic review. *Crit Care* 7(3):R46, 2003.
28. Ho KM, Dobb GJ, Webb SA: A comparison of early gastric and post-pyloric feeding in critically ill patients: a meta-analysis. *Intensive Care Med* Mar 29, 2006 [Epub ahead of print].
29. Haslam D, Fang J: Enteral access for nutrition in the intensive care unit. *Curr Opin Clin Nutr Metab Care* 9(2):155, 2006.
30. Raakow R, Hintze R, Schmidt S, et al: The laparoscopic Janeway gastrostomy. An alternative technique when percutaneous endoscopic gastrostomy is impractical. *Endoscopy* 33:610, 2001.
31. Burns SM, Carpenter R, Blevins C, et al: Detection of inadvertent airway intubation during gastric tube insertion: capnography versus a colorimetric carbon dioxide detector. *Am J Crit Care* 15:1, 2006.
32. Araujo-Preza CE, Melhado ME, Gutierrez PJ, et al: Use of capnography to verify feeding tube placement. *Crit Care Med* 30:2255, 2002.
33. Boivin MA, Levy H: Gastric feeding with erythromycin is equivalent to transpyloric feeding in the critically ill. *Crit Care Med* 29:1916, 2001.
34. Boivin M, Levy H, Hayes J: A multicenter, prospective study of the placement of transpyloric feeding tubes with assistance of a magnetic device. The Magnet-Guided Enteral Feeding Tube Study Group. *JPEN J Parenter Enteral Nutr* 24:304, 2000.
35. Silva CC, Saconato H, Atallah An: Metoclopramide for migration of nasoenteral rube. *Cochrane Database Syst Rev* 4:CD003353, 2002.
36. Phipps LM, Weber MD, Ginder BR, et al: A randomized controlled trial comparing three different techniques of nasojejunal feeding tube placement in critically ill children. *JPEN J Parenter Enteral Nutr* 29(6):420, 2005.
37. Lee AJ, Eve R, Bennett MJ: Evaluation of a technique for blind placement of post-pyloric feeding tubes in intensive care: application in patients with gastric ileus. *Intensive Care Med* 32(4):553, 2006.
38. Foote JA, Kemmeter PR, Prichard PA, et al: A randomized trial of endoscopic and fluoroscopic placement of postpyloric feeding tubes in critically ill patients. *JPEN J Parenter Enteral Nutr* 28(3):154, 2004.
39. Fang JC, Hilden K, Holubkov R, DiSario JA: Transnasal endoscopy vs. fluoroscopy for the placement of nasoenteric feeding tubes in critically ill patients. *Gastrointest Endosc* 62(5):661, 2005.
40. Dranoff JA, Angood PJ, Topazian M: Transnasal endoscopy for enteral feeding tube placement in critically ill patients. *Am J Gastroenterol* 94(10):2902, 1999.
41. Napolitano LM, Wagel M, Heard SO: Endoscopic placement of nasoenteric feeding tubes in critically ill patients: a reliable alternative. *J Laparoendosc Adv Surg Tech* 8:395, 1998.
42. Kulling D, Bauerfeind P, Fried M: Transnasal versus transoral endoscopy for the placement of nasoenteral feeding tubes in critically ill patients. *Gastrointest Endosc* 52:506, 2000.
43. Fang JC, Hilden K, Holubkov R, DiSario JA: Transnasal endoscopy vs. fluoroscopy for the placement of nasoenteric feeding tubes in critically ill patients. *Gastrointest Endosc* 62(5):661, 2005.
44. Vitale MA, Villotti G, D'Alba L, et al: Unsedated transnasal percutaneous endoscopic gastrostomy placement in selected patients. *Endoscopy* 37(1):48, 2005.
45. Ponsky JL, Gauderer MWL, Stellato TA, et al: Percutaneous approaches to enteral alimentation. *Am J Surg* 149:102, 1985.
46. Dormann AJ, Glosemeyer R, Leistner U, et al: Modified percutaneous endoscopic gastrostomy (PEG) with gastropexy—early experience with a new introducer technique. *Z Gastroenterol* 38:933, 2000.
47. Maetani I, Tada T, Ukita T, et al: PEG with introducer or pull method: A prospective randomized comparison. *Gastrointest Endosc* 57(7):837, 2003.
48. Melvin W, Fernandez JD: Percutaneous endoscopic transgastric jejunostomy: a new approach. *Am Surg* 71(3):216, 2005.
49. Fan AC, Baron TH, Rumalla A, Harewood GC: Comparison of direct percutaneous endoscopic jejunostomy and PEG with jejunal extension. *Gastrointest Endosc* 56(6):890, 2002.
50. Shetzline MA, Suhocki PV, Workman MJ: Direct percutaneous endoscopic jejunostomy with small bowel enteroscopy and fluoroscopy. *Gastrointest Endosc* 53(6):633, 2001.
51. Maple JT, Petersen BT, Baron TH, et al: Direct percutaneous endoscopic jejunostomy: outcomes in 307 consecutive attempts. *Am J Gastroenterol* 100(12):2681, 2005.
52. Ho SG, Marchinkow LO, Legiehn GM, et al: Radiological percutaneous gastrostomy. *Clin Radiol* 56:902, 2001.
53. Giuliano AW, Yoon HC, Lomis NN, et al: Fluoroscopically guided percutaneous placement of large-bore gastrostomy and gastrojejunostomy tubes: review of 109 cases. *J Vasc Interv Radiol* 11:239, 2001.
54. Schurink CA, Tuynman H, Scholten P, et al: Percutaneous endoscopic gastrostomy: complications and suggestion to avoid them. *Eur J Gastroenterol Hepatol* 13:819, 2001.
55. Edelman DS: Laparoendoscopic approaches to enteral access. *Semin Laparosc Surg* 8:195, 2001.
56. Shapiro T, Minard G, Kudsk KA: Transgastric jejunal feeding tubes in critically ill patients. *Nutr Clin Pract* 12:164, 1997.
57. Hiebert J, Brown A, Anderson R, et al: Comparison of continuous vs intermittent tube feedings in adult burn patients. *JPEN J Parenter Enteral Nutr* 5:73, 1981.
58. Steevens EC, Lipscomb AF, Poole GV, et al: Comparison of continuous vs. intermittent nasogastric enteral feeding in trauma patients: perceptions and practice. *Nutr Clin Pract* 17(2):118, 2002.
59. Rassias AJ, Ball PA, Corwin HL: A prospective study of tracheopulmonary complications associated with the placement of narrow-bore enteral feeding tubes. *Crit Care* 2:25, 1998.
60. Mullan H, Roubenoff RA, Roubenoff R: Risk of pulmonary aspiration among patients receiving enteral nutrition support. *JPEN J Parenter Enteral Nutr* 16:160, 1992.
61. Maloney JP, Ryan TA: Detection of aspiration in enterally fed patients: A requiem for bedside monitors of aspiration. *JPEN J Parenter Enteral Nutr* 26[6Suppl]S34; 2002.
62. Ringel AF, Jameson GL, Foster ES: Diarrhea in the intensive care patient. *Crit Care Clin* 11:465, 1995.
63. Dodge JA, Yassa JG: Essential fatty acids deficiency after prolonged treatment with elemental diet. *Lancet* 2:192, 1975.
64. McKinlay J, Wildgoose A, Wood W, et al: The effect of system design on bacterial contamination of enteral tube feeds. *J Hosp Infect* 47:138, 2001.
65. Okuma T, Nakamura M, Totake H, et al: Microbial contamination of enteral feeding formulas and diarrhea. *Nutrition* 16:719, 2000.
66. Lucia Rocha Carvalho M, Beninga Morais T, Ferraz Amaral D, et al: Hazard analysis and critical control point system approach in the evaluation of environmental and procedural sources of contamination of enteral feedings in three hospitals. *JPEN J Parenter Enteral Nutr* 24(50):296, 2000.
67. Williams TA, Leslie GD: A review of the nursing care of enteral feeding tubes in critically ill adults. *Intensive Crit Care Nurs* 21(1):5, 2005.
68. Marcuard SP, Stegall KS: Unclogging feeding tubes with pancreatic enzyme. *JPEN J Parenter Enteral Nutr* 14:198, 1990.

John P. Weaver

CHAPTER **17**

Cerebrospinal Fluid Aspiration

This chapter presents guidelines for safe cerebrospinal fluid (CSF) aspiration for the emergency department or the intensive care physician, and provides a basic understanding of the indications, techniques, and potential complications of these procedures.

Physicians and physician extenders under supervision by a physician routinely and safely perform most CSF aspiration procedures. The necessary equipment and sterile supplies are readily accessible in most acute hospital patient care units. Most CSF aspirations are performed without sedation, at times using local anesthesia alone and, when necessary, sedation may be required for an uncooperative patient or part of the pediatric population [1]. Radiographic imaging is needed in situations in which external anatomic landmarks provide inadequate guidance for safe needle placement or when needle placement using external landmarks alone has proved unsuccessful due to anatomic variations caused by trauma, operative scar, congenital defects, or degenerative changes. Fluoroscopy may be used for lumbar puncture, C1-2 puncture, and myelography. Computed tomography (CT) or magnetic resonance imaging (MRI) may be used for stereotactic placement of ventricular catheters. Clinicians should recognize the need for specialized equipment and training in certain cases.

An implanted reservoir or shunt system should not be accessed without prior consultation with a neurosurgeon, despite the apparent simplicity of the procedure itself. Violating implanted systems carries several risks, including infection, which can result in a lengthy hospitalization, prolonged antibiotic course, and several operative procedures for shunt externalization, hardware removal, and insertion of a new shunt system.

Contraindications to lumbar puncture include skin infection at the entry site, anticoagulation or blood dyscrasias, papilledema in the presence of supratentorial masses, posterior fossa lesions, and known spinal subarachnoid block or spinal cord arteriovenous malformations.

CEREBROSPINAL FLUID ACCESS

DIAGNOSTIC PURPOSES

CSF analysis continues to be a major diagnostic tool in many diseases. The most common indication for CSF sampling is the suspicion of a cerebral nervous system (CNS) infection. CSF is also analyzed for the diagnosis of subarachnoid hemorrhage (SAH), demyelinating diseases, CNS spread of neoplasm, and CNS degenerative conditions. CSF access is necessary for neurodiagnostic procedures such as myelography and cisternography, and studies for device patency (tube studies). CSF pressure recording, particularly opening pressure, is important in the di-

agnosis of normal pressure hydrocephalus, benign intracranial hypertension, and head injury.

The diagnostic tests performed on the aspirated CSF depend on the patient's age, history, and differential diagnosis. A basic profile includes glucose and protein values, a blood cell count, Gram's stain, and aerobic and anaerobic cultures. CSF glucose depends on blood glucose levels and is usually equivalent to two thirds of the serum glucose. It is slightly higher in neonates. Glucose is transported into the CSF via carrier-facilitated diffusion, and changes in spinal fluid glucose concentration lag blood levels by about 2 hours. Increased CSF glucose is nonspecific and usually reflects hyperglycemia. Hypoglycorrhachia can be the result of any inflammatory or neoplastic meningeal disorder and reflects increased glucose use by nervous tissue or leukocytes and inhibited transport mechanisms. Elevated lactate levels reflecting anaerobic glycolysis usually accompany the lower glucose concentrations.

CSF protein content is usually less than 0.5% of that in plasma due to blood-brain barrier exclusion. Albumin constitutes up to 75% of CSF protein, and immunoglobulin G (IgG) is the major component of the gamma-globulin fraction. IgG freely traverses a damaged blood-brain barrier. Although often nonspecific, elevated CSF protein is an indicator of CNS pathology. There is a gradient of total protein content in the spinal CSF column with the highest level normally found in the lumbar subarachnoid space at 20 to 50 mg/dL, followed by the cisterna magna at 15 to 25 mg/dL and the ventricles at 6 to 12 mg/dL. A value exceeding 500 mg/dL is compatible with an intraspinal tumor or spinal compression causing a complete subarachnoid block, meningitis, or bloody CSF [2]. Low protein levels are seen in healthy children younger than 2 years of age, pseudotumor cerebri, acute water intoxication, and leukemic patients.

A normal CSF cell count includes no erythrocytes and a maximum of five leukocytes per milliliter. A greater number of cells are normally found in children (up to 10 per milliliter, mostly lymphocytes). CSF cytology can be helpful in identifying cells to diagnose primary or metastatic CNS tumors and inflammatory disorders [3].

Hemorrhage

A *nontraumatic* SAH in the adult population may be due to a ruptured aneurysm. A paroxysmal severe headache is the classic symptom of aneurysm rupture, but atypical headaches reminiscent of migraine are not uncommon. Leblanc [4] reported that up to 50% of patients with a warning "leak" headache are undiagnosed after evaluation by their physician, and 55% of patients with premonitory warning headaches had normal CT findings but all had a positive finding of SAH on lumbar puncture. Lumbar puncture is indicated with such presenting headache if the head CT is not diagnostic and if the clinical history and presentation are atypical. A lumbar puncture should not be performed without prior CT if the patient has any focal neurologic deficits because the neurologic abnormality might indicate the presence of an intracranial hematoma. Intracranial mass lesions can increase the likelihood of downward transtentorial herniation following a lumbar puncture. A SAH can also cause acute obstructive hydrocephalus by intraventricular extension, thereby causing obstruction to CSF flow or by obstruction of the resorptive mechanisms at the arachnoid granulations. In such a case, the CT scan would demonstrate ventriculomegaly, which is best treated by the placement of a ventricular catheter.

A traumatic lumbar puncture presents a diagnostic dilemma, especially in the context of diagnosing suspected SAH. Differentiating characteristics include a decreasing red blood cell count in tubes collected serially during the procedure, the presence of a fibrinous clot in the sample, and a typical ratio of about 1 leukocyte per 700 red blood cells. Xanthochromia is more indicative of SAH and is quickly evaluated by spinning a fresh CSF sample and comparing the color of the supernatant to that of water, or by the use of a spectrophotometer. Spinal fluid accelerates red blood cell hemolysis, and hemoglobin products are released within 2 hours of the initial hemorrhage creating the xanthochromia. Associated findings, such as a slightly depressed glucose level, increased protein, and an elevated opening pressure, are also more suggestive of the presence of an SAH. Another method to differentiate between blood due to intracranial hemorrhage and that due to a traumatic spinal tap has been demonstrated in neonates [5]. The mean corpuscular volume of erythrocytes in the CSF can be compared with that in peripheral blood. The mean corpuscular volume in CSF will be lower than in venous blood in cases of SAH, but the values are similar if the hemorrhage was a traumatic lumbar puncture.

Infection

CSF evaluation is the single most important aspect of the laboratory diagnosis of meningitis. The analysis usually includes a Gram's stain, blood cell count with white cell differential, protein and glucose levels, and aerobic and anaerobic cultures with antibiotic sensitivities. With suspicion of tuberculosis or fungal meningitis, the fluid is analyzed by acid-fast stain, India ink preparation, cryptococcal antigen, and culture in appropriate media. More extensive cultures may be performed in the immunocompromised patient.

Immunoprecipitation tests to identify bacterial antigens for *Streptococcus pneumoniae*, Streptococcus group B, *Hemophilus influenzae*, and *Neisseria meningitidis* (meningococcus) allow rapid diagnosis and early specific treatment. Polymerase chain reaction testing can be performed on CSF for rapid identification of several viruses, particularly those commonly responsible for CNS infections in patients with acquired immunodeficiency syndrome. Polymerase chain reaction tests exist for herpes, varicella zoster, cytomegalovirus, and Epstein-Barr virus, as well as toxoplasmosis and *Mycobacterium tuberculosis* [6]. If the clinical suspicion is high for meningitis, antibiotic therapy should be initiated without delay following CSF collection [7].

Shunt System Failure

A ventriculoperitoneal shunt is the most commonly encountered system. The hardware varies but commonly consists of a ventricular catheter connected to a reservoir and valve mecha-

nism at the skull and a subcutaneous catheter that passes in the neck and anterior chest wall to the peritoneum. The distal tubing may also have been inserted in the jugular vein, the pleura, or even the urinary bladder. Proximal shunt failure of the ventricular catheter may be due to choroid plexus obstruction or cellular debris from CSF infection. Valve or distal tubing obstruction occurs also from cellular debris, from disconnection, poor CSF absorption, or formation of an intraabdominal pseudocyst.

The clinical presentation of an obstructed shunt is variable; it may be slowly progressive, intermittent, or there may be a rapid decline in mentation progressing into a coma. A CT scan should be performed immediately and compared with previous studies because the ventricular system in a shunted patient is often congenitally or chronically abnormal. Ventriculomegaly is a good indicator of a malfunctioning shunt, but noncompliant ventricles may remain small and not vary significantly in size.

Aspiration from the reservoir or valve system of a shunt can be performed to determine patency and to collect CSF to diagnose an infectious process. However, one should remember that shunt aspiration is an invasive procedure that carries a risk of contaminating the system with skin flora. The resultant shunt infection requires a lengthy hospitalization for shunt externalization, antibiotic treatment, and replacement of all hardware. Therefore, CSF collection by shunt tap should be performed very selectively and after other potential sources of infection have been evaluated. When shunt failure is due to distal obstruction, aspiration of CSF may temper neurologic impairment and even be lifesaving until formal shunt revision can be performed. The determination of the need for a shunt tap, as well as the procedure, is best left to a neurosurgeon.

Normal Pressure Hydrocephalus

Serial lumbar punctures or continuous CSF drainage via a lumbar subarachnoid catheter can be used as provocative diagnostic tests to select patients who would benefit from a shunt for CSF diversion. The results have a positive predictive value if the patient's gait improves. Lumbar CSF access may also be used for infusion tests, measurement of CSF production rate, pressure-volume index, and outflow resistance or absorption. Some studies suggest that these values are also predictive of therapeutic CSF diversion [8–10].

Benign Intracranial Hypertension (Pseudotumor Cerebri)

Benign intracranial hypertension occurs in young persons, often obese young women. Intracranial pressure (ICP) is elevated without focal deficits and in the absence of ventriculomegaly or intracranial mass lesions. Etiologic factors for childhood presentation include chronic middle ear infection, dural sinus thrombosis, head injury, vitamin A overdosage, tetracycline exposure, internal jugular venous thrombosis, and idiopathic causes [11]. Some authors have proposed a broader definition of the "pseudotumor cerebri syndrome" based on the underlying pathophysiologic mechanism of the presumed CSF circulation disorder [12].

Lumbar puncture demonstrates an elevated ICP (up to 40 cm H_2O), and CSF dynamics demonstrate an increase in outflow resistance. Serial daily punctures can be therapeutic, with CSF aspirated until closing pressure is within normal limits (less than 20 cm H_2O). In some cases, this can restore the balance between CSF formation and absorption; other cases require medical therapy such as weight loss, steroids, acetazolamide, diuretics, and glycerol. If all these therapeutic interventions fail, placement of a permanent shunting system may be necessary.

Neoplasms

The subarachnoid space can be infiltrated by various primary or secondary tumors, giving rise to symptoms of meningeal irritation. CSF cytology can determine the presence of neoplastic cells, although their complete identification is not always possible. Systemic neoplasms such as melanoma or breast cancer have a greater propensity to metastasize into the CSF spaces than do primary CNS tumors and may even present primarily as meningeal carcinomatosis. Ependymoma, medulloblastoma or primitive neuroectodermal tumor, germinoma, and high-grade glioma are the most commonly disseminated primary tumors. Hematopoietic cancers such as leukemia and lymphoma also frequently infiltrate the subarachnoid spaces with little or no parenchymal involvement. CSF sampling is useful for an initial diagnostic and screening tool in the neurologically intact patient who harbors a tumor type with high risk of CNS relapse. A generous amount of CSF or multiple samples may be required for diagnosis. Cisternal puncture may enhance the diagnosis if the lumbar CSF is nondiagnostic [13]. Acute leukemias that tend to invade the CNS include acute lymphocytic leukemia, acute nonlymphocytic leukemia, acute myelogenous leukemia, acute myelomonocytic leukemia, and acute undifferentiated leukemia [14]. Individual proliferating T and B lymphocytes can also be detected in the CSF and may aid in the differentiation of an opportunistic infection from a leukemic infiltration [15]. CSF analysis for auto antibodies could play a role in the diagnosis of some paraneoplastic syndromes (e.g., anti-Yo titers in paraneoplastic cerebellar degeneration) [16].

Myelography

Lumbar puncture is the most common means of access for lumbar and cervical myelography because the density of contrast material is higher than CSF and may be directed by gravity to the area of interest. Cervical C1-2 puncture may be the usual access route for cervical myelography but is often reserved for patients in whom a successful lumbar puncture is not possible due to extensive arachnoiditis, epidural tumor, severe spinal stenosis, or CSF block.

Other Neurologic Disorders

There is extensive literature on CSF changes in demyelinating diseases, including multiple sclerosis. Typical lumbar puncture findings are normal ICP, normal glucose levels, mononuclear pleocytosis, and elevated protein levels due to increased endothelial permeability. Immunoelectrophoresis reveals elevated IgG and oligoclonal bands [17]. Antibodies against cardiolipin synthetic lecithin, a lectin protein involved in the structural stabilization of myelin, have been detected in the CSF of patients with multiple sclerosis and may constitute a very sensitive and specific diagnostic test [18].

CSF findings described in other disease states include elevated tau protein and decreased β-amyloid precursor protein in Alzheimer's disease and the presence of anti-GM1 antibodies and cytoalbumin dissociation in Guillain-Barré syndrome.

THERAPEUTIC INTERVENTION

Fistulas

CSF leaks occur for a variety of reasons, including nontraumatic and traumatic etiologies. Orthostatic headaches are a characteristic symptom, and CSF rhinorrhea may be evident. Iatrogenic postoperative CSF leaks may occur following surgery at the skull base as a result of dural or bony defects. CSF fistulas following middle cranial fossa or cerebellopontine angle surgery occur infrequently, and CSF usually leaks through the auditory tube to the nasopharynx. Dural closure in the posterior fossa following suboccipital craniectomy is often difficult and not watertight. A fistula in that area usually results in a pseudomeningocele, which is clinically apparent as subcutaneous swelling at the incision site with potential wound breakdown. Leaks following lumbar surgery are unusual but may occur as a result of recent myelography, dural tear, or inadequate dural closure [19]. In pediatric patients, repair of meningoceles or other spina bifida defects are more likely to present with a CSF leak because of dural or fascial defects.

The most common presentation of a CSF fistula follows trauma. Basilar skull fractures that traverse the ethmoid or frontal sinuses can cause CSF rhinorrhea. Fractures along the long axis of the petrous bone usually involve the middle ear, causing the hemotympanum noted on examination and CSF otorrhea if the tympanic membrane is ruptured. Delayed leaks are not uncommon because the fistula can be occluded with adhesions, hematoma, or herniated brain tissue, which temporarily tamponades the defect.

The diagnosis of a leak is often easily made on clinical examination. At times, the nature of a "drainage fluid" is uncertain and laboratory characterization is necessary. Dipping the fluid for glucose is misleading because nasal secretions are positive for glucose. A chloride level often shows a higher value than in peripheral blood, but identification of β_2-transferrin is the most accurate diagnostic for CSF. This protein is produced by neuraminidase in the brain and is uniquely found in the spinal fluid and perilymph [20].

Postural drainage by patient's head elevation is the primary treatment of CSF leak. Placement of a lumbar drainage catheter or daily lumbar punctures can be useful nonoperative approaches, should conservative therapy fail. The use of a continuous lumbar drainage catheter is somewhat controversial because of the potential for intracranial contamination from the sinuses if the intracranial pressure is lowered. To help prevent such complications, the lumbar drain collection bag should be maintained no lower than the patient's shoulder level and the duration of drainage should not exceed 5 days.

Intracranial Hypertension

Intracranial hypertension can cause significant neurologic morbidity or even death. Access to the intracranial CSF space is useful for diagnosis and treatment [21]. A ventriculostomy is commonly used both as an ICP monitor and as a means to treat intracranial hypertension by CSF drainage. An ICP measuring device should be placed following traumatic brain injury for patients who exhibit a Glasgow Coma Scale score less than 8, a motor score less than 6 (not aphasic), diffuse brain edema, hematoma (epidural, subdural, intraparenchymal), cortical contusions, or absent or compressed basal cisterns on initial CT. ICP monitoring can also be indicated in cerebrovascular diseases, including aneurysmal SAH, spontaneous cerebral hematoma, ischemic and hypoxic cerebral insults, and intraventricular hemorrhage. Obstructive hydrocephalus is another major indication for placement of a ventricular catheter for drainage and monitoring. ICP may be elevated due to cerebral edema that surrounds tumors, intracranial hematomas, ischemic brain, and traumatic contusions, or that occurs postoperatively or following cranial radiation therapy. Diffuse brain swelling also occurs in the setting of inflammatory and infectious disorders such as Reye's syndrome or meningitis, or as a result of hyperthermia, carbon dioxide retention, or intravascular congestion.

Drug Therapy

The CSF can be a route of administration for medications such as chemotherapeutic agents and antibiotics. Treatment of lymphoma and leukemia often involves intrathecal injections of various agents, which may be infused through a lumbar route or an intraventricular injection via an implanted reservoir. Meningeal carcinomatosis is treated by intrathecal chemotherapy (e.g., methotrexate). Serial injections of small amounts are performed in an attempt to minimize neurotoxicity, and the use of a ventricular reservoir may be less traumatic for the patient than multiple lumbar punctures [22]. Treatment of meningitis and ventriculitis may include intrathecal antibiotics in addition to systemic therapy. Careful dosage and administration are recommended, especially if the ventricular route is used, as many antibiotics can cause seizures or an inflammatory ventriculitis when given intrathecally.

TECHNIQUES OF CSF ACCESS

There are several techniques for CSF aspiration. All procedures should be performed using sterile technique, and the skin is prepared with antiseptic washing and draped with sterile towels.

LUMBAR PUNCTURE

Lumbar puncture is a common procedure that is readily performed by the general practitioner, rarely requiring radiologic assistance. It can be performed in any hospital or outpatient setting where commercially prepared lumbar puncture trays are available. In patients with advanced spinal degeneration, extensive previous lumbar surgery or congenital defects, the use of fluoroscopic needle placement may be required. C1-2 punctures are seldom required.

In adults, CSF aspirations are adequately performed under local anesthesia using 1% lidocaine without premedication. In the pediatric population, however, sedation is often required and allows for a smoother procedure. This is also true in the case of anxious, confused, or combative adult patients.

Oral or rectal chloral hydrate is often used in children, and moderate sedation using intravenous midazolam and fentanyl can be highly successful in appropriately monitored adult and children if performed by an experienced individual. The application of a topical anesthetic, such as EMLA cream (2.5% lidocaine and 2.5% prilocaine), preceding injection can also be useful. Conversely, it has been demonstrated in a controlled clinical trial that in the neonatal population, injection of a local anesthetic for lumbar puncture is probably not required and does not reduce perceived stress or discomfort [23].

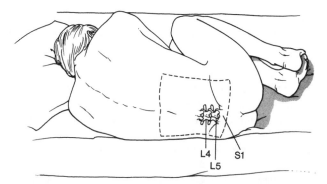

FIGURE 17-1.   Patient in the lateral decubitus position with back at edge of bed and knees, hips, back, and neck flexed. [From Davidson RI: Lumbar puncture, in VanderSalm TJ (ed): *Atlas of Bedside Procedures.* 2nd ed. Boston, Little, Brown, 1988, with permission.]

Figures 17-1 and 17-2 depict some of the steps for lumbar puncture [24]. The patient is placed in the lateral knee-chest position or sitting while leaning forward over a bedside table. The sitting position may be preferred for obese patients in whom adipose tissue can obscure the midline, or in elderly patients with significant lumbar degenerative disease. The local anesthetic is injected subcutaneously using a 25- or 27-gauge needle. A 1.5-inch needle is then inserted through the skin wheal and additional local anesthetic is injected along the midline, thus anesthetizing the interspinous ligaments and muscles. This small anesthetic volume is usually adequate; however, a more extensive field block is accomplished by additional injections on each side of the interspinous space near the lamina [25].

The point of skin entry is midline at the level of the superior iliac crests, which is usually between the spinous processes of L3-4. Lower needle placement at L4-5 or L5-S1 is required in children and neonates to avoid injury to the conus medullaris, which lies more caudal than in adults. The needle is advanced with the stylet or obturator in place to maintain needle patency and prevent iatrogenic intraspinal epidermoid tumors [2]. The

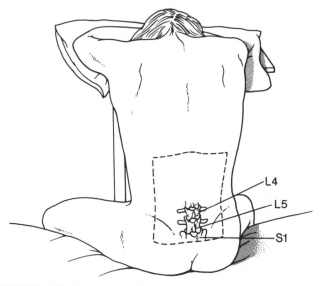

FIGURE 17-2.   Patient sitting on the edge of the bed leaning on bedside stand. [From Davidson RI: Lumbar puncture, in VanderSalm TJ (ed): *Atlas of Bedside Procedures.* 2nd ed. Boston, Little, Brown, 1988, with permission.]

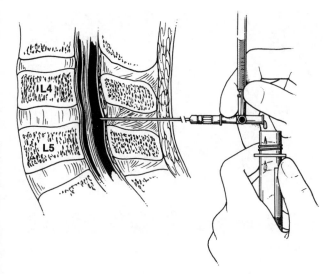

FIGURE 17-3. The spinal needle is advanced to the spinal subarachnoid space and cerebrospinal fluid samples collected after opening pressure is measured. [From Davidson RI: Lumbar puncture, in VanderSalm TJ (ed): *Atlas of Bedside Procedures.* 2nd ed. Boston, Little, Brown, 1988, with permission.]

bevel of the needle should be parallel to the longitudinal fibers of the dura and spinal column. The needle should be oriented rostrally at an angle of about 30 degrees to the skin and virtually aiming toward the umbilicus. When properly oriented, the needle will pass through the following structures before entering the subarachnoid space: skin, superficial fascia, supraspinous ligament, interspinous ligament, ligamentum flavum, epidural space with its fatty areolar tissue and internal vertebral plexus, dura, and arachnoid membrane (Fig. 17-3). The total depth will vary from less than 1 inch in the very young patient to as deep as 4 inches in the obese adult. The kinesthetic sensations of passing through the ligaments into the epidural space followed by dural puncture are quite consistent and recognized with practice. Once intradural, the bevel of the needle is redirected in a cephalad direction in order to improve CSF flow. A needle no smaller than a 22-gauge spinal needle should be used for pressure measurement. The opening pressure is best measured with the patient's legs relaxed and extended partly from the knee-chest position. Pressure measurements may be difficult in children and may be estimated using CSF flow rate [26].

Once CSF is collected, the closing pressure is measured prior to needle withdrawal. It is best to replace the stylet in the needle prior to exiting the subarachnoid space. CSF pressure measurements are not accurate if performed in the sitting position due to the hydrostatic pressure of the CSF column above the entry point or if a significant amount of CSF was lost when the stylet is first withdrawn. If necessary, the pressure could be measured by reclining the patient to the lateral position once entry in the CSF space has been secured. A coaxial needle was found to be helpful in morbidly obese patients [27].

Although a lumbar puncture is typically safe, there are a number of potential complications and risks involved. Hemorrhage is uncommon but can be seen in association with bleeding disorders and anticoagulation therapy. Spinal SAH has been reported in such conditions, resulting in blockage of CSF outflow with subsequent back and radicular pain, sphincter disturbances, and even paraparesis [28]. Spinal subdural hematoma is like-

wise very infrequent, but it is associated with significant morbidity that may require prompt surgical intervention. Infection by introduction of skin flora into the subarachnoid spaces, causing meningitis, is uncommon and preventable if aseptic techniques are used. Risks of infection are increased in serial taps or placement of lumbar catheters for the treatment of CSF fistulas.

Postural headache is the most common complication following lumbar puncture. Its reported frequency varies from 1% to 70% [29]. It is thought to be due to excessive leakage of CSF into the paraspinous spaces, resulting in intracranial hypotension with stretching and expansion of the pain-sensitive intracerebral veins. MRI has demonstrated a reduced CSF volume following lumbar puncture but no significant brain displacement and no correlation with headache [30]. Psychological factors and previous history of headaches seem to strongly influence the patient's risk of and tolerance to headache [31]. A smaller needle size, parallel orientation to the dural fibers, and a paramedian approach are associated with a decreased risk, and stylet reinsertion prior to withdrawal of the spinal needle has also been reported to decrease the risk of headache after lumbar puncture [29].

The choice of needle type has been the subject of literature debate. Several needle tip designs are available, including the traditional Quincke needle with a beveled cutting tip, the Sprotte needle with a pencil point and side hole, and the Whitacre needle, which is similar to the Sprotte but with a smaller side hole [32]. The cost of a Whitacre or Sprotte atraumatic spinal needle is several times that of a Quincke needle. However, the use of an atraumatic needle seems to be adequate for the performance of a diagnostic lumbar puncture and is probably associated with a lower risk of a postdural puncture headache [33].

Postdural puncture headache typically develops within 72 hours and lasts 3 to 5 days. Conservative treatment consists of bed rest, hydration, and analgesics. Nonphenothiazine antiemetics are administered if the headache is associated with nausea. If the symptoms are more severe, methylxanthines (caffeine or theophylline) are prescribed orally or parenterally. These agents are successful in up to 85% of patients [34]. Several other pharmacologic agents are discussed in the literature, but none seems to be as effective as caffeine. If the headache persists or is unaffected, an epidural blood patch is then recommended because it is one of the most effective treatments for this condition [35]. Epidural injection of other agents, such as saline, dextran, or adenocorticotropic hormone, has also been described and may be valuable under certain conditions (e.g., sepsis or acquired immunodeficiency syndrome) [36].

Other parameters controlling needle choice include the purpose of the procedure and whether an injection is to be performed. If a pressure reading is an important part of the procedure, a larger-gauge needle is necessary, especially if an atraumatic tip is to be used. CSF flow rate is also slow in the smaller-size atraumatic needle, and a 20-gauge needle will probably be required for large-volume drainage [33]. Needles as small as 26 or 27 gauge can be used for aspiration or therapeutic infusion. Injection through an atraumatic spinal needle has to be very carefully performed as the needle hole is lateral and not directly at the tip.

An uncommon sequela of lumbar puncture or continuous CSF drainage is hearing loss. Drainage decreases ICP, which is transmitted to the perilymph via the cochlear aqueduct and can cause hearing impairment [37]. The rate of occurrence of this complication is reported to be 0.4% but is probably higher because it goes unrecognized and seems reversible. There are a few documented cases of irreversible hearing loss [38].

Transient sixth-nerve palsy has also been reported, probably due to nerve traction following significant CSF removal. Neurovascular injury can occur uncommonly in the setting of a subarachnoid block due to spinal tumors. In this situation, CSF drainage leads to significant traction and spinal coning with subsequent neurologic impairment [39,40].

LATERAL CERVICAL (C1-2) PUNCTURE

The C1-2 or lateral cervical puncture was originally developed for percutaneous cordotomy. It may be used for myelography or aspiration of CSF if the lumbar route is inaccessible. It is most safely performed with fluoroscopic guidance, although that is not always necessary. The puncture is performed with the patient supine, the head and neck flexed, and the lateral neck draped. The skin entry point is 1 cm caudal and 1 cm dorsal to the tip of the mastoid process. The site is infiltrated with a local anesthetic, and the spinal needle is introduced and directed toward the junction of the middle and posterior thirds of the bony canal to avoid an anomalous vertebral or posterior inferior cerebellar artery that may lie in the anterior half of the canal. The stylet should be removed frequently to check for CSF egress. When the procedure is performed under fluoroscopy, the needle is seen to be perpendicular to the neck and just under the posterior ring of C1. The same sensation is recognized when piercing the dura as in a lumbar puncture, and the bevel is then directed cephalad in a similar fashion. Complications of the lateral cervical puncture include injury to the spinal cord or the vertebral artery and irritation of a nerve root, causing local pain and headache.

CISTERNAL PUNCTURE

A cisternal puncture provides CSF access via the cisterna magna when other routes are not possible. A preoperative lateral skull radiograph is performed to ensure normal anatomy. The patient is positioned sitting with the head slightly flexed. The hair is shaved in the occipital region and the area prepared, draped, and infiltrated with lidocaine. The entry point is in the midline between the external occipital protuberance in the upper margin of the spinous process of C2 or via an imaginary line through both external auditory meati [5]. The spinal needle is directed through a slightly cephalad course and usually strikes the occipital bone. It is then redirected more caudally in a stepwise fashion until it passes through the atlanto-occipital membrane and dura, producing a "popping" sensation. The cisterna magna usually lies 4 to 6 cm deep to the skin; the needle should not be introduced beyond 7 to 7.5 cm from the skin, to prevent injury to the medulla or the vertebral arteries. The procedure can be performed relatively safely in a cooperative patient as the cisterna magna is a large CSF space; however, it is rarely practiced due to the greater potential morbidity.

ASPIRATION OF RESERVOIRS AND SHUNTS

In-line subcutaneous reservoirs in ventriculoatrial or ventriculoperitoneal shunting systems are located proximal to the unidirectional valve and can be accessed percutaneously. The reservoirs are usually button-sized, measuring approximately 7 to

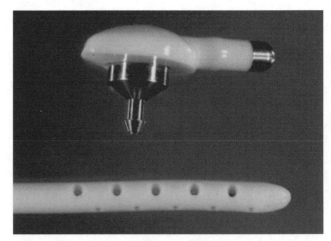

FIGURE 17-4.   Close-up view of ventricular reservoir in the calvarial burr hole, the funneled base connected directly to the proximal end of the ventricular catheter. The distal perforated end is shown.

10 mm in diameter and 2 mm in height. They can be located in the burr hole directly connected to the ventricular catheter (Fig. 17-4) or as an integral part of the valve system (Fig. 17-5). Indications for reservoir taps have been previously discussed.

The procedure can be performed in any hospital or outpatient setting. Gloves, mask, antiseptic solution, razor, sterile drapes, 23- or 25-gauge needle (short hub or butterfly), tuberculin syringe, and sterile collection tubes are readied. The patient can be in any comfortable position that allows access to the reservoir. Sedation may be required for toddlers but is otherwise unnecessary. Reference to a skull radiograph may be helpful in localization. The reservoir is palpated, overlying hair is shaved, and the skin is cleansed. Local anesthesia is usually not required. The use of topical anesthetic creams is occasionally considered, but this does require shaving of a larger area of the scalp. The needle is inserted perpendicular to the skin and into the reservoir, to a total depth of 2 to 5 mm. A manometer is then connected to the needle or butterfly tubing for pressure measurement. Drug injection or CSF collection is performed.

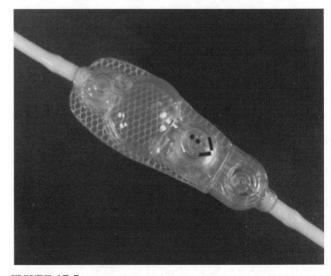

FIGURE 17-5.   A domed reservoir in series in one type of shunt valve. The large, clear-domed area for puncture lies immediately proximal to the one-way valve.

A "dry tap" usually indicates faulty placement or catheter obstruction. Occasionally, an old reservoir may have retracted into the burr hole and not be palpable or may be too calcified for needle penetration. Older shunting systems may not even have a reservoir. Risks and complications of shunt aspiration include improper insertion, contamination with skin flora, introduction of blood in the shunt system, and choroid plexus hemorrhage due to vigorous aspiration. Although the aspiration technique is quite simple, it is always best to consult a neurosurgeon.

Lumboperitoneal Shunt

Lumboperitoneal shunts are placed via percutaneous insertion of a lumbar subarachnoid catheter or through a small skin incision. They are tunneled subcutaneously around the patient's flank to the abdomen, where the distal catheter enters the peritoneal cavity through a separate abdominal incision. A reservoir or valve or both may be used and are located on the lateral aspect of the flank. Careful palpation between the two incisions usually reveals the tubing path and reservoir placement in the nonobese patient. Aspiration is simple after the patient is placed in lateral decubitus position. A pillow under the dependent flank may be of assistance. The same technique as described for a ventricular shunt is then performed. Fluid aspiration should be particularly gentle as an additional risk of this procedure is nerve root irritation.

Ventricular Reservoirs

Ventricular reservoirs are inserted as part of a blind system consisting of a catheter located in a CSF space, usually the lateral ventricle, and without distal run-off. Such systems are placed for CSF access purposes only, such as for instillation of antibiotics or chemotherapeutic agents, or CSF aspiration for treatment and monitoring. The reservoirs do not divert or shunt CSF. Ommaya reservoirs are dome-shaped structures (Fig. 17-6) with a diameter of 1 to 2 cm and have a connecting port placed at their base or side. They are placed subcutaneously and attached to a

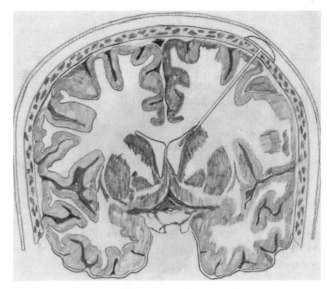

FIGURE 17-7. Coronal section through the brain at the level of the frontal horns, illustrating the subgaleal/epicalvarial location at the reservoir, with the distal perforated part of the catheter lying within the ventricle.

ventricular subarachnoid catheter (Fig. 17-7). Aspiration technique is essentially the same as from a shunt reservoir; however, the Ommaya reservoir is often larger and differs in shape from many shunt reservoirs. It is accessed, preferably, with a 25-gauge needle or butterfly. CSF is allowed to flow by gravity if possible; a volume equal to that to be instilled is removed and held for analysis or reinjection. The antibiotic or chemotherapeutic agent is injected; 1 mL of CSF or sterile saline can be used to flush the dose into the ventricle, or gentle barbotage of the reservoir may be performed to achieve the same goal. Risks and complications are essentially the same as in shunt aspirations (i.e., infection, bleeding, improper insertion), with the addition of chemical ventriculitis or arachnoiditis.

VENTRICULOSTOMY

A ventriculostomy is a catheter placed in the lateral ventricle for CSF drainage or ICP monitoring and treatment. It is performed by a neurosurgeon in the operating room or at the bedside in the intensive care unit or emergency department. It is usually performed through the nondominant hemisphere and into the frontal horn of the lateral ventricle. An alternate approach is to cannulate the occipital horn or trigone through an occipital entry point located 6 cm superior to the inion and 4 cm from the midline. Premedication is not necessary unless the patient is very anxious or combative. Radiographic guidance is typically not required unless the procedure is being performed stereotactically. CT or MRI stereotaxy is needed if the ventricles are very small, as in diffuse brain swelling or slit ventricle syndrome. Complications of ventriculostomy placement include meningitis or ventriculitis, scalp wound infection, intracranial hematoma or cortical injury, and failure to cannulate the ventricle.

LUMBAR DRAINAGE

Continuous CSF drainage via a lumbar catheter is useful in the treatment of CSF fistulas and as a provocative test to demonstrate the potential effects of shunting in normal pressure

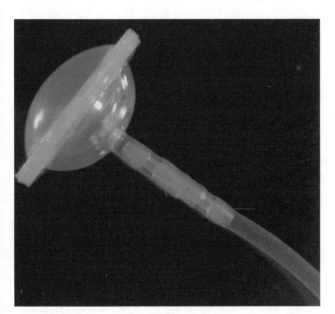

FIGURE 17-6. Close-up view of a ventricular (Ommaya) double-domed reservoir, the caudal half of which is designed to lie within the burr hole.

hydrocephalus or ventriculomegaly of various etiologies. Commercially available lumbar drainage kits are closed sterile systems that drain into a replaceable collection bag. Catheter placement is performed just as in lumbar puncture; however, a large-bore Touhy needle is used, through which the catheter is threaded once CSF return has been confirmed. Needle orientation follows the same guidelines as discussed for a lumbar puncture and is even more important in the case of this large-gauge needle. Epidural catheter kits could also be used, although the catheters tend to be slightly stiffer and have a narrower diameter. Complications include hemorrhage in the epidural or subarachnoid space, infection, inability to aspirate CSF, CSF leak, nerve root irritation, and, most ominously, a supratentorial subdural hematoma secondary to overdrainage. This complication tends to be more common in elderly individuals. The potential for overdrainage is significant because of the large diameter of the catheter and because the amount of drainage depends on the cooperation of the patient and the nursing staff.

SUMMARY

Of the various techniques available for CSF access, lumbar puncture is the procedure most commonly and safely performed by the general practitioner. Other techniques are described that may require the assistance of a radiologist, neurologist, anesthesiologist, or neurosurgeon.

REFERENCES

1. Friedman AG, Mulhern RK, Fairclough D, et al: Midazolam premedication for pediatric bone marrow aspiration and lumbar puncture. *Med Pediatr Oncol* 19:499, 1992.
2. Wood J: Cerebrospinal fluid: techniques of access and analytical interpretation, in Wilkins R, Rengachary S (eds): Neurosurgery. 2nd ed. New York, McGraw Hill, 1996; p 165.
3. Bigner SH: Cerebrospinal fluid cytology: current status and diagnostic applications. *J Neuropathol Exp Neurol* 51:235, 1992.
4. Leblanc R: The minor leak preceding subarachnoid hemorrhage. *J Neurosurg* 66:35, 1981.
5. Yurkadok M, Kocabas CN: CSF erythrocyte volume analysis: a simple method for the diagnosis of traumatic tap in newborn infants. *Pediatr Neurosurg* 17:199, 1991–1992.
6. D'Arminio-Monteforte A, Cinque P, Vago L, et al: A comparison of brain biopsy and CSF PCR in the diagnosis of CNS lesions in AIDS patients. *J Neurol* 244:35, 1997.
7. Greenlee JE: Approach to diagnosis of meningitis: cerebrospinal fluid evaluation. *Infect Dis Clin North Am* 4:583, 1990.
8. Albeck MJ, Borgesen SE, Gjerris F, et al: Intracranial pressure and cerebrospinal fluid outflow conductance I healthy subjects. *J Neurosurg* 74:597, 1991.
9. Lundar T, Nornes H: Determination of ventricular fluid outflow resistance in patients with ventriculomegaly. *J Neurol Neurosurg Psychiatry* 53:896, 1990.
10. Tans JT, Poortvliet DC: Reduction of ventricular size after shunting for normal pressure hydrocephalus related to CSF dynamics before shunting. *J Neurol Neurosurg Psychiatry* 51:521, 1988.
11. Dhiravibulya K, Ouvrier R, Johnston I, et al: Benign intracranial hypertension in childhood: a review of 23 patients. *J Paediatr Child Health* 27:304, 1991.
12. Johnston I, Hawke S, Halmagyi J, et al: The pseudotumor syndrome: disorders of cerebrospinal fluid circulation causing intracranial hypertension without ventriculomegaly. *Arch Neurol* 48:740, 1991.
13. Rogers LR, Duchesneau PM, Nunez C, et al: Comparison of cisternal and lumbar CSF examination in leptomeningeal metastasis. *J Neurol* 42:1239, 1992.
14. Bigner SH, Johnston WWW: The cytopathology of cerebrospinal fluid, I. Non-neoplastic condition, lymphoma and leukemia. *Acta Cytol* 25:335, 1981.
15. Thomas RS, Beuche W, Felgenhauer K: The proliferation rate of T and B lymphocytes in cerebrospinal fluid. *J Neurol* 238:27, 1991.
16. Furneaux HM, Rosenblum MK, Dalmau J, et al: Selective expression of Purkinje cell antigens in tumor tissue in patients with paraneoplastic cerebellar degeneration. *N Engl J Med* 322:1844, 1990.
17. Fishman RA. *Cerebrospinal Fluid in Diseases of the Nervous System.* 2nd ed. Philadelphia, WB Saunders, 1992.
18. Zanetta JP, Tranchant C, Kuchler-Bopp S, et al: Presence of anti-CSL antibodies in the cerebrospinal fluid of patients: a sensitive and specific test in the diagnosis of multiple sclerosis. *J Neuroimmuol* 52:175, 1994.
19. Agrillo U, Simonetti G, Martino V: Postoperative CSF problems after spinal and lumbar surgery: general review. *J Neurosurg Sci* 35:93, 1991.
20. Nandapalan V, Watson ID, Swift AC: β_2-Transferrin and CSF rhinorrhea. *Clin Otolaryngol* 21:259, 1996.
21. Lyons MK, Meyer FB: Cerebrospinal fluid physiology and the management of increased intracranial pressure. *Mayo Clin Proc* 65:684, 1990.
22. Nakagawa H, Murasawa A, Kubo S, et al: Diagnosis and treatment of patients with meningeal carcinomatosis. *J Neurooncol* 13:81, 1992.
23. Porter FL, Miller JP, Cole FS, et al: A controlled clinical trial of local anesthesia for lumbar punctures in newborns [see comments]. *Pediatrics* 88:663, 1991.
24. Davidson RI: Lumbar puncture, in VanderSalm TJ (ed): *Atlas of Bedside Procedures.* 2nd ed. Boston, Little, Brown, 1988.
25. Wilkinson HA: Technical note: Anesthesia for lumbar puncture. *JAMA* 249:2177, 1983.
26. Ellis RW III, Strauss LC, Wiley JM, et al: A simple method of estimating cerebrospinal fluid pressure during lumbar puncture. *Pediatrics* 89:895, 1992.
27. Johnson JC, Deeb ZL: Coaxial needle technique for lumbar puncture in the morbidly obese patient. *Radiology* 179:874, 1991.
28. Scott EW, Cazenave CR, Virapongse C: Spinal subarachnoid hematoma complicating lumbar puncture: diagnosis and management. *Neurosurgery* 25:287, 1989.
29. Strupp M, Brandt T: Should one reinsert the stylet during lumbar puncture? *N Engl J Med* 336:1190, 1997.
30. Grant F, Condon B, Hart I, et al: Changes in intracranial CSF volume after lumbar puncture and their relationship to post-LP headache. *J Neurol Neurosurg Psychiatry* 54:440, 1991.
31. Lee T, Maynard N, Anslow P, et al: Post-myelogram headache: physiological or psychological? *Neuroradiology* 33:155, 1991.
32. Peterman S: Post myelography headache: a review. *Radiology* 200:765, 1996.
33. Carson D, Serpell M: Choosing the best needle for diagnostic lumbar puncture. *Neurology* 47:33, 1996.
34. Leibold RA, Yealy DM, Coppola M, et al: Post-dural puncture headache: characteristics, management and prevention. *Ann Emerg Med* 22:1863, 1993.
35. Choi A, Laurito CE, Cunningham FE: Pharmacologic management of post-dural headache. *Ann Pharmacother* 30:831, 1996.
36. Barrios-Alarcon J, Aldrete JA, Paragas-Tapia D: Relief of post-lumbar puncture headache with epidural dextran 40: a preliminary report. *Reg Anesth* 14:78, 1989.
37. Walsted A, Salomon G, Thomsen J: Hearing decrease after loss of cerebrospinal fluid: a new hydrops model? *Acta Otolaryngol* 111:468, 1991.
38. Michel O, Brusis T: Hearing loss as a sequel of lumbar puncture. *Ann Otol Rhinol Laryngol* 101:390, 1992.
39. Wong MC, Krol G, Rosenblum MK: Occult epidural chloroma complicated by acute paraplegia following lumbar puncture. *Ann Neurol* 31:110, 1992.
40. Mutoh S, Aikou I, Ueda S: Spinal coning after lumbar puncture in prostate cancer with asymptomatic vertebral metastasis: a case report. *J Urol* 145:834, 1991.

Philip J. Ayvazian

CHAPTER **18**

Percutaneous Suprapubic Cystostomy

Percutaneous suprapubic cystotomy is used to divert urine from the bladder when standard urethral catheterization is impossible or undesirable [1–10]. The procedure for placement of a small-diameter catheter is rapid, safe, and easily accomplished at the bedside under local anesthesia. This chapter will first address methods for urethral catheterization before discussing the percutaneous approach.

URETHRAL CATHETERIZATION

Urethral catheterization remains the principal method for bladder drainage. The indications for the catheter should be clarified because they influence the type and size of catheter to be used. A history and physical examination with particular attention to the patient's genitourinary system is important.

Catheterization may be difficult with male patients in several instances. Patients with lower urinary tract symptoms (e.g., urinary urgency, frequency, nocturia, decreased stream, and hesitancy) may have benign prostatic hypertrophy. These patients may require a larger-bore catheter, such as a 20 or 22 French (Fr). When dealing with urethral strictures, a smaller-bore catheter should be used, such as a 12 or 14 Fr. Patients with a history of prior prostatic surgery such as transurethral resection of the prostate, open prostatectomy, or radical prostatectomy may have an irregular bladder neck as a result of contracture after surgery. The use of a coudé-tip catheter, which has an upper deflected tip, may help in negotiating the altered anatomy after prostate surgery. The presence of a high-riding prostate or blood at the urethral meatus suggests urethral trauma. In this situation, urethral integrity must be demonstrated by retrograde urethrogram before urethral catheterization is attempted.

Urethral catheterization for gross hematuria requires large catheters such as the 22 or 24 Fr, which have larger holes for irrigation and removal of clots. Alternatively, a three-way urethral catheter may be used to provide continuous bladder irrigation to prevent clotting. Large catheters impede excretion of urethral secretions, however, and can lead to urethritis or epididymitis if used for prolonged periods.

TECHNIQUE

In male patients, after the patient is prepared and draped, 10 mL of a 2% lidocaine hydrochloride jelly is injected retrograde into the urethra. Anesthesia of the urethral mucosa requires 5 to 10 minutes after occluding the urethral meatus either with a penile clamp or manually to prevent loss of the jelly. The balloon

of the catheter is tested, and the catheter tip is covered with a water-soluble lubricant. After stretching the penis upward and perpendicular to the body, the catheter is inserted into the urethral meatus. The catheter is advanced up to the hub to ensure its entrance into the bladder. To prevent urethral trauma, the balloon is not inflated until urine is observed draining from the catheter. Irrigation of the catheter with normal saline helps verify the position. A common site of resistance to catheter passage is the external urinary sphincter within the membranous urethra, which may contract voluntarily. Any other resistance may represent a stricture, necessitating urologic consultation. In patients with prior prostate surgery, an assistant's finger placed in the rectum may elevate the urethra and allow the catheter to pass into the bladder.

In female patients, short, straight catheters are preferred. Typically, a smaller amount of local anesthesia is used. Difficulties in catheter placement occur after urethral surgery or vulvectomy, or with vaginal atrophy or morbid obesity. In these cases, the meatus is not visible and may be retracted under the symphysis pubis. Blind catheter placement over a finger located in the vagina at the palpated site of the urethral meatus may be successful.

When urologic consultation is obtained, other techniques for urethral catheterization can be used. Flexible cystoscopy may be performed to ascertain the reason for difficult catheter placement and for insertion of a guidewire. A urethral catheter then can be placed over the guidewire by the Seldinger technique. Filiforms and followers are useful for urethral strictures.

INDICATIONS

On occasion, despite proper technique (as outlined previously), urethral catheterization is unsuccessful. These are the instances when percutaneous suprapubic cystotomy is necessary. Undoubtedly, the most common indication for percutaneous suprapubic cystotomy is for the management of acute urinary retention in men. Other indications for a percutaneous suprapubic cystotomy in the intensive care unit are listed in Table 18-1.

CONTRAINDICATIONS

The contraindications to percutaneous suprapubic cystotomy are listed in Table 18-2. An inability to palpate the bladder or distortion of the pelvic anatomy from previous surgery or trauma makes percutaneous entry of the bladder difficult. In these situations, the risks of penetrating the peritoneal cavity become

159

TABLE 18-1.   Indications for Percutaneous Cystotomy

Unsuccessful urethral catheterization in the setting of acute
  urinary retention
After prostatic surgery
Presence of urethral trauma
After antiincontinence procedures
Prostatic bilobar hyperplasia
Urethral stricture
Severe hypospadias
Periurethral abscess
Presence of severe urethral, epididymal, or prostate infection

substantial. The bladder may not be palpable if the patient is in
acute renal failure with oliguria or anuria, has a small contracted
neurogenic bladder, or is incontinent. When the bladder is not
palpable, it can be filled in a retrograde manner with saline to
distend it. In men, a 14 Fr catheter is placed in the fossa navic-
ularis just inside the urethral meatus, and the balloon is filled
with 2 to 3 mL of sterile water to occlude the urethra. Saline is injected slowly into the catheter until the bladder is palpable; then
the suprapubic tube may be placed. In patients with a contracted
neurogenic bladder, it is impossible to adequately distend the
bladder by this approach. For these patients, ultrasonography is
used to locate the bladder and allow the insertion of a 22-gauge
spinal needle. Saline is instilled into the bladder via the needle
to distend the bladder enough for suprapubic tube placement.
(Fig. 18-1)

In patients with previous lower abdominal surgery, ultrasonographic guidance is often necessary before a percutaneous cystotomy can be performed safely. Previous surgery can lead to
adhesions that can hold a loop of intestine in the area of insertion. Other relative contraindications include patients with
coagulopathy, a known history of bladder tumors, or active
hematuria and retained clots. In patients with bladder tumors,
percutaneous bladder access should be avoided because tumor
cell seeding can occur along the percutaneous tract. Suprapubic cystotomy tubes are small in caliber and therefore do not
function effectively with severe hematuria and retained clots.
Instead, open surgical placement of a large-caliber tube is necessary if urethral catheterization is impossible.

TECHNIQUE

There are two general types of percutaneous cystotomy tubes
that range in size from 8 to 14 Fr. The first type uses an obturator with a preloaded catheter. Examples include the Stamey
catheter (Cook Urological, Spencer, IN) and the Bonanno
catheter (Beckton Dickinson and Co., Franklin Lakes, NJ) [11].
The Stamey device is a polyethylene Malecot catheter with a luer
lock hub that fits over a hollow needle obturator (Fig. 18-2A).
When the obturator is locked to the hub of the catheter, the

TABLE 18-2.   Contraindications to Percutaneous Cystotomy

Nonpalpable bladder
Previous lower abdominal surgery
Coagulopathy
Known bladder tumor
Clot retention

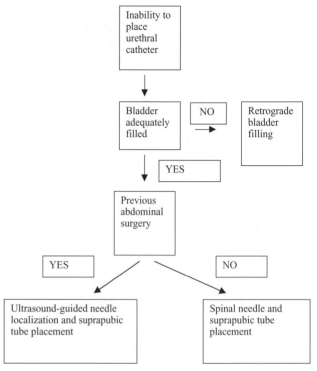

FIGURE 18-1.   Algorithm for percutaneous suprapubic tube placement.

Malecot flanges are pulled inward (closed), and the system is
ready for use. The Bonanno catheter uses a flexible 14-Fr Teflon
tube, which is inserted over a hollow 18-gauge obturator (Fig.
18-2B). The obturator locks into the catheter hub and extends
beyond the catheter tip. When the obturator is withdrawn,
the tube pigtails in the bladder. One advantage to the Stamey

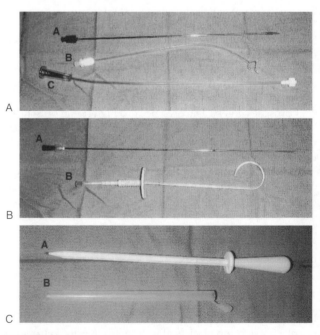

FIGURE 18-2.   **A:** Stamey suprapubic cystostomy trocar set (*A* is
the obturator, *B* is the Malecot catheter, and *C* is the drainage tube).
B: Bonanno catheter set (*A* is the obturator and *B* is the catheter).
C: Lawrence suprapubic catheter (*A* is the trocar and *B* is the sheath).

catheter is that the flanges provide a secure retaining system. The Bonanno catheter generally induces fewer bladder spasms, however, and is better tolerated.

The second type of percutaneous cystotomy tube consists of a trocar and sheath, which are used to penetrate the abdominal wall and bladder. One of the most popular systems is the Lawrence suprapubic catheter (Rusch, Duluth, GA). This system allows a standard Foley catheter to be placed after removal of the trocar (Fig. 18-2C).

The patient is placed in the supine position; a towel roll may be placed under the hips to extend the pelvis. Trendelenburg position may help to move the abdominal contents away from the bladder. The bladder is palpated to ensure that it is distended. The suprapubic region is shaved (with clippers, not a razor), prepared with a 2% chlorhexidine or 10% povidone-iodine solution, and draped with sterile towels. The insertion site is several centimeters above the symphysis pubis in the midline: This approach avoids the epigastric vessels. In obese patients with a large abdominal fat pad, the fold is elevated. The needle should be introduced into the suprapubic crease, where the fat thickness is minimal. One percent lidocaine is used to anesthetize the skin, subcutaneous tissues, rectus fascia, and retropubic space. A 22-gauge spinal needle with a 5-mL syringe is directed vertically and advanced until urine is aspirated. If the bladder is smaller or if the patient had previous pelvic surgery, the needle is directed at a 60-degree caudal angle. Insertion of the cystotomy tube is predicated on the feasibility of bladder puncture and after the angle and depth of insertion is established with the spinal needle (Fig. 18-3).

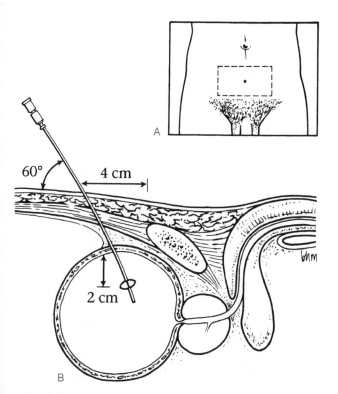

FIGURE 18-3.   Technique of suprapubic trocar placement. **A:** Area to be shaved, prepared, and draped before trocar placement. **B:** Position of the Stamey trocar in the bladder. The angle, distance from the pubis, and position of the catheter in relation to the bladder wall are demonstrated.

At the site of bladder puncture, a small 2-mm incision is made with a no. 11 blade. The catheter mounted on the obturator is advanced in toward the bladder. Two hands are used to grasp the system to provide a forceful, but controlled, thrust through the abdominal wall. One hand can be positioned on the obturator at a site marking the depth of the bladder. A syringe attached to the end of the obturator is used to aspirate urine and confirm obturator placement. Once the bladder is penetrated, the entire system is advanced 2 to 3 cm. This prevents the catheter tip from withdrawing into the retropubic space when the bladder decompresses. After unlocking the obturator from the catheter, the obturator acts as a guide while the catheter is advanced into the bladder. When using a Stamey catheter, the catheter can be gently withdrawn until the Malecot flanges meet resistance against the anterior bladder wall. The Stamey catheter is then advanced 2 cm back into the bladder to allow for movement. This maneuver pulls the catheter away from the bladder trigone and helps reduce bladder spasms.

The same general technique applies to placement of the Lawrence suprapubic catheter system. After the bladder is penetrated, urine appears at the hub of the suprapubic catheter introducer (trocar plus sheath). The trocar is then removed, and a Foley catheter is inserted. The Foley catheter balloon is inflated to secure it in the bladder. Pulling the tab at the top of the peel-away sheath allows the remaining portion of the sheath to be removed away from the catheter.

The patency of the catheter is assessed by irrigating the bladder after decompression. The catheter can be fixed with a simple nylon suture and sterile dressing. The Bonanno catheter contains a suture disc. The Lawrence suprapubic catheter does not require extra fixation because the balloon on the Foley catheter secures it in place.

SUPRAPUBIC CATHETER CARE

Bladder spasms occur commonly after suprapubic catheter placement. When using a Stamey catheter or a Foley catheter, bladder spasms can be prevented by withdrawing the tube until it meets the anterior bladder wall and then advancing 2 cm back into the bladder. Persistent bladder spasms can be treated with anticholinergic therapy (e.g., oxybutynin and hyoscyamine). This medication should be discontinued before removing the suprapubic tube to prevent urinary retention.

A suprapubic tube that ceases to drain is usually caused by kinking of the catheter or displacement of the catheter tip into the retropubic space. If necessary, suprapubic catheters may be replaced using either an exchange set (available for Stamey catheters) or by dilating the cystotomy tract. Closure of the percutaneous cystotomy tract is generally prompt after the tube is removed. Prolonged suprapubic tube use can lead to a mature tract, which may take several days to close. If the tract remains open, bladder decompression via a urethral catheter may be required.

COMPLICATIONS

Placement of suprapubic cystotomy tubes is generally safe with infrequent complications. Possible complications are listed in Table 18-3 [12,13]. Bowel complications are severe but rare with this procedure [14]. Penetration of the peritoneal cavity or bowel perforation produces peritoneal or intestinal symptoms

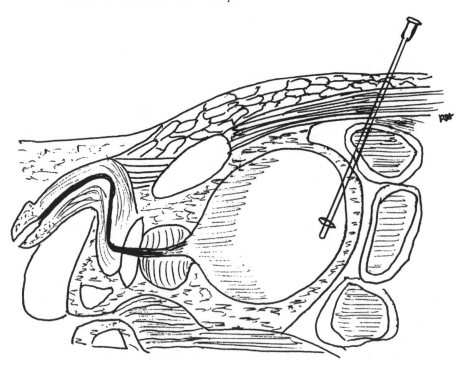

FIGURE 18-4. Placement of the suprapubic tube can perforate entrapped bowel.

and signs. This complication can be avoided by attempting the procedure only on well-distended bladders and using a mid-line approach no more than 4 cm above the pubis.

In patients who have had previous lower abdominal or pelvic surgery, an ultrasound should be used to properly place the suprapubic tube and rule out entrapped bowel (Fig. 18-4). Patients who develop peritoneal symptoms and signs require a full evaluation of not only the location of the suprapubic tube (by a cystogram) but also of the cystotomy tract. A kidney-ureter-bladder radiograph and computed tomography scans may be required.

Hematuria is the most common complication after suprapubic tube placement. Rarely, this requires open cystotomy for placement of a large-caliber tube for irrigation. Hematuria can occur secondary to laceration of a submucosal vessel or rapid decompression of a chemically distended bladder. It can be avoided by gradual bladder decompression.

Complications associated with the catheter include loss of a portion of the catheter in the bladder, calcification of the catheter, or bladder stone formation. These complications can be avoided by preventing prolonged catheter use. Beyond 4 weeks, evaluation and replacement or removal must be considered.

When chronically distended bladders are decompressed, patients are at risk for postobstructive diuresis. Patients who are

TABLE 18-3. Complications of Percutaneous Cystotomy

Peritoneal and bowel perforation
Hematuria
Retained or calcified catheter
Bladder stones
Postobstructive diuresis
Hypotension
Bladder perforation

at greatest risk include those with azotemia, peripheral edema, congestive heart failure, and mental status changes. Patients with postobstructive diuresis (i.e., urine outputs greater then 200 mL per hour) require frequent monitoring of vital signs and intravenous fluid replacement.

Hypotension rarely occurs after suprapubic tube placement. It may be caused by a vasovagal response or relief of pelvic veins compressed by bladder distention. Fluid administration alleviates this complication.

Another rare but possible complication is a through-and-through bladder perforation. This is treated conservatively with bladder decompression.

REFERENCES

1. Hilton P, Stanton SL: Suprapubic catheterization. *Br Med J* 281:1261, 1980.
2. Sethia KK, Selkon JB, Berry AR, et al: Prospective randomized controlled trial of urethral versus suprapubic catheterization. *Br J Surg* 74:624, 1987.
3. Carter HB: Instrumentation and endoscopy, in Walsh PC, Retnik AB, Vaughan ED, et al (eds): *Campbell's Urology*. Philadelphia, WB Saunders, 1998.
4. O'Brien WM: Percutaneous placement of a suprapubic tube with peel away sheath introducer. *J Urol* 145:1015, 1991.
5. Chiou RK, Morton JJ, Engelsgjerd JS, et al: Placement of large suprapubic tube using peel-away introducer. *J Urol* 153:1179, 1995.
6. Meessen S, Bruhl P, Piechota HJ: A new suprapubic cystostomy trocar system. *Urology* 56: 315, 2000.
7. Lee MJ, Papanicolaou N, Nocks BN, et al: Fluoroscopically guided percutaneous suprapubic cystostomy for long-term bladder drainage: an alternative to surgical cystostomy. *Radiology* 188:787, 1993.
8. Aguilera PA, Choi T, Durham BA: Ultrasound-guided suprapubic cystostomy catheter placement in the emergency department. *J Emerg Med* 26(3):319, 2004.
9. Irby PB, Stoller ML: Percutaneous suprapubic cystostomy. *J Endourol* 7(2):125, 1993.
10. Lawrentschuk N, Lee D, Marriott P, et al: Suprapubic stab cystostomy: a safer technique. *Urology* 62(5):932, 2003.
11. Bonanno PJ, Landers DE, Rock DE: Bladder drainage with the suprapubic catheter needle. *Obstet Gynecol* 35:807, 1970.
12. Drutz HP, Khosid HI: Complications with Bonanno suprapubic catheters. *Am J Obstet Gynecol* 149:685, 1984.
13. Dogra PN, Goel R: Complication of percutaneous suprapubic cystostomy. *Int Urol Nephrol* 36(3):343, 2004.
14. Hebert DB, Mitchell GW: Perforation of the ileum as a complication of suprapubic catheterization. *Obstet Gynecol* 62:662, 1983.

Bonnie J. Bidinger
Maria E. Abruzzo
Eric W. Jacobson

CHAPTER **19**

Aspiration of the Knee and Synovial Fluid Analysis

Arthrocentesis is a safe and relatively simple procedure that involves the introduction of a needle into the joint space to remove synovial fluid. It constitutes an essential part of the evaluation of any arthritis of unknown cause, frequently with the intent to rule out a septic process [1–3].

Ropes and Bauer [4] first categorized synovial fluid as *inflammatory* or *noninflammatory* in 1953, terms that are still used today. Hollander et al. [5] and Gatter and McCarty [6] coined the term *synovianalysis* to describe the process of joint fluid analysis in 1961 and were instrumental in establishing the critical role of synovial fluid analysis to diagnose certain forms of arthritis. Septic arthritis and crystalline arthritis can be diagnosed by synovial fluid analysis alone. They may present similarly but require markedly different treatments, thus necessitating early arthrocentesis and prompt synovial fluid analysis.

INDICATIONS

Arthrocentesis is performed for diagnostic and therapeutic purposes. The main indication for arthrocentesis is to assist in the evaluation of arthritis of unknown cause. In the intensive care unit, it is most commonly performed in the setting of acute monoarthritis or oligoarthritis (presenting with one to three inflamed joints) to rule out septic arthritis. Many types of inflammatory arthritis mimic septic arthritis. Synovial fluid analysis is useful in differentiating the various causes of inflammatory arthritis [4,7] (Table 19-1). Therefore, patients presenting with monoarthritis or oligoarthritis of recent onset require prompt arthrocentesis with subsequent synovial fluid analysis, preferably before initiation of treatment.

Arthrocentesis is also used for therapeutic purposes. In a septic joint, serial joint aspirations are required to remove accumulated inflammatory or purulent fluid. This allows serial monitoring of the total white blood cell count, Gram's stain, and culture to assess response to treatment and accomplishes complete drainage of a closed space. Inflammatory fluid contains many destructive enzymes that contribute to cartilage and bony degradation; removal of the fluid may slow this destructive process [8,9]. Additionally, arthrocentesis allows for injection of long-acting corticosteroid preparations into the joint space, which may be a useful treatment for various inflammatory and noninflammatory forms of arthritis [10,11].

Before performing arthrocentesis, it must be ascertained that the true joint is inflamed and an effusion is present. This requires a meticulous physical examination to differentiate arthritis from periarticular inflammation. Bursitis, tendinitis, and cellulitis all may mimic arthritis. In the knee, the examination begins with assessment of swelling. A true effusion may cause bulging of the parapatellar gutters and the suprapatellar pouch [12]. The swelling should be confined to the joint space. To check for small effusions, the bulge test is performed [13]. Fluid is stroked from the medial joint line into the suprapatellar pouch and then from the suprapatellar pouch down along the lateral joint line. If a bulge of fluid is noted at the medial joint line, a small effusion is present (Fig. 19-1). If a large effusion is suspected, a patellar tap is performed [14]. The left hand is used to apply pressure to the suprapatellar pouch while the right hand taps the patella against the femur with sharp downward pressure. If the patella is ballottable, an effusion is probably present. Comparison with the opposite joint is helpful. Many texts describe joint examination and assessment for fluid in the knee and other joints [12–15].

CONTRAINDICATIONS

Absolute contraindications to arthrocentesis, in general, include local infection of the overlying skin or other periarticular structures and severe coagulopathy [1–3,11]. If coagulopathy is present and septic arthritis is suspected, every effort should be made to correct the coagulopathy (with fresh-frozen plasma or alternate factors) before joint aspiration. Therapeutic anticoagulation is not an absolute contraindication, but every effort should be made to avoid excessive trauma during aspiration in this circumstance. Known bacteremia is a contraindication because inserting a needle into the joint space disrupts capillary integrity, allowing joint space seeding [16]. However, if septic arthritis is strongly suspected, joint aspiration is indicated. The presence of articular instability (e.g., that seen with badly damaged joints) is a relative contraindication, although the presence of a large presumed inflammatory fluid may still warrant joint aspiration.

TABLE 19-1.   Common Causes of Noninflammatory and Inflammatory Arthritides

Noninflammatory	Inflammatory
Osteoarthritis	Rheumatoid arthritis
Trauma/internal derangement	Spondyloarthropathies
Avascular necrosis	Psoriatic arthritis
Hemarthrosis	Reiter's syndrome/reactive
Malignancy	arthritis
Benign tumors	Ankylosing spondylitis
Osteochondroma	Ulcerative colitis/regional
Pigmented villonodular synovitis	enteritis
	Crystal-induced arthritis
	Monosodium urate (gout)
	Calcium pyrophosphate
	dihydrate (pseudogout)
	Hydroxyapatite
	Infectious arthritis
	Bacterial
	Mycobacterial
	Fungal
	Connective tissue diseases
	Systemic lupus erythematosus
	Vasculitis
	Scleroderma
	Polymyositis
	Hypersensitivity
	Serum sickness

COMPLICATIONS

The major complications of arthrocentesis are iatrogenically induced infection and bleeding, both of which are extremely rare [1]. The risk of infection after arthrocentesis has been estimated to be less than 1 in 10,000 [17]. Hollander [18] reported an incidence of less than 0.005% in 400,000 injections. Strict adherence to aseptic technique reduces the risk of postarthrocentesis infection. Significant hemorrhage is also extremely rare. Correction of prominent coagulopathy before arthrocentesis reduces this risk.

Another potential complication of arthrocentesis is direct injury to the articular cartilage by the needle. This is not quantifiable, but any injury to cartilage could be associated with degenerative change over time. To avoid cartilaginous damage, the needle should be pushed in only as far as necessary to obtain

fluid, and excessive movement of the needle during the procedure should be avoided.

Other complications include discomfort from the procedure itself; allergic reactions to the skin preparation or local anesthetic [19]; and, in the case of steroid injection, postinjection flare and local soft tissue atrophy from the glucocorticoid [20].

TECHNIQUE

Joint aspiration is easily learned. A sound knowledge of the joint anatomy, including the bony and soft tissue landmarks used for joint entry, is needed. Strict aseptic technique must be followed to minimize risk of infection, and relaxation of the muscles surrounding the joint should be encouraged because muscular contraction can impede the needle's entry into the joint.

Most physicians in the intensive care unit can aspirate the knee because it is one of the most accessible joints. Other joints should probably be aspirated by an appropriate specialist, such as a rheumatologist or an orthopaedic surgeon. Certain joints are quite difficult to enter blindly and are more appropriately entered using radiologic guidance, such as with fluoroscopy or computed tomography; these include the hip, sacroiliac, and temporomandibular joints. Many texts describe in detail the aspiration technique of other joints [3,18,20,21]. The technique for knee aspiration is as follows:

1. Describe the procedure to the patient, including the possible complications, and obtain written informed consent.
2. Collect all items needed for the procedure (Table 19-2).
3. With the patient supine and the knee fully extended, examine the knee to confirm the presence of an effusion, as described previously.
4. Identify landmarks for needle entry. The knee may be aspirated from a medial or lateral approach. The medial approach is more commonly used and is preferred when small effusions are present. Identify the superior and inferior borders of the patella. Entry should be halfway between the borders just inferior to the undersurface of the patella (Fig. 19-2). The entry site may be marked with pressure from the end of a ballpoint pen with the writing tip retracted. An indentation mark should be visible.
5. Cleanse the area with 2% chlorhexidine in 70% isopropyl alcohol and allow the area to dry. Practice universal

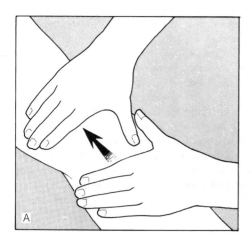

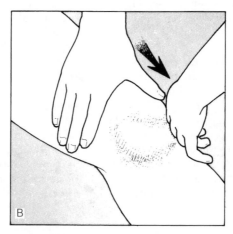

FIGURE 19-1. The bulge test. **A:** Milk fluid from the suprapatellar pouch into the joint. **B:** Slide hand down the lateral aspect of the joint line and watch for a bulge medial to the joint.

TABLE 19-2. Arthrocentesis Equipment

Procedure	Equipment
Skin preparation and local anesthesia	2% chlorhexidine in 70% isopropyl alcohol Ethyl chloride spray For local anesthesia—1% lidocaine; 25-gauge, 1.5-in needle; 22-gauge, 1.5-in needle; 5-mL syringe Sterile sponge/cloth
Arthrocentesis	Gloves 20- to 60-mL syringe (depending on size of effusion) 18- to 22-gauge, 1.5-in needle Sterile sponge/cloth Sterile clamp Sterile bandage
Collection	15-mL anticoagulated tube (with sodium heparin or ethylenediaminetetraacetic acid) Sterile tubes for routine cultures Slide, cover slip

precautions: wear gloves at all times while handling any body fluid, although they need not be sterile for routine knee aspiration. Do not touch the targeted area once it has been cleaned.

6. Apply local anesthesia. A local anesthetic (1% lidocaine) may be instilled with a 25-gauge, 1.5-inch needle into the subcutaneous skin. Once numbing has occurred, deeper instillation of the local anesthetic to the joint capsule can be performed. Some physicians may use ethyl chloride as an alternative anesthetic. However, this agent provides only superficial anesthesia of the skin. To use, spray ethyl chloride directly onto the designated area; stop when the first signs of freezing are evident in order to limit potential for skin damage.

7. To enter the knee joint, use an 18- to 22-gauge, 1.5-inch needle with a 20- to 60-mL syringe. Use a larger gauge needle particularly if septic arthritis is suspected because the aspirated fluid may be purulent and more difficult to aspirate.

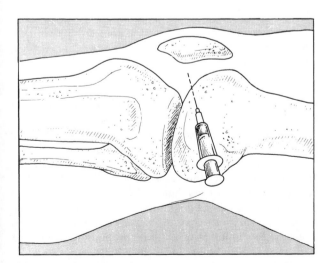

FIGURE 19-2. Technique of aspirating the knee joint. The needle enters halfway between the superior and inferior borders of the patella and is directed just inferior to the patella.

Use a quick thrust through the skin and on through the capsule to minimize pain. Avoid hitting periosteal bone, which causes significant pain, or cartilage, which causes cartilaginous damage. Aspirate fluid to fill the syringe. If the fluid appears purulent or hemorrhagic, try to tap the joint dry, which will remove mediators of inflammation that may perpetuate an inflammatory or destructive process. If the syringe is full and more fluid remains, a sterile hemostat may be used to clamp the needle, thus stabilizing it, while switching syringes. When the syringes have been switched, more fluid can be withdrawn. The syringes must be sterile.

Conversely, effusions are sometimes difficult to aspirate. Reasons for this include increased fluid viscosity, fibrin and other debris impeding flow through the needle, loculated fluid, and use of a needle with an inappropriately small gauge. Additionally, the fluid may not be accessible by the approach being used [22]. At times, one can obtain a small drop of joint fluid by using continuous suction as the needle is withdrawn from the joint space [20]. This small specimen can then be sent for Gram's stain, culture, and if possible, crystal analysis.

8. When the fluid has been obtained, quickly remove the needle and apply pressure to the needle site with a piece of sterile gauze. When bleeding has stopped, remove the gauze, clean the area with alcohol, and apply an adhesive bandage. If the patient is receiving anticoagulation therapy or has a bleeding diathesis, apply prolonged pressure.

9. Document the amount of fluid obtained and perform gross examination, noting the color and clarity. A string sign may be performed at the bedside to assess fluid viscosity (see the following section). Send fluid for cell count with differential count, Gram's stain, routine culture, specialized cultures for *Gonococcus, Mycobacterium,* and fungus, if indicated, and polarized microscopic examination for crystal analysis. Other tests, such as glucose and complement determinations, are generally not helpful. Use an anticoagulated tube to send fluid for cell count and crystal analysis. Sodium heparin and ethylenediaminetetraacetic acid are appropriate anticoagulants. Lithium heparin and calcium oxalate should be avoided because they can precipitate out of solution to form crystals, thus potentially giving a false-positive assessment for crystals [6,23]. Fluid may be sent for Gram's stain and culture in the syringe capped with a blunt tip, or in a sterile red-top tube.

SYNOVIAL FLUID ANALYSIS

Synovial fluid analysis is identical for all joints and begins with bedside observation of the fluid. The color, clarity, and viscosity of the fluid are characterized. Synovial fluid is divided into noninflammatory versus inflammatory types based on the total nucleated cell count. A white blood cell count less than or equal to 2,000 per mm^3 is defined as a *noninflammatory fluid*, and a count greater than 2,000 per mm^3 is defined as an *inflammatory fluid*. Table 19-3 shows how fluid is divided into major categories based on appearance and cell count. Table 19-1 lists causes for noninflammatory and inflammatory effusions.

TABLE 19-3. Joint Fluid Characteristics

Characteristic	Normal	Noninflammatory	Inflammatory	Septic
Color	Clear	Yellow	Yellow or opalescent	Variable—may be purulent
Clarity	Transparent	Transparent	Translucent	Opaque
Viscosity	Very high	High	Low	Typically low
Mucin clot	Firm	Firm	Friable	Friable
White blood cell count per mm^3	200	200–2,000	2,000–100,000	>50,000, usually >100,000
Polymorphonuclear cells (%)	<25	<25	>50	>75
Culture	Negative	Negative	Negative	Usually positive

GROSS EXAMINATION

Color

Color and clarity should be tested using a clear glass tube. Translucent plastic, as used in most disposable syringes, interferes with proper assessment [1].

Normal synovial fluid is colorless. Noninflammatory and inflammatory synovial fluid appears yellow or straw-colored. Septic effusions frequently appear purulent and whitish. Depending on the number of white blood cells present, pure pus may be extracted from a septic joint. Hemorrhagic effusions appear red or brown. If the fluid looks like pure blood, the tap may have aspirated venous blood. The needle is removed, pressure is applied, and the joint is reentered from an alternate site. If the same bloody appearance is noted, the fluid is a hemorrhagic effusion and probably not related to the trauma of the aspiration. If any question remains, the hematocrit of the effusion is compared with that of peripheral blood. The hematocrit in a hemorrhagic effusion is typically lower than that of peripheral blood. In the case of a traumatic tap, the hematocrit of the fluid should be equal to that of peripheral blood. For causes of a hemorrhagic effusion, refer to Table 19-4.

Clarity

The clarity of synovial fluid depends on the number and types of cells or particles present. Clarity is tested by reading black print on a white background through a glass tube filled with the synovial fluid.

If the print is easily read, the fluid is transparent. This is typical of normal and noninflammatory synovial fluid. If the black print can be distinguished from the white background, but is not clear, the fluid is translucent. This is typical of inflammatory effusions. If nothing can be seen through the fluid, it is opaque. This occurs with grossly inflammatory, septic, and hemorrhagic fluids (see Table 19-3).

TABLE 19-4. Causes of a Hemorrhagic Effusion

Trauma (with or without fracture)
Hemophilia and other bleeding disorders
Anticoagulant therapy
Tumor (metastatic and local)
Hemangioma
Pigmented villonodular synovitis
Ehlers-Danlos syndrome
Scurvy

Viscosity

The viscosity of synovial fluid is a measure of the hyaluronic acid content. Hyaluronic acid is one of the major substances in synovial fluid that gives it a viscous quality. Degradative enzymes such as hyaluronidase are released in inflammatory conditions, thus destroying hyaluronic acid and other proteinaceous material, resulting in a thinner, less-viscous fluid. Highly viscous fluid, on the other hand, can be seen in myxedematous effusions/hypothyroid effusions.

Viscosity can be assessed at the bedside using the string sign [1]. A drop of fluid is allowed to fall from the end of the needle or syringe and the length of the continuous string that forms estimated. Normal fluid typically forms at least a 6-cm continuous string. Inflammatory fluid does not form a string; instead, it drops off the end of the needle or syringe like water dropping from a faucet. Again, universal precautions should always be used when handling synovial fluid.

The mucin clot, another measure of viscosity, estimates the presence of intact hyaluronic acid and hyaluronic acid–protein interactions. This test is performed by placing several drops of synovial fluid in 5% acetic acid and then mixing with a stirring stick. A good mucin clot forms in normal, noninflammatory fluid. The fluid remains condensed in a clot resembling chewed gum. A poor mucin clot is seen with inflammatory fluid; the fluid disperses diffusely within the acetic acid.

CELL COUNT AND DIFFERENTIAL

The cell count should be obtained as soon as possible after arthrocentesis, as a delay of even several hours may cause an artificially low white blood cell count [24]. The total white blood cell count of synovial fluid differentiates noninflammatory from inflammatory fluid, as noted previously. In general, the higher the total white blood cell count, the more likely the joint is to be infected. This is not absolute, however, and there is considerable overlap. For instance, a total white cell count above 100,000 per mm^3 may be seen in conditions other than infection [25], whereas a total white blood cell count of 50,000 per mm^3 may be due to infection, crystalline disease, or a systemic inflammatory arthropathy [19]. The technique for the cell count is identical to that used with peripheral blood. The fluid may be diluted with normal saline for a manual count, or an automated counter may be used. Viscous fluid with excessive debris may clog a counter or give falsely elevated results, thus making the manual procedure somewhat more accurate.

The differential white blood cell count is also performed using the technique used for peripheral blood, typically using Wright's stain. The differential is calculated based on direct visualization. The differential count includes cells typically seen in peripheral blood, such as polymorphonuclear cells, monocytes, and lymphocytes, as well as cells localized to the synovial space. In general, the total white blood cell count and the polymorphonuclear cell count increase with inflammation and infection [25]. Septic fluid typically has a differential of greater than 75% polymorphonuclear cells (see Table 19-3).

In addition to distinguishing polymorphonuclear cells from monocytes and lymphocytes, Wright's stain can detect other cells in synovial fluid that can be useful in establishing a diagnosis. For instance, iron-laden chondrocytes, which are seen in hemochromatosis, may be picked up by Wright's stain, as may be fat droplets and bone marrow spicules, which are suggestive for trauma or a fracture into the joint [22].

CRYSTALS

All fluid should be assessed for the presence of crystals. As with cell count, crystal analysis should be performed as soon as possible after arthrocentesis. A delay is associated with a decreased yield [24]. One drop of fluid is placed on a slide and covered with a cover slip; this is examined for crystals using a compensated polarized light microscope. The presence of intracellular monosodium urate (MSU) or calcium pyrophosphate dihydrate (CPPD) crystals confirms a diagnosis of gout or pseudogout, respectively. MSU crystals are typically long and needle-shaped: They may appear to pierce through a white blood cell. The crystals are negatively birefringent, appearing yellow when parallel with the plane of reference. Typically, CPPD crystals are small and rhomboid. The crystals are weakly positively birefringent, appearing blue when oriented parallel to the plane of reference. Rotating the stage of the microscope by 90 degrees and thereby the orientation of the crystals (now perpendicular to the plane of reference) changes their color: MSU crystals turn blue and CPPD crystals turn yellow. Refer to Tables 19-5 and 19-6

TABLE 19-5.   Classification of Hyperuricemia

Primary hyperuricemia
  Idiopathic
  Enzymatic defects (e.g., hypoxanthine guanine phosphoribosyl-
    transferase deficiency)
Secondary hyperuricemia
  Increased production of uric acid
    Increased de novo purine synthesis
    Excessive dietary purine intake
    Increased nucleic acid turnover (myeloproliferative/
      lymphoproliferative disorders, psoriasis, hemolytic anemia,
      ethyl alcohol abuse)
  Decreased renal excretion of uric acid
    Medications
      Diuretics
      Low-dose salicylates
      Pyrazinamide
      Ethambutol
      Cyclosporine
    Chronic renal failure
    Hyperacidemia (lactic acidosis, ketoacidosis, starvation,
      ethyl alchohol abuse)
    Lead nephropathy

TABLE 19-6.   Conditions Associated with Calcium Pyrophosphate Dihydrate Deposition Disease

Hereditary
Sporadic (idiopathic)
Aging
Metabolic diseases
  Hyperparathyroidism
  Hypothyroidism
  Hypophosphatemia
  Hypomagnesemia
  Hemochromatosis
Amyloidosis
Trauma

for a classification of hyperuricemia and conditions associated with CPPD deposition disease.

In addition to MSU and CPPD crystals, other less-common crystals may induce an inflammatory arthropathy: Basic calcium crystals (e.g., hydroxyapatite) and oxalate crystals are two such types. Hydroxyapatite crystals can incite acute articular and periarticular inflammation, much like MSU crystals in gout. Clinically, this is difficult to distinguish between septic arthritis and cellulitis, respectively [26]. On light microscopy, however, crystals appear as clumps of shiny nonbirefringent globules and with alizarin red S stain, the clumps appear red-orange [26,27]. If hydroxyapatite is suspected, alizarin red S stain must be requested specifically from the laboratory as it is not a routine component of the crystal analysis. Calcium oxalate crystals can also induce an inflammatory arthritis: This is generally seen in patients on long-term hemodialysis [28–30] but may also be seen in young patients with primary oxalosis [26]. Clinically, arthritis secondary to calcium oxalate deposition often appears like the other crystalline arthropathies [30] and therefore can only be differentiated by synovianalysis. In this case, synovial fluid typically reveals characteristic bipyramidal crystals as well as polymorphic forms [26].

The yield for all crystals can be increased by spinning the specimen and examining the sediment. If the fluid cannot be examined immediately, it should be refrigerated to preserve the crystals. It is important to note that even in the presence of crystals, infection must be considered because crystals can occur concomitantly with a septic joint.

Other crystals include cryoimmunoglobulins in patients with multiple myeloma and essential cryoglobulinemia [31], and cholesterol crystals in patients with chronic inflammatory arthropathies, such as rheumatoid arthritis. Cholesterol crystals are a nonspecific finding and appear as platelike structures with a notched corner.

GRAM'S STAIN AND CULTURE

The Gram's stain is performed as with other body fluids. It should be performed as soon as possible to screen for the presence of bacteria. It has been reported that the sensitivity of synovial fluid Gram's stain in septic arthritis ranges between 50% and 75% for nongonococcal infection and less than 10% for gonococcal infection [19]. Specificity is much higher; this suggests that a positive Gram's stain, despite a negative culture, should be considered evidence of infection [19]. In fact, it is not uncommon for only the Gram's stain to be positive in the setting of infection [19]. However, the absence of bacteria by Gram's stain does not rule out a septic process.

Synovial fluid in general should be cultured routinely for aerobic and anaerobic bacterial organisms. A positive culture confirms septic arthritis. In certain circumstances (e.g., in chronic monoarticular arthritis), fluid may be cultured for the presence of mycobacteria, fungus, and spirochetes. If disseminated gonorrhea is suspected, the laboratory must be notified because the fluid should be plated directly onto chocolate agar or Thayer-Martin medium. Just as Gram's stain of synovial fluid in gonococcal infection is often negative, so too is synovial fluid culture [32]. Synovial fluid culture is positive approximately 10% to 50% of the time, versus 75% to 95% of the time for nongonococcal infection [19]. However, cultures of genitourinary sites and mucosal sites in gonococcal infection are positive approximately 80% of the time [33]. Therefore, when suspicion of gonococcal arthritis is high (e.g., in a young, healthy, sexually active individual with a dermatitis-arthritis syndrome), the diagnosis must often be confirmed by a positive culture from the urethra, cervix, rectum, or pharynx [32].

In addition to documenting infection and identifying a specific organism, synovial fluid culture can be useful in determining antibiotic sensitivities and subsequent treatment. Furthermore, serial synovial fluid cultures can help in assessing response to therapy. For example, a negative follow-up culture associated with a decrease in synovial fluid polymorphonuclear cell count is highly suggestive of improvement.

Other studies on synovial fluid (e.g., glucose, protein, lactate dehydrogenase, complement, immune complexes) generally are not helpful. Specifically, in a study by Shmerling et al. [34], the investigators observed that synovial fluid glucose and protein were "highly inaccurate." The synovial fluid glucose and protein misclassified effusions as inflammatory versus noninflammatory 50% of the time. In contrast, synovial fluid cell count and differential were found to be reliable and complementary; sensitivity and specificity of cell count was 84% for both and for the differential was 75% and 92%, respectively [34]. Although synovial fluid lactate dehydrogenase was also found to be accurate, it did not offer any additional information above and beyond the cell count and differential. A more recent critical appraisal of synovial fluid analysis was conducted by Swan et al. [35] in 2002. Through a detailed survey of the literature, the authors confirmed the diagnostic value of synovial fluid analysis in cases of acute arthritis when an infectious or crystalline etiology is suspected, and also in cases of intercritical gout. The usefulness of other synovial fluid assays was not supported by the literature [35].

Of note, there are special stains for synovial fluid that can be helpful when the clinical picture correlates; these include Congo red staining for amyloid arthropathy. Amyloid deposits display an apple-green birefringence with polarized light [36,37]. Prussian blue stain for iron deposition may reveal iron in synovial lining cells in hemochromatosis [22]. However, neither of these studies should be considered a routine component of synovial fluid analysis.

REFERENCES

1. Gatter RA. *A Practical Handbook of Joint Fluid Analysis.* Philadelphia, Lea & Febiger, 1984.
2. Stein R. *Manual of Rheumatology and Outpatient Orthopedic Disorders.* Boston, Little, Brown, 1981.
3. Krey PR, Lazaro DM. *Analysis of Synovial Fluid.* Summit, NJ, CIBA-GEIGY, 1992.
4. Ropes MW, Bauer W. *Synovial Fluid Changes in Joint Disease.* Cambridge, MA, Harvard University Press, 1953.
5. Hollander JL, Jessar RA, McCarty DJ: Synovianalysis: an aid in arthritis diagnosis. *Bull Rheum Dis* 12:263, 1961.
6. Gatter RA, McCarty DJ: Synovianalysis: a rapid clinical diagnostic procedure. *Rheumatism* 20:2, 1964.
7. Schumacher HR: Synovial fluid analysis. *Orthop Rev* 13:85, 1984.
8. Greenwald RA: Oxygen radicals inflammation and arthritis: pathophysiological considerations and implications for treatment. *Semin Arthritis Rheum* 20:219, 1991.
9. Robinson DR, Tashjian AH, Levine L: Prostaglandin E2 induced bone resorption by rheumatoid synovia: a model for bone destruction in RA. *J Clin Invest* 56:1181, 1975.
10. Hollander JL, Brown EM Jr, Jessar RA, et al: Hydrocortisone and cortisone injected into arthritic joints. *JAMA* 147:1629, 1951.
11. Gray RG, Tenenbaum J, Gottlieb NL: Local corticosteroid injection treatment in rheumatic disorders. *Semin Arthritis Rheum* 10:231, 1981.
12. Polley HF, Hunder GG: *Rheumatologic Interviewing and Physical Examination of the Joints.* 2nd ed. Philadelphia, WB Saunders, 1978.
13. Doherty M, Hazelman BL, Hutton CW, et al. *Rheumatology Examination and Injection Techniques.* London, WB Saunders, 1992.
14. Hoppenfeld S. *Physical Examination of the Spine and Extremities.* Norwalk, CT, Appleton-Century-Crofts, 1976.
15. Hoder KG, Hunder GG: History and physical examination of the musculoskeletal system, in Harris ED Jr, Budd RC, Firestein GS, et al (eds): *Kelley's Textbook of Rheumatology.* 7th ed. Philadelphia, Elsevier Saunders, 2005; p 483.
16. McCarty DJ Jr: A basic guide to arthrocentesis. *Hosp Med* 4:77, 1968.
17. Gottlieb NL, Riskin WG: Complications of local corticosteroid injections. *JAMA* 243:1547, 1980.
18. Hollander JL: Intrasynovial steroid injections, in Hollander JL, McCarty DL Jr (eds): *Arthritis and Allied Conditions.* 8th ed. Philadelphia, Lea & Febiger, 1972; p 517.
19. Shmerling RH: Synovial fluid analysis. A critical reappraisal. *Rheum Dis Clin North Am* 20(2):503, 1994.
20. Wise C: Arthrocentesis and injection of joints and soft tissues, in Harris ED Jr, Budd RC, Firestein GS, et al (eds): *Kelley's Textbook of Rheumatology.* 7th ed. Philadelphia, Elsevier Saunders, 2005; p 692.
21. Canoso JJ: Aspiration and injection of joints and periarticular tissues, in Hochberg MC, Silman AJ, Smolen JS, et al (eds): *Rheumatology.* 3rd ed. London, Philadelphia, Elsevier, 2003; p 233.
22. Schumacher HR Jr: Synovial fluid analysis, in Katz WA (ed): *Diagnosis and Management of Rheumatic Diseases.* 2nd ed. Philadelphia, JB Lippincott, 1988.
23. Tanphaichitr K, Spilberg I, Hahn B: Lithium heparin crystals simulating calcium pyrophosphate dihydrate crystals in synovial fluid [letter]. *Arthritis Rheum* 9:966, 1976.
24. Kerolus G, Clayburne G, Schumacher HR Jr: Is it mandatory to examine synovial fluids promptly after arthrocentesis? *Arthritis Rheum* 32:271, 1989.
25. Krey PR, Bailen DA: Synovial fluid leukocytosis: a study of extremes. *Am J Med* 67:436, 1979.
26. Reginato AJ, Schumacher HR Jr: Crystal-associated arthropathies. *Clin Geriatr Med* 4(2):295, 1988.
27. Paul H, Reginato AJ, Schumacher HR: Alizarin red S staining as a screening test to detect calcium compounds in synovial fluid. *Arthritis Rheum* 26:191, 1983.
28. Hoffman G, Schumacher HR, Paul H, et al: Calcium oxalate microcrystalline associated arthritis in end stage renal disease. *Ann Intern Med* 97:36, 1982.
29. Reginato AJ, Feweiro JL, Barbazan AC, et al: Arthropathy and cutaneous calcinosis in hemodialysis oxalosis. *Arthritis Rheum* 29:1387, 1986.
30. Schumacher HR, Reginato AJ, Pullman S: Synovial fluid oxalate deposition complicating rheumatoid arthritis with amyloidosis and renal failure. Demonstration of intracellular oxalate crystals. *J Rheumatol* 14:361, 1987.
31. Dornan TL, Blundell JW, Morgan AG: Widespread crystallization of paraprotein in myelomatosis. *QJM* 57:659, 1985.
32. Sack K: Monoarthritis: differential diagnosis. *Am J Med* 102[1A]:30S, 1997.
33. Mahowald ML: Gonococcal arthritis, in Hochberg MC, Silman AJ, Smolen JS, et al (eds): *Rheumatology.* 3rd ed. London, Mosby, 2003; p 1067.
34. Shmerling RH, Delbanco TL, Tosteson ANA, et al: Synovial fluid tests. What should be ordered? *JAMA* 264:1009, 1990.
35. Swan A, Amer H, Dieppe P: The value of synovial fluid assays in the diagnosis of joint disease: a literature survey. *Ann Rheum Dis* 61(6):493, 2002.
36. Lakhanpal S, Li CY, Gertz MA, et al: Synovial fluid analysis for diagnosis of amyloid arthropathy. *Arthritis Rheum* 30(4):419, 1987.
37. Gordon OA, Pruzanski W, Ogryzlo MA: Synovial fluid examination for the diagnosis of amyloidosis. *Ann Rheum Dis* 32:428, 1973.

Mark Dershwitz

CHAPTER **20**

Anesthesia for Bedside Procedures

When a patient in an intensive care unit (ICU) requires a bedside procedure, it is usually the attending intensivist, as opposed to a consultant anesthesiologist, who directs the administration of the necessary hypnotic, analgesic, and/or paralytic drugs. Furthermore, unlike in the operating room, the ICU usually has no equipment for the administration of gaseous (e.g., nitrous oxide) or volatile (e.g., isoflurane) anesthetics. Anesthesia for bedside procedures in the ICU is thus accomplished via a technique involving total intravenous anesthesia (TIVA).

COMMON PAIN MANAGEMENT PROBLEMS IN ICU PATIENTS

DOSING OF AGENT

Selecting the proper dose of an analgesic to administer is problematic for several reasons, including difficulty in assessing the effectiveness of pain relief, pharmacokinetic differences between the critically ill and other patients, and normal physiologic changes associated with aging.

Assessing the Effectiveness of Pain Relief

Critically ill patients often are incapable of communicating their feelings because of delirium, obtundation, or endotracheal intubation. This makes psychological evaluation quite difficult, as surrogate markers of pain intensity, (e.g., tachycardia, hypertension, and diaphoresis) are inherent in the host response to critical illness.

Pharmacokinetic Considerations

Most of the vasopressors and vasodilators administered in the ICU by continuous intravenous (IV) infusion have relatively straightforward pharmacokinetic (PK) behavior: They are water-soluble molecules that are bound very little to plasma proteins. In contrast, the hypnotics and opioids used in TIVA have high lipid solubility and most are extensively bound to plasma proteins, causing their PK behavior to be far more complex. Figure 20-1 shows the disappearance curves of fentanyl and nitroprusside after bolus injection. The fentanyl curve has three phases: a very rapid phase (with a half-life of 0.82 minutes) lasting about 10 minutes, during which the plasma concentration decreases more than 90% from its peak value; an intermediate phase (with a half-life of 17 minutes) lasting from about 10 minutes to an hour; and finally a terminal, very slow phase (with a half-life of 465 minutes) beginning about an hour after bolus injection. After a single bolus injection of fentanyl, the terminal phase occurs at plasma concentrations below which there is a pharmacologic effect. However, after multiple bolus injections or a continuous infusion, this latter phase occurs at therapeutic

plasma concentrations. Thus, fentanyl behaves as a short-acting drug after a single bolus injection but as a very long-lasting drug after a continuous infusion of more than an hour in duration (i.e., fentanyl accumulates). Thus, it is inappropriate to speak of *the* half-life of fentanyl.

The disappearance curve of nitroprusside has two phases: A very rapid phase (with a half-life of 0.89 minute) lasting about 10 minutes, during which the plasma concentration decreases more than 85% from its peak value, and a terminal phase (with a half-life of 14 minutes). It may be slightly slower in offset as compared with fentanyl during the initial 10 minutes after a bolus injection, but it does not accumulate at all even after a prolonged infusion.

The PK behavior of the lipid-soluble hypnotics and analgesics given by infusion may be described by their context-sensitive half-times. This concept may be defined as follows: When a drug is given as an IV bolus followed by an IV infusion designed to maintain a constant plasma drug concentration, the time required for the plasma concentration to fall by 50% after termination of the infusion is the context-sensitive half-time (CSHT) [1]. Figure 20-2 depicts the CSHT curves for the medications most likely to be used for TIVA in ICU patients.

PK behavior in critically ill patients is unlike that in normal subjects for several reasons. Because ICU patients frequently have renal and/or hepatic dysfunction, drug excretion is significantly impaired. Hypoalbuminemia, common in critical illness, decreases protein binding and increases free drug concentration [2]. Because free drug is the only moiety available to tissue receptors, decreased protein binding increases the pharmacologic effect for a given plasma concentration. Alterations in intravascular and extravascular volume status are common in ICU patients and can also affect drug concentration. It is therefore more important in the ICU patient that the doses of medications used for TIVA are individualized for a particular patient.

Physiologic Changes Associated with Aging

People 65 years of age and older comprise the fastest growing segment of the population and constitute the majority of patients in many ICUs. Aging leads to (a) a decrease in total body water and lean body mass; (b) an increase in body fat and, hence, an increase in the volume of distribution of lipid-soluble drugs; and (c) a decrease in drug clearance rates, due to reductions in liver mass, hepatic enzyme activity, liver blood flow, and renal excretory function. There is a progressive, age-dependent increase in pain relief and electroencephalographic suppression among elderly patients receiving the same dose of opioid as younger patients. There is also an increase in CNS depression in elderly patients following administration of identical doses of benzodiazepines.

169

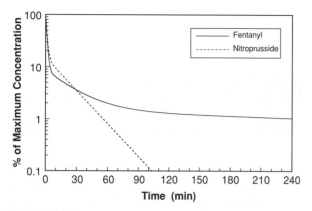

FIGURE 20-1. The time courses, on a semilogarithmic scale, of the plasma concentrations of fentanyl [29] and nitroprusside [30] following a bolus injection. Each concentration is expressed as the percentage of the peak plasma concentration. The fentanyl curve has three phases with half-lives of 0.82, 17, and 465 minutes. The nitroprusside curve has two phases with half-lives of 0.89 and 14 minutes.

SELECTION OF AGENT

Procedures performed in ICUs today span a spectrum that extends from those associated with mild discomfort (e.g., esophagogastroscopy) to those that are quite painful (e.g., orthopaedic manipulations, wound debridement, tracheostomy) (Table 20-1). Depending on their technical difficulty, these procedures can last from minutes to hours. To provide a proper anesthetic, medications should be selected according to the nature of the procedure and titrated according to the patient's response to surgical stimulus. In addition, specific disease states should be considered in order to maximize safety and effectiveness.

Head Trauma

Head-injured patients require a technique that provides effective yet brief anesthesia, so that the capacity to assess neurologic status is not lost for extended periods of time. In addition, the technique must not adversely affect cerebral perfusion pressure. If the effects of the anesthetics dissipate too rapidly, episodes of agitation and increased intracranial pressure may occur that jeopardize cerebral perfusion. In contrast, if the medications

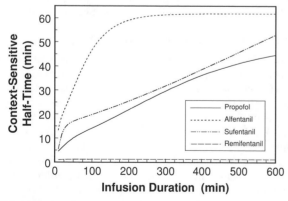

FIGURE 20-2. The context-sensitive half-times for propofol [31], alfentanil [32], sufentanil [33], and remifentanil [34] as a function of infusion duration.

TABLE 20-1. Bedside Procedures and Associated Levels of Discomfort

Mildly to moderately uncomfortable
  Transesophageal echocardiography[a]
  Transtracheal aspiration
  Thoracentesis[a]
  Paracentesis[a]
Moderately to severely uncomfortable
  Endotracheal intubation[a]
  Flexible bronchoscopy[a]
  Thoracostomy[a]
  Bone marrow biopsy
  Colonoscopy
  Peritoneal dialysis catheter insertion[a]
  Peritoneal lavage[a]
  Percutaneous gastrostomy[a]
  Percutaneous intraaortic balloon insertion[a]
Extremely painful
  Rigid bronchoscopy
  Debridement of open wounds
  Dressing changes
  Orthopaedic manipulations
  Tracheostomy[a]
  Pericardiocentesis/pericardial window[a]
  Open lung biopsy
  Ventriculostomy[a]

---

[a]Procedures in which the level of discomfort may be significantly mitigated by the use of local anesthesia.

---

last too long, there may be difficulty in making an adequate neurologic assessment following the procedure.

Coronary Artery Disease

Postoperative myocardial ischemia following cardiac and noncardiac surgery strongly predicts adverse outcome [3]. Accordingly, sufficient analgesia should be provided during and after invasive procedures to reduce plasma catecholamine and stress hormone levels.

Renal and/or Hepatic Failure

The association between sepsis and acute renal failure has been recognized for many years. Risk of an adverse drug reaction is at least 3 times higher in azotemic patients than in those with normal renal function. This risk is magnified by excessive unbound drug or drug metabolite(s) in the circulation and changes in the target tissue(s) induced by the uremic state.

Liver failure alters the volumes of distribution of many drugs by impairing synthesis of the two major plasma-binding proteins, albumin and α_1-acid glycoprotein. In addition, reductions in hepatic blood flow and hepatic enzymatic activity decrease drug clearance rates.

CHARACTERISTICS OF SPECIFIC AGENTS USED FOR BEDSIDE PROCEDURES

HYPNOTICS

The characteristics of the hypnotics are listed in Table 20-2. When rapid awakening is desired, propofol or etomidate are the hypnotic agents of choice. Ketamine may be useful when a longer duration of anesthesia is needed. Midazolam is rarely used alone as a hypnotic; however, its profound anxiolytic and

TABLE 20-2.   Characteristics of Intravenous Hypnotic Agents[a]

	Propofol	*Etomidate*	*Ketamine*	*Midazolam*	*Fospropofol*[b]
Bolus dose (mg/kg)	1–2	0.2–0.3	1–2	0.05–0.1	5–12
Onset	Fast	Fast	Fast	**Intermediate**	**Intermediate**
Duration	Short	Short	Intermediate	Intermediate	Short
Cardiovascular effects	↓	**None**	↑	Minimal	↓
Respiratory effects	↓	↓	**Minimal**	↓	↓
Analgesia	None	None	**Profound**	None	None
Amnesia	Mild	Mild	**Profound**	**Profound**	Mild

[a]The listed doses should be reduced 50% in elderly patients. Entries in bold type indicate noteworthy differences among the drugs.
[b]These parameters are based on a single study in normal volunteers [18]. The behavior of this investigational medication in critically ill patients requires further investigation.

amnestic effects render it useful in combination with other agents.

Propofol

DESCRIPTION.   Propofol is a hypnotic agent associated with pleasant emergence and little hangover. It has essentially replaced thiopental for induction of anesthesia, especially in outpatients. It is extremely popular because it is readily titratable and has more rapid onset and offset kinetics than midazolam. Thus, patients emerge from anesthesia more rapidly after propofol than after midazolam, a factor that may make propofol the preferred agent for sedation and hypnosis in general, and in particular for patients with altered level of consciousness.

The CSHT for propofol is about 10 minutes following a 1-hour infusion, and the CSHT increases about 5 minutes for each additional hour of infusion for the first several hours, as shown in Figure 20-2. Thus, the CSHT is about 20 minutes after a 3-hour infusion. The CSHT rises much more slowly for infusions longer than a day; a patient who is sedated (but not rendered unconscious) with propofol for 2 weeks will recover in approximately 3 hours [4]. This rapid recovery of neurologic status makes propofol a good sedative in ICU patients, especially those with head trauma, who may not tolerate mechanical ventilation without pharmacologic sedation.

Even though recovery following termination of a continuous infusion is faster with propofol than with midazolam, a comparative trial showed that the two drugs were roughly equivalent in effectiveness for overnight sedation of ICU patients [5]. For long-term sedation (e.g., more than 1 day), however, recovery is significantly faster in patients given propofol.

In spontaneously breathing patients sedated with propofol, respiratory rate appears to be a more predictable sign of adequate sedation than hemodynamic changes. The ventilatory response to rebreathing carbon dioxide during a maintenance propofol infusion is similar to that induced by other sedative drugs (i.e., propofol significantly decreases the slope of the carbon dioxide response curve). Nevertheless, spontaneously breathing patients anesthetized with propofol are able to maintain normal end-tidal carbon dioxide values during minor surgical procedures.

Bolus doses of propofol in the range of 1 to 2 mg per kg induce loss of consciousness within 30 seconds. Maintenance infusion rates of 100 to 200 μg per kg per minute are adequate

in younger subjects, whereas doses should be reduced by 20% to 50% in elderly individuals.

ADVERSE EFFECTS

Cardiovascular.   Propofol depresses ventricular systolic function and lowers afterload but has no effect on diastolic function [6,7]. Vasodilation results from calcium channel blockade. In patients undergoing coronary artery bypass surgery, propofol (2 mg per kg IV bolus) produced a 23% fall in mean arterial blood pressure, a 20% increase in heart rate, and a 26% decrease in stroke volume. In pigs, propofol caused a dose-related depression of sinus node and His-Purkinje system functions, but had no effect on atrioventricular node function or on the conduction properties of atrial and ventricular tissues. In patients with coronary artery disease, propofol administration may be associated with a reduction in coronary perfusion pressure and increased myocardial lactate production [8].

Neurologic.   Propofol may improve neurologic outcome and reduce neuronal damage by depressing cerebral metabolism. Propofol decreases cerebral oxygen consumption, cerebral blood flow, and cerebral glucose use in humans and animals to the same degree as reported for thiopental and etomidate [9]. Propofol frequently causes pain when injected into a peripheral vein. Injection pain is less likely if the injection site is located proximally on the arm or if the injection is made via a central venous catheter.

Metabolic.   The emulsion used as the vehicle for propofol contains soybean oil and lecithin and supports bacterial growth; iatrogenic contamination leading to septic shock is possible. Currently available propofol preparations contain ethylenediaminetetraacetic acid (EDTA), metabisulfite, or benzyl alcohol as a bacteriostatic agent. Because EDTA chelates trace metals, particularly zinc, serum zinc levels should be measured daily during continuous propofol infusions. Hyperlipidemia may occur, particularly in infants and small children. Accordingly, triglyceride levels should be monitored daily in this population whenever propofol is administered continuously for more than 24 hours. An investigational water-soluble prodrug of propofol, fospropofol, may be available in the future (see later discussion).

Etomidate

DESCRIPTION.   Etomidate has onset and offset PK characteristics similar to propofol and it has an unrivaled cardiovascular profile, even in the setting of cardiomyopathy [10]. Not only does etomidate lack significant effects on myocardial contractility, but baseline sympathetic output and baroreflex regulation of sympathetic activity are well preserved. Etomidate depresses in a dose-related manner cerebral oxygen metabolism and blood flow without changing the intracranial volume-pressure relationship.

Etomidate is particularly useful (rather than thiopental or propofol) in certain patient subsets: hypovolemic patients, multiple trauma victims with closed-head injury, and those with low ejection fraction, severe aortic stenosis, left main coronary artery disease, or severe cerebral vascular disease. Etomidate may be contraindicated in patients with established or evolving septic shock because of its inhibition of cortisol synthesis [11]. The coadministration of a glucocorticoid with etomidate may be logical, but this regimen has not been evaluated by clinical trials.

ADVERSE EFFECTS
Metabolic. Etomidate, when given by prolonged infusion, may increase mortality associated with low plasma cortisol levels [12]. Even single doses of etomidate can produce adrenal cortical suppression lasting 24 hours or more in healthy patients undergoing elective surgery [13]. These effects are more pronounced as the dose is increased or if continuous infusions are used for sedation. Etomidate-induced adrenocortical suppression occurs because the drug blocks a key step in the metabolic pathway in adrenal steroidogenesis. It is also noteworthy that etomidate causes the highest incidence of postoperative nausea and vomiting of any of the IV anesthetic agents.

Ketamine

DESCRIPTION. Ketamine induces a state of sedation, amnesia, and marked analgesia in which the patient experiences a strong feeling of dissociation from the environment. It is unique among the hypnotics in that it reliably induces unconsciousness by the intramuscular route. Ketamine is rapidly metabolized by the liver to norketamine, which is pharmacologically active. Ketamine is both slower in onset and offset as compared with propofol or etomidate following IV infusion.

Many clinicians consider ketamine to be the analgesic of choice in patients with a history of bronchospasm. In the usual dosage, it decreases airway resistance, probably by blocking norepinephrine uptake, which in turn stimulates β-adrenergic receptors in the lungs. In contrast to many β-agonist bronchodilators, ketamine is not arrhythmogenic when given to asthmatic patients receiving aminophylline.

Ketamine may be safer than other hypnotics or opioids in unintubated patients because it depresses airway reflexes and respiratory drive to a lesser degree. It may be particularly useful for procedures near the airway, where physical access and ability to secure an airway is limited (e.g., gunshot wounds to the face). Because ketamine increases salivary and tracheobronchial secretions, an anticholinergic (e.g., 0.2 mg glycopyrrolate) should be given prior to its administration. In patients with borderline hypoxemia despite maximal therapy, ketamine may be the drug of choice as ketamine does not inhibit hypoxic pulmonary vasoconstriction.

Another major feature that distinguishes ketamine from most other IV anesthetics is that it stimulates the cardiovascular system (i.e., raises heart rate and blood pressure). This action appears to result both from direct stimulation of the CNS with increased

sympathetic nervous system outflow and from blockade of norepinephrine reuptake in adrenergic nerves.

Because pulmonary hypertension is a characteristic feature of acute respiratory distress syndrome, drugs that increase right ventricular afterload should be avoided. In infants with either normal or elevated pulmonary vascular resistance, ketamine does not affect pulmonary vascular resistance as long as constant ventilation is maintained, a finding also confirmed in adults.

Cerebral blood flow does not change when ketamine is injected into cerebral vessels. In mechanically ventilated pigs with artificially produced intracranial hypertension in which intracranial pressure (ICP) is on the shoulder of the compliance curve, 0.5 to 2.0 mg per kg IV ketamine does not raise ICP; likewise, in mechanically ventilated preterm infants, 2 mg per kg IV ketamine does not increase anterior fontanelle pressure, an indirect monitor of ICP [14,15]. Unlike propofol and etomidate, however, ketamine does not lower cerebral metabolic rate. It is relatively contraindicated in patients with an intracranial mass, with increased ICP, or who have suffered recent head trauma.

ADVERSE EFFECTS
Psychological. Emergence phenomena following ketamine anesthesia have been described as floating sensations, vivid dreams (pleasant or unpleasant), hallucinations, and delirium. These effects are more common in patients older than 16 years, in females, after short operative procedures, after large doses (greater than 2 mg per kg IV), and after rapid administration (greater than 40 mg per minute). Precurrent or concurrent treatment with benzodiazepines or propofol usually minimizes or prevents these phenomena [16].

Cardiovascular. Because ketamine increases myocardial oxygen consumption, there is risk of precipitating myocardial ischemia in patients with coronary artery disease if ketamine is used alone. On the other hand, combinations of ketamine plus diazepam, ketamine plus midazolam, or ketamine plus sufentanil are well tolerated for induction in patients undergoing coronary artery bypass surgery. Repeated bolus doses are often associated with tachycardia. This can be reduced by administering ketamine as a constant infusion.

Ketamine produces myocardial depression in the isolated animal heart. Hypotension has been reported following ketamine administration in hemodynamically compromised patients with chronic catecholamine depletion.

Neurologic. Ketamine does not lower the minimal electroshock seizure threshold in mice. When administered with aminophylline, however, a clinically apparent reduction in seizure threshold is observed.

Midazolam

DESCRIPTION. Although capable of inducing unconsciousness in high doses, midazolam is more commonly used as a sedative. Along with its sedating effects, midazolam produces anxiolysis, amnesia, and relaxation of skeletal muscle.

Anterograde amnesia following midazolam (5 mg IV) peaks 2 to 5 minutes after IV injection and lasts 20 to 40 minutes. Because midazolam is highly (95%) protein-bound (to albumin), drug effect is likely to be exaggerated in ICU patients. Recovery from midazolam is prolonged in obese and elderly patients and following continuous infusion because it accumulates to a significant degree. In patients with renal failure, active conjugated metabolites of midazolam may accumulate and delay recovery. Although flumazenil may be used to reverse excessive sedation or respiratory depression from midazolam, its duration of action is only 15 to 20 minutes. In addition, flumazenil may precipitate acute anxiety reactions or seizures, particularly in patients receiving chronic benzodiazepine therapy.

Midazolam causes dose-dependent reductions in cerebral metabolic rate and cerebral blood flow, suggesting that it may be beneficial in patients with cerebral ischemia.

Due to its combined sedative, anxiolytic, and amnestic properties, midazolam is ideally suited both for brief, relatively painless procedures (e.g., endoscopy) and for prolonged sedation (e.g., during mechanical ventilation).

ADVERSE EFFECTS

Respiratory. Midazolam (0.15 mg per kg IV) depresses the slope of the carbon dioxide response curve and increases the dead space–tidal volume ratio and arterial P_{CO_2}. Respiratory depression is even more marked and prolonged in patients with chronic obstructive pulmonary disease. Midazolam also blunts the ventilatory response to hypoxia.

Cardiovascular. Small (less than 10%) increases in heart rate and small decreases in systemic vascular resistance are frequently observed after administration of midazolam. It has no significant effects on coronary vascular resistance or autoregulation.

Neurologic. Because recovery of cognitive and psychomotor function may be delayed for up to 24 hours, midazolam as the sole hypnotic may not be appropriate in situations where rapid return of consciousness and psychomotor function are a high priority.

Fospropofol

Fospropofol is a water-soluble prodrug of propofol. Fospropofol is metabolized to propofol by the action of alkaline phosphatase. The peak hypnotic effect occurs in about 10 minutes following a bolus injection. The kinetic disposition of liberated propofol differs from that of injected propofol emulsion, with the former being slower for reasons that are as yet unexplained [17,18].

Apparent advantages of an aqueous solution of fospropofol are the reduced risk of bacterial contamination as compared with propofol emulsion and the absence of a lipid load that has been associated with organ toxicity during long-term infusions of propofol emulsion. Whether the new medication causes less pain on injection remains to be determined. It may find utility for sedation in the intensive care unit.

OPIOIDS

Morphine

DESCRIPTION. Pain relief by morphine and its surrogates is relatively selective in that other sensory modalities (touch, vibration, vision, hearing) are not obtunded. Opioids blunt pain by (a) inhibiting pain processing by the dorsal horn of the spinal cord, (b) decreasing transmission of pain by activating descending inhibitory pathways in the brainstem, and (c) altering the emotional response to pain by actions on the limbic cortex.

Various types of opioid receptors (denoted by Greek letters) have been discovered in the CNS. The classic pharmacologic effects of morphine-like analgesia and ventilatory depression are mediated by μ receptors. Other μ effects include sedation, euphoria, tolerance and physical dependence, decreased gastrointestinal motility, biliary spasm, and miosis. The κ receptor shares a number of effects with the μ receptor, including analgesia, sedation, and ventilatory depression. The δ receptor is responsible for mediating some of the analgesic effects of the endogenous opioid peptides, especially in the spinal cord. Few of the clinically used opioids have significant activity at δ receptors at the usual analgesic doses.

Morphine is a substrate for the P-glycoprotein, a protein responsible for the transport of many molecules out of cells. The combination of slow CNS penetration due to lower lipid solubility and rapid efflux accounts for the slow onset of morphine's CNS effects. Peak analgesic effects may not occur for over an hour after IV injection; hence, the plasma profile of morphine does not parallel its clinical effects [19].

Morphine is unique among the opioids in causing significant histamine release after IV injection that occurs almost immediately. The beneficial effect of giving morphine to a patient with acute pulmonary edema is far more related to this hemodynamic effect rather than to its analgesic and sedating effects.

ADVERSE EFFECTS

Gastrointestinal. Constipation, nausea, and/or vomiting are well-described side effects of morphine administration. Reduced gastric emptying and bowel motility (both small and large intestine), often leading to adynamic ileus, appear to be mediated both peripherally (by opioid receptors located in the gut) and centrally (by the vagus nerve).

Cardiovascular. Hypotension is not unusual following morphine administration, especially if it is given rapidly (i.e., 5 to 10 mg per minute). In patients pretreated with both H_1- and H_2-antagonists, the hypotensive response following morphine administration is significantly attenuated, despite comparable increases in plasma histamine concentrations. These data strongly implicate histamine as the mediator of these changes.

Respiratory. Morphine administration is followed by a dose-dependent reduction in responsiveness of brainstem respiratory centers to carbon dioxide. Key features of this phenomenon include a reduction in the slope of the ventilatory and occlusion pressure responses to carbon dioxide, a rightward shift of the minute ventilatory response to hypercarbia, and an increase in resting end-tidal carbon dioxide and the apneic threshold (i.e., the P_{CO_2} value below which spontaneous ventilation is not initiated without hypoxemia). The duration of these effects often exceeds the time course of analgesia. In addition to blunting the carbon dioxide response, morphine decreases hypoxic ventilatory drive. Morphine administration in renal failure patients has been associated with prolonged respiratory depression secondary to persistence of its active metabolite, morphine-6-glucuronide [20].

The administration of small doses of IV naloxone (40 μg) to patients in order to reverse the ventilatory depressant effect of morphine may produce some adverse effects. Anecdotal reports describe the precipitation of vomiting, delirium, arrhythmias, pulmonary edema, cardiac arrest, and sudden death subsequent to naloxone administration in otherwise healthy patients after surgery. Furthermore, the duration of action of naloxone is shorter than any of the opioids it may be used to antagonize (except remifentanil). Recurring ventilatory depression therefore remains a distinct possibility and in the spontaneously breathing patient is a source of potential morbidity.

Reversal with a mixed opioid agonist-antagonist such as nalbuphine or butorphanol appears to be safer than with naloxone. Mixed opioid agonist-antagonist agents may either increase or decrease the opioid effect, depending on the dose administered, the particular agonist already present, and the amount of agonist remaining.

For bedside procedures in the ICU, many of these problems can be obviated by using a shorter-acting opioid.

Neurologic. Morphine has little effect on cerebral metabolic rate or cerebral blood flow when ventilation is controlled. Morphine may affect cerebral perfusion pressure adversely by lowering mean arterial pressure.

Fentanyl and Its Congeners

DESCRIPTION. Fentanyl, alfentanil, sufentanil, and remifentanil enter and leave the CNS much more rapidly than morphine, thereby causing a much faster onset of effect after IV administration. The only significant difference among these agents is their PK behavior.

Fentanyl may be useful when given by intermittent bolus injection (50 to 100 μg), but when given by infusion its duration becomes prolonged [21]. Alfentanil, originally marketed as an "ultra-short" duration medication, is not; Figure 20-2 shows that its CSHT is almost an hour after a 2-hour infusion. Thus, for TIVA in ICU patients in whom rapid emergence is desirable, sufentanil or remifentanil are the preferred choices for continuous infusion. When the procedure is expected to be followed by postoperative pain, sufentanil is preferred. Figure 20-2 shows that its CSHT is similar to that of propofol for infusions of up to 10 hours. When the procedure is expected to be followed by minimal postoperative pain (e.g., bronchoscopy), remifentanil is preferred. Its CSHT is about 4 minutes, regardless of the duration of the infusion.

Remifentanil owes its extremely short duration to rapid metabolism by tissue esterases, primarily in skeletal muscle [22]. Its PK behavior is unchanged in the presence of severe hepatic [23] or renal [24] failure.

Sufentanil infusion for TIVA may be initiated with a 0.5- to 1.5-μg per kg bolus followed by an infusion at 0.01 to 0.03 μg per kg per minute. If given with a propofol infusion, the two infusions may be stopped simultaneously as governed by the curves in Figure 20-2. Remifentanil infusion for TIVA may be initiated with a 0.5- to 1.5-μg per kg bolus followed by an infusion at 0.05 to 0.5 μg per kg per minute. The remifentanil infusion should be continued until after the procedure is completed; if the patient is expected to have postoperative pain, another opioid should be given because the remifentanil effect will dissipate within a few minutes.

ADVERSE EFFECTS
Cardiovascular. Although fentanyl, sufentanil, alfentanil, and remifentanil do not affect plasma histamine concentrations, bolus doses can be associated with hypotension, especially when infused rapidly (i.e., less than 1 minute). This action is related to medullary vasomotor center depression and vagal nucleus stimulation.

Neurologic. Fentanyl and sufentanil have been reported to increase ICP in ventilated patients following head trauma. Fen-

tanyl, sufentanil, and alfentanil may adversely affect cerebral perfusion pressure by lowering mean arterial pressure. All of the fentanyl derivatives may cause chest wall rigidity when a large bolus is given rapidly. This effect may be mitigated by neuromuscular blocking agents as well as by coadministration of a hypnotic agent.

NEUROMUSCULAR BLOCKING AGENTS

There are two pharmacologic classes of neuromuscular blocking (NMB) agents: depolarizing agents (e.g., succinylcholine) and nondepolarizing agents (e.g., vecuronium, cisatracurium). Succinylcholine is an agonist at the nicotinic acetylcholine receptor of the neuromuscular junction. Administration of succinylcholine causes an initial intense stimulation of skeletal muscle, manifested as fasciculations, followed by paralysis due to continuing depolarization. Nondepolarizing agents are competitive antagonists of acetylcholine at the neuromuscular junction; they prevent acetylcholine, released in response to motor nerve impulses, from binding to its receptor and initiating muscle contraction. Distinctions among the nondepolarizing agents are made based on PK differences as well as by their cardiovascular effects. Table 20-3 summarizes the NMB agents.

NMB agents are used to facilitate endotracheal intubation and to improve surgical conditions by decreasing skeletal muscle tone. Prior to intubation, the administration of an NMB agent will result in paralysis of the vocal cords, increasing the ease with which the endotracheal tube may be inserted and decreasing the risk of vocal cord trauma. During surgery, the decrease in skeletal muscle tone may aid in surgical exposure (as during abdominal surgery), decrease the insufflation pressure needed during laparoscopic procedures, and make joint manipulation easier during orthopaedic surgery. NMB agents should *not* be used to prevent patient movement, which is indicative of inadequate anesthesia. Dosing of NMB agents should be based on monitoring evoked twitch response; ablation of two to three twitches of the train-of-four is sufficient for the majority of surgical procedures and permits easy reversal.

Succinylcholine

DESCRIPTION. Succinylcholine has the fastest onset and shortest duration of the NMB agents. A dose of 1 mg per kg of succinylcholine will result in fasciculations within seconds, and excellent intubating conditions in less than a minute. Succinylcholine is usually considered the drug of choice when the airway must be quickly secured, such as when the patient has a full stomach or has symptomatic gastroesophageal reflux.

A small dose (e.g., 0.5 mg of vecuronium) of a nondepolarizing agent given before succinylcholine will prevent the fasciculations caused by succinylcholine. There is a delay in onset (to about 1.5 minutes) of the peak effect of succinylcholine when it is given following a small dose of a nondepolarizing agent.

Succinylcholine is metabolized by plasma cholinesterase, a circulating enzyme. In most people, its duration of action will be about 5 to 10 minutes. There are a number of inherited abnormalities of plasma cholinesterase, which may prolong the duration of succinylcholine. If a patient is deficient in plasma cholinesterase but has normal renal function, succinylcholine will be eliminated unchanged with a half-life of about 20 to 30 minutes.

TABLE 20-3. Characteristics of the Neuromuscular Blocking Agents

Drug	Indication	Dose (mg/kg)	Onset (min)	Time to 25% Recovery (min)
Succinylcholine	Routine intubation	1	0.7	10
	Rapid sequence intubation			
Rocuronium	Rapid sequence intubation in a patient in whom succinylcholine is contraindicated	0.6	1.5	40
		1.2	1.1	70
Cisatracurium	Intubation and/or maintenance for a case of up to several hours in duration	0.1	3	40
		0.2	2	60
Vecuronium	Intubation and/or maintenance for a case of up to several hours in duration	0.1	2	50
Pancuronium	Maintenance of long-term muscle paralysis by infusion at a rate of 0.025–0.050 mg/kg/hr	0.1	3	90

ADVERSE EFFECTS

Neurologic. Succinylcholine may trigger malignant hyperthermia in genetically susceptible persons. Its use in the pediatric population is controversial because of the possibility that a child may have a genetically determined myopathy, associated with malignant hyperthermia, that has not yet become symptomatic.

Succinylcholine may cause a malignant rise in the extracellular potassium concentration in patients with major acute burns, upper or lower motor neuron lesions, prolonged immobility, massive crush injuries, and various myopathies. Although the usual doses of succinylcholine cause a transient increase in the plasma potassium concentration of about 0.5 mEq/L, preexisting hyperkalemia is generally not a contraindication to its use.

Cardiovascular. Succinylcholine often causes transient tachycardia due to its vagolytic effect. Interestingly, a second dose of succinylcholine, given prior to the complete dissipation of the first dose, may cause bradycardia or asystole. Preceding such a second dose with a dose of atropine or glycopyrrolate will prevent this vagomimetic effect.

Nondepolarizing NMB Agents

DESCRIPTION. Vecuronium, rocuronium, and cisatracurium are commonly used to facilitate intubation in persons in whom succinylcholine is contraindicated. They are also used for maintenance of muscle paralysis for surgical procedures lasting up to several hours. These three agents are essentially devoid of cardiovascular effects, and the choice among them is usually made on the basis of desired PK parameters as listed in Table 20-3. Vecuronium and rocuronium are metabolized by the liver; their durations may be increased in persons with hepatic dysfunction or decreased in persons taking medications that induce hepatic cytochrome P450 (e.g., phenytoin). Cisatracurium is metabolized both enzymatically (by plasma cholinesterase) and by nonenzymatic ester hydrolysis that occurs at physiologic pH; the drug is supplied at an acidic pH, and kept refrigerated prior to use, to prevent this nonenzymatic degradation. The PK of cisatracurium is thus affected less by coexisting disease (e.g., hepatic or renal dysfunction) or by interaction with concomitantly administered medications.

Pancuronium is a longer-lasting NMB agent. In the ICU, it may be used for longer-term therapy to facilitate mechanical ventilation. Pancuronium has a vagolytic effect that may cause tachycardia and that may persist throughout its administration. Doses of these medications are listed in Table 20-3.

ADVERSE EFFECTS. Any patient receiving NMB agents should be properly sedated. Longer-term therapy with NMB agents may cause muscle weakness persisting for months afterward. The risk factors for developing such a myopathy are coadministration with a glucocorticoid and long duration of NMB therapy [25]. It is controversial whether NMB agents in the steroidal class (pancuronium, vecuronium, rocuronium) have a higher propensity of causing myopathy than the NMB agents in the benzylisoquinoline class (atracurium, cisatracurium, mivacurium).

Reversal of Muscle Paralysis

When there is no longer any need for muscle paralysis, it is reasonable to permit the agent to wear off *as long as the patient remains properly sedated until muscle strength has recovered.* Adequate recovery of muscle strength is indicated by the absence of fade using the double-burst mode of the evoked twitch response.

Alternatively, pharmacologic reversal of muscle paralysis may be achieved by the administration of an anticholinesterase such as neostigmine, 0.04 to 0.06 mg per kg. To counter the parasympathomimetic effects of neostigmine, glycopyrrolate, 0.008 to 0.012 mg per kg, is given concomitantly.

PRACTICAL CONSIDERATIONS FOR TIVA

Electing to perform common procedures (e.g., tracheostomy, percutaneous gastrostomy) in the ICU instead of the operating room represents a potential cost savings of tremendous scope. Not only does this strategy eradicate costly operating room time and support resources, it eliminates misadventures that sometimes occur in hallways and on elevators. Cost analyses estimate an average overall cost reduction of 50% or more compared with traditional operative procedures [26]. TIVA represents the most cost-effective method of facilitating this.

In most patients, safe and effective TIVA may be achieved via the infusions of propofol plus sufentanil or propofol plus remifentanil. Premedication with midazolam decreases the required propofol doses and decreases the likelihood of recall for intraoperative events. Bolus doses should not be used in hemodynamically unstable patients, and lower bolus doses should be used in elderly individuals. NMB agents are also given if needed.

The opioid infusion rate is titrated to minimize signs of inadequate analgesia (e.g., tachycardia, tachypnea, hypertension, sweating, mydriasis), although differentiation of pain from the sympathetic responses to critical illness is difficult. The propofol infusion rate is titrated to the end point of loss of consciousness; the new depth of anesthesia monitors (bispectral index or patient state index) facilitate locating this end point more accurately. Loss of consciousness should be achieved prior to the initiation of muscle paralysis. It is possible for patients to be completely aware of intraoperative events at times when there is no change in hemodynamics or any manifestation of increased sympathetic activity [27,28]. Hence, administering an opioid to blunt incisional pain without inducing loss of consciousness with a hypnotic is inappropriate.

The following additional points deserve consideration in this context:

1. In subhypnotic doses, propofol is less effective than midazolam in producing amnesia. In the absence of coadministration of a benzodiazepine, propofol must cause unconsciousness in order to reliably prevent recall. Prompt treatment of patient responses (movement, tachycardia, hypertension) is important.

2. Medications infused for TIVA should be given via a carrier IV fluid running continuously at a rate of at least 50 mL per hour. This method not only helps deliver medication into the circulation, it also serves as another monitor of occlusion of the drug delivery system. Occlusion of the infusion line for more than a few minutes may lead to patient awareness.

3. In order to take advantage of the known CSHT values for the TIVA agents, communication with the surgeon during the procedure is important in order to anticipate the optimum time for stopping the infusions. The sufentanil and propofol infusions are stopped in advance of the end of the procedure, while remifentanil is infused until the procedure is complete.

4. To maintain reasonably constant propofol and sufentanil blood concentrations, the maintenance infusion rates should be decreased during the procedure because the plasma concentrations increase over time at constant infusion rates. An approximate guideline is a 10% reduction in the infusion rate every 30 minutes.

5. Strict aseptic technique is especially important during the handling of propofol.

REFERENCES

1. Hughes MA, Glass PSA, Jacobs JR: Context-sensitive half-time in multicompartment pharmacokinetic models for intravenous anesthetic drugs. *Anesthesiology* 76:334, 1992.
2. Koch-Weser J, Sellers EM: Binding of drugs to serum albumin. *N Engl J Med* 294:311, 1976.
3. Mangano DT, Browner WS, Hollenberg M: Association of perioperative myocardial ischemia with cardiac morbidity and mortality in men undergoing noncardiac surgery. *N Engl J Med* 323:1781, 1990.
4. Barr J, Egan TD, Sandoval NF, et al: Propofol dosing regimens for ICU sedation based upon an integrated pharmacokinetic-pharmacodynamic model, *Anesthesiology* 95:324, 2001.
5. Ronan KP, Gallagher TH, Hamby BG: Comparison of propofol and midazolam for sedation in intensive care unit patients. *Crit Care Med* 23:286, 1995.
6. Pagel PS, Warltier DC: Negative inotropic effects of propofol as evaluated by the regional preload recruitable stroke work relationship in chronically instrumented dogs. *Anesthesiology* 78:100, 1993.
7. Pagel PS, Schmeling WT, Kampine JP, et al: Alteration of canine left ventricular diastolic function by intravenous anesthetics in vivo: ketamine and propofol. *Anesthesiology* 76:419, 1992.
8. Mayer N, Legat K, Weinstabl C, et al: Effects of propofol on the function of normal, collateral-dependent, and ischemic myocardium. *Anesth Analg* 76:33, 1993.
9. Van Hemelrijck J, Fitch W, Mattheussen M, et al: Effect of propofol on cerebral circulation and autoregulation in baboons. *Anesth Analg* 71:49, 1990.
10. Goading JM, Wang JT, Smith RA, et al: Cardiovascular and pulmonary responses following etomidate induction of anesthesia in patients with demonstrated cardiac disease. *Anesth Analg* 58:40, 1979.
11. Jackson WJ: Should we use etomidate as an induction agent for endotracheal intubation in patients with septic shock? A critical appraisal. *Chest* 127:1031, 2005.
12. Ledingham IM, Finlay WEI, Watt I, et al: Etomidate and adrenocortical function. *Lancet* 1:1434, 1983.
13. Fragen RJ, Shanks CA, Molteni A, et al: Effects of etomidate on hormonal responses to surgical stress. *Anesthesiology* 61:652, 1984.
14. Pfenninger E, Dick W, Ahnefeld FW: The influence of ketamine on both normal and raised intracranial pressure of artificially ventilated animals. *Eur J Anaesthesiol* 2:297, 1985.
15. Friesen RH, Thieme RE, Honda AT, et al: Changes in anterior fontanel pressure in preterm neonates receiving isoflurane, halothane, fentanyl, or ketamine. *Anesth Analg* 66:431, 1987.
16. White PF: Pharmacologic interactions of midazolam and ketamine in surgical patients. *Clin Pharmacol Ther* 31:280, 1982.
17. Gibiansky E, Struys MMRF, Gibiansky L, et al: Aquavan® injection, a water-soluble prodrug of propofol, as a bolus injection: a phase I dose-escalation comparison with Diprivan® (Part 1). *Anesthesiology* 103:718, 2005.
18. Struys MMRF, Vanluchene ALG, Gibiansky E, et al: Aquavan® injection, a water-soluble prodrug of propofol, as a bolus injection: a phase I dose-escalation comparison with Diprivan® (Part 2). *Anesthesiology* 103:730, 2005.
19. Dershwitz M, Walsh JL, Morishige RJ, et al: Pharmacokinetics and pharmacodynamics of inhaled versus intravenous morphine in healthy volunteers. *Anesthesiology* 93:619, 2000.
20. Aitkenhead AR, Vater M, Achola K, et al: Pharmacokinetics of single-dose intravenous morphine in normal volunteers and patients with end-stage renal failure. *Br J Anaesth* 56:813, 1984.
21. Shafer SL, Varvel JR: Pharmacokinetics, pharmacodynamics, and rational opioid selection. *Anesthesiology* 74:53, 1991.
22. Dershwitz M, Rosow CE: Remifentanil: an opioid metabolized by esterases. *Exp Opin Invest Drugs* 5:1361, 1996.
23. Dershwitz M, Hoke JF, Rosow CE, et al: Pharmacokinetics and pharmacodynamics of remifentanil in volunteer subjects with severe liver disease. *Anesthesiology* 84:812, 1996.
24. Hoke JF, Shlugman D, Dershwitz M, et al: Pharmacokinetics and pharmacodynamics of remifentanil in subjects with renal failure compared to healthy volunteers. *Anesthesiology* 87:533, 1997.
25. Leatherman JW, Fluegel WL, David WS, et al: Muscle weakness in mechanically ventilated patients with severe asthma. *Am J Respir Crit Care Med* 153:1686, 1996.
26. Barba CA, Angood PB, Kauder DR, et al: Bronchoscopic guidance makes percutaneous tracheostomy a safe, cost effective, and easy to teach procedure. *Surgery* 118:879, 1995.
27. Ausems ME, Hug CC Jr, Stanski DR, et al: Plasma concentrations of alfentanil required to supplement nitrous oxide anesthesia for general surgery. *Anesthesiology* 65:362, 1986.
28. Philbin DM, Rosow CE, Schneider RC, et al: Fentanyl and sufentanil anesthesia revisited: how much is enough? *Anesthesiology* 73:5, 1990.
29. Shafer SL, Varvel JR, Aziz N, et al: Pharmacokinetics of fentanyl administered by computer-controlled infusion pump. *Anesthesiology* 73:1091, 1990.
30. Vesey CJ, Sweeney B, Cole PV: Decay of nitroprusside. II: in vivo. *Br J Anaesth* 64:704, 1990.
31. Shafer A, Doze VA, Shafer SL: Pharmacokinetics and pharmacodynamics of propofol infusions during general anesthesia. *Anesthesiology* 69:348, 1988.
32. Scott JC, Stanski DR: Decreased fentanyl and alfentanil dose requirements with age. A simultaneous pharmacokinetic and pharmacodynamic evaluation. *J Pharmacol Exp Ther* 240:159, 1987.
33. Hudson RJ, Bergstrom RG, Thomson IR, et al: Pharmacokinetics of sufentanil in patients undergoing abdominal aortic surgery. *Anesthesiology* 70:426, 1989.
34. Egan TD, Lemmens HJM, Fiset P, et al: The pharmacokinetics of the new short acting opioid remifentanil (GI87084B) in healthy adult male volunteers. *Anesthesiology* 79:881, 1993.

Young H. Kim
Ducksoo Kim

CHAPTER **21**

Interventional Radiology: Drainage Techniques

Image-guided percutaneous drainage is a safe and widely accepted first-line treatment for infected or symptomatic fluid collections in the body. Image guidance for drainage is most commonly performed with computed tomography (CT) and ultrasonography (US). Compared with surgery, especially in critically ill patients, percutaneous drainage is less invasive, safer, faster, and more cost-effective.

GENERAL AIMS

The aim of the radiologist is to identify the source of infection or any symptomatic fluid collection, to triage the patients, and to perform image-guided aspiration or catheter drainage procedures to establish diagnosis, relive the symptom, or provide treatment in a safe and timely manner.

DIAGNOSTIC IMAGING

CT scan is commonly the first-line imaging modality for establishing the diagnosis. Concomitant use of intravenous contrast and oral contrast increase diagnostic ability and accuracy. When there is suspicion of bowel leakage, administration of water-soluble contrast is mandatory. CT provides excellent axial anatomic information of the patient. However, need for intravenous contrast use and radiation exposure is the main limiting factors. US is easy to perform, with no radiation exposure and no need for contrast use, and provides high diagnostic yield when performed by experienced radiologists. In addition to operator dependency, air in the bowel loops, deeply situated lesions, and large-body habitus of the patient limits use of US as first-line diagnostic or therapeutic modality.

INDICATIONS

Needle aspiration can be performed to determine the nature of the fluid collection or alleviate symptoms in a noninfected collection such as a pleural effusion or ascites. A catheter drainage procedure is performed in patients with fluid collections that are infected or causing pressure symptoms with the use of 8 to 14 French (Fr) catheters [1]. Percutaneous catheter drainage can be a curative or temporary measure, with a subsequent surgical treatment depending on the nature and extent of underlying disease [2]. Inflammation with concomitant infection of the organ (appendicitis, diverticulitis, and cholecystitis) or any

fluid accumulation with or without infection can be an indication for drainage. No clear size criteria exist for the abscess to be drained. Usually, abscesses larger than 3 to 4 cm in their greatest diameter or an infected fluid collection that does not respond to initial antibiotic treatment can be an indication for a percutaneous drainage procedure. Indication, as well as requests for an image-guided drainage procedure for both diagnostic and therapeutic purposes, is increasing because of technical progress and improved success of procedures [3,4]. The most common indications for catheter drainage are outlined in Table 21-1.

CONTRAINDICATIONS

Absolute contraindications are coagulopathy unresponsive to therapy and absence of a safe access route. An uncooperative patient is problematic, but can be treated under general anesthesia or deep sedation. Transgression of major vessels should always be avoided. Transgression of spleen, pancreas, bowel loops, and pleural space should be avoided. Transenteric (jejunum, ileum) routes are considered a contraindication to catheter drainage, but have become a relative contraindication for needle aspiration procedures. Splenic biopsy and percutaneous drainage of splenic abscess can be performed cautiously, especially when the coagulation profile is normal [5]. Liver, kidney, and stomach may be transgressed during needle aspiration or catheter drainage when there is no direct route available. Transrectal, transvaginal, and transgluteal approaches have become regarded as safe routes for deep pelvic fluid collection [6–8].

RISKS, BENEFITS, AND ALTERNATIVES

The overall complications rate is 5% to 10%. Mortality ranges from 1% to 6% and is usually a consequence of sepsis or multiorgan failure. The benefits of the drainage in 70% to 90% of cases rest in avoiding the need of a more invasive surgical intervention [9]. When there is no safe access available, surgery should be considered. Medical observation may also be considered, especially for certain pancreatic pseudocysts, with 30% of them known to resolve spontaneously. Abscesses smaller than 3 cm in their greatest diameter can be treated successfully with antibiotics alone and thus may not require percutaneous drainage [2].

TABLE 21-1.   Indications for Catheter Drainage

Inflammation
  Appendicitis
  Diverticulitis
  Infected pancreatic pseudocyst
  Cholecystitis
  Tuboovarian abscess
Postsurgical collections
  Anastomotic leak
  Hematoma
  Abscess
  Biloma
  Seroma
  Urinoma
  Lymphocele

PREPROCEDURE PREPARATION

Review of the most recent radiologic imaging is essential for the evaluation of locations, extent, and relationship of fluid to vital structures. Imaging modality is chosen based on the location of the lesion and operator experience. The safest and most minimally invasive route should be selected based on the two-dimensional or three-dimensional CT images, even when US-guided procedure is performed. Recent previous intravenous contrast-enhanced CT scans should always be available throughout the procedure for exact anatomic localization. Check coagulation profiles for their appropriate level before the procedure: Prothrombin time (less than 15 seconds), partial thromboplastin time (less than 35 seconds), platelet count (more than 75,000 per mL), and international normalized ratio (less than 1.5). Laboratory work is required within 2 to 3 days prior to the date of the examination to ensure that the patient's condition has not changed.

Prior to the procedure, anticoagulants should be stopped. For example, aspirin should be stopped a week before; heparin, 6 hours prior to the procedure; and Coumadin, several days before as directed by the referring physician. Discontinuation of anticoagulant is a difficult decision because the interruption of anticoagulant therapy may increases the risk of thromboembolism. The most common indications for Coumadin therapy are atrial fibrillation, the presence of a mechanical heart valve, and venous thromboembolism [10,11]. Discontinuation of anticoagulant should be directed by the referring physician and by weighing risks and benefits of the procedure to be done. Oral intake, except some medications, should be stopped 4 to 6 hours before the procedure. Nothing by mouth is important for prevention of possible aspiration/asphyxia from vomitus during the procedure and for limiting air introduction into the gastrointestinal tract, which can limit US examination. Oral contrast can be provided 60 to 90 minutes before the procedure and at the CT scan room before the procedure in order to visualize bowel loops. In most of the cases, prior intravenous and oral contrast-enhanced CT scans are used for planning the approach to the collection. Repeat use of contrast at the time of procedure is not required. Obtain intravenous access for hydration and medication with 20-gauge or larger catheter. Antibiotic coverage in patients with an abscess before the procedure is important to reduce septic complications.

EQUIPMENT

Portable US is now widely used for diagnostic and interventional procedures at the bedside for reasons of its portability and ability to identify and characterize fluid collections. CT is more commonly used for drainage procedures. US-guided procedures done in the intensive care unit or CT-guided procedures done in the CT room require the assistance of a technologist and qualified nurse. Drainage of the gallbladder is performed using combined use of US for localization and fluoroscopy with contrast to confirm cystic duct or bile duct patency. The nursing staff assists in monitoring the patient during the procedure and administers adequate analgesic and anxiolytic medication. Sterile aspiration kits contain lidocaine, needles, blade, syringes, and test tubes. Depending on the clinical situation, aerobic and anaerobic culture bottles should be available. Needles, catheters, and guidewires of various sizes according to the planned technique, method, and modality should be available to radiologist.

PATIENT CONSENT AND TIME-OUT

Consent from patient or legal proxy must be obtained after explanation of the risks, benefits, or alternatives of the procedure. A time-out should be performed to identify the patient, review patient allergies, and acknowledge the procedure to be performed.

ANESTHESIA AND MONITORING

Available options for analgesia and anesthesia include local anesthesia, local anesthesia with moderate sedation, and general anesthesia. Local anesthesia with moderate sedation is appropriate for most patients undergoing diagnostic and interventional procedures and is provided by the radiology care team (radiologist and certified nurse). Subcutaneous infiltration of 5 to 10 mL 1% lidocaine with a 25-gauge needle is most commonly used for local anesthesia. A wide selection of sedatives and analgesics is available. We routinely use midazolam, 0.5 to 2 mg, and fentanyl, 25 to 150 μg. General anesthesia is appropriate for an unstable or uncooperative patient or when there is potential for airway obstruction as a result of the procedure. Except for simple procedures such as paracentesis or thoracentesis in a stable patient, continuous monitoring of the patient is mandatory. Heart rate, blood pressure, electrocardiogram, and pulse oximetry should be monitored and recorded every 5 minutes during the procedure.

STERILE TECHNIQUE

Procedure should be completed with strict sterile technique including an antiseptic surgical scrub preparation. The radiologist and assisting staff must wear a sterile gown and gloves and uncontaminated hat and mask. Preparation of the patient's skin prior to procedure should include at least 10 cm surrounding the insertion site. The preferred antiseptic is a chlorhexidine-based preparation, 10% povidone iodine or 70% alcohol. A sterile drape that is large enough to prevent accidental contamination during insertion and allows good visualization of the insertion site is ideal.

PROCEDURES

GENERAL CONSIDERATIONS

CT and US are excellent modalities for identifying potential areas before the drainage procedure. A well-circumscribed fluid collection with enhancing mature wall is better suited for drainage procedures. Selection of CT or US should be made depending on the location of the fluid collection. US is best suited when the collection is superficial (pleural, peritoneal or gallbladder). CT is best used when the fluid is located deep in the peritoneum or in the retroperitoneum. The position of the patient is determined to assure shortest safe access to the collection, comfort of the patient, and convenience of the operator. Determination of the skin entry site is important because it affects the angle and depth of needle insertion. US allows real-time monitoring of the path of the needle and may shorten the procedure time. CT visualizes the needle and catheter related to the target lesion clearly, although repeated CT scanning is required to assure the needle passes along the planned course.

DIAGNOSTIC OR THERAPEUTIC ASPIRATION

Needle aspiration with 22- or 20-gauge needle is a very safe procedure. Usually, local anesthesia with 1% lidocaine is sufficient for the patient. Withdraw 5 to 10 mL of fluid for Gram's stain and culture and sensitivity for any catheter drainage procedures and, in addition, amylase for suspected pancreatic leak. Additional fluid (20 to 100 mL) may be necessary for cytologic analysis.

For the viscous fluid or hematoma, a larger-bore needle (16- or 18-gauge) should be used.

CATHETER SELECTION

Commercial drainage catheters come in a wide variety of sizes and materials, and should be determined based on their cost, comfort, flexibility, size of lumen and side holes, tip configuration, surface coating and ease of tracking (ability to follow guidewire), material durability, kink resistance, and securing mechanism. Use the largest catheter that can be safely placed. Drainage of cysts, seromas, urinomas, and noninfected fluid collections may be accomplished with a 7 to 10 Fr catheter. However, removal of necrotic debris or hematoma may require 14 to 16 Fr, or more. Abscesses can be easily drained with a 10 to 12 Fr catheter. Multiple catheters may be needed for large collections or multiloculated collections. Aspirates from all collections should be obtained through separate sterile procedures to avoid cross-contamination [12].

THERAPEUTIC CATHETER DRAINAGE

The catheter is introduced by using either the trocar or the Seldinger technique (Fig. 21-1). The trocar technique is one-step procedure that involves the use of a catheter with a stylet. The Seldinger technique involves the following steps: the placement of a needle into the collection, insertion of a guidewire through the needle and removal of the needle, and dilation of the tract and placement of a catheter over the guidewire with subsequent removal of the guidewire. When the fluid collection

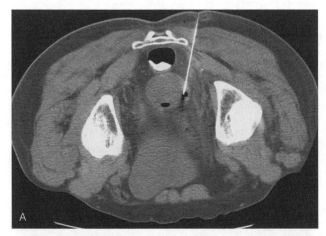

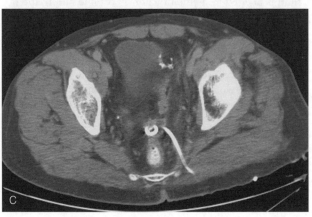

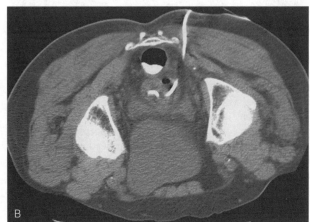

FIGURE 21-1. Computed tomography (CT)-guided transgluteal catheter drainage of a pelvic abscess from perforated sigmoid diverticulitis in a 65-year-old man. **A:** CT scan obtained in prone position demonstrates a localizing needle placed in the pelvic abscess. **B:** CT scan obtained after satisfactory position of catheter with a Seldinger technique. **C:** Follow-up CT scan obtained after 1 week following catheter drainage shows near-complete resolution of pelvis abscess.

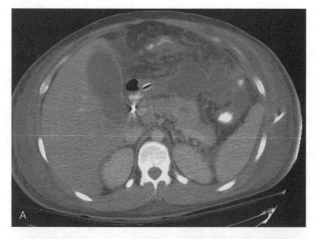

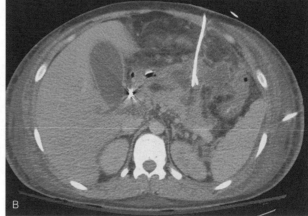

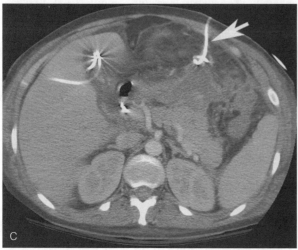

FIGURE 21-2.   Catheter placement and catheter dislodgement. **A:** Computed tomography (CT) scan obtained in a 45-year-old patient with acute pancreatitis complicated with peripancreatic infected fluid collection. **B:** CT scan obtained after satisfactory position of drainage catheter in peripancreatic fluid. **C:** CT scan obtained 3 days after catheter placement due to sudden decrease of drainage and sustained fever demonstrates pigtail catheter (*arrow*) positioned superior to the fluid collection.

is superficial, large, and easily accessible, the trocar technique is preferred. This technique is easier to perform that the Seldinger technique but has the risk of more serious complications due to unintentional injury to bowel or vessel. The tandem trocar technique involves initial CT-guided placement of a 21- to 22-gauge spinal needle into the fluid collection. This needle provided an externally and internally visible guide, ensuring that the catheter is correctly inserted parallel to the needle. The Seldinger technique involves the insertion of an 18- to 21-gauge sheathed needle into the abscess. The sheath allows the needle to be exchanged for a 0.035-inch guidewire, over which dilators are inserted and serial dilatation is performed. Next, the catheter is placed over the 0.35-inch wire and secured. The wire is then removed [8]. It is very important to maintain guidewire access during drainage procedure. If it is lost, reentry may be difficult due to decompression of the abscess. Drainage of the fluid should be minimized before the catheter placement into the fluid collection is completed.

FIXING THE CATHETER

Most catheters have a self-locking mechanism and usually consists of a string that threads through the catheter to its tip. When the string is pulled and fixed in position, the tension retains the pigtail catheter in a fixed, rounded position. In addition, the catheter is fixed to the skin with a one-sided locking device to

prevent accidental dislodgement of the drainage catheter. Dislodgement of drainage catheters is the most common postprocedural complication (Fig. 21-2). Attach a bag for gravity drainage and place a stopcock at the catheter's external end for routine irrigation. A Pleur-Evac type of device should be used for intrapleural collections to prevent tension pneumothorax.

MANAGEMENT OF THE CATHETER

Gentle irrigation of the catheter with 10 to 20 mL of saline using a sterile technique every 8 to 24 hours depending on viscosity of fluid is needed to maintain patency. Volume and frequency of catheter flushes should be adjusted based on cavity size, drainage quality, and quantity. Input and output of the saline should be calculated. Catheter output should be monitored daily. Simple abscess treatment is usually completed within 1 to 2 weeks. A more complex abscess or enteric fistula may require weeks to months, and cholecystostomy catheter removal requires a minimum of 3 weeks of drainage to allow adequate time for a well-formed mature tract to develop [13].

PATIENT RESPONSE

With adequate drainage, defervescence occurs usually within 24 to 48 hours, but may take up to 4 to 5 days. Persistent fever may suggest an undrained abscess, which should be evaluated with a repeat CT or US examination. If necessary, catheter repositioning or additional catheterization may be required. Some researchers have demonstrated that both multilocular, septated and viscous fluid may be successfully treated percutaneously. Use of lytic agents such as urokinase in these situations may shorten the treatment time and improve the clinical course [14].

REMOVAL OF THE CATHETER

The timing of catheter removal is determined by the abatement of clinical symptoms and signs of infection, and less than 10 mL per day of drainage for 2 consecutive days. A repeat CT scan or US to document the absence of a residual collection may be performed prior to catheter removal. In case of a sterile collection (hematoma or seroma), even if incompletely drained, early catheter removal is recommended in order to prevent infection [6]. Removal of the catheter should be done after release of the self-locking mechanism, which is easily achieved by untying the string or by cutting the catheter.

CLINICAL OUTCOME AND COMPLICATIONS

The success rate of percutaneous abscess drainage, without need of any further surgical intervention, is 70% to 90%, and depends on the location and type of abscess. Reasons of treatment failure include improper catheter position, catheter dislodgement, premature catheter removal, organized hematoma, associated fistula, immature abscess, or multiloculated fluid collection. The rate of complications of percutaneous drainage is 5% to 10%. The rate of major complications is 5% to 7%, and includes bleeding, infection, perforation, infection of initially sterile collection, septicemia (associated with disseminated intravascular coagulation or hypotension), bowel fistula, empyema, and death. The rate of minor complications is 3% to 5%, and includes transient fever, entry site skin infection, and catheter malfunction. Mortality within 30 days of the procedure is 1% to 6%, and is

related to sepsis or multiple organ failure rather than the procedure itself.

Patients who need placement of a drainage catheter should be evaluated and treated before and after the procedures in a cooperative fashion with the referring intensive care unit services. Frequent communication about the clinical course of the patient in conjunction with the quality and quantity of drainage is essential. Follow-up CT, US, and fluoroscopy with contrast studies are performed to further monitor the status of drainage, especially if the patient is not clinically improving or the infection is not resolving.

REFERENCES

1. Jaffe TA, Nelson RC, Delong DM, et al: Practice pattern in percutaneous image-guided intraabdominal abscess drainage: survey of academic and private practice centers. *Radiology* 233:750, 2004.
2. Siewert B, Tye G, Kruskal J, et al: Impact of CT-guided drainage in the treatment of diverticular abscesses: size matters. *AJR Am J Roentgenol* 186:680, 2006.
3. Mueller PR, vanSonnenberg E: Interventional radiology in the chest and abdomen. *N Eng J Med* 322:1364, 1990.
4. Hahn PF, Gervais DA, O'Neill MJ, et al: Nonvascular interventional procedures: analysis of a 10-year database containing more than 21,000 cases. *Radiology* 220:730, 2001.
5. Lucey BC, Boland GW, Maher MM, et al: Percutaneous nonvascular splenic intervention: a 10-year review. *AJR Am J Roentgenol* 179:1591, 2002.
6. vanSonnenberg E, D'Agostino HB, Casola G, et al: US-guided transvaginal drainage of pelvic abscesses and fluid collections. *Radiology* 181:53, 1991.
7. Kuligowska E, Keller E, Ferrucci JT: Treatment of pelvic abscesses: value of one-step sonographically guided transrectal needle aspiration and lavage. *AJR Am J Roentgenol* 164:201, 1995.
8. Harisinghani MG, Gervais DA, Maher MM, et al: Transgluteal approach for percutaneous drainage of deep pelvic abscesses: 154 cases. *Radiology* 228:701, 2003.
9. Kandarpa K, Saini S: Handbook of interventional radiologic procedures, in Kandarpa K, Aruny JE (eds): *Handbook of Interventional Radiology*. 2nd ed. Boston, Little, Brown & Company, 1996; p 258.
10. Hirsh J, Dalen JE, Deykin D, et al: Oral anticoagulants: mechanism of action, clinical effectiveness, and optimal therapeutic range. *Chest* 108(Suppl):231S, 1995.
11. Becker RC, Ansell J: Antithrombotic therapy: an abbreviated reference for clinicians. *Arch Intern Med* 155:149, 1995.
12. Heneghan JP, Everts RJ, Nelson RC: Multiple fluid collections: CT- or US-guided aspiration-evaluation of microbiologic results and implications for clinical practice. *Radiology* 212:669, 1999.
13. Wise JN, Gervais DA, Akman A, et al: Percutaneous cholecystostomy catheter removal and incidence of clinically significant bile leaks: a clinical approach to catheter management. *AJR Am J Roentgenol* 184:1647, 2005.
14. Lahorra JM, Haaga JR, Stellato T, et al: Safety of intracavitary urokinase with percutaneous abscess drainage. *AJR Am J Roentgenol* 160:171, 1993.

John A. Paraskos
Alan A. Orquiola

CHAPTER **22**

Cardiopulmonary Resuscitation

HISTORY

Since the introduction of cardiopulmonary resuscitation (CPR), we have been forced to rethink our definitions of life and death. Although sporadic accounts of attempted resuscitations are recorded from antiquity [1–3], until recently no rational quarrel could be found with the sixth century BC poetic fragment of Ibycus, "You cannot find a medicine for life once a man is dead" [4]. Until 1960, successful resuscitation was largely limited to artificial ventilation for persons who had undergone respiratory arrest due to such causes as near-drowning, smoke inhalation, and aspiration. Such attempts were likely to succeed if performed before cardiac arrest had resulted from hypoxia and acidosis. Emergency thoracotomy with "open heart massage" was rarely resorted to and was occasionally successful if definitive therapy was readily available [5]. Electrical reversal of ventricular fibrillation (VF) by externally applied electrodes was described in 1956 by Zoll et al. [6]. This ability to reverse a fatal arrhythmia without opening the chest challenged the medical community to develop a method of sustaining adequate ventilation and circulation long enough to bring the electrical defibrillator to the patient's aid. By 1958, adequate rescue ventilation became possible with the development of the mouth-to-mouth technique described by Safar et al. [7,8] and Elam et al. [9]. In 1960, Kouwenhoven et al. [10] described "closed chest cardiac massage," thus introducing the modern era of CPR. The simplicity of this technique—"all that is needed are two hands"—has led to its widespread dissemination. The interaction of this technique of sternal compression with mouth-to-mouth ventilation was developed as basic CPR. The first national conference on CPR was sponsored by the National Academy of Sciences in 1966 [11]. Instruction in CPR for both professionals and the public soon followed through community programs in basic life support (BLS) and advanced cardiac life support (ACLS). Standards for both BLS and ACLS were set in 1973 [12] and were updated in 1979 [13], 1985 [14], 1992 [15], 2000 [16], and 2005 [17].

For some individuals with adequately preserved cardiopulmonary and neurologic systems, the cessation of breathing and cardiac contraction may be reversed if CPR and definitive care are quickly available. If other systems are also spared, prolonged and vigorous life may ensue. The short period during which the loss of vital signs may be reversed is often referred to as *clinical death*. For clinical death to be reversed, however, ventilation and circulation must be restored before irreversible damage to vital structures occurs. The state of irreversible death is referred to as *biologic death*. In difficult circumstances, the best single criterion

(medical and legal) for the ultimate death of the functioning integrated human individual (i.e., the person) is brain death [18–23]. By this criterion, we can make decisions as to the appropriateness of continuing "life-sustaining" techniques.

EFFICACY

The value of standardized CPR continues to undergo considerable scrutiny. Unfortunately, it appears that its efficacy is limited. CPR does not seem to go beyond short-term sustaining of viability until definitive therapy can be administered. This was the stated goal of Kouwenhoven et al. [10]. The benefit of rapid initiation of CPR has been demonstrated in numerous studies [24–29]. Data from prehospital care systems in Seattle showed that 43% of patients found in VF were discharged from the hospital if CPR (i.e., BLS) was applied within 4 minutes and defibrillation (i.e., ACLS) within 8 minutes. If either was delayed, survival rates were much lower. Survival rates for patients in asystole or with pulseless electrical activity (PEA) were much lower [30–33]. In a Miami study, none of the patients found in bradyarrhythmia or asystole survived, whereas 23% of those in VF were eventually discharged [34,35]. Perhaps one of the benefits of the early initiation of CPR is the prolongation of VF, which increases the likelihood that ACLS with attempts at defibrillation will be successful. If the onset of CPR is delayed, or if the time to defibrillation is longer than 10 minutes, the probability is greater that the patient will be in asystole or in *fine* VF and will convert to asystole.

Even though patients experiencing cardiac arrest in the hospital can be expected to receive CPR and definitive therapy well within the 4- and 8-minute time frames, older studies determined that their chances of being discharged alive were generally worse than for out-of-hospital patients. This was thought to be due to serious underlying medical problems [36–40]. A more recent study suggests that when in-hospital cardiac arrests due to VF or ventricular tachycardia (VT) are witnessed and defibrillation is conducted rapidly, survival to discharge is excellent [41].

In 1967, Pantridge and Geddes [42] introduced the mobile intensive care unit (ICU) in Belfast, Ireland. Since then, emergency medical transport programs have spread throughout the world. In recent decades, there has been a move to further approximate the mobile ICU of Pantridge and Geddes by adding the capability of defibrillation to the emergency medical service system [43–46]. This is already in place in most metropolitan areas. Recognizing the importance of early defibrillation, it is imperative that all first-response systems provide this necessary service, either by using emergency medical technicians capable of performing defibrillation or by equipping and training emergency personnel with automatic or semiautomatic defibrillators [47–50]. The development of inexpensive, small, lightweight, easy-to-use, voice-prompted defibrillators would allow early access to defibrillation, before the arrival of emergency medical services (EMS) [51,52]. Where these have been made available, and where first-responders have been trained in their use, survival rates have been dramatically improved [53–55].

Although the current approach is modestly successful for VF, CPR techniques have most likely not yet been optimized, and further improvement is greatly needed [56]. Cardiac output has been measured at no better than 25% of normal during conventional CPR in humans [57–60]. In animal models, myocardial perfusion and coronary flow have been measured at 1% to 5% of normal [61–63]. Cerebral blood flow has been estimated to be 3% to 15% of normal when CPR is begun immediately [64–66], but it decreases progressively as CPR continues [67,68] and intracranial pressures rise [69,70]. Despite these pessimistic findings, complete neurologic recovery has been reported in humans even after prolonged administration of CPR [71].

Researchers continue to evaluate new approaches and techniques, and further refinements in the delivery of CPR can be expected. Although research in this area must be enthusiastically encouraged, assiduous attention to research methods and their applicability to humans is required to prevent an overly hasty and potentially injurious change in the current guidelines. The wide variety of experimental methods and models makes evaluation of apparently contradictory research results difficult. Animal preparations for research in resuscitative techniques have limited application to humans, largely because of differences in size and configuration of the thoracic cage. Before new basic CPR techniques can be endorsed with any confidence, they must have been demonstrated to improve either survival or neurologic outcome. In addition, they must be simple to apply in an arrest and, optimally, they should be simple to teach and applicable by one rescuer without undue effort.

MECHANISMS OF BLOOD FLOW DURING RESUSCITATION

Any significant improvement in CPR technique would seem to require an understanding of the mechanism by which blood flows during CPR. However, there is no unanimity among researchers in this area. It is of interest that significant advances seem to have been made by research groups holding very different ideas concerning the basic mechanism of blood flow during CPR. Indeed, it is possible that several mechanisms are operative; which of these is most important may vary according to a patient's size and chest configuration.

CARDIAC COMPRESSION THEORY

In 1960, when Kouwenhoven et al. [10] reported on the efficacy of closed chest cardiac massage, most researchers accepted the theory that blood is propelled by compressing the heart trapped between the sternum and the vertebral column. According to this theory, during sternal compression the intraventricular pressures would be expected to rise higher than the pressures elsewhere in the chest. With each sternal compression, the semilunar valves would be expected to open and the atrioventricular (AV) valves to close. With sternal release, the pressure in the ventricles would be expected to fall and the AV valves to open, allowing the heart to fill from the lungs and systemic veins. Indeed, an echocardiographic study using minipigs has shown such valve motion, and a transesophageal echocardiographic study in humans also supports this theory [72,73]. Although some animal studies have demonstrated pressure changes consistent with this theory [74], most have not [75]. If the cardiac compression mechanism were operative, ventilation would best be interposed between sternal compressions so as not to interfere with cardiac compression. Also, the faster the sternal compression, the higher the volume of blood flow, assuming that the ventricles could fill adequately. The theory of cardiac compression was first brought into question in 1962, when Weale and Rothwell-Jackson [76] demonstrated that during chest compression there is a rise in venous pressure almost equal to that of the arterial pressure. The following year, Wilder et al. [77] showed that ventilating synchronously with chest compression produced higher arterial pressures than alternating ventilation and compression. It was more than a decade, however, before more data confirmed these initial findings.

THORACIC PUMP THEORY

In 1976, Criley et al. [78] reported that during cardiac arrest, repeated forceful coughing is capable of generating systolic pressures comparable with those of normal cardiac activity. This finding strongly suggested that high intrathoracic pressures are capable of sustaining blood flow, independent of sternal compression. Subsequently, Niemann et al. [79] proposed that the propulsion of blood during sternal compression is due to the same mechanism of increased intrathoracic pressure. Studies using pressure measurements [80,81] and angiography [82] support this hypothesis, as do most echocardiographic studies [83,84]. According to this theory, the heart serves only as a conduit during CPR. Forward flow is generated by a pressure gradient between intrathoracic and extrathoracic vascular structures. Flow to the arterial side is favored by functional venous valves and greater compressibility of veins, compared to arteries, at their exit points from the thorax [75,82,85,86]. The thoracic pump theory provides the rationale for experimental attempts at augmenting forward flow by increasing intrathoracic pressure.

EXPERIMENTAL AND ALTERNATIVE TECHNIQUES OF CPR

Several experimental and alternate techniques of CPR are presented in Table 22-1 [64,66,74,87–106].

INTERPOSED ABDOMINAL COMPRESSION CPR

Interposed abdominal compression CPR was developed by Ralston et al. [107] and Babbs et al. [108]. This technique includes manual compression of the abdomen by an extra rescuer during the relaxation phase of chest compression (Fig. 22-1).

TABLE 22-1.   Experimental and Alternate Techniques of Cardiopulmonary
Resuscitation (CPR)

Researcher [Reference]	Technique	Notes
Taylor et al. (1977) [87]	Longer compression	Proposed use of longer duration to 40%–50% of the duration compression-relaxation cycle.
Chandra et al. (1980) [64,88]	Simultaneous chest compression and lung inflation	High airway pressures of 60–110 mm Hg are used to augment carotid flow, requiring intubation and a mechanical ventilator. Its use has not met with universal success [89,90].
Harris et al. (1967) [91,92] Redding (1971) [93] Koehler et al. (1983) [66] Chandra et al. (1981) [94]	Abdominal binding	Abdominal binding increases intrathoracic pressure by redistributing blood into the thorax during CPR. Studies have demonstrated adverse effects on coronary perfusion [95], cerebral oxygenation [96], and canine resuscitation [107].
Ralston et al. (1982) [107]	Interposed abdominal	Abdominal compression is released when the sternum is compressed. Higher oxygen delivery and cerebral and myocardial blood flows are reported [97,98]. One study suggests an improved survival and neurologic outcome [100].
Barranco et al. (1990) [101]	Simultaneous chest	Simultaneous chest and abdominal compression provided higher intrathoracic pressures in compression in humans.
Maier et al. (1984) [74]	High-impulse CPR	At compression rates of 150/min (with moderate force and brief duration), cardiac output in dogs increased as the coronary flow remained as high as 75% of prearrest values. High impulse and high compression rates can result in rescuer fatigue and increased injury.
Cohen et al. (1993) [102]	Active compression	Forceful rebound using a plungerlike device resulted in improved hemodynamics [103]. Clinical results are equivocal [104,105].
Halperin et al. (1986) [106]	Vest inflation	Circumferential chest pressure with an inflatable vest showed improved hemodynamics and survival in dogs [106].

The mid-abdomen is compressed at a point halfway between the xiphoid process and the umbilicus with a force of approximately 100 mm Hg of external pressure. This pressure is estimated to be equivalent to that required to palpate the aortic pulse in a subject with a normal pulse. Two randomized clinical trials have demonstrated a statistically significant improvement in outcome measures for in-hospital cardiac arrest [109,110], but no improvement has been shown for out-of-hospital arrest [111]. Based on these findings, interposed abdominal compression CPR is recommended as an option for in-hospital cardiac arrest when sufficient personnel trained in the technique are available. However, it should be emphasized that the safety and efficacy of interposed abdominal compression CPR in patients with recent abdominal surgery, pregnancy, or aortic aneurysm has not been studied.

OPEN CHEST CPR

One of the first forms of successful CPR was open chest CPR. It was shown to be effective when definitive care was rapidly available and is associated with survival rates, largely in operating room arrests, ranging from 16% to 37% [5,112,113]. Mechanistically, open chest CPR clearly involves cardiac compression without use of a thoracic gradient. Weale and Rothwell-Jackson [76] demonstrated lower venous pressures and higher arterial pressures than with closed chest compression. There is considerable evidence that open chest CPR may be more efficacious than closed chest CPR in terms of cardiac output and cerebral and myocardial preservation [114,115]. One study has suggested increased return of spontaneous circulation with open chest CPR [116]. Clearly, some patients with penetrating chest trauma are not likely to respond to chest compression and are candidates for open chest CPR [59,117,118]. Several studies suggest a benefit from thoracotomy in these patients [119–121]. If open chest CPR is to be used, it should be used early in the sequence [122,123]. Patients with blunt chest and abdominal trauma may also be candidates for open chest CPR. Obviously, this technique should not be attempted unless adequate facilities and trained personnel are available.

CARDIOPULMONARY BYPASS FOR UNRESPONSIVE ARREST

Cardiopulmonary bypass is certainly not a form of routine life support; however, it has been considered as a possible adjunct to artificial circulation. It is an indispensable adjunct to cardiac surgery and is being used more frequently for invasive

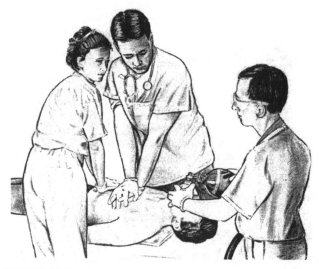

FIGURE 22-1.   Interposed abdominal compression cardiopulmonary resuscitation. It is more convenient when the interposed chest and abdominal compressions are performed from opposite sides of the patient. [From Guidelines 2000 for cardiopulmonary resuscitation and emergency cardiovascular care. *Circulation* 102[Suppl 8]:I-1, 2000, with permission. Copyright 2000, American Heart Association.]

procedures as a standby in case of sudden cardiac collapse. Cardiopulmonary bypass has been used in arrests unresponsive to standard methods of CPR [124]. In dog models, bypass has been shown capable of providing near-normal end-organ blood flow with improved "resuscibility" and neurologic status [125–129]. Emergency bypass can be instituted with femoral artery and vein access, without thoracotomy [130]. Further study of its use in humans will be necessary before it can be recommended for wider use in cardiac arrest. Its potential use is restricted to centers capable of providing this technological level of treatment. The cost necessitates careful consideration of the potential to save the patient.

INFECTIOUS DISEASES AND CPR

The fear provoked by the spread of human immunodeficiency virus (HIV) may lead to excessive caution when dealing with strangers; it has clearly decreased the willingness of both the lay public and health professionals to learn and perform CPR. The effect of this fear on CPR is serious and must be addressed at some length [131].

The public's fear can be counteracted only by continued education and by stressing the facts. Health care workers have more opportunities for exposure to patients with HIV and their concerns must be adequately addressed [132].

Saliva has not been implicated in the transmission of HIV even after bites, percutaneous inoculation, or contamination of open wounds with saliva from HIV-infected patients [133–138]. Hepatitis B–positive saliva has also not been demonstrated to be infectious when applied to oral mucous membranes or through contamination of shared musical instruments or CPR training manikins used by hepatitis B carriers. However, it is not impossible that the mouth-to-mouth technique might result in the exchange of blood between patient and rescuer if there are open lesions or trauma to the buccal mucosa or lips. Diseases such as tuberculosis, herpes, and respiratory viral infections are potentially spread during mouth-to-mouth ventilation. Infections thought to have been transmitted by CPR include *Helicobacter pylori* [139], *Mycobacterium tuberculosis* [140], meningococcus [141], herpes simplex [142], *Shigella* [143], *Streptococcus* [144], *Salmonella* [145], and *Neisseria gonorrhea* [146]. There have been no cases reported of transmission of HIV, hepatitis B virus, hepatitis C virus, or cytomegalovirus [146]. The impact of these facts is different for lay people and health care professionals, and different for those carrying infection and for those at risk of infection [147].

IMPLICATIONS FOR RESCUERS WITH KNOWN OR POTENTIAL INFECTION

Potential rescuers who know or highly suspect that they are infected with a serious pathogenic organism should not perform mouth-to-mouth ventilation if another rescuer is available who is less likely to be infectious or if the circumstances allow for any other immediate and effective method of ventilation, such as using mechanical ventilation devices.

IMPLICATIONS FOR HEALTH CARE PROFESSIONALS

Although the probability of a rescuer becoming infected with HIV during CPR seems minimal, all those called on to provide CPR in the course of their employment should have ready access to mechanical ventilation devices. Bag-valve mask devices should be available as initial ventilation equipment, and early endotracheal intubation should be encouraged when equipment and trained professionals are available. Masks with one-way valves and plastic mouth and nose covers with filtered openings are available and provide some protection from transfer of oral fluids and aerosols. S-shaped mouthpieces, masks without one-way valves, and handkerchiefs provide little, if any, barrier protection and should not be considered for routine use. With these guidelines in mind, health care professionals are reminded that they have a special moral and ethical, and in some instances legal, obligation to provide CPR, especially in the setting of their occupational duties.

IMPLICATIONS FOR MANIKIN TRAINING IN CARDIOPULMONARY RESUSCITATION

The guidelines of the American Heart Association (AHA) specify that students or instructors should not actively participate in CPR training sessions with manikins if they have dermatologic lesions on their hands or in oral or circumoral areas, if they are known to be infected with hepatitis or HIV, or if they have reason to believe that they are in the active stage of any infectious process. In routine ventilation training, instructors should not allow participants to exchange saliva by performing mouth-to-mouth ventilation in sequence without barrier mouthpieces. Special plastic mouthpieces and specialized manikins protect against such interchange of mucus.

TRAINING IN CPR FOR PEOPLE WITH CHRONIC INFECTIONS

If a potentially infectious person is to be trained in CPR, common-sense precautions should be taken to protect other participants from any risk of infection. The chronically infected individual should be given a separate manikin for practice that is adequately disinfected before anyone else uses it. The chronically infected trainee should be made aware of the preceding guidelines for potential rescuers with infections. In addition, the potential risk of infection for the immunocompromised rescuer should not be ignored.

An agency that requires successful completion of a CPR course as a prerequisite for employment must decide whether to waive its requirement for an employee who is unable to complete a CPR course for whatever reason. That agency also must determine whether a chronically infected person should continue to work in a situation in which CPR administration is a duty of employment.

STANDARD PROCEDURES AND TEAM EFFORT

The distinctive function of the ICU is to serve as a locus of concentrated expertise in medical and nursing care, life-sustaining technologies, and treatment of complex multiorgan system derangement. Historically, it was the development of effective treatment for otherwise rapidly fatal arrhythmias during acute myocardial infarction that impelled the medical community to establish ICUs [148]. Rapid response by medical personnel has been facilitated by constant professional attendance and the development of widely accepted guidelines for resuscitation. Each member of the professional team is expected to respond in accordance with these guidelines.

The skills necessary to perform adequately during a cardiac or respiratory arrest and to interface smoothly with ACLS techniques cannot be learned from reading texts and manuals. CPR courses taught according to AHA guidelines allow hands-on experience that approximates the real situation and tests the psychomotor skills needed in an emergency. All those who engage in patient care should be trained in BLS. Those whose duties require a higher level of performance should be trained in ACLS as well. As these skills deteriorate with disuse, they need to be updated. It is worth noting that there is no "certification" in BLS or ACLS. Issuance of a "card" is neither a license to perform these techniques nor a guarantee of skill, but simply an acknowledgment that an individual attended a specific course and passed the required tests. If employers or government agencies require such a card of their health workers, it is by their own mandate.

The ensuing discussion of BLS and ACLS techniques follows the recommendations and guidelines established by the AHA and presented in a supplement to volume 112 of *Circulation* [17].

BASIC LIFE SUPPORT FOR ADULTS WITH AN UNOBSTRUCTED AIRWAY

BLS is meant to support the circulation and respiration of those who have experienced cardiac or respiratory arrest. After recognizing and ascertaining its need, definitive help is summoned without delay and CPR is initiated.

RESPIRATORY ARREST

Respiratory arrest may result from airway obstruction, near-drowning, stroke, smoke inhalation, drug overdose, electrocution, or physical trauma. In the ICU, pulmonary congestion, respiratory distress syndrome, and mucous plugs are frequent causes of primary respiratory arrests. The heart usually continues to circulate blood for several minutes, and the residual oxygen in the lungs and blood may keep the brain viable. Early intervention by opening the airway and providing ventilation may prevent cardiac arrest and may be all that is required to restore spontaneous respiration. In the intubated patient, careful suctioning of the airway and attention to the ventilator settings are required.

CARDIAC ARREST

Cardiac arrest results in rapid depletion of oxygen in vital organs. After 6 minutes, brain damage is expected to occur, except in cases of hypothermia (e.g., near-drowning in cold water). Therefore, early bystander CPR (within 4 minutes) and rapid ACLS with attempted defibrillation (within 8 minutes) are essential in improving survival and neurologic recovery rates [49,149].

The sequence of steps in CPR may summarized as the ABCs of CPR: *a*irway, *b*reathing, and *c*irculation. This mnemonic is useful in teaching the public, but it should be remembered that each step is preceded by *assessment* of the need for intervention: Before opening the airway, the rescuer determines unresponsiveness; before breathing, the rescuer determines breathlessness; before circulation, the rescuer determines pulselessness (Table 22-2).

ASSESSMENT AND DETERMINATION OF UNRESPONSIVENESS AND ALERTING OF EMERGENCY MEDICAL SERVICES

A person who has undergone cardiac arrest may be found in an apparently unconscious state (i.e., an unwitnessed arrest), or may be observed to suddenly lapse into apparent unconsciousness (i.e., a witnessed arrest). In either case, the rescuer must react promptly to assess the person's responsiveness by attempting to wake and communicate with the person by tapping or gently shaking and shouting. The rescuer should summon nearby staff for help. If no other person is immediately available, the rescuer should call hospital emergency line for the resuscitation team to respond (e.g., "code blue").

In an optimally functioning ICU, nearly all arrests should be witnessed. Early recognition of cardiac and respiratory arrests is facilitated by electronic monitoring of cardiac rhythm and often of respiratory rate and hemodynamic measurements. Video monitors often extend visual monitoring. Unfortunately, it is quite possible for a patient to become lost behind this profusion of electronic signals, the dependability of which varies widely. For several precious minutes, a heart with PEA continues to provide a comforting electronic signal, while the brain suffers hypoxic damage. A high frequency of false alarms due to loose electrodes or other artifacts may dangerously raise the threshold of awareness and prolong the response time of the ICU team. The overall efficacy of the monitoring devices, therefore, depends highly on meticulous skin preparation and care of electrodes, transducers, pressure cables, and the like.

Sudden apparent loss of consciousness, occasionally with seizures, may be the first signal of arrest and requires prompt reaction. After determining unresponsiveness, the pulse is assessed. If the carotid pulse cannot be palpated in 5 to 10 seconds, and a defibrillator is not immediately available, a precordial thump may be performed by striking the lower third of the sternum with the fist, from a height of approximately 8 inches (or the span of the stretched fingers of one hand). If the pulse does not return and a defibrillator is not immediately available, the rescuer should proceed with establishing the airway (see the next section). If a defibrillator is immediately available, it should be used instead of a precordial thump; this is expected to be the case in a monitored arrest in an ICU.

OPENING THE AIRWAY AND DETERMINING BREATHLESSNESS

After establishing unresponsiveness and positioning the individual on his or her back (Fig. 22-2), the next step is to open the airway and check for spontaneous breathing (see Chapter 1). In a monitored arrest with VF or tachycardia, this step is taken after initial attempts to defibrillate. Meticulous attention to establishing an airway and supplying adequate ventilation is essential to any further resuscitative effort. The team leader must carefully monitor the adequacy of ventilation.

The head tilt–chin lift maneuver (Figs. 22-3 and 22-4) is usually successful in opening the airway. The head is tilted backward by a hand placed on the forehead. The fingers of the other hand are positioned under the mandible, and the chin is lifted upward. The teeth are almost approximated, but the mouth is not allowed to close. Because considerable cervical hyperextension occurs, this method should be avoided in patients with cervical injuries or suspected cervical injuries.

TABLE 22-2.   Summary of Basic Life Support ABCD Maneuvers for Infants, Children, and Adults (Newborn Information Not Included)[a]

Maneuver	Adult Lay Rescuer: 8 years HCP: Adolescent and older	Child Lay Rescuers: 1 to 8 years HCP: 1 year to adolescent	Infant Under 1 year of age
Airway	Head tilt–chin lift (HCP: suspected trauma, use jaw thrust)		
Breathing Initial	2 breaths at 1 sec/breath	2 effective breaths at 1 sec/breath	
HCP: Rescue breathing without chest compressions	10 to 12 breaths/min (approximate)	12 to 20 breaths/min (approximate)	
HCP: Rescue breaths for CPR with advanced airway	8 to 10 breaths/min (approximate)		
Foreign body airway obstruction	Abdominal thrusts		Back slaps and chest thrusts
Circulation HCP: Pulse check (≤10 sec)	Carotid		Brachial or femoral
Compression landmarks	Lower half of sternum, between nipples		Just below nipple line (lower half of sternum)

Compression method:
  Push hard and fast
  Allow complete recoil
	Heel of one hand, other hand on top	Heel of one hand or as for adults	2 or 3 fingers
			HCP (2 rescuers): 2 thumb–encircling hands

Compression depth	$1^{1}/_{2}$ to 2 in	Approximately one-third to one-half the depth of the chest	
Compression rate	Approximately 100/min		
Compression-ventilation ratio	30:2 (one or two rescuers)	30:2 (single rescuer) HCP: 15:2 (2 rescuers)	
Defibrillation AED	Use adult pads Do not use child pads	Use AED after 5 cycles of CPR (out of hospital). Use pediatric system for child 1 to 8 years if available **HCP: For sudden collapse (out of hospital) or in-hospital arrest use AED as soon as available**	No recommendation for infants <1 year of age

Note: Maneuvers used by only health care providers are indicated by "HCP." AED, automatic external defibrillator.

[a]Adapted from ECC Committee, Subcommittees and Task Forces of the American Heart Association. 2005 American Heart Association Guidelines for Cardiopulmonary Resuscitation and Emergency Cardiovascular Care. *Circulation* 112[24 Suppl]:IV1-203, 2005.

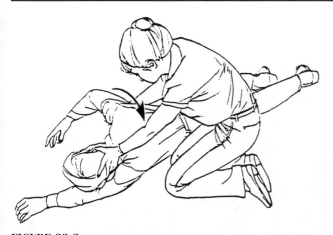

FIGURE 22-2.   The patient must be supine on a firm, flat surface. [From Guidelines for cardiopulmonary resuscitation and emergency cardiac care. Emergency Cardiac Care Committee and Subcommittees, American Heart Association. *JAMA* 268:2171, 1992, with permission. Copyright 1992, American Medical Association.]

The jaw-thrust maneuver (Fig. 22-5) provides the safest initial approach to opening the airway of a patient with a cervical spine injury; it usually allows excellent airway opening with a minimum of cervical extension. The angles of the mandible are grasped using both hands and lifting upward, thus tilting the head gently backward.

After opening the airway, the rescuer should take 3 to 5 seconds to determine whether there is spontaneous air exchange. This is accomplished by placing an ear over the patient's mouth and nose while watching to see if the patient's chest and abdomen rise and fall ("look, listen, and feel;" see Fig. 22-4). If the rescuer fails to see movement, hear respiration, or feel the rush of air against the ear and cheek, rescue breathing should be initiated.

RESCUE BREATHING

If spontaneous breathing is absent, rescue breathing with an airway-mask-bag unit must be initiated (see Chapter 1). If

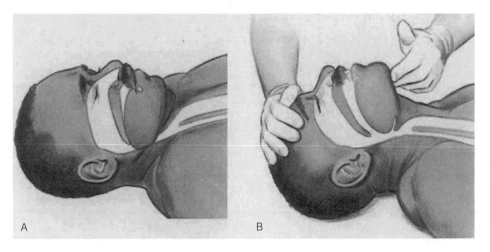

FIGURE 22-3. Opening the airway. **A:** Airway obstruction caused by tongue and epiglottis. **B:** Opening the airway with the head tilt–chin lift maneuver. [From *BLS for Healthcare Providers*, American Heart Association, 2006, with permission. Copyright 2006, American Heart Association.]

equipment is immediately available and the rescuer is trained, intubation and ventilatory adjuncts should be used initially. Each breath should be delivered during 1 second, allowing the patient's lungs to deflate between breaths. Thereafter, the rate of ten to 12 breaths per minute is maintained for as long as is necessary, with tidal volumes of approximately 700 mL. Delivering the breath during 1 second helps to prevent gastric insufflation. Melker et al. [150,151] demonstrated airway pressures well in excess of those required to open the lower esophageal sphincter when quick breaths are used to ventilate patients. If the patient wears dentures, they are usually best left in place to assist in forming an adequate seal.

If air cannot be passed into the patient's lungs, another attempt at opening the airway should be made. The jaw-thrust maneuver may be necessary. If subsequent attempts at ventilation are still unsuccessful, the patient should be considered to have an obstructed airway and attempts should be made to dislodge a potential foreign body obstruction.

DETERMINING PULSELESSNESS

In the adult, the absence of a central pulse is best determined by palpating the carotid artery (Fig. 22-6), although rarely the carotid pulse may be absent because of localized obstruction. If a pulse is not felt after 10 seconds of careful searching, chest compression is initiated, unless electrical countershock for ventricular arrhythmia or artificial pacing for asystole is immediately available. Although lay rescuers are no longer expected to perform a pulse check because it has been shown that checking the carotid pulse by a lay person is an inaccurate method of confirming the presence or absence of circulation [152], it is the position of the AHA that *health care providers* should continue

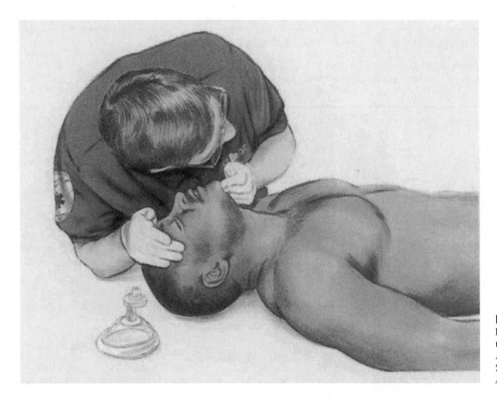

FIGURE 22-4. Determining breathlessness. Open the airway and "look, listen, and feel." [From *BLS for Healthcare Providers*, American Heart Association, 2006, with permission. Copyright 2006, American Heart Association.]

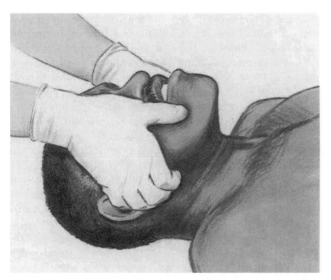

FIGURE 22-5. Jaw-thrust maneuver: opening the airway with minimal extension of the neck. [From *BLS for Healthcare Providers*, American Heart Association, 2006, with permission. Copyright 2006, American Heart Association.]

to be taught and to perform a pulse check. Therefore, rescuers should start CPR if the victim is unconscious (unresponsive), not moving and not breathing [153].

CHEST COMPRESSION

Artificial circulation depends on adequate chest compression through sternal depression. Recent recommendations of CPR are "push hard at a rate of 100 compressions per minute, allow full chest recoil and minimize interruptions in chest compressions" [153]. The safest manner of depressing the sternum is with the heel of the rescuer's hand at the nipple line, with the fingers kept off the rib cage (Fig. 22-7). It is usually most effective to cover the heel of one hand with the heel of the other, the heels being parallel to the long axis of the sternum. If the rescuer's hands are placed either too high or too low on the sternum, or if the fingers are allowed to lie flat against the rib cage, broken ribs and organ laceration can result. Although it is important to allow the chest to recoil to its normal position after each compression, it is not advisable to lift the hands from the chest or change their position.

The rescuer's elbows should be kept locked and the arms straight, with the shoulders directly over the patient's sternum (Fig. 22-7). This position allows the rescuer's upper body to provide a perpendicularly directed force for sternal depression. The sternum is depressed 1.5 to 2.0 inches (4 to 5 cm) at a rate of approximately 100 compressions per minute. In large patients, a slightly greater depth of sternal compression may be needed to generate a palpable carotid or femoral pulse. At the end of each compression, pressure is released, and the sternum is allowed to return to its normal position. Equal time should be allotted to compression and relaxation with smooth movements, avoiding jerking or bouncing the sternum. Manual and automatic chest compressors are available for fatigue-free sternal compression and are used by some EMS crews and emergency room and ICU personnel. Whether using hinged manually operated devices or compressed air-powered plungers, the rescuer must be constantly vigilant about proper placement and adequacy of sternal compression. An experimental device using a plungerlike suction device may improve flow by facilitating sternal rebound and thoracic vascular filling; this has been referred to as *active compression-decompression CPR* [108,109].

Ventilation and sternal compression should not be interrupted except under special circumstances. Warranted interruptions include execution of ACLS procedures (e.g., endotracheal intubation, placement of central venous lines) or an absolute need to move the patient. Even in these limited circumstances, interruption of CPR should be minimized. In a retrospective analysis of the VF waveform, interruption of CPR was associated with the decreased probability of conversion of VF to another rhythm [154].

TWO-RESCUER CPR

The combination of artificial ventilation and circulation can be delivered more efficiently and with less fatigue by two rescuers. One rescuer, positioned at the patient's side, performs sternal compressions while the other, positioned at the patient's head, maintains an open airway and performs ventilation. This technique should be mastered by all health care workers called on to perform CPR. Lay people have not been routinely taught this method, in the interest of improving retention of basic skills. The compression rate for two-rescuer CPR, as for one-rescuer CPR, is approximately 100 compressions per minute. The new recommendation of the compression to ventilation ratio is 30 to 2.

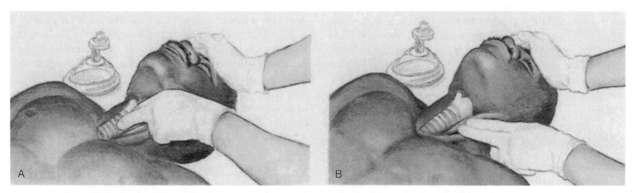

FIGURE 22-6. Determining pulselessness. **A:** Feeling the laryngeal cartilage. **B:** Fingers slide into groove between trachea and sternocleidomastoid muscle, searching for carotid pulse. [From *BLS for Healthcare Providers*, American Heart Association, 2006, with permission. Copyright 2006, American Heart Association.]

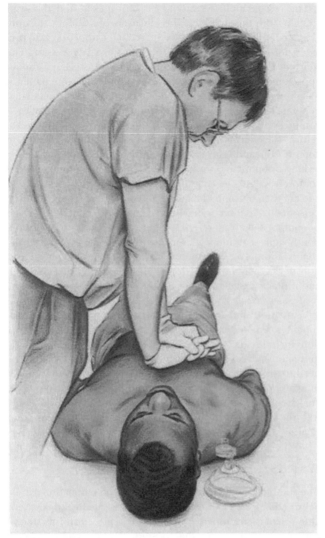

FIGURE 22-7. External chest compression. Proper position of the rescuer: place heel of hand on the breast bone at the nipple line with shoulders directly over the patient's sternum and elbows locked. [From *BLS for Healthcare Providers*, American Heart Association, 2006, with permission. Copyright 2006, American Heart Association.]

In an animal model of cardiac arrest, a compression-ventilation ratio of 30 to 2 was associated with significantly shorter time to return of spontaneous circulation [155]. The only exception to this recommendation is when two health care workers are providing CPR to a child or infant (except newborns); in this instance, a 15 to 2 compression to ventilation ratio should be used [153]. When the rescuer performing compressions is tired, the two rescuers should switch responsibilities with the minimum possible delay.

COMPLICATIONS OF BLS PROCEDURES

Proper application of CPR should minimize serious complications, but serious risks are inherent in BLS procedures and should be accepted in the context of cardiac arrest. Awareness of these potential complications is important to the postresuscitative care of the arrest patient.

Gastric distention and regurgitation are common complications of artificial ventilation without endotracheal intubation. These complications are more likely to occur when ventilation pressures exceed the opening pressure of the lower esophageal sphincter [156,157]. In mask ventilation, 1 second should be allowed for air delivery. Although an esophageal obturator airway may decrease the threat of distention and regurgitation during its use, the risk is increased at the time of its removal. To obviate this risk, the trachea should be intubated and protected with an inflated cuff before the esophageal cuff is deflated and the esophageal obturator removed.

Complications of sternal compression and manual thrusts include rib and sternal fractures, costochondral separation, flail chest, pneumothorax, hemothorax, hemopericardium, subcutaneous emphysema, mediastinal emphysema, pulmonary contusions, bone marrow and fat embolism, and lacerations of the esophagus, stomach, inferior vena cava, liver, or spleen [158–160]. Although rib fractures are common during CPR, especially in the elderly, no serious sequelae are likely unless tension pneumothorax occurs and is ignored. The more serious complications are unlikely to occur in CPR if proper hand position is maintained and exaggerated depth of sternal compression is avoided. Overzealous or repeated abdominal or chest thrusts for relief of airway obstruction are more likely to cause fractures or lacerations. For this reason, abdominal thrust is not recommended for the infant younger than 1 year.

MONITORING THE EFFECTIVENESS OF BASIC LIFE SUPPORT

The effectiveness of rescue effort is assessed regularly by the ventilating rescuer, who notes the chest motion and the escape of expired air. The adequacy of circulation is assessed by noting an adequate carotid pulse with sternal compressions.

Animal studies suggest that the best guides to the efficacy of ongoing CPR efforts are aortic diastolic pressure and myocardial perfusion pressure (aortic diastolic minus right atrial diastolic) [61,161–165]. In instrumented patients for whom systemic arterial pressure (with or without central venous pressure) is available, attempts should be made to optimize myocardial perfusion pressure during CPR.

Pupillary response, if present, is a good indicator of cerebral circulation. However, fixed and dilated pupils should not be accepted as evidence of irreversible or biologic death. Ocular diseases, such as cataracts, and a variety of drugs (e.g., atropine and ganglion-blocking agents) interfere with the pupillary light reflex. The decision to cease BLS should be made only by the physician in charge of the resuscitation effort; this decision should not be made until it is obvious that the patient's cardiovascular system will not respond with return of spontaneous circulation to adequate administration of ACLS, including electrical and pharmacologic interventions. Remediable problems, such as airway obstruction, severe hypovolemia, and pericardial tamponade should also have been reasonably excluded by careful attention to ACLS protocols.

PEDIATRIC RESUSCITATION

Most infants and children who require resuscitation have had a primary respiratory arrest. Cardiac arrest results from the ensuing hypoxia and acidosis; therefore, the focus of pediatric resuscitation is airway maintenance and ventilation. The outcomes for CPR in children with cardiac arrest are poor because the cessation of cardiac activity is usually the manifestation of prolonged hypoxia. Brain damage is, therefore, all too common. Respiratory arrest, if treated before cessation of cardiac activity has supervened, carries a much better prognosis [166,167]. It is for this reason that it is recommended to provide the initial steps of CPR for infants and children before taking the time to telephone for emergency assistance. The first minute of CPR will allow opening of the airway and the beginning of artificial ventilation. If an obstructed airway is found, attempts at dislodging a foreign body should not be delayed. In children with a history of cardiac disease or arrhythmias, or in previously healthy children who are witnessed to have a sudden collapse, a primary arrhythmic event is more likely, and immediate activation of the emergency medical service system may be beneficial.

Effective techniques for ventilation and chest compression vary with the child's size. Infant procedures are applicable to patients who are smaller than an average child of 1 year. Child techniques are applicable to patients who are of a size similar to the average child of 1 to 8 years. Adult techniques are appropriate for patients who appear larger than the typical child of 8 years of age.

If the child is found to be apneic, he or she is placed in the supine position and the head tilt–chin lift maneuver is used to open the airway (Fig. 22-8). Overextension of the neck is unnecessary and is best avoided. Some believe overextension of the child's flexible neck may obstruct the trachea; however, there are no data to support this. The jaw-thrust maneuver should be used if an adequate airway is not obtained with the head tilt–chin lift maneuver or if neck injury is suspected.

Artificial ventilation of the infant requires the rescuer's mouth to cover both the mouth and nose to make an effective seal. If the child's face is too large to allow a tight seal to be made over both nose and mouth, the mouth alone is covered, as for the adult.

The lung volume of the pediatric patient is small enough that a "puff" of air from the airway-mask-bag unit apparatus might be adequate to inflate the lungs. However, the smaller diameter of the tracheobronchial tree and any pulmonary disease that may be contributing to the arrest usually provide considerable resistance to airflow. Therefore, a surprising amount of inspiratory pressure may be needed to move adequate air into the lungs. This is especially true for the child who may have edematous respiratory passages. Accordingly, adequacy of ventilation must be monitored by observing the rising and falling of the chest and feeling and listening for the exhaled air from the child's mouth and nose. Excessive ventilatory volumes may exceed esophageal opening pressure and cause gastric distention.

Gastric decompression is dangerous and should be avoided until the patient has been intubated and the cuff inflated to protect the respiratory tract from aspiration. If the gastric distention is so severe that ventilation is greatly compromised, the child's body should be turned to one side before pressure on the abdomen is applied. It is preferable to use a gastric tube with suction whenever possible.

The ventilation rate for infants is approximately 20 breaths per minute (one every 3 seconds), whereas the rate for the child can be 12 to 20 breaths per minute (one every 3 to 5 seconds). Adolescents are ventilated at the adult rate of ten to 12 breaths per minute (one every 5 seconds). If artificial circulation is not necessary, more rapid ventilatory rates are acceptable.

Artificial circulation is instituted in the absence of a palpable pulse. The pulse of the larger child can easily be detected at the carotid artery, as in the adult. The neck of the infant, however, is too short and fat for reliable palpation of the carotid artery. Palpation of the precordium is also unreliable; some infants have no precordial impulse in spite of adequate cardiac output. It is recommended, therefore, that the presence of an infant's pulse be determined by palpating the brachial artery between the elbow and the shoulder.

To apply chest compression in an infant, the rescuer's index finger is placed on the sternum, just below the intermammary line. The proper area for compression is one fingerbreadth below the intermammary line on the lower sternum, at the location of the middle and ring fingers (Fig. 22-9). Using two or three fingers, the sternum is compressed approximately one-third to one-half the depth of the thorax. Alternatively, for chest compressions in the infant, the *two thumb–encircling hands* technique

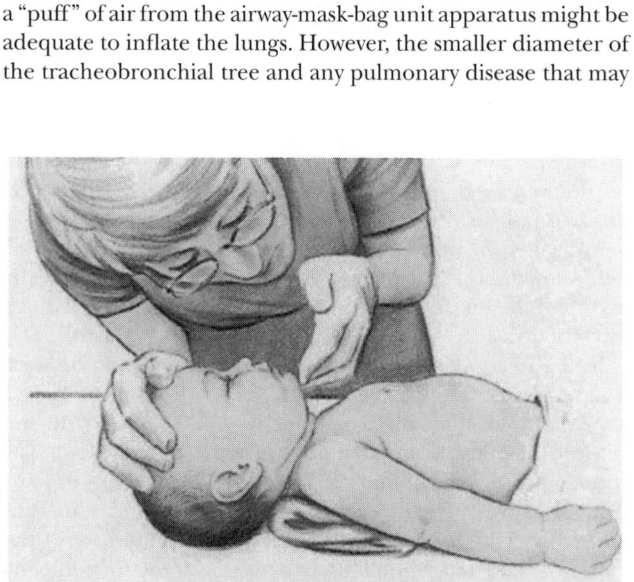

FIGURE 22-8. Head tilt–chin lift in the infant: Opening the airway. [From *BLS for Healthcare Providers*, American Heart Association, 2006, with permission. Copyright 2006, American Heart Association.]

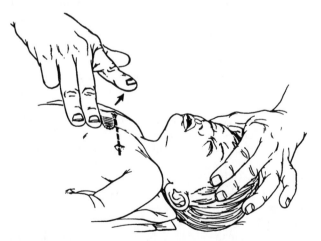

FIGURE 22-9. Locating finger position for sternal compression in the infant, using an imaginary line between the nipples. [From Standards and guidelines for cardiopulmonary resuscitation (CPR) and emergency cardiac care (ECC). *JAMA* 255:2843, 1986, with permission. Copyright 1986, American Medical Association.]

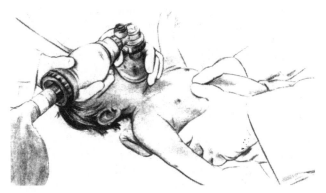

FIGURE 22-10. Chest compression in the infant using the two thumb-encircling hands technique (two rescuers are required). [From Guidelines 2000 for cardiopulmonary resuscitation and emergency cardiovascular care. *Circulation*102[Suppl 8]:I-1, 2000, with permission. Copyright 2000, American Heart Association.]

may be used when two rescuers are available (Fig. 22-10). The frequency of sternal compressions for infants and children is 100 per minute. During one-rescuer support, the ratio of compression to ventilation is 30 to 2 for infants and children [153].

OBSTRUCTED AIRWAY

An unconscious patient can experience airway obstruction when the tongue falls backward into the pharynx. Alternatively, the epiglottis may block the airway when the pharyngeal muscles are lax. In the sedated or ill patient, regurgitation of stomach contents into the pharynx is a frequent cause of respiratory arrest. Blood clots from head and facial injuries are another source of pharyngeal and upper airway obstruction. Even otherwise healthy people may have foreign body obstruction from poorly chewed food, large wads of gum, and so forth. The combination of attempting to swallow unchewed food, drinking alcohol, and laughing is particularly conducive to pharyngeal obstruction. Children's smaller airways are likely to obstruct with small nuts or candies. Children are also prone to airway obstruction by placing toys or objects such as marbles or beads in their mouths.

Persons who experience partial obstruction with reasonable gas exchange should be encouraged to continue breathing efforts with attempts at coughing. A patient whose obstruction is so severe that air exchange is obviously markedly impaired (cyanosis with lapsing consciousness) should be treated as having complete obstruction.

Persons who experience complete obstruction may still be conscious. They are unable to cough or vocalize. A subdiaphragmatic abdominal thrust (Heimlich maneuver) may force air from the lungs in sufficient quantity to expel a foreign body from the airway [168,169].

If the person is still standing, the rescuer stands behind the person and wraps his or her arms around the person's waist. The fist of one hand is placed with the thumb side against the person's abdomen in the mid-line, slightly above the umbilicus and well below the xiphoid process (Fig. 22-11). The fist is grasped with the other hand and quickly thrust inward and upward. It may be necessary to repeat the thrust six to ten times to clear the airway. Each thrust should be a separate and distinct movement.

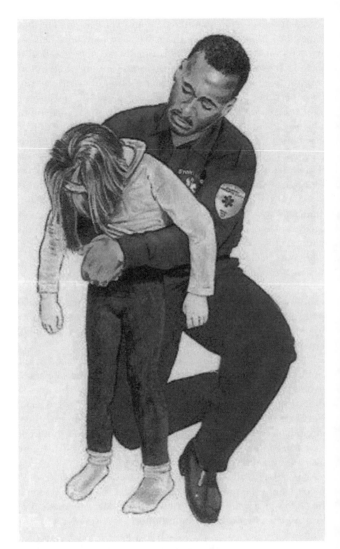

FIGURE 22-11. Abdominal thrust with conscious patient standing: rescuer standing behind individual with foreign body airway obstruction. [From *BLS for Healthcare Providers*, American Heart Association, 2006, with permission. Copyright 2006, American Heart Association.]

If the patient is unconscious or lying down, he or she should be positioned face up in the supine position. The rescuer kneels beside or astride the person's thighs and places the heel of one hand against the person's abdomen, slightly above the navel and well below the xiphoid process. The other hand is placed directly on top of the first and pressed inward and upward with a quick forceful thrust.

In the unconscious patient, a finger sweep should be used to attempt to dislodge the foreign body if it remains lodged after multiple subdiaphragmatic abdominal thrusts. With the face up, the person's mouth is opened by grasping the lower jaw and tongue with the thumb and fingers. The jaw is lifted upward (tongue-jaw lift). The index finger of the other hand is inserted down along the inside of the cheek, deeply to the base of the tongue. A hooking action is used to maneuver the foreign body into the mouth where it can be removed. Blind finger sweeps should be avoided in infants and children because it is more likely that a foreign object or swollen epiglottis will be pushed further into the airway. The tongue-jaw lift should be used and may in itself partially relieve the obstruction. If a foreign body is visualized, however, it should be grasped and removed.

If attempted rescue breathing in an arrested patient fails to move air into the lungs, an obstructed airway must be presumed to be present. It may simply be due to the tongue or epiglottis, rather than a foreign body. If the airway remains closed after repositioning the head, other maneuvers to open the airway, including the jaw thrust and tongue-jaw lift, must be used. If the airway remains obstructed, subdiaphragmatic abdominal thrusts are used, as described previously. Careful suction and direct visualization are also used when available.

Chest thrusts may be substituted for abdominal thrusts in patients in advanced stages of pregnancy, in patients with severe ascites, or in the markedly obese. The fist is placed in mid-sternum for the erect and conscious patient. For the supine patient, the hand is positioned on the lower sternum, as for external cardiac compression. Each thrust is delivered slowly and distinctly.

If attempts at dislodging a foreign body or relieving airway obstruction fail, special advanced procedures are necessary to provide oxygenation until direct visualization, intubation, or tracheostomy is accomplished.

ADVANCED CARDIAC LIFE SUPPORT IN ADULTS

The use of adjunctive equipment, more specialized techniques, and pharmacologic and electrical therapy in the treatment of a person who has experienced cardiac or respiratory arrest is generally referred to as *ACLS*. These techniques and their interface with BLS and the EMS are considered in the AHA's ACLS teaching program. An improvement in survival after in-hospital cardiac arrest has been demonstrated after medical house officers were trained in ACLS [170]. An in-depth discussion is available in the ACLS text published by the AHA.

The focus of the following sections is on the techniques and medications used in the initial resuscitative efforts. The demarcation from therapies more commonly reserved for the ICU is often indistinct; indeed, it is expected to vary with the experience of the prehospital team and the degree of physician supervision. In general, most ACLS measures should be applied by trained personnel operating within an EMS system in the community, in transport, or in the hospital setting.

AIRWAY AND VENTILATORY SUPPORT

Oxygenation and optimal ventilation are prerequisites for successful resuscitation (see Chapter 1). Supplemental oxygen should be administered as soon as it becomes available, beginning with 100%. In the postresuscitation period, the amount of administered oxygen may be decreased as guided by the arterial blood partial pressure of oxygen.

Emergency ventilation commonly begins with the combined use of a mask and oral airway. Mouth-to-mask ventilation is very effective as long as an adequate seal is maintained between the mask and face. Most masks are best fitted by flaring the top and molding it over the bridge of the nose. The inflated rim is then carefully molded to the cheeks as the mask is allowed to recoil. Relatively firm pressure is required to maintain the seal. Masks with one-way valves also provide a measure of isolation from the patient's saliva and breath aerosol. Bag-valve-mask ventilation requires strong hands and a self-inflating bag. The bag should

be connected to a gas reservoir and to oxygen so that 100% oxygen delivery can be approximated. It cannot be overemphasized that the success of this method depends on airway patency and an adequate seal between the mask and face. Equally important is adequate compression of the bag to deliver the required tidal volume. It is advisable that everyone who uses this technique practice on a recording ventilating manikin to assess the adequacy of the method in his or her hands. Many people will discover that their hands are not large enough or strong enough to deliver 700 mL of air. Some may have to squeeze the bag between their elbow and chest wall to supply adequate ventilation. If two people are available to ventilate, one should secure the mask while the other uses both hands to attend to the bag.

The mask design should include the following features:

- The use of transparent material, which allows the rescuer to assess lip color and to observe vomitus, mucus, or other obstructing material in the patient's airway.
- A cushioned rim around the mask's perimeter to conform to the patient's face and to facilitate a tight seal.
- A standard 15- to 22-mm connector, which allows the use of additional airway equipment.
- A comfortable fit to the rescuer's hand.
- An oxygen insufflation inlet, which allows oxygen supplementation during mouth-to-mask ventilation.
- A one-way-valve, which allows some protection during mouth-to-mask ventilation.
- Availability in appropriate sizes and shapes, for various-sized faces. Most adults will be accommodated by a standard medium-sized (no. 4) oval-shaped mask.

Ventilating bags must be designed to include the following features:

- A self-refilling bag, which allows operation independent of a fresh gas source.
- A fresh gas inlet, which allows ambient air or supplemental oxygen to flow into the reservoir bag through a valve inlet.
- A nipple for oxygen connection, located near the gas inlet valve.
- A reservoir bag that is easy to clean and sterilize without damaging.
- Availability in pediatric and adult sizes.
- A nonrebreathing valve directing flow to the patient during inhalation and to the atmosphere during exhalation. The valve casing should be transparent to allow visual inspection of its function. It should be easy to clean and assemble. A pop-off feature is often present to prevent inadvertently high airway pressures; however, such valves should have provision to override the pop-off feature because higher airway pressures are sometimes required to ventilate lungs with unusually high resistances, especially in children.
- Reservoir tubing that can be attached to the fresh gas inlet valve, which allows an accumulation of oxygen to refill the reservoir bag during the refill cycle. Such a reservoir allows delivered oxygen to approach 100%; without it, the self-refilling bag can deliver only 40% to 50% oxygen.

Oxygen-powered resuscitators allow the pressure of compressed oxygen tanks at 50 psi to drive lung inflation. They are usually triggered by a manual control button, and the oxygen can be delivered through a mask or tube for ease of ventilation.

These devices deliver oxygen at a flow rate of 100 L per minute and allow airway pressures of 60 cm H_2O. However, when used with masks and unprotected airways (not separated from the esophagus by an inflated cuff), these devices are likely to cause gastric distention and poor ventilation. They are not as reliable as mouth-to-mask or valve-bag-mask ventilation. When used in adults, they should be recalibrated to deliver flows of no more than 40 L per minute to avoid opening the lower esophageal sphincter. A relief valve that opens at approximately 60 cm H_2O and vents any excess volume into the atmosphere should be present. In addition, an alarm that sounds whenever the relief valve pressure is exceeded should be present. This alarm warns the rescuer that the patient requires higher inspiratory pressures and may not be adequately ventilated. Barotrauma is likely to occur in infants and children. Children often have high airway resistances and are difficult to ventilate with these resuscitators. These devices should be avoided in general and should not be used with infants or children.

Endotracheal intubation is required if the patient cannot be rapidly resuscitated or when adequate spontaneous ventilation does not resume quickly. Experienced personnel should attempt intubation. The patient should be hyperventilated before each attempt, and resuscitative efforts should not be interrupted for more than 30 seconds with each attempt. Cricoid pressure should be applied, when possible, by a second person during endotracheal intubation to protect against regurgitation of gastric contents. The prominence inferior to that of the thyroid cartilage is the cricoid cartilage. Downward pressure should be applied with the thumb and index finger (Fig. 22-12) until the cuff of the endotracheal tube is inflated [156,171].

Once the patient is intubated and the trachea is protected from regurgitation, faster inspiratory flow rates are possible. However, hyperventilation should be avoided. Checking arterial blood gases will assist in the determination of an adequate minute ventilation. Increasing the respiratory rate may be detrimental [172].

The laryngeal mask airway (LMA) has been effective for maintaining airway patency during anesthesia since 1988 and has been accepted as one of the adjuncts for airway control and ventilation during CPR. The LMA provides a more stable and consistent means of ventilation than bag-mask ventilation [173–175]. The current research concludes that regurgitation is less common with LMA than with the bag-mask, and although it cannot provide complete protection from aspiration, it is less frequent when used as the first-line airway device [173,176–178]. Multiple studies have documented the advantages of LMA for its relative ease with insertion and ease of use by a variety of personnel: nurses, medical students, respiratory therapists, and EMS, many with little prior experience using the device [177–180]. Studies have shown that inexperienced personnel achieved an 80% to 94% success rate on the first placement attempts and achieved 98% and 94% on subsequent attempts of adult and pediatric cases, respectively. The LMA provides adequate and effective ventilation when measured against endotracheal intubation [174,180]. Additionally, less equipment and training are needed to insert the device successfully. It may also have advantages over the endotracheal tube when patient airway access is obstructed, the patient has an unstable neck injury, or when suitable positioning of the patient for endotracheal intubation is unattainable [181–183]. LMA insertion has been successful when attempts at endotracheal intubation by experts were unsuccessful [174,179,180]. Endotracheal tubes can be fiberoptically inserted through an established LMA.

Contraindications for LMA use include the patient with an increased risk of aspiration pneumonitis [184–188]. Examples of such situations include morbid obesity, pregnancy, recent food ingestion, gastrointestinal obstruction, and hiatal hernia. Despite these considerations, oxygenation and ventilation during cardiac arrest receive top priority and the LMA should be used if it is the fastest and efficient means of providing airway patency [189].

If attempts at relieving an obstructed airway have failed, several advanced techniques may be used to secure the airway until intubation or tracheostomy is successfully performed. In transtracheal catheter ventilation, a catheter is inserted over a needle through the cricothyroid membrane (Fig. 22-13). The needle is removed and intermittent jet ventilation initiated [190]. In cricothyrotomy, an opening is made in the cricothyroid membrane with a knife [190–193]. Tracheostomy, if still necessary, is best performed in the operating room by a skilled

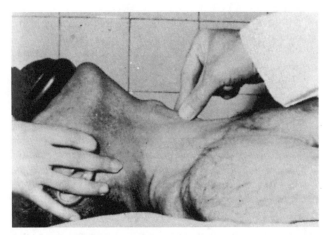

FIGURE 22-12. Cricoid pressure: Application of downward pressure over the cricoid with neck extended. [From BA Sellick: Cricoid pressure to control regurgitation of stomach contents during induction of anaesthesia. *Lancet* 2:404, 1961, with permission.]

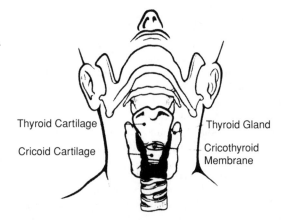

Thyroid Cartilage

Cricoid Cartilage

Thyroid Gland

Cricothyroid Membrane

FIGURE 22-13. Landmarks for locating the cricothyroid membrane for use of transtracheal catheter ventilation or cricothyrotomy. [From *Textbook of Advanced Cardiac Life Support*. Chicago, American Heart Association, 1987, with permission. Copyright American Heart Association.]

surgeon after the airway has already been secured by one of the aforementioned techniques.

CIRCULATORY SUPPORT

Chest compression should not be unduly interrupted while adjunctive procedures are instituted. The rescuer coordinating the resuscitation effort must ensure that adequate pulses are generated by the compressor. The carotid or femoral pulse should be evaluated every few minutes.

Mechanical chest compressors seem useful in the hands of experienced resuscitators. It is important that such devices be correctly calibrated to provide a stroke of 1.5 to 2.0 inch. The position of the press on the sternum must be checked frequently to ensure adequate compression with a minimum of damage. The press may be a manually operated hinged device or may be powered by compressed gas (usually 100% oxygen). The plunger is mounted on a backboard and is associated with a time–pressure-cycled ventilator. This device is programmed to deliver CPR using a compression duration that is 50% of the cycle length. Such units allow the patient to be harnessed to the backboard, fixing the location of the plunger. When used properly, with careful monitoring of patient position, this device facilitates CPR during transport. An acceptable electrocardiogram (ECG) can often be recorded with the compressor in operation, and defibrillation can be delivered during the downstroke of chest compression, without delays in CPR.

Electrocardiographic monitoring is necessary during resuscitation to guide appropriate electrical and pharmacologic therapy. Until ECG monitoring allows diagnosis of the rhythm, the patient should be assumed to be in VF (see section Ventricular Fibrillation and Pulseless Ventricular Tachycardia).

Most defibrillators currently marketed have built-in monitoring circuitry in the paddles or pads ("quick-look"). On application of the defibrillator paddles, the patient's ECG is displayed on the monitor screen. This facilitates appropriate initial therapy. For continuous monitoring beyond the first few minutes, a standard ECG monitoring unit should be used.

Electrocardiographic monitoring must never be relied on without frequent reference to the patient's pulse and clinical condition. What appears on the monitor screen to be VF or asystole must not be treated as such unless the patient is found to be without a pulse. An apparently satisfactory rhythm on the monitor must be accompanied by an adequate pulse and blood pressure.

DEFIBRILLATION

Electrical defibrillation is the definitive treatment for most cardiac arrests. It should be delivered as early as possible and repeated frequently until VF or pulseless VT has been terminated.

Electrical defibrillation involves passing an electrical current through the heart and causing synchronous depolarization of the myofibrils. As the myofibrils repolarize, the opportunity arises for the emergence of organized pacemaker activity.

Proper use of the defibrillator requires special attention to the following:

1. *Selection of proper energy levels* (see Clinical Settings section). This lessens myocardial damage and arrhythmias occasioned by unnecessarily high energies. For biphasic de-

fibrillators, the energy should be 120 to 200 J. For the monophasic defibrillators, the energy should be 360 J [77].
2. *Proper asynchronous mode.* The proper mode must be selected if the rhythm is VF. The synchronizing switch must be deactivated or the defibrillator will dutifully await the R wave that will never come. For rapid pulseless VT (approximately 150 to 200 beats per minute), it is best not to attempt synchronization with the R wave because this increases the likelihood of delivering the shock on the T wave. If the countershock should fall on the T wave and induce VF, another unsynchronized countershock must be delivered promptly after confirming pulselessness.
3. *Proper position of the paddles or pads.* This allows the major energy of the electrical arc to traverse the myocardium. The anterolateral position requires that one paddle or pad be placed to the right of the upper sternum, just below the clavicle. The other paddle or pad is positioned to the left of the nipple in the left midaxillary line. In the anteroposterior position, one paddle or pad is positioned under the left scapula with the patient lying on it. The anterior paddle or pad is positioned just to the left of the lower sternal border.
4. *Adequate contact between paddles or pads and skin.* This should be ensured, using just enough electrode paste to cover the paddle face without spilling over the surrounding skin. The rescuer should hold the paddles with firm pressure (approximately 25 pounds). The pressure should be delivered using the forearms; leaning into the paddles should be avoided for fear that the rescuer may slip. If defibrillator electrode paddles are used, the skin must be carefully prepared according to the manufacturer's directions.
5. *No contact with anyone other than the patient.* The rescuer must be sturdily balanced on both feet and not standing on a wet floor. CPR must be discontinued with no one remaining in contact with the patient. It is the responsibility of the person defibrillating to check the patient's surroundings, ensure the safety of all participants, loudly announce the intention to countershock, and depress both buttons. The use of an automatic or semiautomatic defibrillator does not decrease the operator's need for diligence.
6. If no skeletal muscle twitch or spasm has occurred, the equipment, contacts, and synchronizer switch used for elective cardioversions should be rechecked.

Electrical energy delivered in a biphasic waveform is clearly superior to monophasic waveforms for implantable defibrillators [194], but there is a paucity of evidence to show that one waveform is superior over another with regard to return of spontaneous circulation or survival to hospital discharge [77]. External defibrillators are now available with biphasic waveforms.

ELECTRONIC PACEMAKER

Pacemaker therapy requiring positioning of transvenous or transthoracic electrodes is time-consuming, technically demanding, and usually interferes with adequate performance of CPR. External pacing equipment often allows myocardial capture with some discomfort and skeletal muscle contraction [195]. Obviously, this is unimportant during asystole or bradycardic cardiac arrest. Unfortunately, pacing does not produce a perfusing rhythm in most cases of cardiac arrest [196–198].

Patients who respond to emergency pacing are those with severe bradycardias or conduction block who have reasonably well-preserved myocardial function [199].

VENOUS ACCESS

Venous access with a reliable intravenous (IV) route must be established early in the course of the resuscitative effort to allow for the administration of necessary drugs and fluids. However, initial defibrillation attempts and CPR should not be delayed for the placement of an IV line. Peripheral venous access through antecubital veins is often more convenient because it is less likely to interfere with other rescue procedures. Cannulation of such veins may be difficult, however, because of venous collapse or constriction. A large-bore catheter system should be used because needles in the vein are apt to become dislodged during CPR. A long catheter may be threaded into the central circulation. Alternatively, the extremity may be elevated for 10 to 20 seconds and 20 mL of flush solution used to help entry of the drug into the central circulation [200]. Lower extremity peripheral veins should be avoided because it is questionable whether drugs enter into the central circulation from such veins during CPR [82,201].

Central venous access offers a more secure route for drug administration and should be attempted if initial resuscitative efforts are not successful. Femoral vein cannulation is apparently difficult to achieve during CPR [202], and flow into the thorax is slower than with upper torso access. If the femoral vein is successfully cannulated, a long line should be placed into the vena cava above the level of the diaphragm. Internal jugular or subclavian routes are preferable, but long line placement should not be allowed to delay defibrillation attempts or interfere with CPR. They should be placed by experienced operators.

Although central lines may be associated with an increased incidence of complications for patients receiving fibrinolytic therapy, they are not an absolute contraindication to its use.

In infants and children as well as adults, the intraosseous route is easy to achieve and is very effective for venous access. Special kits to achieve intraosseous access in the adult are now available.

Drugs such as epinephrine, atropine, and lidocaine can be administered via the endotracheal tube if there is delay in achieving venous access. However, this route requires a higher dose to achieve an equivalent blood level [203–205], and a sustained duration of action (a "depot effect") can be expected if there is a return in spontaneous circulation [204,205]. It is suggested that 2.0 to 2.5 times the IV dose be administered when using the endotracheal route. Delivery of the drug to the circulation is facilitated by diluting the drug to 10 mL of normal saline or distilled water and delivering it through a catheter positioned beyond the tip of the endotracheal tube. Stop chest compressions, spray the solution quickly down the endotracheal tube, and give several quick insufflations before reinitiating chest compressions. Intracardiac injection of epinephrine is to be avoided.

CORRECTION OF HYPOXIA

Hypoxia should be corrected early during CPR with administration of the highest possible oxygen concentration. Inadequate perfusion, decreased pulmonary blood flow, pulmonary edema, atelectasis, and ventilation-perfusion mismatch all contribute to the difficulty in maintaining adequate tissue oxygenation.

Inadequate tissue oxygenation results in anaerobic metabolism, the generation of lactic acid, and the development of metabolic acidosis.

CORRECTION OF ACIDOSIS

Correction of acidosis must be considered when the arrest has lasted for more than several minutes. *Metabolic acidosis* develops because of tissue hypoxia and conversion to anaerobic metabolism. *Respiratory acidosis* occurs because of apnea or hypoventilation with intrapulmonary ventilation-perfusion abnormalities; the marked decrease in pulmonary blood flow that exists even with well-performed CPR also contributes.

Sodium bicarbonate reacts with hydrogen ions to buffer metabolic acidosis by forming carbonic acid and then carbon dioxide and water. Each 50 mEq of sodium bicarbonate generates 260 to 280 mm Hg of carbon dioxide, which can be eliminated only through the expired air. Because carbon dioxide of exhaled gas during CPR is decreased, the carbonic acid generated by sodium bicarbonate cannot be effectively eliminated. Paradoxic intracellular acidosis is likely to result, and arterial blood gases may not correctly reflect the state of tissue acidosis [206,207]. The sodium and osmolar load of bicarbonate is high; excessive administration results in hyperosmolarity, hypernatremia, and worsened cellular acidosis. With these concerns in mind, the AHA guidelines suggest that sodium bicarbonate be avoided until successful resuscitation has reestablished a perfusing rhythm [208]. In the postresuscitative state, the degree of acidosis can be better estimated from blood gases and the acidemia corrected with hyperventilation and possibly bicarbonate administration. Sodium bicarbonate is of questionable value in treating the metabolic acidosis during cardiac arrest; it has not been shown to facilitate ventricular defibrillation or survival in cardiac arrest [209,210]. In any case, bicarbonate should not be used during cardiac arrest until at least 10 minutes have passed, the patient is intubated, and the patient has not responded to initial defibrillatory and drug intervention. An exception is the patient with known preexisting hyperkalemia in whom administration of bicarbonate is recommended. The use of bicarbonate may also be of value in patients who have a known preexisting bicarbonate-responsive acidosis or a tricyclic antidepressant overdosage, or to alkalinize the urine in drug overdosage. When bicarbonate is used, 1 mEq per kg may be given as the initial dose. When possible, further therapy should be guided by the calculated base deficit. To avoid iatrogenically induced alkalosis, complete correction of the calculated base deficit should be avoided.

VOLUME REPLACEMENT

Increased central volume is often required during CPR, especially if the initial attempts at defibrillation have failed. PEA is particularly likely to be caused either by acute severe hypovolemia (e.g., exsanguination) or by a cardiovascular process for which volume expansion may be a lifesaving temporizing measure (e.g., pericardial tamponade, pulmonary embolism, and septic shock). The usual clues for hypovolemia, such as collapsed jugular and peripheral veins and evidence of peripheral vasoconstriction, are unavailable during cardiac arrest; furthermore, dry mucous membranes and absence of normal secretions (tears, saliva) are unreliable in acute hypovolemia. Most physical findings of tamponade, pulmonary embolism, or septic shock are absent during arrest. Therefore, one must be guided by an appropriate clinical history and have a low threshold to administer volume during CPR.

Simple crystalloids, such as 5% dextrose in water (D_5W), are inappropriate for rapid expansion of the circulatory blood volume. Isotonic crystalloids (0.9% saline, Ringer's lactate), colloids, or blood are necessary for satisfactory volume expansion. Crystalloids are more readily available, easier to administer, and less expensive than colloids. They are also free of the potential to cause allergic reactions or infections. Colloids are more likely to sustain intravascular volume and oncotic pressure. Some studies have suggested shorter resuscitation times and better survival with colloids as opposed to crystalloids [211].

If the patient has a weak pulse, simple elevation of the legs may help by promoting venous return to the central circulation. In profound hypovolemia with subsequent arrest, medical antishock garments (medical antishock trouser suits) may ameliorate the hypovolemia until fluid administration or surgical intervention can supervene. Volume challenges should be given as needed until pulse and blood pressure have been restored or until there is evidence of volume overload. In the postresuscitative phase, pulmonary artery and central venous catheterization are usually needed to adequately monitor volume replacement. Fluid replacement is guided by the patient's clinical course, urine output, and catheterization data. The goal is to achieve optimal cardiac output and perfusion pressure without excessive fluid expansion or pulmonary congestion.

DRUG THERAPY

SYMPATHOMIMETIC DRUGS AND VASOPRESSORS

Sympathomimetic drugs either act directly on adrenergic receptors or act indirectly by releasing catecholamines from nerve endings. Most useful during cardiac emergencies are the adrenergic agents, which include the endogenous biogenic amines epinephrine, norepinephrine, and dopamine, and the synthetic agent isoproterenol and its derivative dobutamine [212–214].

Epinephrine

Epinephrine is a naturally occurring catecholamine that has both α and β activity. Although epinephrine is the pressor agent used most frequently during CPR, the evidence that it improves the outcome in humans is scant.

Indications for the use of epinephrine include all forms of cardiac arrest because its α-vasoconstrictive activity is important in raising the perfusion pressure of the myocardium and brain. The importance of α-adrenergic activity during resuscitation has been noted in several studies [215–217], whereas administration of pure β agonists (e.g., isoproterenol or dobutamine) has been shown to be ineffective [218,219]. The β action of epinephrine is theoretically useful in asystole and bradycardic arrests by increasing heart rate. The β effect has also been touted to convert asystole to VF or to convert "fine" VF to "coarse." Coarse or wide-amplitude VF is easier to convert to a perfusing rhythm than fine or small-amplitude VF. However, this primarily may be due to the shorter time course of the arrest in patients still manifesting wide-amplitude rather than small-amplitude VF.

Epinephrine is best administered intravenously. As soon as possible after failed ventricular defibrillation attempts (or if de-

fibrillation is not an option), an adult in cardiac arrest should be given a 1-mg dose at a 1 to 10,000 dilution (10 mL). It should be given in the upper extremity or centrally (see the earlier discussion in the section Venous Access), and may be repeated every 5 minutes. If a peripheral line is used, the drug should be administered rapidly and this should be followed by a 20-mL bolus of IV fluid and elevation of the extremity. It should not be administered in the same IV line as an alkaline solution. If an IV line has not been established, the endotracheal route may be used, but the intracardiac route should be avoided because it is prone to serious complications such as intramyocardial injection, coronary laceration, and pneumothorax. An IV titration of 1 to 4 μg per minute can also be given for inotropic and pressor support. Brown et al. [220,221] published data using a swine model that strongly suggest that doses of epinephrine 10 times those prescribed previously may be more advantageous during arrest. Martin et al. [222] demonstrated a drop in end-tidal partial pressure of carbon dioxide during CPR in a canine model with high-dose epinephrine. This occurred despite a rise in coronary perfusion pressure and may be due to pulmonary vascular shunting or a further diminution of cardiac output. Early results with the use of high-dose epinephrine in humans were modestly encouraging [223–225], but two multicenter trials have failed to demonstrate an improvement in survival or neurologic outcome [226,227].

Risks in the use of epinephrine and other α agonists include tissue necrosis from extravasation and inactivation from admixture with bicarbonate.

Norepinephrine

Norepinephrine is a potent α agonist with β activity. Its salutary α effects during CPR are similar to those of epinephrine [228,229]. However, there are no data to support the belief that it is superior to epinephrine during an arrest.

The major effect of norepinephrine is on the blood vessels. Initial coronary vasoconstriction usually gives way to coronary vasodilatation, probably as a result of increased myocardial metabolic activity. In a heart with compromised coronary reserve, this may cause further ischemia. During cardiac arrest, its usefulness, like that of epinephrine, is most likely due to peripheral vasoconstriction with an increase in perfusion pressure. In patients with spontaneous circulation who are in cardiogenic shock (when peripheral vasoconstriction is often already extreme), its effect is more difficult to predict. Norepinephrine also causes considerable renal and mesenteric vasoconstriction, whereas dopamine at low infusion rates causes vasodilatation in these vascular beds.

Indications for the use of norepinephrine during cardiac arrest are similar to those for epinephrine, although there does not appear to be any reason to prefer it to epinephrine. Norepinephrine appears to be most useful in the treatment of shock caused by inappropriate decline in peripheral vascular resistance such as septic shock and neurogenic shock. It is administered by IV infusion, titrated to an adequate perfusion pressure. Four to 8 mg of the bitartrate (2 to 4 mg of the base) should be diluted in 500 mL D_5W or 5% dextrose in normal saline. If 8 mg of the bitartrate is diluted to 500 mL, 1 mL will contain 16 μg per mL; a microdrip administration set may be used to deliver 1 mL in 60 drops. After observing the response to an initial dose of 2 μg per minute, the dose is adjusted to maintain a low normal blood pressure (85 to 90 mm Hg systolic, or somewhat higher in a previously hypertensive individual). An average effective adult dose is 2 to 12 μg per minute. Higher doses are needed in some people. Norepinephrine should not be administered in the same IV line as an alkaline solution. After the patient has been transferred to a critical care unit, the drug may be continued for several days, but should be gradually tapered when possible. Abrupt termination of the infusion (as may occur in transport) may lead to sudden severe hypotension.

Precautions to the use of norepinephrine include its inappropriate use in hypovolemic shock and in patients with already severe vasoconstriction. Intraarterial pressure monitoring is strongly recommended when using norepinephrine because indirect blood pressure measurement is often incorrect in patients with severe vasoconstriction. In patients with myocardial ischemia or infarction, the myocardial oxygen requirements are increased by all catecholamines, but especially by norepinephrine because of its marked afterload-increasing properties. Unless the increased oxygen delivery occasioned by the rise in perfusion pressure outweighs the increase in myocardial oxygen requirement caused by the afterload increase, norepinephrine is likely to have deleterious effects. Heart rate, rhythm, ECG evidence for ischemia, direct systemic and pulmonary pressures, urine output, and cardiac output should be closely monitored when using this drug in patients with myocardial ischemia or infarction. Extravasation of norepinephrine in superficial tissues is apt to result in ischemic necrosis and sloughing. Therefore, norepinephrine should be administered through a catheter well advanced into the vein. If extravasation does occur, 5 to 10 mg of phentolamine in 10 to 15 mL of saline should be infiltrated as soon as possible into the area of extravasation.

Isoproterenol

This synthetic catecholamine has almost pure β-adrenergic activity. Its cardiac activity includes potent inotropic and chronotropic effects, both of which will increase the myocardium's oxygen demand. In addition to bronchodilatation, the arterial beds of the skeletal muscles, kidneys, and gut dilate, resulting in a marked drop in systemic vascular resistance. Cardiac output can be expected to increase markedly unless the increased myocardial oxygen demand results in substantial myocardial ischemia. Systolic blood pressure is usually maintained because of the rise in cardiac output, but the diastolic and mean pressures usually decrease. As a result, coronary perfusion pressure drops at the same time that the myocardial oxygen requirement is increased. This combination can be expected to have deleterious effects in patients with ischemic heart disease, especially during cardiac arrest. The main clinical usefulness of isoproterenol is in its ability to stimulate pacemakers within the heart.

Indications for isoproterenol are primarily in the setting of atropine-resistant, hemodynamically significant bradyarrhythmias, including profound sinus and junctional bradycardia, as well as various forms of high-degree AV block. It should be used only as an interim measure, until effective transcutaneous or IV pacing can be instituted. If the aortic diastolic pressure is already low, epinephrine is likely to be better tolerated as a stimulus to pacemakers. *Under no circumstances should isoproterenol be used during cardiac arrest* [196].

Isoproterenol is administered by titration of an IV solution. One mg of isoproterenol (Isuprel) is diluted with either 250 mL D$_5$W (4 mg per mL) or 500 mL D$_5$W (2 mg per mL). The infusion rate should be only rapid enough to effect an adequate perfusing heart rate (2 to 20 μg per minute, or 0.05 to 0.5 μg per kg per minute). Depending on the adequacy of cardiac reserve, a target heart rate as low as 50 to 55 beats per minute may be satisfactory. Occasionally, more rapid rates are necessary.

Precautions in the use of isoproterenol are largely due to the increase in myocardial oxygen requirement, with its potential for provoking ischemia; *this effect, coupled with the possibility of dropping the coronary perfusion pressure, makes isoproterenol a dangerous selection in the coronary patient.* The marked chronotropic effects may cause tachycardia and may provoke serious ventricular arrhythmias, including VF. Isoproterenol is usually contraindicated if tachycardia is already present, especially if the arrhythmia may be secondary to digitalis toxicity. If significant hypotension develops with its use, it may be combined with another β agonist with α activity. However, switching to dopamine or epinephrine is usually preferable; better yet is the use of pacing for rate control.

Dopamine

This naturally occurring precursor of norepinephrine has α-, β-, and dopamine-receptor stimulating activity. The dopamine-receptor activity dilates renal and mesenteric arterial beds at low doses (1 to 2 μg per kg per minute) which may not produce an increase in heart rate or blood pressure. These effects cannot be blocked with either β- or α-blocking agents. At doses from 2 to 10 μg per kg per minute, dopamine exerts primarily β-adrenergic activity, with an increase in contractile force and heart rate. At doses of 10 μg per kg per minute and greater, the α-adrenergic activity becomes more and more prominent, causing peripheral vasoconstriction and constriction of renal and splanchnic arterial beds. At doses greater than 20 μg per kg per minute, α activity is likely to overcome dopaminergic effects and lower renal and mesenteric blood flow.

Indications for the use of dopamine are primarily significant hypotension and cardiogenic shock. Its dopaminergic effects may be useful in early shock, with decreasing urine output; it may be started at low doses along with volume expansion.

Dopamine is administered by IV titration. A 200-mg ampule is diluted to 250 or 500 mL in D$_5$W or 5% dextrose in normal saline for a concentration of 800 or 400 mg per mL. Dopamine should not be administered in the same IV line as an alkaline solution. For hypotension, the initial infusion rate is usually 2 to 5 μg per kg per minute, which is increased until a satisfactory response is achieved in blood pressure and urine output. As with all catecholamine infusions, the lowest infusion rate that results in satisfactory perfusion should be the goal of therapy. Rarely, a patient may need in excess of 20 μg per kg per minute. Urine output, cardiac output, systemic vascular resistance, and left ventricular filling pressure monitoring is necessary for optimal control of the hemodynamic response.

Precautions for dopamine are similar to those for other catecholamines. Tachycardia or ventricular arrhythmias may require reduction in dosage or discontinuation of the drug. If significant hypotension occurs from the dilating activity of dopaminergic or β-active doses, small amounts of an α-active drug may be added. Dopamine may increase myocardial ischemia. Sloughing may occur if dopamine extravasates into subcutaneous tissues. If this occurs, phentolamine should be infiltrated into the area of extravasation, as for norepinephrine extravasation.

Dobutamine

Dobutamine is a potent synthetic β-adrenergic agent that differs from isoproterenol in that tachycardia is less problematic. Unless ischemia supervenes, cardiac output will increase, as will renal and mesenteric blood flow.

Dobutamine is indicated primarily for the short-term enhancement of ventricular contractility in the patient with heart failure. It may be used for postresuscitative stabilization of the arrest patient or for the patient with heart failure refractory to other drugs. It also may be used in combination with IV nitroprusside, which lowers peripheral vascular resistance and thereby left ventricular afterload. Whereas nitroprusside lowers peripheral resistance, dobutamine maintains the perfusion pressure by augmenting the cardiac output.

Dobutamine is administered by slow-titrated IV infusion. A dose as low as 0.5 μg per kg per minute may prove to be effective, but the usual dose range is 2.5 to 10.0 μg per kg per minute. A 250-mg vial is dissolved in 10 mL of sterile water and then to 250 or 500 mL D_5W, for a concentration of 1 or 0.5 μg per mL. Dobutamine should not be administered in the same IV line as alkaline solutions.

Precautions for dobutamine are similar to those for other β agonists. Dobutamine may cause tachycardia, ventricular arrhythmias, myocardial ischemia, and extension of infarction. It must be used with caution in patients with coronary artery disease.

Vasopressin

Vasopressin is not a catecholamine but a naturally occurring antidiuretic hormone. In high doses, it is a powerful constrictor of smooth muscles and as such has been studied as an adjunctive therapy for cardiac arrest in an attempt to improve perfusion pressures and organ flows. Animal studies have suggested better hemodynamics, organ flow, and acid-base status compared to epinephrine [230,231]. A combination of epinephrine and vasopressin did not improve myocardial blood flow and actually decreased cerebral blood flow in a swine model [228]. It is reported that of eight patients with in-hospital arrest who were given 40 U of IV vasopressin after they had failed to respond to initial defibrillation and epinephrine administration, all had return in spontaneous circulation, and three were discharged neurologically intact [232]. Vasopressin may be especially useful in prolonged cardiac arrest as it remains effective as a vasopressor even in severe acidosis [233,234]. It may be used as a first agent in arrest in lieu of epinephrine or as the second agent if the first dose of epinephrine failed to cause a return in pulse.

ANTIARRHYTHMIC AGENTS

Antiarrhythmics have been thought to play an important role in stabilizing the rhythm in many resuscitation situations; however, the data in support of their value are scanty. Although lidocaine, bretylium, and procainamide had been considered useful in counteracting the tendency to ventricular arrhythmias, convincing evidence of benefit to their use for pulseless VT and VF is wanting. Based on recent studies, amiodarone has gained considerable acceptance for the emergency treatment of refractory VT and VF.

Amiodarone

Amiodarone is a benzofurane derivative that is structurally similar to thyroxine and contains a considerable level of iodine. Gastrointestinal absorption is slow; therefore, when given orally, the onset of action is delayed while the drug slowly accumulates in adipose tissue. The mean elimination half-life is 64 days (range, 24 to 160 days). IV administration allows rapid onset of action, with therapeutic blood levels achieved within 600 mg given over 24 hours.

Amiodarone decreases myocardial contractility, and it also causes vasodilatation, which counterbalances the decrease in contractility. In general, it is therefore well tolerated, even by those with myocardial dysfunction.

Amiodarone given intravenously has been successful in terminating a variety of reentrant and nonreentrant supraventricular and ventricular rhythms [235,236]. In a major study of out-of-hospital cardiac arrest due to ventricular arrhythmias refractory to shock, patients were initially treated with either amiodarone (246 patients) or placebo (258 patients). Patients given amiodarone had a higher incidence of bradycardia (41% vs. 25%) and hypotension (59% vs. 48%), but also a higher rate of survival to hospital admission (44% vs. 34%) [237]. This study did not demonstrate an increase in survival to hospital discharge or in neurologic status. Based on this study, amiodarone has been given status as an option for use after defibrillation attempts and epinephrine in refractory ventricular arrhythmias during cardiac arrest (class IIb). It also is an optional choice for ventricular rate control in rapid atrial arrhythmias in patients with impaired left ventricular function when digitalis has proved ineffective. Other optional uses are for control of hemodynamically stable VT, polymorphic VT, preexcited atrial arrhythmias, and wide-complex tachycardia of uncertain origin. It may also be useful for chemical cardioversion of atrial fibrillation or as an adjunct to electrical cardioversion of refractory paroxysmal supraventricular tachycardia (PSVT) and atrial fibrillation or flutter.

Administration in cardiac arrest (pulseless VT or VF) is by rapid IV infusion of 300 mg diluted in 20 to 30 mL of saline or D_5W. Supplementary infusions of 150 mg may be used for recurrent or refractory VT or VF.

Administration for rhythms with a pulse is by IV infusion of 150 mg given during 10 minutes, followed by infusion of 1 mg per minute for 6 hours, and then 0.5 mg per minute. Supplemental infusions of 150 mg may be given for recurrent or resistant arrhythmias to a total maximum dose of 2 g during 24 hours.

Lidocaine

This antiarrhythmic agent has been used for ventricular arrhythmias, such as premature ventricular complexes and VT. Premature ventricular complexes are not unusual in apparently healthy people and most often are benign. Even in the patient with chronic heart disease, premature ventricular complexes and nonsustained VT are usually asymptomatic, and controversy exists concerning the need to treat under these circumstances. The situation is very different for patients with myocardial ischemia or recent myocardial infarction, who are much more likely to progress from premature ventricular complexes to sustained VT or VF. Such patients are often treated with antiarrhythmic agents such as lidocaine. There is some evidence for the efficacy of prophylactic lidocaine in reducing primary VF in patients with acute myocardial infarction [238,239]. However, the toxic-to-therapeutic ratio is not favorable enough to warrant its routine use in patients with suspected acute myocardial infarction [240–244].

Lidocaine is of indeterminate efficacy but is an acceptable alternative because of its established use, historical suggestion of efficacy, and suppression of hemodynamically compromising premature ventricular complexes or hemodynamically stable VT. Its routine prophylactic use is not recommended for patients with suspected myocardial infarction. Correction of the underlying cause of the ventricular irritability (e.g., myocardial ischemia, hypoxemia, hypercarbia, electrolyte imbalance, digitalis excess) must also be addressed for successful management of the arrhythmia.

Administration of lidocaine begins with an IV bolus. The onset of action is rapid. Its duration of action is brief but may be prolonged by continuous infusion. A solution of lidocaine, typically 20 mg per mL (2%), should be prepared for IV administration. Prefilled syringes are available for bolus injection. (See the section Ventricular Fibrillation and Pulseless Ventricular Tachycardia for current dosing recommendations.) If the patient has suffered an acute myocardial infarction and has had ventricular arrhythmias, the infusion is continued for hours to days and tapered slowly. If the cause of the arrhythmia has been corrected, the infusion may be tapered more rapidly.

Precautions should be taken against excessive accumulation of lidocaine. The dosage should be reduced in patients with low cardiac output, congestive failure, hepatic failure, and age older than 70 years because of the decreased liver metabolism of the drug. Toxic manifestations are usually neurologic and can vary from slurred speech, tinnitus, sleepiness, and dysphoria to localizing neurologic symptoms. Frank seizures may occur with or without preceding neurologic symptoms and may be controlled with short-acting barbiturates or diazepam. Conscious patients should be warned about possible symptoms of neurologic toxicity and asked to report them immediately if they occur. Enlisting the patient's aid may also allay the fear that could otherwise develop from unexpected neurologic symptoms. The fear surrounding intensive cardiac care is great enough without allowing the patient to assume the worst should such symptoms develop. Excessive blood levels can significantly depress myocardial contractility.

Procainamide

Procainamide hydrochloride is an antiarrhythmic agent with quinidinelike activity. Like quinidine, it is useful in suppressing a wide variety of ventricular and supraventricular arrhythmias. It is effective against reentrant as well as ectopic arrhythmogenic mechanisms. It has somewhat less vagolytic effect than quinidine and does not cause the rise in digoxin level seen with quinidine. Procainamide is sometimes of use in the critical care setting for the suppression of ventricular arrhythmias not effectively treated by amiodarone or lidocaine or in patients who cannot be treated with either of these two agents. It may also be used in patients with supraventricular arrhythmias causing hemodynamic compromise or worsening ischemia.

Procainamide is administered either orally or by IV injection. For serious arrhythmias in the critical care setting, IV injection is preferable. An infusion of 20 mg per minute (0.3 mg per kg per minute) is given up to a loading dose of 17 mg per kg (1.2 g for a 70-kg patient) or until the arrhythmia is suppressed, hypotension develops, or the QRS widens by 50% of its original

width. A maintenance infusion may then be started at 1 to 4 mg per minute. The dosage should be lowered in the presence of renal failure. Blood levels of procainamide and its metabolite N-acetyl procainamide should be monitored in patients with renal failure or patients who are receiving more than 3 mg per minute for more than 24 hours. Infusions as low as 1.4 mg per kg per hour may be needed in patients with renal insufficiency.

Precautions in the use of procainamide include its production of systemic hypotension, disturbance in AV conduction, and decreased ventricular contractility. IV infusion must be carefully monitored, with frequent blood pressure determinations and measurement of ECG intervals PR, QRS, and QT. Hypotension usually responds to slowing the infusion rate. If the QRS interval increases by more than 50% of its initial width, procainamide infusion should be discontinued. Widened QRS signifies toxic blood levels and may herald serious AV conduction abnormalities and asystole. This is particularly true of patients with digitalis intoxication and those with antecedent AV conduction abnormalities. A marked decrease in QT interval may predispose a patient to torsades de pointes. Patients who have ventricular arrhythmias of the torsades variety or ventricular arrhythmias associated with bradycardias should not be treated with procainamide.

Adenosine

Adenosine is an endogenous purine nucleoside that depresses AV nodal conduction and sinoatrial nodal activity. Because of the delay in AV nodal conduction, adenosine is effective in terminating arrhythmias that use the AV node in a reentrant circuit (e.g., PSVT) [245]. In supraventricular tachycardias, such as atrial flutter or atrial fibrillation, or atrial tachycardias that do not use the AV node in a reentrant circuit, blocking transmission through the AV node may prove helpful in clarifying the diagnosis [246]. However, the use of adenosine in wide-complex tachycardia of uncertain origin to discriminate between VT and supraventricular tachycardia with aberrancy is discouraged. The half-life of adenosine is less than 5 seconds because it is rapidly metabolized.

Administration is by IV bolus of 6 mg given during 1 to 3 seconds, followed by a 20-mL saline flush. An additional dose of 12 mg may be given if no effect is seen within 1 to 2 minutes. Patients taking theophylline may need higher doses [247].

Side effects caused by adenosine are transient and may include flushing, dyspnea, and anginalike chest pain (even in the absence of coronary disease). Sinus bradycardia and ventricular ectopy are common after terminating PSVT with adenosine, but the arrhythmias are typically so short-lived as to be clinically unimportant. The reentrant tachycardia may recur after the effect of adenosine has dissipated and may require additional doses of adenosine or a longer-acting drug, such as verapamil or diltiazem.

Theophylline and other methylxanthines, such as theobromine and caffeine, block the receptor responsible for adenosine's electrophysiologic effect; therefore, higher doses may be required in their presence. Dipyridamole and carbamazepine, on the other hand, potentiate and may prolong the effect of adenosine; therefore, other forms of therapy may be advisable [247].

Verapamil and Diltiazem

Unlike other calcium channel-blocking agents, verapamil and diltiazem increase refractoriness in the AV node and significantly slow conduction. This action may terminate reentrant tachycardias that use the AV node in the reentrant circuit (e.g., PSVT). These drugs may also slow the ventricular response in patients with atrial flutter or fibrillation and even in patients with multifocal atrial tachycardia. They should be used only in patients in whom the tachycardia is known to be supraventricular in origin.

Administration of verapamil is by IV bolus of 2.5 to 5.0 mg during 2 minutes. In the absence of a response, additional doses of 5 to 10 mg may be given at 15- to 30-minute intervals to a maximum of 20 mg. The maximum cumulative dose is 20 mg. Diltiazem may be given as an initial dose of 0.25 mg per kg with a follow-up dose of 0.35 mg per kg, if needed [248,249]. A maintenance infusion of 5 to 15 mg per hour may be used to control the rate of ventricular response in atrial fibrillation.

Verapamil and diltiazem should be used for arrhythmias known to be supraventricular in origin and in the absence of preexcitation. Both verapamil and diltiazem may decrease myocardial contractility and worsen congestive heart failure or even provoke cardiogenic shock in patients with significant left ventricular dysfunction. They should be used with caution, therefore, in patients with known cardiac failure or suspected diminished cardiac reserve, and in the elderly. If worsened failure or hypotension develops after the use of these agents, calcium should be administered, as described in section Other Agents.

Magnesium

Cardiac arrhythmias and even sudden cardiac death have been associated with magnesium deficiency [250]. Hypomagnesemia decreases the uptake of intracellular potassium and may precipitate VT or fibrillation. Routine use of magnesium in cardiac arrest or after myocardial infarction is not recommended. Magnesium may be of value for patients with torsades de pointes, even in the absence of hypomagnesemia.

Magnesium is administered intravenously. For rapid administration during VT or VF with suspected or documented hypomagnesemia, 1 to 2 g may be diluted in 100 mL of D_5W and given during 1 to 2 minutes. A 24-hour infusion of magnesium may be used for periinfarction patients with documented hypomagnesemia. A loading dose of 1 to 2 g is diluted in 100 mL D_5W and slowly given during 5 minutes to 1 hour, followed by an infusion of 0.5 to 1 g per hour during the ensuing 24 hours. Clinical circumstances and the serum magnesium level dictate the rate and duration of the infusion. Hypotension or asystole may occur with rapid administration.

OTHER AGENTS

Additional drugs occasionally found useful or necessary during resuscitation or in the immediate postresuscitation period include atropine, calcium, nitroprusside, and nitroglycerine; these agents are discussed in the following sections. Many other drugs may be required in particular circumstances and are discussed in other parts of this text. An incomplete list of these drugs includes beta-blockers, ibutilide, propafenone, flecainide, sotalol, digoxin, antibiotics, thiamine, thyroxine, morphine, naloxone, adrenocorticoids, fibrinolytic agents, anticoagulants, antiplatelet agents, and dextrose.

Atropine Sulfate

Atropine is a vagolytic drug of use in increasing heart rate by stimulating pacers and facilitating AV conduction suppressed by excessive vagal tone.

Atropine is indicated primarily in bradycardias causing hemodynamic difficulty or associated with ventricular arrhythmias (see Fig. 22-17). Atropine may be useful in AV block at the nodal level. It is also used in asystole and bradycardic arrests in the hope that decreased vagal tone will allow the emergence of an effective pacemaker [251].

Atropine is administered by IV bolus. If a rapid, full vagolytic response is desired, as in asystole or bradycardic arrest, 1 mg should be administered intravenously at once. If a satisfactory response has not occurred within several (3 to 5) minutes, additional 1-mg doses should be given in a bolus, to a maximum dose of 3 mg (0.04 mg per kg) [252]. For bradycardia with a pulse, the initial dose should be 0.5 mg repeated every 5 minutes until the desired effect is obtained, to a maximum dose of 3 mg (0.04 mg per kg). Atropine may be given by the endotracheal route at doses 2.5 times the IV dose.

Precautions for atropine include the requirement that an inordinately rapid heart rate not be produced. Patients with ischemic heart disease are likely to have worsened ischemia or ventricular arrhythmias if the rate is too rapid. Uncommonly, a patient will have a paradoxic slowing of rate with atropine; this is more likely to occur with smaller first doses and is caused by a central vagal effect. This effect is rapidly counteracted by additional atropine. In this situation, the next dose of atropine should be given immediately. If additional atropine does not correct the problem, the patient may require judicious use of isoproterenol or pacemaker therapy.

Calcium

Calcium's positive inotropic effect has led to its use in cardiac arrest. The contractile state of the myocardium depends in part on the intracellular concentration of the calcium ion. Transmembrane calcium flux serves an important regulatory function in both active contraction and active relaxation. The use of calcium in cardiac arrest is based on an early report by Kay and Blalock [253] in which several pediatric cardiac surgical patients were successfully resuscitated, apparently with the aid of calcium. However, several field studies have failed to demonstrate an improvement in survival or neurologic outcome with the use of calcium versus a control [254–256]. In addition, many patients are found during arrest to have severely hypercalcemic blood levels after usual doses of calcium [257,258]. This is apparently due to the markedly contracted volume of distribution of the ion in the arrested organism. In addition, calcium has the theoretic disadvantage of facilitating postanoxic tissue damage, especially in the brain and heart. Digitalis toxicity may be exacerbated by the administration of calcium.

Calcium is indicated only in those circumstances in which calcium has been shown to be of benefit [251,259]: Calcium channel blocker toxicity, severe hyperkalemia, severe hypocalcemia, arrest after multiple transfusions with citrated blood, fluoride toxicity, and while coming off heart-lung bypass after cardioplegic arrest.

Calcium is available as calcium chloride, calcium gluceptate, and calcium gluconate. The gluconate salt is unstable and less frequently available. The chloride salt provides the most direct source of calcium ion and produces the most rapid effect. The gluceptate and gluconate salts require hepatic degradation to release the free calcium ion. Calcium chloride is, therefore, the best choice. It is highly irritating to tissues and must be injected into a large vein with precautions to avoid extravasation. Calcium chloride is available in a 10% solution. An initial dose of 250 to 500 mg may be administered slowly during several minutes. It may be repeated as necessary at 10-minute intervals, if strong indications exist.

Precautions for calcium use include the need for slow injection without extravasation. If bicarbonate has been administered through the same line, it must be cleared before introducing the calcium. If the patient has a rhythm, rapid injection may result in bradycardia. Calcium salts must be used with caution in patients receiving digitalis.

Sodium Nitroprusside

This is a rapidly acting dilator of both arteries and veins. Systemic arterial dilatation decreases impedance to left ventricular outflow (afterload reduction), thereby diminishing resistance to left ventricular ejection and improving cardiac output. Venous dilatation simultaneously provides preload reduction by withholding blood from the central circulation and reducing left ventricular filling pressure and volume. Myocardial oxygen consumption drops and subendocardial blood flow may rise as the ventricular wall stress is lowered. In addition, the lowered left ventricular filling pressures cause a decrease in pulmonary capillary pressure and pulmonary congestion. Although vasodilators are most commonly used in the critical care unit, they are occasionally needed in the emergency room to aid in the stabilization of the resuscitated patient with severe left ventricular dysfunction.

Nitroprusside is indicated in any situation in which cardiac output is severely reduced, causing either cardiogenic shock with elevated systemic vascular resistance or pulmonary congestion from elevated left ventricular filling pressure. Patients with aortic or mitral regurgitation or a left-to-right shunt from a ventricular septal rupture are apt to respond especially well to nitroprusside infusion. Nitroprusside has also become a preferred treatment for patients in hypertensive crisis.

Nitroprusside is administered by IV infusion. The onset of action is rapid, so that the effects of dose change become apparent within several minutes. For patients with severe left ventricular failure, infusion should begin at 10 μg per minute, with increments of 5 to 10 μg per minute at 5-minute intervals. Most patients respond to a total dose of 50 to 100 μg per minute, although an occasional patient requires a significantly higher dose. Patients in hypertensive crisis may be started at 50 μg per minute and may require as much as 400 to 1,000 μg per minute. Nitroprusside is available in 50-μg vials of dihydrate. The drug should be dissolved in 5 mL of D_5W and diluted to a volume of 250 to 1,000 mL in D_5W. Because of the instability of the reconstituted solution, it is recommended that it be used within 4 hours. The solution should be wrapped in opaque material because nitroprusside will deteriorate more rapidly with exposure to light.

Precautions for nitroprusside include hypotension, usually secondary to excessive dosage. Although most patients with hypotension cannot tolerate nitroprusside, some can be given nitroprusside with volume repletion. Nitroprusside is converted to thiocyanate by a hepatic enzyme, and the thiocyanate is cleared by the kidneys. Signs and symptoms of thiocyanate toxicity include nausea, tinnitus, blurred vision, delirium, elevated superior vena cava, or mixed venous oxygen saturation and a lactic acidosis. Nitroprusside should be discontinued if the latter two signs are observed.

Nitroglycerin

Like nitroprusside, nitroglycerin is a vasodilator that may prove useful in the emergency treatment of the postresuscitation patient. It may be given sublingually, transdermally, or intravenously, depending on the situation and desired dose. Unlike nitroprusside, nitroglycerin is a more potent dilator of venous capacitance vessels than of arterioles; therefore, it is more a preload reducer than an afterload reducer. Coronary dilatation does occur and may be particularly beneficial in patients with coronary spasm and acute ischemia. Myocardial ischemia is reversed through the lowering of preload and myocardial oxygen consumption as well as by coronary dilatation.

Sublingual or transdermal nitroglycerin is indicated for angina. The sublingual route is preferable. For persistent or frequently recurring ischemia unrelieved by other routes of administration, an infusion of nitroglycerin is often effective. It is useful for suspected coronary spasm. An infusion of nitroglycerin may also be used for preload reduction in patients with left ventricular failure. It may be given together with an infusion of nitroprusside, especially if ischemia has not been reversed by the hemodynamic effects of nitroprusside alone.

Nitroglycerin is administered by a sublingual tablet or spray (0.3 to 0.4 mg) or by a transdermal patch or ointment. For rapid effect, the sublingual route should be used. It may be repeated every 3 to 5 minutes, if pain relief or ST-segment deviation has not occurred. If ischemia persists, an infusion should be started and titrated to achieve the desired result. A 50-mg bolus of nitroglycerin may be given before the initiation of an IV drip. Two 20-mg vials may be diluted in 250 mL D_5W for a concentration of 160 μg per mL. The infusion is started at 10 to 20 mg per minute and increased by 5 to 10 μg every 5 to 10 minutes until the desired effect is achieved (e.g., fall in left ventricular pressure to 15 to 18 mm Hg, relief of chest pain, or return of ST segments to baseline). Although most patients respond to 50 to 200 μg per minute, an occasional patient will require 500 μg per minute or more; however, the maintenance of high plasma levels of nitroglycerine may induce tolerance. *Whenever possible, intermittent dosing with nitrate-free periods is recommended, and the use of the lowest effective dose is advised.*

Precautions for nitroglycerin use include hypotension and syncope, especially if the patient has had an acute myocardial infarction, is volume-depleted, has restriction to either left ventricular filling (e.g., pericardial constriction or tamponade, hypertrophic disease, mitral stenosis, pulmonic stenosis, or pulmonary hypertension), or obstruction to left ventricular outflow (e.g., aortic stenosis, pulmonic stenosis, or hypertrophic obstructive cardiomyopathy). Rapid titration of IV nitroglycerin in patients with left ventricular failure requires careful hemodynamic monitoring to ensure efficacy and safety. The hypotensive patient may be placed in the Trendelenburg position and given volume replacement. Rarely, a patient with severe obstructive coronary disease develops worsened ischemia with nitroglycerin through a coronary steal mechanism. If ischemia is persistent in spite of maximal tolerated nitroglycerin dose, attempts should be made to decrease the dose, and other modalities of therapy, including heparin or cardiac catheterization, should be considered with a view to early revascularization.

CLINICAL SETTINGS

The procedures involved in the resuscitation of a person who has experienced cardiovascular or respiratory collapse are all part of a continuum progressing from the initial recognition of the problem and the institution of CPR to intervention with defibrillators, drugs, pacemakers, transport, and postresuscitative evaluation and care (Figs. 22-14 through 22-17). The following sections focus on the pharmacologic and electrical interventions appropriate to various clinical settings common in cardiac arrest.

VENTRICULAR FIBRILLATION AND PULSELESS VENTRICULAR TACHYCARDIA

Electrical defibrillation is the most important intervention in treating these arrhythmias (see Chapter 6). The sooner it is administered, the more likely it is to succeed. If a defibrillator is not immediately available and an adult cardiac arrest is witnessed, a precordial thump is recommended by some authors [260,261]; however, no recommendation for or against its use is made in the recent AHA guidelines. Many witnessed arrests in the emergency room will be in monitored patients; the rescuer, however, must never rely solely on the monitored signal but must always confirm the need for CPR by determining the absence of a pulse. Quick-look paddles or pads should confirm the diagnosis of VF or VT and a countershock should

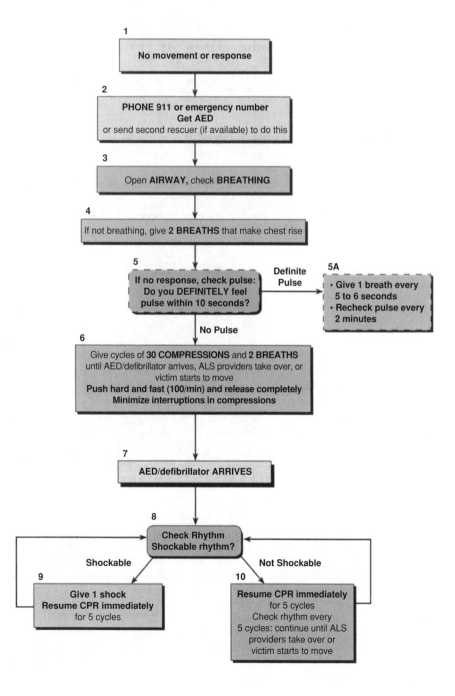

FIGURE 22-14. Adult basic life support healthcare provider algorithm. [From *Circulation* 112[Suppl 24]:IV-19-34, 2005, with permission. Copyright 2005, American Heart Association guidelines for cardiopulmonary resuscitation and emergency cardiovascular care.]

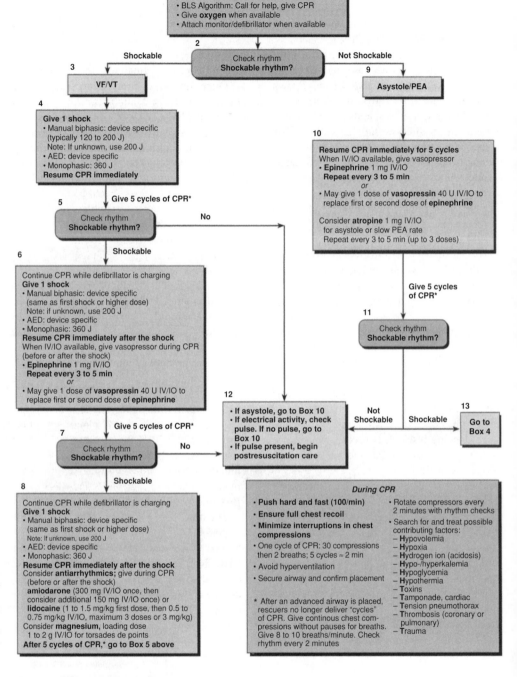

FIGURE 22-15. Advanced cardiac life support pulseless arrest algorithm. [From *Circulation* 112[Suppl 24]:IV-58-66, 2005, with permission. Copyright 2005, American Heart Association guidelines for cardiopulmonary resuscitation and emergency cardiovascular care.]

be attempted (120 to 200 J for biphasic defibrillators and 360 J for monophasic defibrillators). CPR should be resumed without rechecking the rhythm or a pulse. After 2 minutes or about five cycles of CPR, the rhythm should be rechecked. If VF or VT is still present, another shock is applied at the same energy level. CPR is again resumed immediately, and if an IV line is available, vasopressors (epinephrine, 1 mg IV, or intraosseous [IO] every 3 to 5 minutes, or vasopressin 40 units, IV/IO) are administered. After another five cycles of CPR, the rhythm is checked again. If VF or VT is still present, another shock is applied.

After the second shock, if the patient remains in VF or VT, consideration should be given to the administration of an antiarrhythmic agent: amiodarone (300 mg IV/IO once with an additional dose of 150 mg IV/IO if necessary) or lidocaine (1.0 to 1.5 mg per kg IV/IO followed by additional doses of 0.5 to 0.75 mg per kg, if necessary, up to a total dose of 3 mg per kg).

Adequacy of ventilation should be assessed with an arterial blood gas determination, if possible. Sodium bicarbonate is of questionable value during cardiac arrest but should be administered if the patient is known to have preexisting hyperkalemia.

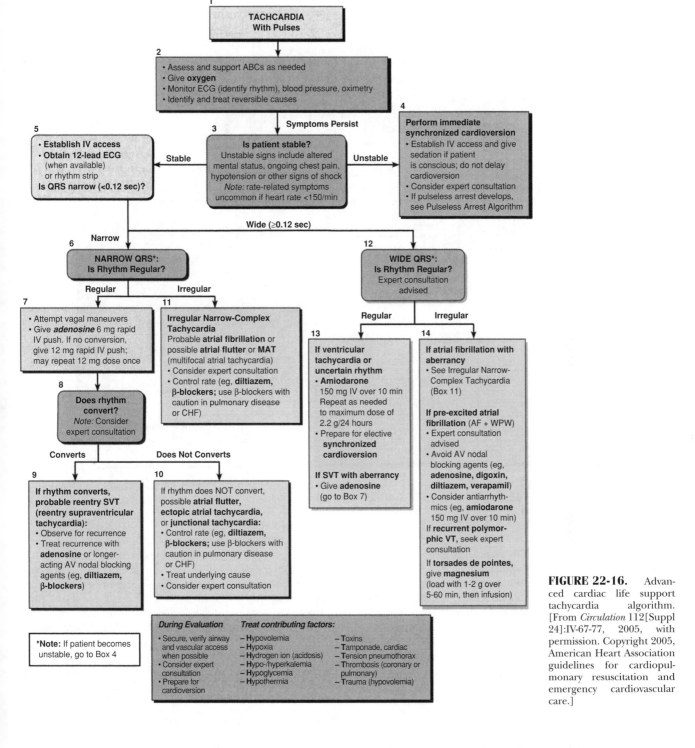

1
TACHCARDIA
With Pulses

2
- Assess and support ABCs as needed
- Give **oxygen**
- Monitor ECG (identify rhythm), blood pressure, oximetry
- Identify and treat reversible causes

Symptoms Persist

3
Is patient stable?
Unstable signs include altered mental status, ongoing chest pain, hypotension or other signs of shock
Note: rate-related symptoms uncommon if heart rate <150/min

5
- **Establish IV access**
- **Obtain 12-lead ECG** (when available) or rhythm strip
Is QRS narrow (<0.12 sec)?

Stable   Unstable

4
Perform immediate synchronized cardioversion
- Establish IV access and give sedation if patient is conscious; do not delay cardioversion
- Consider expert consultation
- If pulseless arrest develops, see Pulseless Arrest Algorithm

Narrow   Wide (≥0.12 sec)

6
NARROW QRS*:
Is Rhythm Regular?

Regular   Irregular

12
WIDE QRS*:
Is Rhythm Regular?
Expert consultation advised

Regular   Irregular

7
- Attempt vagal maneuvers
- Give **adenosine** 6 mg rapid IV push. If no conversion, give 12 mg rapid IV push; may repeat 12 mg dose once

11
Irregular Narrow-Complex Tachycardia
Probable **atrial fibrillation** or possible **atrial flutter** or MAT (multifocal atrial tachycardia)
- Consider expert consultation
- Control rate (eg, **diltiazem, β-blockers;** use β-blockers with caution in pulmonary disease or CHF)

8
Does rhythm convert?
Note: Consider expert consultation

Converts   Does Not Converts

13
If ventricular tachycardia or uncertain rhythm
- **Amiodarone** 150 mg IV over 10 min Repeat as needed to maximum dose of 2.2 g/24 hours
- Prepare for elective **synchronized cardioversion**

If SVT with aberrancy
- Give **adenosine** (go to Box 7)

14
If atrial fibrillation with aberrancy
- See Irregular Narrow-Complex Tachycardia (Box 11)

If pre-excited atrial fibrillation (AF + WPW)
- Expert consultation advised
- Avoid AV nodal blocking agents (eg, **adenosine, digoxin, diltiazem, verapamil**)
- Consider antiarrhythmics (eg, **amiodarone** 150 mg IV over 10 min)
If recurrent polymorphic VT, seek expert consultation
If torsades de pointes, give **magnesium** (load with 1-2 g over 5-60 min, then infusion)

9
If rhythm converts, probable reentry SVT (reentry supraventricular tachycardia):
- Observe for recurrence
- Treat recurrence with **adenosine** or longer-acting AV nodal blocking agents (eg, **diltiazem, β-blockers**)

10
If rhythm does NOT convert, possible **atrial flutter, ectopic atrial tachycardia,** or **junctional tachycardia:**
- Control rate (eg, **diltiazem, β-blockers;** use β-blockers with caution in pulmonary disease or CHF)
- Treat underlying cause
- Consider expert consultation

*Note: If patient becomes unstable, go to Box 4

During Evaluation
- Secure, verify airway and vascular access when possible
- Consider expert consultation
- Prepare for cardioversion

Treat contributing factors:
- Hypovolemia
- Hypoxia
- Hydrogen ion (acidosis)
- Hypo-/hyperkalemia
- Hypoglycemia
- Hypothermia
- Toxins
- Tamponade, cardiac
- Tension pneumothorax
- Thrombosis (coronary or pulmonary)
- Trauma (hypovolemia)

FIGURE 22-16. Advanced cardiac life support tachycardia algorithm. [From *Circulation* 112[Suppl 24]:IV-67-77, 2005, with permission. Copyright 2005, American Heart Association guidelines for cardiopulmonary resuscitation and emergency cardiovascular care.]

ASYSTOLE

Asystole is obviously the end result of any pulseless rhythm. When asystole is the presenting rhythm, it is often the termination of untreated VF. In the prehospital setting, many cases of asystole are related to delayed initiation of BLS or ACLS. Primary asystole associated with increased parasympathetic tone is less common but does occur. Whether this rhythm occurs as the initial rhythm or follows on VT or fibrillation, it carries a very

poor prognosis. Less than 1% to 2% of patients can be expected to revert successfully to a perfusing rhythm. Even more rarely will such patients leave the hospital with reasonable neurologic integrity or significant long-term survival; their best hope lies in the early discovery and treatment of a reversible cause for cardiovascular collapse, such as hypovolemia. Occasionally, asystole develops due to excessive vagal tone, such as is seen with induction of anesthesia, during surgical procedures, or with stimulation of the carotid body, bladder, biliary, or gastrointestinal tract.

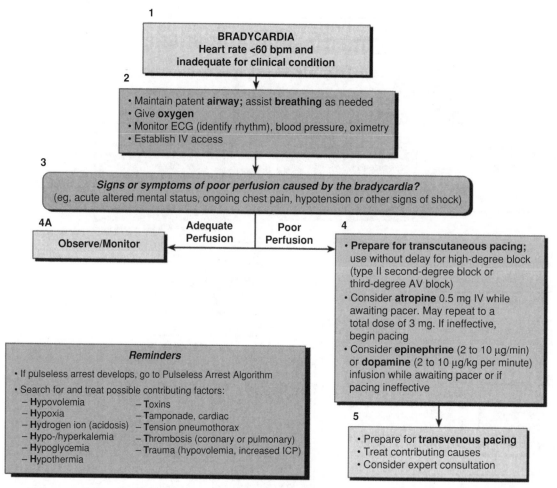

FIGURE 22-17. Bradycardia algorithm. [From *Circulation* 112[Suppl 24]:IV-67-77, 2005, with permission. Copyright 2005, American Heart Association guidelines for cardiopulmonary resuscitation and emergency cardiovascular care.]

Unfortunately, most patients with asystole have severe coronary artery disease and are unlikely to be saved.

In patients with apparent asystole, CPR is initiated and an IV line is established as soon as possible (Fig. 22-15). Either epinephrine (1 mg IV/IO and repeated every 3 to 5 minutes) or vasopressin (1 dose of 40 U IV/IO to replace the first or second dose of epinephrine) is administered. Atropine at a dose of 1 mg IV/IO may also be considered. After five cycles of CPR, the rhythm is rechecked. If asystole persists, the aforementioned sequence is repeated

It has been demonstrated that VF may masquerade as asystole in several leads and for minutes at a time [262]. It is therefore important to check at least two different lead configurations at 90-degree orientation to confirm the diagnosis of asystole. Routine shocking of asystole, however, is discouraged because of the possibility of increasing parasympathetic tone [263,264] and thus decreasing further any chance of return of spontaneous rhythm. No improvement in survival has been demonstrated with the use of shocks for presumed asystole [265,266].

As in other forms of arrest, neither sodium bicarbonate nor calcium has been shown to be of benefit; these agents should be considered only under specific circumstances (see previous discussion).

Temporary artificial pacing is of no likely benefit in primary or postcountershock asystole. Pacing with endocardial, percutaneous transthoracic, or external transcutaneous electrodes has led to pitifully few long-term survivals in these cases [196–198].

The use of isoproterenol in an attempt to stimulate pacemakers through its β-adrenergic agonist effects has not proved beneficial. Indeed, its peripheral β stimulation produces a decrease in arterial resistance and perfusion pressure that is likely to be detrimental, whereas α agonists seem to increase myocardial and cerebral perfusion [215–218,267,268].

PULSELESS ELECTRICAL ACTIVITY

PEA is present when an arrest patient is found to have organized ECG ventricular complexes (QRS) not associated with a palpable pulse (Fig. 22-15). Pulseless VT is not considered a form of PEA. Electromechanical dissociation is a form of PEA in which the QRS is unaccompanied by any evidence of ventricular contraction and the emergency response is the same. Bradysystolic rhythms and severe wide-complex bradycardias may be considered along with PEA. These arrhythmias may be associated with specific clinical states that, if reversed early, may lead to the return of a pulse. It is best, therefore, to consider them together. When PEA is encountered, severe hypovolemia, hypoxia, acidosis, hyperkalemia or hypokalemia, hypoglycemia, hypothermia, drug overdose, cardiac tamponade, massive pulmonary embolism, tension pneumothorax, and severe myocardial contractile dysfunction should be considered.

With the diagnosis of PEA, CPR is initiated and, as soon as possible, volume is administered in the form of IV crystalloid or colloid. If PEA is indeed caused by intravascular volume depletion, a fluid challenge may return a pulse. As described in section Asystole, vasopressors should be administered every 3 to 5 minutes if a pulse has not returned. In bradycardic PEA, atropine is given as in asystole. Bicarbonate is used for preexisting hyperkalemia and is acceptable for known preexisting bicarbonate-responsive acidosis, tricyclic overdose, to alkalinize the urine with other drug overdoses, and in intubated and well-ventilated patients with prolonged arrest intervals.

In patients at high risk for pericardial effusions (i.e., patients hospitalized with known malignancy, severe renal failure, recent myocardial infarction, or recent cardiac catheterization), pericardiocentesis should be attempted early in the course of CPR if the patient is not responding to volume administration and α agonists. In prehospital arrests, pericardial tamponade is rare, but an attempt at pericardiocentesis is warranted if there is no favorable response to volume or α agonists. Echocardiography, when available, almost always confirms or excludes the possibility of tamponade and may be useful in delineating the volume status as well as the function of the ventricles.

SPECIAL SITUATIONS

Patients who have nearly drowned in cold water may recover after prolonged periods of submersion. Apparently, the hypothermia and the bradycardia of the diving reflex may serve to protect against organ damage [269–271]. Successful resuscitation has been described after considerable periods of submersion [270,271]. Because it is often difficult for bystanders and rescuers to estimate the duration of submersion, in most cases it is warranted to initiate CPR at the scene, unless physical evidence exists of irreversible death, such as putrefaction or dependent rubor.

Hypothermia may occur with environmental exposures other than cold-water drowning. The body's ability to maintain temperature is diminished by alcohol, sedation, antidepressants, neurologic problems, and advanced age. Because of the associated bradycardia and oxygen-sparing effects, prolonged hypothermia and arrest may be tolerated with complete recovery. A longer period may be needed to establish breathlessness and pulselessness because of profound bradycardia and slowed respiratory rate. Resuscitative efforts should not be abandoned until near-normal temperature has been reestablished [272].

Electrical shock and lightning strike may lead to tetanic spasm of respiratory muscles or convulsion, causing respiratory arrest. VF or asystole may occur from the electrical shock or after prolonged respiratory arrest. Before initiating assessment and CPR, the potential rescuer must ascertain whether the person who has been shocked is still in contact with the electrical energy and that live wires are not in dangerous proximity. If the individual is located at the top of a utility pole, CPR is best instituted after the person is lowered to the ground [273].

Open-chest CPR with thoracotomy should be applied early in cases of penetrating chest trauma associated with cardiac arrest (see previous discussion). In such patients, thoracotomy by trained personnel allows for the relief of pericardial tamponade and possible control of exsanguinating hemorrhage. Well-equipped trauma centers should have multidisciplinary teams that can provide early, definitive surgical treatment. The unanswered question is whether another subgroup of patients who have not responded to conventional ACLS techniques (including defibrillation attempts and drugs) would benefit from thoracotomy and open-chest CPR. Animal studies suggest that survival may be improved over closed-chest compression if open–chest CPR is used within the first 15 minutes of arrest [274–276]. If open-chest CPR is delayed until 20 minutes or more of closed-chest CPR, there is no improvement in outcome despite improved hemodynamics. In patients with out-of-hospital arrest in whom open-chest CPR was attempted after 30 minutes of conventional CPR, survival did not improve [277].

Open-chest CPR may also be indicated in blunt trauma with cardiac arrest and cardiac arrest due to hypothermia, pulmonary embolism, pericardial tamponade, or abdominal hemorrhage in which initiation of conventional therapy and closed-chest CPR is not proving effective. In the aforementioned cases, the decision to use open-chest CPR presupposes quick availability of definitive surgical intervention. Early surgical exploration is indicated in penetrating abdominal trauma with deterioration and cardiac arrest in which aortic cross-clamping may provide temporary control of abdominal hemorrhage.

Induced therapeutic hypothermia (32°C to 34°C) for 12 to 24 hours improves survival and neurologic outcome in comatose patients who have survived an out-of-hospital VF arrest [278,279]. Hypothermia may also be beneficial for in-hospital arrests. Lower cardiac index and hyperglycemia tend to occur more frequently in hypothermic patients. Shivering must be prevented to reduce metabolic rate.

REFERENCES

1. Paraskos JA: Biblical accounts of resuscitation. *J Hist Med Allied Sci* 47:310, 1992.
2. Paraskos JA: History of CPR and the role of the national conference. *Ann Emerg Med* 22:274, 1993.
3. Safar P: History, in Safar P, Bircher N (eds): *Cardiopulmonary Cerebral Resuscitation*. London, WB Saunders, 1988; p 7.
4. Ibycus: "Chrysippus," quoted in Strauss MB (ed): *Familiar Medical Quotations*. Boston, Little, Brown and Company, 1968.
5. Stephenson HE Jr: *Cardiac Arrest and Resuscitation*. St. Louis, Mosby, 1958.
6. Zoll PM, Linenthal AJ, Gibson W, et al: Termination of ventricular fibrillation in man by externally applied electrical countershock. *N Engl J Med* 254:727, 1956.
7. Safar P: Mouth to mouth airway. *Anesthesiology* 18:904, 1957.
8. Safar P, Escarraga L, Elam JO: A comparison of the mouth to mouth and mouth to airway methods of artificial respiration with the chest pressure arm-lift method. *N Engl J Med* 258:671, 1958.
9. Elam JO, Green DG, Brown ES, et al: Oxygen and carbon dioxide exchange and energy cost of expired air resuscitation. *JAMA* 167:328, 1958.
10. Kouwenhoven WB, Jude JR, Knickerbocker GG: Closed chest cardiac massage. *JAMA* 173:1064, 1960.
11. Cardiopulmonary resuscitation: statement by the Ad Hoc Committee on Cardiopulmonary Resuscitation of the Division of Medical Sciences, National Academy of Sciences—National Research Council. *JAMA* 198:372, 1966.
12. Standards for cardiopulmonary resuscitation (CPR) and emergency cardiac care (ECC). *JAMA* 227[Suppl]:833, 1974.
13. Standards and guidelines for cardiopulmonary resuscitation (CPR) and emergency cardiac care (ECC). *JAMA* 244:453, 1980.
14. Standards and guidelines for cardiopulmonary resuscitation (CPR) and emergency cardiac care (ECC). *JAMA* 255:2843, 1986.
15. Emergency Cardiac Care Committee and Subcommittees, American Heart Association. Guidelines for cardiopulmonary resuscitation and emergency cardiac care. *JAMA* 268:2171, 1992.

16. Guidelines 2000 for cardiopulmonary resuscitation and emergency cardiac care. *Circulation* 102[Suppl 8]:I-1, 2000.

17. ECC Committee, Subcommittees and Task Forces of the American Heart Association. 2005 American Heart Association Guidelines for Cardiopulmonary Resuscitation and Emergency Cardiovascular Care. *Circulation* 112[24 Suppl]:IV1-203, 2005.

18. A definition of irreversible coma: report of the Ad Hoc Committee of the Harvard Medical School to Examine the Definition of Brain Death. *JAMA* 205:337, 1968.

19. An appraisal of the criteria of cerebral death. A summary statement: a collaborative study. *JAMA* 237:982, 1976.

20. Guidelines for the determination of death: report of the medical consultants on the diagnosis of death to the President's Commission for the Study of Ethical Problems in Medicine and Biomedical and Behavioral Research. *JAMA* 246:2184, 1981.

21. *Kansas Session Laws of 1970*, cha378.

22. *Commonwealth v Golston*, 366 NE 2d 744 (1977).

23. Wijdicks EFM: The diagnosis of brain death. *N Engl J Med* 344:1215, 2001.

24. Lund I, Skulberg A: Resuscitation of cardiac arrest outside hospitals: experience with a mobile intensive care unit in Oslo. *Acta Anaesthesiol Scand Suppl* 53:13, 1973.

25. Copley DP, Mantle JA, Roger WJ, et al: Improved outcome for prehospital cardiopulmonary collapse with resuscitation by bystanders. *Circulation* 56:902, 1977.

26. Cummins RO, Eisenberg MS, Hallstrom AP, et al: Survival of out-of-hospital cardiac arrest with early initiation of cardiopulmonary resuscitation. *Am J Emerg Med* 3:114, 1985.

27. Weaver WD, Cobb LA, Hallstrom AP, et al: Considerations for improving survival from out-of-hospital cardiac arrest. *Ann Emerg Med* 15:1181, 1986.

28. Holmberg M, Holmberg S, Herlitz J: Effect of bystander cardiopulmonary resuscitation in out-of-hospital cardiac arrest patients in Sweden. *Resuscitation* 47:59, 2000.

29. Rewers M, Tilgreen RE, Crawford ME, et al: One-year survival after out-of-hospital cardiac arrest in Copenhagen according to the 'Utstein style.' *Resuscitation* 47:137, 2000.

30. Eisenberg MS, Bergner L, Hallstrom A: Cardiac resuscitation in the community: Importance of rapid provision and implications for program planning. *JAMA* 241:1905, 1979.

31. Weaver WD, Copass MK, Bufi D, et al: Improved neurologic recovery and survival after early defibrillation. *Circulation* 69:943, 1984.

32. Doig CJ, Sandham JD: A 2-year prospective cohort study of cardiac resuscitation in a major Canadian hospital. *Clin Invest Med* 23:132, 2000.

33. Zoch TW, Desbiens NA, DeStefano F, et al: Short- and long-term survival after cardiopulmonary resuscitation. *Arch Intern Med* 160:1969, 2000.

34. Myerburg RJ, Conde CA, Sung RJ, et al: Clinical electrophysiologic and hemodynamic profile of patients resuscitated from prehospital cardiac arrest. *Am J Med* 68:568, 1980.

35. Myerburg RJ, Kessler KM, Zaman L, et al: Survivors of prehospital cardiac arrest. *JAMA* 247:1485, 1982.

36. Camarata SJ, Weil MH, Hanashiro PK, et al: Cardiac arrest in the critically ill: 1. A study of predisposing causes in 132 patients. *Circulation* 44:688, 1971.

37. Hahn RG, Hutchinson JC, Conte JE: Cardiopulmonary resuscitation in a university hospital, an analysis of survival and cost. *West J Med* 131:344, 1979.

38. DeBard ML: Cardiopulmonary resuscitation: analysis of six years' experience and review of the literature. *Ann Emerg Med* 10:408, 1981.

39. Bedell SE, Delbanco TL, Cook EF, et al: Survival after cardiopulmonary resuscitation in the hospital. *N Engl J Med* 309:569, 1983.

40. Lemire JG, Johnson AL: Is cardiac resuscitation worthwhile? A decade of experience. *N Engl J Med* 286:970, 1972.

41. Spearpoint KG, McLean CP, Zideman DA: Early defibrillation and the chain of survival in 'in-hospital' adult cardiac arrest; minutes count. *Resuscitation* 44:165, 2000.

42. Pantridge JF, Geddes JS: A mobile intensive care unit in the management of myocardial infarction. *Lancet* 2:271, 1967.

43. Tweed WA, Bristow G, Donen N: Resuscitation from cardiac arrest: assessment of a system providing only basic life support outside of hospital. *Can Med Assoc J* 122:297, 1980.

44. Vertesi L, Wilson L, Glick N: Cardiac arrest: comparison of paramedic and conventional ambulance services. *Can Med Assoc J* 128:809, 1983.

45. Stults KR, Brown DD, Schug VL, et al: Prehospital defibrillation performed by emergency medical technicians in rural communities. *N Engl J Med* 310:219, 1984.

46. Smith JP, Bodai BI: The urban paramedic's scope of practice. *JAMA* 253:544, 1985.

47. Stults KR, Brown DD, Kerber RE: Efficacy of an automated external defibrillator in the management of out-of-hospital cardiac arrest: validation of the diagnostic algorithm and initial clinical experience in a rural environment. *Circulation* 73:701, 1986.

48. Weaver WD, Hill D, Fahrenbruch CE, et al: Use of the automatic external defibrillator in the management of out-of-hospital cardiac arrest. *N Engl J Med* 319:661, 1988.

49. Eisenberg MS, Copass MK, Hallstrom AP, et al: Treatment of out-of-hospital cardiac arrest with rapid defibrillation by emergency medical technicians. *N Engl J Med* 302:1379, 1980.

50. Emergency Cardiac Care Committee: automatic external defibrillators and advanced cardiac life support: a new initiative from the American Heart Association. *Am J Emerg Med* 9:91, 1991.

51. Cobb LA, Eliastam M, Kerber RE, et al: Report of the American Heart Association task force on the future of cardiopulmonary resuscitation. *Circulation* 85:2346, 1992.

52. Weisfeldt ML, Kerber RE, McGoldrick RP: Public access defibrillation: a statement from the American Heart Association Task Force on Automatic External Defibrillation. *Circulation* 92:2763, 1995.

53. O'Rourke RA: Saving lives in the sky. *Circulation* 96:2775, 1997.

54. Kern KB, Paraskos JA: 31st Bethesda Conference: Task Force 1: cardiac arrest. *J Am Coll Cardiol* 35:832, 2000.

55. Valenzuela TD, Roe DJ, Nichol G, et al: Outcomes of rapid defibrillation by security officers after cardiac arrest in casinos. *N Engl J Med* 343:1206, 2000.

56. Paraskos JA: External compression without adjuncts. *Circulation* 74[Suppl]:IV-33, 1986.

57. MacKenzie GJ, Taylor SH, McDonald AH, et al: Haemodynamic effects of external cardiac compression. *Lancet* 1:1342, 1964.

58. DelGuercio LRM, Coomaraswamy RP, State D: Cardiac output and other hemodynamic variables during external cardiac massage in man. *N Engl J Med* 269:1398, 1963.

59. Del Guercio LRM, Feind NR, Cohn JD, et al: Comparison of blood flow during external and internal cardiac massage in man. *Circulation* 31[Suppl 1]:171, 1965.

60. Oriol A, Smith HJ: Hemodynamic observations during closed-chest cardiac massage. *Can Med Assoc J* 98:841, 1968.

61. Ditchey RV, Winkler JV, Rhodes CA: Relative lack of coronary blood flow during closed-chest resuscitation in dogs. *Circulation* 66:297, 1982.

62. Niemann JT, Rosborough JP, Ung S, et al: Coronary perfusion pressure during experimental cardiopulmonary resuscitation. *Ann Emerg Med* 11:127, 1982.

63. Luce JM, Ross BK, O'Quin RJ, et al: Regional blood flow during cardiopulmonary resuscitation in dogs using simultaneous and non-simultaneous compression and ventilation. *Circulation* 67:258, 1983.

64. Chandra N, Weisfeldt ML, Tsitlik J, et al: Augmentation of carotid flow during cardiopulmonary resuscitation by ventilation at high airway pressure simultaneous with chest compression. *Am J Cardiol* 48:1053, 1981.

65. Jackson RE, Joyce K, Danosi SF, et al: Blood flow in the cerebral cortex during cardiac resuscitation in dogs. *Ann Emerg Med* 13:657, 1984.

66. Koehler RC, Chandra N, Guerci AD, et al: Augmentation of cerebral perfusion by simultaneous chest compression and lung inflation with abdominal binding after cardiac arrest in dogs. *Circulation* 67:266, 1983.

67. Stajduhar K, Steinberg R, Sotosky M, et al: Cerebral blood flow and common carotid artery blood flow during open-chest CPR in dogs. *Ann Emerg Med* 13:385, 1984.

68. Sharff JA, Pantley G, Noel E: Effect of time on regional organ perfusion during two methods of cardiopulmonary resuscitation. *Ann Emerg Med* 13:649, 1984.

69. Guerci A, Chandra N, Levin H, et al: Hemodynamic determinants of intracranial pressure during resuscitation. *Circulation* 64:IV-304, 1981.

70. Bircher N, Safar P: Open-chest CPR. an old method whose time has returned. *Am J Emerg Med* 2:568, 1984.

71. Krug JJ: Cardiac arrest secondary to Addison's disease. *Ann Emerg Med* 15:735, 1986.

72. Deshmukh HG, Weil MH, Rackow EC, et al: Echocardiographic observations during cardiopulmonary resuscitation: a preliminary report. *Crit Care Med* 13:904, 1985.

73. Pell AC, Guly UM, Sutherland GR, et al: Mechanism of closed chest cardiopulmonary resuscitation investigated by transesophageal echocardiography. *J Accid Emerg Med* 11:139, 1994.

74. Maier GW, Tyson GS Jr, Olsen CO, et al: The physiology of external cardiac massage: high-impulse cardiopulmonary resuscitation. *Circulation* 70:86, 1984.

75. Weisfeldt ML, Chandra N: Physiology of cardiopulmonary resuscitation, in Creger WP (ed): *Annual Review of Medicine. Selected Topics in Clinical Sciences.* Palo Alto, CA, Annual Reviews, 1981; p 437(vol 32).

76. Weale FE, Rothwell-Jackson RL: The efficiency of cardiac massage. *Lancet* 1:990, 1962.

77. Wilder RJ, Weir D, Rush BF, et al: Methods of coordinating ventilation and closed chest cardiac massage in the dog. *Surgery* 53:186, 1963.

78. Criley JM, Blaufuss AJ, Kissel GL: Cough-induced cardiac compression. *JAMA* 236:1246, 1976.

79. Niemann JT, Rosborough JP, Brown D, et al: Cough-CPR. documentation of systemic perfusion in man and in an experimental model—A "window" to the mechanism of blood flow in external CPR. *Crit Care Med* 8:141, 1980.

80. Rudikoff MT, Maughan WL, Effron M, et al: Mechanisms of blood flow during cardiopulmonary resuscitation. *Circulation* 61:345, 1980.

81. Weisfeldt ML, Chandra N, Tsitlik J: Increased intrathoracic pressure—not direct heart compression—causes the rise in intrathoracic vascular pressures during CPR in dogs and pigs. *Crit Care Med* 9:377, 1981.

82. Niemann JT, Rosborough JP, Hausknecht M, et al: Pressure-synchronized cineangiography during experimental cardiopulmonary resuscitation. *Circulation* 64:985, 1981.

83. Rich S, Wix HL, Shapiro EP: Clinical assessment of heart chamber size and valve motion during cardiopulmonary resuscitation by two-dimensional echocardiography. *Am Heart J* 102:368, 1981.

84. Werner JA, Greene HL, Janko CL, et al: Visualization of cardiac valve motion in man during external chest compression using two-dimensional echocardiography: implications regarding the mechanism of blood flow. *Circulation* 63:1417, 1981.

85. Babbs CF: New versus old theories of blood flow during CPR. *Crit Care Med* 8:191, 1980.

86. Fisher J, Vaghaiwalla F, Tsitlik J, et al: Determinants and clinical significance of jugular venous valve competence. *Circulation* 65:188, 1982.

87. Taylor GJ, Tucker WM, Greene HL, et al: Importance of prolonged compression during cardiopulmonary resuscitation in man. *N Engl J Med* 296:1515, 1977.

88. Chandra N, Rudikoff M, Weisfeldt ML: Simultaneous chest compression and ventilation at high airway pressure during cardiopulmonary resuscitation. *Lancet* 1:175, 1980.

89. Bircher N, Safar P: Comparison of standard and "new" closed-chest CPR and open-chest CPR in dogs. *Crit Care Med* 9:384, 1981.

90. Sanders AB, Ewy GA, Alferness CA, et al: Failure of one method of simultaneous chest compression, ventilation, and abdominal binding during CPR. *Crit Care Med* 10:509, 1982.

91. Harris LC Jr, Kirimli B, Safar P: Augmentation of artificial circulation during cardiopulmonary resuscitation. *Anesthesiology* 28:730, 1967.

92. Harris LC Jr, Kirimli B, Safar P: Ventilation–cardiac compression ratios in CPR. *Anesthesiology* 28:806, 1967.

93. Redding JS: Abdominal compression in cardiopulmonary resuscitation. *Anesth Analg* 50:668, 1971.

94. Chandra N, Snyder LD, Weisfeldt ML: Abdominal binding during cardiopulmonary resuscitation in man. *JAMA* 246:351, 1981.

95. Niemann JT, Rosborough JP, Ung S, et al: Hemodynamic effects of continuous abdominal binding during cardiac arrest and resuscitation. *Am J Cardiol* 53:269, 1984.

96. Bircher N, Safar P: Cerebral preservation during cardiopulmonary resuscitation. *Crit Care Med* 13:185, 1985.

97. Voorhees WD, Babbs CF, Niebauer MJ: Improved oxygen delivery during cardiopulmonary resuscitation with interposed abdominal compressions. *Ann Emerg Med* 12:128, 1983.

98. Voorhees WD, Ralston SH, Babbs CF: Regional blood flow during cardiopulmonary resuscitation with abdominal counterpulsation in dogs. *Am J Emerg Med* 2:123, 1984.

99. Babbs CF, Schoenlein WE, Lowe MW: Gastric insufflation during IAC-CPR and standard CPR in a canine model. *Am J Emerg Med* 3:99, 1985.

100. Sack JB, Kesselbrenner MB, Bregman D: Survival from in-hospital cardiac arrest with interposed abdominal counterpulsation during cardiopulmonary resuscitation. *JAMA* 267:379, 1992.

101. Barranco F, Lesmes A, Irles JA, et al: Cardiopulmonary resuscitation with simultaneous chest and abdominal compression: comparative study in humans. *Resuscitation* 20:67, 1990.

102. Cohen TV, Goldner BG, Maccaro PC, et al: A comparison of active compression–decompression cardiopulmonary resuscitation for cardiac arrest occurring in the hospital. *N Engl J Med* 329:1918, 1993.

103. Shultz JJ, Coffeen P, Sweeney M, et al: Evaluation of standard and active compression-decompression CPR in an acute human model of ventricular fibrillation. *Circulation* 89:684, 1994.

104. Stiell IG, Hebert PC, Wells GA, et al: The Ontario Trial of active compression-decompression cardiopulmonary resuscitation for in-hospital and pre-hospital cardiac arrest. *JAMA* 275:1417, 1996.

105. Plaisance P, Lurie KG, Vicaut E, et al: French Active Compression-Decompression Cardiopulmonary Resuscitation Study Group. A comparison of standard cardiopulmonary resuscitation and active compression-decompression resuscitation for out-of-hospital cardiac arrest. *N Engl J Med* 341:569, 1999.

106. Halperin HR, Guerci AD, Chandra N, et al: Vest inflation without simultaneous ventilation during cardiac arrest in dogs: improved survival from prolonged cardiopulmonary resuscitation. *Circulation* 74:1407, 1986.

107. Ralston SH, Babbs CF, Niebauer MJ: Cardiopulmonary resuscitation with interposed abdominal compression in dogs. *Anesth Analg* 61:645, 1982.

108. Babbs CF, Ralston SH, Geddes LA: Theoretical advantages of abdominal counterpulsation in CPR as demonstrated in a simple electrical model of the circulation. *Ann Emerg Med* 13:660, 1984.

109. Sack JB, Kesselbrenner MB, Bregman D: Survival from in-hospital cardiac arrest with interposed abdominal counterpulsation during cardiopulmonary resuscitation. *JAMA* 267:379, 1992.

110. Ward KR, Sullivan RJ, Zelenak RR, et al: A comparison of interposed abdominal compression CPR and standard CPR by monitoring end-tidal PCO_2. *Ann Emerg Med* 18:831, 1989.

111. Mateer JR, Steuven HA, Thompson BM, et al: Pre-hospital IAC-CPR versus standard CPR: paramedic resuscitation of cardiac arrests. *Am J Emerg Med* 3:143, 1985.

112. Stephenson HE Jr, Reid C, Hinton JW: Some common denominators in 1200 cases of cardiac arrest. *Ann Surg* 137:731, 1953.

113. Turk LN, Glenn WW: Cardiac arrest—results of attempted resuscitation in 42 cases. *N Engl J Med* 251:795, 1954.

114. Bartlett RL, Stewart NJ, Raymond J, et al: Comparative study of three methods of resuscitation: closed-chest manual, and direct mechanical ventricular assistance. *Ann Emerg Med* 13:773, 1984.

115. Bircher N, Safar P: Manual open-chest cardiopulmonary resuscitation. *Ann Emerg Med* 13:770, 1984.

116. Takino M, Okada Y: The optimum timing of resuscitative thoracotomy for non-traumatic out-of-hospital cardiac arrest. *Resuscitation* 26:69, 1993.

117. Shocket E, Rosenblum R: Successful open cardiac massage after 75 minutes of closed chest massage. *JAMA* 200:157, 1967.

118. Sykes MK, Ahmed N: Emergency treatment of cardiac arrest. *Lancet* 2:347, 1963.

119. Bodai BI, Smith JP, Ward RE, et al: Emergency thoracotomy in the management of trauma—A review. *JAMA* 249:1891, 1983.

120. Cogbill TH, Moore EE, Milikan JS, et al: Rationale for selective application of emergency department thoracotomy in trauma. *J Trauma* 23:453, 1983.

121. Danne PD, Finelli F, Champion HR: Emergency bay thoracotomy. *J Trauma* 24:796, 1984.

122. Kern KB, Sanders AB, Badylak SF, et al: Long-term survival with open-chest cardiac massage after ineffective closed-chest compression in a canine model. *Circulation* 75:498, 1987.

123. Kern KB, Sanders AB, Janas W, et al: Limitations of open-chest cardiac massage after prolonged, untreated cardiac arrest in dogs. *Ann Emerg Med* 20:761, 1991.

124. Long WB, Rosenblum S, Grady IP: Successful resuscitation of bupivacaine-induced cardiac arrest using cardiopulmonary bypass. *Anesth Analg* 69:403, 1989.

125. Pretto E, Safar P, Saito R, et al: Cardiopulmonary bypass after prolonged cardiac arrest in dogs. *Ann Emerg Med* 16:611, 1987.

126. Levine R, Gorayeb M, Safar P, et al: Emergency cardiopulmonary bypass after cardiac arrest and prolonged closed-chest CPR in dogs. *Ann Emerg Med* 16:620, 1987.

127. Martin GB, Nowak RM, Carden DL, et al: Cardiopulmonary bypass vs CPR as treatment for prolonged canine cardiopulmonary arrest. *Ann Emerg Med* 16:628, 1987.

128. Carden DL, Martin GB, Nowak RM, et al: The effect of cardiopulmonary bypass resuscitation on cardiac arrest induced lactic acidosis in dogs. *Resuscitation* 17:153, 1989.

129. Beyersdorf F, Acar C, Buckberg GD, et al: Studies on prolonged acute regional ischemia: IV. Aggressive surgical treatment for intractable ventricular fibrillation after myocardial infarction. *J Thorac Cardiovasc Surg* 98:557, 1989.

130. Hartz R, LoCicero J III, Sanders JH Jr, et al: Clinical experience with portable cardiopulmonary bypass in cardiac arrest patients. *Ann Thorac Surg* 50:437, 1990.

131. Ornato JP, Hallagan LF, McMahon SB, et al: Attitudes of BCLS instructors about mouth-to-mouth resuscitation during the AIDS epidemic. *Ann Emerg Med* 19:151, 1990.

132. Block AJ: The physician's responsibility for the care of AIDS patients: an opinion. *Chest* 94:1283, 1988.

133. Fox PC, Wolff A, Yeh CK, et al: Saliva inhibits HIV-1 infectivity. *J Am Dent Assoc* 116:635, 1988.

134. Freidland GH, Saltzman BR, Rogers MF, et al: Lack of transmission of HTLV III/LAV infection to household contacts of patients with AIDS or AIDS-related complex with oral candidiasis. *N Engl J Med* 314:344, 1986.

135. Marcus R: Surveillance of health care workers exposed to blood from patients infected with the human immunodeficiency virus. *N Engl J Med* 319:1118, 1988.

136. Sande MH: Transmission of AIDS: the case against casual contagion. *N Engl J Med* 314:380, 1986.

137. Recommendations for Prevention of HIV Transmission in Health Care Settings. *MMWR Morb Mortal Wkly Rep* 36[Suppl 2]:3S, 1987.

138. Update: Universal Precautions for Prevention of Transmission of Human Immunodeficiency Virus, Hepatitis B Virus, and Other Bloodborne Pathogens in Health Care Settings. *MMWR Morb Mortal Wkly Rep* 37(24):377, 1988.

139. Simmons M, Deao D, Moon L, et al: Bench evaluation: three face-shield CPR barrier devices. *Respir Care* 40:618, 1995.

140. Exhaled-air pulmonary resuscitators (EAPRS), and disposable manual pulmonary resuscitators (DMPRS). *Health Devices* 18:333, 1989.

141. Feldman HA: Some recollections of the meningococcal disease: the first Harry F. Dowling lecture. *JAMA* 220:1107, 1972.

142. Hendricks AA, Shapiro EP: Primary herpes simplex infection following mouth-to-mouth resuscitation. *JAMA* 243:257, 1980.

143. Todd MA, Bell JS: Shigellosis from cardiopulmonary resuscitation [letter]. *JAMA* 243:331, 1980.

144. Valenzuela TD, Hooten TM, Kaplan EL, et al: Transmission of "toxic strep" syndrome from an infected child to a firefighter during CPR. *Ann Emerg Med* 20:90, 1991.

145. Ahmad F, Senadhira DC, Charters J, et al: Transmission of salmonella via mouth-to-mouth resuscitation [letter]. *Lancet* 335:787, 1990.

146. Mejicano GC, Maki DG: Infections acquired during cardiopulmonary resuscitation: estimating the risk and defining strategies for prevention. *Ann Intern Med* 129:813, 1998.

147. Risk of infection during CPR training and rescue: supplemental guidelines. *JAMA* 262:2714, 1989.

148. Adgey AAJ, Geddes JS, Webb SW, et al: Acute phase of myocardial infarction. *Lancet* 2:501, 1971.

149. Thompson RG, Hallstrom AP, Cobb LA: Bystander-initiated cardiopulmonary resuscitation in the management of ventricular fibrillation. *Ann Intern Med* 90:737, 1979.

150. Melker R, Cavallaro D, Krischer J: One-rescuer CPR—a reappraisal of present recommendations for ventilation. *Crit Care Med* 9:423, 1981.

151. Melker RJ: Asynchronous and other alternative methods of ventilation during CPR. *Ann Emerg Med* 13:758, 1984.

152. Bahr J, Klingler H, Panzer W, et al: Skills of the lay people in checking the carotid pulse. *Resuscitation* 35:23, 1997.

153. 2005 American Heart Association guidelines for cardiopulmonary resuscitation and emergency cardiovascular care. *Circulation*. 2005; 112:III-5–III-16

154. Eftestol T, Sunde K, Steen PA: Effects of interrupting precordial compressions on the calculated probability of defibrillation success during out-of-hospital cardiac arrest. *Circulation* 105:2270; 2002.

155. Dorph E, Wik L, Stromme TA, et al: Oxygen delivery and return of spontaneous circulation with ventilation: compression ratio 2:30 versus chest compressions only CPR in pigs. *Resuscitation* 60:309, 2004.

156. Salem MR, Wong AY, Mani M, et al: Efficacy of cricoid pressure in preventing gastric inflation during bag-mask ventilation in pediatric patients. *Anesthesiology* 40:96, 1974.

157. Melker RJ: Alternative methods of ventilation during respiratory and cardiac arrest. *Circulation* 74[Suppl]:IV-63, 1986.

158. Krischer JP, Fine EG, Davis JH, et al: Complications of cardiac resuscitation. *Chest* 92:287, 1987.

159. Nagel EL, Fine EG, Krischer JP, et al: Complications of CPR. *Crit Care Med* 9:424, 1981.

160. Powner DJ, Holcombe PA, Mello LA: Cardiopulmonary resuscitation-related injuries. *Crit Care Med* 12:54, 1984.

161. Crile G, Dolley DH: Experimental resuscitation of dogs killed by anesthetics and asphyxia. *J Exp Med* 6:713, 1906.

162. Sanders AB, Ewy GA, Taft TV: Prognosis and therapeutic importance of the aortic diastolic pressure in resuscitation from cardiac arrest. *Crit Care Med* 12:871, 1984.

163. Michael JR, Guerci AD, Koehler RC, et al: Mechanisms by which epinephrine augments cerebral and myocardial perfusion during cardiopulmonary resuscitation in dogs. *Circulation* 69:822, 1984.

164. Ralston SH, Voorhees WD, Babbs CF: Intrapulmonary epinephrine during prolonged cardiopulmonary resuscitation: improved regional blood flow and resuscitation in dogs. *Ann Emerg Med* 13:79, 1984.

165. Paradis NA, Martin GB, Rivers EP, et al: Coronary perfusion pressure and the return of spontaneous circulation in humans. *JAMA* 263:1106, 1990.

166. Ludwig S, Kettrick RG, Parker M: Pediatric cardiopulmonary resuscitation. *Clin Pediatr* 23:71, 1984.

167. Torphy DE, Minter MG, Thompson BM: Cardiorespiratory arrest and resuscitation of children. *Am J Dis Child* 138:1099, 1984.

168. Heimlich HJ, Hoffman KA, Canestri FR: Food-choking and drowning deaths prevented by external subdiaphragmatic compression: physiological basis. *Ann Thorac Surg* 20:188, 1975.

169. Heimlich HJ, Uhtley MH: The Heimlich maneuver. *Clin Symp* 31:22, 1979.

170. Lowenstein SR, Sabyan EM, Lassen CF, et al: Benefits of training physicians in advanced cardiac life support. *Chest* 89:512, 1986.

171. Sellick BA: Cricoid pressure to control regurgitation of stomach contents during induction of anæsthesia. *Lancet* 2:404, 1961.

172. Aufderheide TP, Lurie KG: Death by hyperventilation: a common and life-threatening problem during cardiopulmonary resuscitation. *Crit Care Med* 32[Suppl]:S345, 2004.

173. Stone BJ, Chantler PJ, Baskett PJ: The Incidence of regurgitation during :cardiopulmonary resuscitation: a comparison between the bag valve mask and laryngeal mask airway. *Resuscitation* 38:3, 21998.

174. The use of the laryngeal mask airway by nurses during cardiopulmonary resuscitation: results of a multicentre trial. *Anesthesia* 49:3, 1994.

175. Roberts I, Allsop P, Dickinson M, et al: Airway management training using the Laryngeal Mask Airway; a comparison of two different training programmes. *Resuscitation* 33:211, 1997.

176. Kokkinis K: The use of the Laryngeal Mask Airway in CPR. *Resuscitation* 27:9, 1994.

177. Lack A: Regurgitation using the Laryngeal Mask Airway. *Anesthesia* 48:734, 1993.

178. Davies PR, Tighe SQ, Greenslade GL, et al: Laryngeal mask airway and tracheal tube insertion by unskilled personnel. *Lancet* 336:997, 1990.

179. Leach A, Alexander CA, Stone B, et al: The laryngeal mask in cardiopulmonary resuscitation in a district general hospital: a preliminary communication. *Resuscitation* 25:245, 1993.

180. Samarkandi AH, Seraj MA, Dawlatly A, et al: The role of laryngeal mask airway in cardiopulmonary resuscitation. *Resuscitation* 28:103, 1994.

181. Flaishon R, Sotman A, Ben-Abraham R, et al: Antichemical protective gear prolongs time to successful airway management: a randomized, crossover study in humans. *Anesthesiology* 100:260, 2004.

182. Goldik Z, Bornstein J, Eden A, et al: Airway management by physicians wearing anti-chemical warfare gear: comparison between laryngeal mask airway and endotracheal intubation. *Eur J Anesthesiol* 19:166, 2002.

183. Pennant JH, Pace NA, Gajraj NM, et al: Role of the laryngeal mask airway in the immobile cervical spine. *J Clin Anesthesiol* 5:226, 1993.

184. Griffin RM, Hatcher IS: Aspiration pneumonia and the laryngeal mask airway. *Anesthesia* 45:1039, 1990.

185. Leach AB, Alexander CA: The laryngeal mask—an overview. *Eur J Anaesthesiol Suppl* 4:19, 1991.

186. Nanji GM, Maltby JR: Vomiting and aspiration pneumonitis with the laryngeal mask airway. *Canada J. Anaesthesia* 39:69, 1992.

187. Young TM: The laryngeal mask in dental anaesthesia. *Eur J Anaesthesiol Suppl* 4:53, 1991.

188. Beveridge ME: Laryngeal mask anaesthesia for repair of cleft palate. *Anaesthesia* 44:656, 1989.

189. Reed AP: Current concepts in airway management for cardiopulmonary resuscitation (subject review). *Mayo Clinic Proc* 70:1172, 1995.

190. Smith RB, Babinski M, Klain M, et al: Percutaneous transtracheal ventilation. *J Am Coll Emerg Phys* 5:765, 1976.

191. McGill J, Clinton JE, Ruiz E: Cricothyrotomy in the emergency department. *Ann Emerg Med* 11:361, 1982.

192. Simon RR, Brenner BE: Emergency cricothyroidotomy in the patient with massive neck swelling: Part 1: Anatomical aspects. *Crit Care Med* 11:114, 1983.

193. Simon RR, Brenner BE, Rosen MA: Emergency cricothyroidotomy in the patient with massive neck swelling: Part 2: Clinical aspects. *Crit Care Med* 11:119, 1983.

194. Fain E, Sweeney M, Franz M: Improved internal defibrillation efficacy with biphasic waveform. *Am Heart J* 117:358, 1989.

195. Zoll PM, Zoll RH, Falk RH, et al: External noninvasive temporary cardiac pacing: clinical trials. *Circulation* 71:937, 1985.

196. Falk RH, Jacobs L, Sinclair A, et al: External non-invasive cardiac pacing in out-of-hospital cardiac arrest. *Crit Care Med* 11:779, 1983.

197. Hedges JR, Syverud SA, Dalsey WC: Developments in transcutaneous and transthoracic pacing during bradyasystolic arrest. *Ann Emerg Med* 13:822, 1984.

198. Hedges JR, Syverud SA, Dalsey WC, et al: Prehospital trial of emergency transcutaneous cardiac pacing. *Circulation* 76:1337, 1987.

199. Clinton JE, Zoll PM, Zoll R, et al: Emergency noninvasive external pacing. *J Emerg Med* 2:155, 1985.

200. Emerman CL, Pinchak AC, Hancock D, et al: Effect of injection site on circulation times during cardiac arrest. *Crit Care Med* 16:1138, 1988.

201. Kuhn GJ, White BC, Swetnam RE, et al: Peripheral vs central circulation times during CPR: a pilot study. *Ann Emerg Med* 10:417, 1981.

202. Jastremski MS, Matthias HD, Randell PA: Femoral venous catheterization during cardiopulmonary resuscitation: a critical appraisal. *J Emerg Med* 1:387, 1984.

203. Ralston SH, Tacker WA, Showen L, et al: Endotracheal versus intravenous epinephrine during electromechanical dissociation with CPR in dogs. *Ann Emerg Med* 14:1044, 1985.

204. Hoernchen U, Schuettler J, Stoeckel H, et al: Endobronchial instillation of epinephrine during cardiopulmonary resuscitation. *Crit Care Med* 15:1037, 1987.

205. Haehnel J, Lindner KH, Ahnefeld FW: Endobronchial administration of emergency drugs. *Resuscitation* 17:261, 1989.

206. Weil MH, Grundler W, Yamaguchi M, et al: Arterial blood gases fail to reflect acid-base status during cardiopulmonary resuscitation: a preliminary report. *Crit Care Med* 13:884, 1985.

207. Weil MH, Ruiz CE, Michaels S, et al: Acid-base determinants of survival after cardiopulmonary resuscitation. *Crit Care Med* 13:888, 1985.

208. Jaffe A: Cardiovascular pharmacology I. *Circulation* 74[Suppl]:IV-70, 1986.

209. Guerci AD, Chandra N, Johnson E, et al: Failure of sodium bicarbonate to improve resuscitation from ventricular fibrillation in dogs. *Circulation* 74[Suppl]:IV-75, 1986.

210. Dybrik T, Strand T, Steen PA: Buffer therapy during out-of-hospital cardiopulmonary resuscitation. *Resuscitation* 29:89, 1995.

211. Shoemaker WC, Schluchter M, Hopkins JA, et al: Fluid therapy in emergency resuscitation: clinical evaluation of colloid and crystalloid regimens. *Crit Care Med* 9:367, 1981.

212. Otto CW, Yakaitis RW, Blitt CD: Mechanism of action of epinephrine in resuscitation from asphyxial arrest. *Crit Care Med* 9:364, 1981.

213. Otto CW, Yakaitis RW, Redding JS, et al: Comparison of dopamine, dobutamine, and epinephrine in cardiopulmonary resuscitation. *Crit Care Med* 9:366, 1981.

214. Otto CW: Cardiovascular pharmacology II: the use of catecholamines, pressor agents, digitalis, and corticosteroids in CPR and emergency cardiac care. *Circulation* 74[Suppl]: IV-80, 1986.

215. Redding JS, Pearson JW: Evaluation of drugs for cardiac resuscitation. *Anesthesiology* 24:203, 1963.

216. Redding JS, Pearson JW: Resuscitation from ventricular fibrillation: drug therapy. *JAMA* 203:255, 1968.

217. Otto CW, Yakaitis RW, Redding JS, et al: Comparison of dopamine, dobutamine, and epinephrine in CPR. *Crit Care Med* 9:640, 1981.

218. Otto CW, Yakaitis RW, Ewy GA: Effect of epinephrine on defibrillation in ischemic ventricular fibrillation. *Am J Emerg Med* 3:285, 1985.

219. Niemann JT, Haynes KS, Garner D, et al: Postcountershock pulseless rhythms: response to CPR, artificial cardiac pacing, and adrenergic agonists. *Ann Emerg Med* 15:112, 1986.

220. Brown CG, Katz SE, Werman HA, et al: The effect of epinephrine versus methoxamine on regional myocardial blood flow and defibrillation rates following a prolonged cardiorespiratory arrest in a swine model. *Am J Emerg Med* 5:362, 1987.

221. Brown CG, Taylor RB, Werman HA, et al: Myocardial oxygen delivery/consumption during cardiopulmonary resuscitation: a comparison of epinephrine and phenylephrine. *Ann Emerg Med* 17:302, 1988.

222. Martin GB, Gentile NT, Paradis NA, et al: Effect of epinephrine on end-tidal carbon dioxide monitoring during CPR. *Ann Emerg Med* 19:396, 1990.

223. Koscove EM, Paradis NA: Resuscitation from cardiac arrest using high-dose epinephrine therapy. *JAMA* 259:3031, 1988.

224. Gonzalez ER, Ornato JP, Garnett AR, et al: Dose-dependent vasopressor response to epinephrine during CPR in human beings. *Ann Emerg Med* 18:920, 1989.

225. Martin D, Werman HA, Brown CG: Four case studies: high-dose epinephrine in cardiac arrest. *Ann Emerg Med* 19:322, 1990.

226. Stiell IG, Hebert PC, Weitzman BN, et al: High-dose epinephrine in adult cardiac arrest. *N Engl J Med* 327:1045, 1992.

227. Brown CG, Martin DR, Pepe PE, et al: A comparison of standard-dose and high-dose epinephrine in cardiac arrest outside the hospital. *N Engl J Med* 327:1051, 1992.

228. Robinson LA, Brown CG, Jenkins J, et al: The effect of norepinephrine versus epinephrine on myocardial hemodynamics during CPR. *Ann Emerg Med* 18:336, 1989.

229. Brown CG, Robinson LA, Jenkins J, et al: The effect of norepinephrine versus epinephrine on regional cerebral blood flow during cardiopulmonary resuscitation. *Am J Emerg Med* 7:278, 1989.

230. Lindner KH, Brinkmann A, Pfenninger EG, et al: Effect of vasopressin on hemodynamic variables, organ blood flow, and acid-base status in a pig model of cardiopulmonary resuscitation. *Anesth Analg* 77:427, 1993.

231. Lindner KH, Prengel AW, Pfenninger EG, et al: Vasopressin improves vital organ flow during closed-chest cardiopulmonary resuscitation in pigs. *Circulation* 91:215, 1995.

232. Wenzel V, Lindner KH, Augenstein S: Vasopressin combined with epinephrine decreases cerebral perfusion compared with vasopressin alone during CPR in pigs. *Stroke* 29:1467, 1998.

233. Lindner KH, Prengel AW, Brinkmann A, et al: Vasopressin administration in refractory cardiac arrest. *Ann Intern Med* 124:1061, 1996.

234. Fox AW, May RE, Milch WE: Comparison of peptide and non-peptide receptor-mediated responses in rat-tail artery. *J Cardiovasc Pharmacol* 20:282, 1992.

235. Waxman HL, Groh WC, Marchlinski FE, et al: Amiodarone for control of sustained ventricular tachyarrhythmias: clinical and electrophysiologic effects in 51 patients. *Am J Cardiol* 50:1066, 1982.

236. McGovern B, Ruskin JN: The efficacy of amiodarone for ventricular arrhythmias can be predicted with clinical electrophysiologic studies. *Int J Cardiol* 3:71, 1983.

237. Kudenchuk PJ, Cobb LA, Copass M, et al: Amiodarone for resuscitation after out-of-hospital cardiac arrest due to ventricular fibrillation. *N Engl J Med* 341:871, 1999.

238. DeSilva RA, Hennekens CH, Lown B, et al: Lignocaine prophylaxis in acute myocardial infarction: an evaluation of randomised trials. *Lancet* 2:855, 1981.

239. Koster RW, Dunning AJ: Intramuscular lidocaine for prevention of lethal arrhythmias in the prehospital phase of acute myocardial infarction. *N Engl J Med* 313:1105, 1985.

240. Carruth JE, Silverman ME: Ventricular fibrillation complicating acute myocardial infarction: reasons against the routine use of lidocaine. *Am Heart J* 104:545, 1982.

241. Dunn HM, McComb LM, Kinney CD, et al: Prophylactic lidocaine in the early phase of suspected myocardial infarction. *Am Heart J* 110:353, 1985.

242. MacMahon S, Collins R, Peto R, et al: Effects of prophylactic lidocaine in suspected acute myocardial infarction: an overview of results from the randomized controlled trials. *JAMA* 260:1910, 1988.

243. American College of Cardiology/American Heart Association Task Force on Assessment of Diagnostic and Therapeutic Cardiovascular Procedures: guidelines for the early management of patients with acute myocardial infarction. *Circulation* 82:664, 1990.

244. Gunnar RM, Passamani ER, Bourdillon PD, et al: Guidelines for the early management of patients with acute myocardial infarction: a report of the American College of Cardiology/American Heart Association Task Force on Assessment of Diagnostic and Therapeutic Cardiovascular Procedures. *J Am Coll Cardiol* 16:249, 1990.

245. DiMarco JP, Sellers TD, Berne RM, et al: Adenosine: electrophysiologic effects and

therapeutic use for terminating paroxysmal supraventricular tachycardia. *Circulation* 68:1254, 1983.

246. DiMarco JP, Sellers TD, Lerman BB, et al: Diagnostic and therapeutic use of adenosine in patients with supraventricular tachyarrhythmias. *J Am Coll Cardiol* 6:417, 1985.

247. Parker RB, McCollam PL: Adenosine in the episodic treatment of paroxysmal supraventricular tachycardia. *Clin Pharmacol* 9:261, 1990.

248. Salerno DM, Dias VC, Kleiger RE, et al: Efficacy and safety of intravenous diltiazem for treatment of atrial fibrillation and atrial flutter. *Am J Cardiol* 63:1046, 1989.

249. Ellenbogen KA, Dias VC, Plumb VJ, et al: A placebo-controlled trial of continuous intravenous diltiazem infusion for 24-hour heart rate control during atrial fibrillation and atrial flutter: a multicenter study. *J Am Coll Cardiol* 18:891, 1991.

250. Teo KK, Yusuf S, Collins R, et al: Effects of intravenous magnesium in suspected acute myocardial infarction: overview of randomised trials. *BMJ* 303:1499, 1991.

251. Paraskos JA: Cardiovascular pharmacology III atropine, calcium, calcium blockers, and beta blockers. *Circulation* 74[Suppl]:IV-86, 1986.

252. Chamberlain DA, Turner P, Sneddon JM: Effects of atropine on heart rate in healthy man. *Lancet* 2:12, 1967.

253. Kay JH, Blalock A: The use of calcium chloride in the treatment of cardiac arrest in patients. *Surg Gynecol Obstet* 93:97, 1951.

254. Stueven HA, Thompson BM, Aprahamian C, et al: Use of calcium in prehospital cardiac arrest. *Ann Emerg Med* 12:136, 1983.

255. Stueven HA, Thompson BM, Aprahamian C, et al: Calcium chloride: reassessment of use in asystole. *Ann Emerg Med* 13:820, 1984.

256. Harrison EE, Amey BD: Use of calcium in electromechanical dissociation. *Ann Emerg Med* 13:844, 1984.

257. Carlon GC, Howland WS, Kahn RC, et al: Calcium chloride administration in normocalcemic critically ill patients. *Crit Care Med* 8:209, 1980.

258. Dembo DH: Calcium in advanced life support. *Crit Care Med* 9:358, 1981.

259. Thompson BM, Stueven HA, Tonsfeldt DJ: Calcium: limited indications, some danger. *Circulation* 74[Suppl]:IV-90, 1986.

260. Caldwell G, Millar G, Quinn E, et al: Simple mechanical methods of cardioversion: a defense of the precordial thump and cough version. *BMJ* 291:627, 1985.

261. Pennington JE, Taylor J, Lown B: Chest thump for reverting ventricular tachycardia. *N Engl J Med* 283:1192, 1970.

262. Ewy GA, Dahl CF, Zimmerman M, et al: Ventricular fibrillation masquerading as ventricular standstill. *Crit Care Med* 9:841, 1981.

263. Brown DC, Lewis AJ, Criley JM: Asystole and its treatment: the possible role of the parasympathetic nervous system in cardiac arrest. *JACEP* 8:448, 1979.

264. Vassale M: On the mechanism underlying cardiac standstill: factors determining success or failure of escape pacemakers in the heart. *JACEP* 5:35B, 1985.

265. Thompson BM, Brooks RC, Pionkowski RS, et al: Immediate countershock treatment of asystole. *Ann Emerg Med* 13:827, 1984.

266. Stults K, Brown D, Kerber R: Should ventricular asystole be cardioverted? [abstract]. *Circulation* 76[Suppl]:IV-12, 1987.

267. Michael JR, Guerci AD, Koehler RC, et al Mechanisms by which epinephrine augments cerebral and myocardial perfusion during cardiopulmonary resuscitation in dogs. *Circulation* 69:822, 1984.

268. Sanders AB: The roles of methoxamine and norepinephrine in electromechanical dissociation. *Ann Emerg Med* 13:835, 1984.

269. Scholander PF: The master switch of life. *Sci Am* 209:92, 1963.

270. Siebke H, Rod T, Breivik H, et al: Survival after 40 minutes submersion without cerebral sequelae. *Lancet* 1:1275, 1975.

271. Southwick FS, Dalgish PH: Recovery after prolonged asystolic cardiac arrest in profound hypothermia. A case report and literature review. *JAMA* 243:1250, 1980.

272. Steinman AM: The hypothermic code: CPR controversy revisited. *J Emerg Med Serv JEMS* 10:32, 1983.

273. Gordon AS, Ridolpho PF, Cole JE. *Definitive Studies on Pole-Top Resuscitation.* Camarillo, CA, Research Resuscitation Laboratories, Electric Power Research Institute, 1983.

274. Sanders AB, Kern KB, Ewy GA, et al: Improved resuscitation from cardiac arrest with open-chest CPR in dogs. *Crit Care Med* 9:384, 1981.

275. Sanders AB, Kern KB, Atlas M, et al: Importance of the duration of inadequate coronary perfusion pressure in resuscitation from cardiac arrest. *J Am Coll Cardiol* 6:113, 1985.

276. Safar P, Abramson NS, Angelos M, et al: Emergency cardiopulmonary bypass for resuscitation from prolonged cardiac arrest. *Am J Emerg Med* 8:55, 1990.

277. Geehr EC, Lewis FR, Auerbach PS: Failure of open-heart massage to improve survival after prehospital non-traumatic cardiac arrest [letter]. *N Engl J Med* 314:1189, 1986.

278. The hypothermia after cardiac arrest study group: mild therapeutic hypothermia to improve the neurologic outcome after cardiac arrest. *N Engl J Med* 346:549, 2000.

279. Benard SA, Gray TW, Buist MD, et al: Treatment of comatose survivors of out-of-hospital cardiac arrest with induced hypothermia. *N Engl J Med* 346:557, 2000.

Mario De Pinto
W. Thomas Edwards

CHAPTER **23**

Management of Pain in the Critically Ill Patient

Pain is a major problem for patients hospitalized in intensive care units (ICUs) [1–5]. In a study by Whipple et al., [1] assessing pain treatment in 17 patients with multiple trauma wounds, whereas 95% of house staff and 81% of nurses reported adequate analgesia, 74% of patients rated their pain as either moderate or severe.

Ineffectiveness of opioid analgesia in the intensive care setting is related more to the manner in which the medications are used than to the properties of the analgesics themselves [6]. Pain is frequently treated inappropriately because of fears of depressing spontaneous ventilation [7], inducing opioid dependence, and precipitating cardiovascular instability. Moreover, the methods for assessing pain, the techniques for aggressively treating it, and the beneficial results of effective pain management are often poorly understood by many clinicians [8–15].

During the past 2 decades, researchers have discovered that the persistence of severe, inadequately treated pain can lead to anatomic and physiologic changes in the nervous system [16]. The ability of neural tissue to change in response to repeated incoming stimuli, a property known as *neuroplasticity*, can lead to the development of chronic, disabling pain when acute pain is poorly treated. Furthermore, the stress response after surgery and trauma, which includes cytokine and acute-phase reactants release, elevated levels of catecholamines, cortisol, growth and adrenocorticotropic hormones, activation of the renin-angiotensin system, impaired coagulability, and an altered immune response, accounts for a large portion of the mortality in critically ill patients [17]. In several studies, inadequately treated acute pain has been shown to increase this response, resulting in higher morbidity and mortality [18,19]. Another important aspect to consider is the psychological effect that poorly treated acute pain has on patients when the most acute phase of their disease is over. Prolonged, severe anxiety stemming from uncontrolled pain after traumatic injury has been deemed to be a cause of posttraumatic stress disorder [20].

Revised standards for pain management evaluation and treatment have been developed by the Joint Commission of Healthcare Organizations and have become part of all hospital evaluations since 2001 [21]. One critical part of the process required by the Joint Commission of Healthcare Organizations is the assessment of the effectiveness of each intervention and modification of the treatment plan when an appropriate level of analgesia is not achieved [22]. Particular attention has also been dedicated to the need of staff education as well as to the development of a

system in each institution to deliver pain treatments promptly; in particular, staff education has been shown to be effective in improving pain control [23,24].

A correct and successful management of acute pain is based on the following fundamental principles:

- Pain is a subjective phenomenon; always believe the patient when he or she says, "I have pain," whether the observer thinks that the amount of pain reported is appropriate [25].
- Establishing the correct cause of the patient's pain before initiating treatment is of paramount importance.
- Pharmacologic treatment should be based on establishing and maintaining adequate drug levels at active sites to achieve and maintain appropriate levels of analgesia and anxiolysis.
- Continually reevaluate the therapy for its effectiveness and modify the approach, using different treatment modalities as needed.
- Always consider the possibility of using regional analgesia techniques (neuraxial and peripheral nerve blockade) whenever possible. Regional analgesia, when used appropriately and effectively, helps reduce the total amount of opioid analgesics necessary to achieve adequate pain control and subsequently the development of potentially dangerous side effects.

ACUTE PAIN PATHWAYS

Acute pain begins with damage to the skin or deeper structures. Algogens, produced or released locally, stimulate peripheral nociceptors. The signal is propagated along the nociceptor fibers into the dorsal horn of the spinal cord, or, in the case of the cranial nerves, into the sensory nuclei. Modulation, either amplification or attenuation, of the signal can take place before the signal is transmitted into pain-specific areas of the brain and cerebral cortex. An increase in the excitability of spinal neurons and central sensitization will cause an increase in the response to painful stimuli [25]. Reflexes are generated all along the pain pathway, resulting in responses that can be beneficial (e.g., withdrawal from a noxious stimulus) or deleterious (e.g., sympathetic discharge causing neuroendocrine changes characteristic of the stress response) to the injured organism [26]. One of the reflex responses associated with trauma or surgery is increased muscle tone and localized spasm, which increases oxygen consumption and lactic acid production. Increased sympathetic outflow causes tachycardia and increased stroke volume, cardiac work, and myocardial oxygen consumption. Supraspinal reflex responses to pain result in hypothalamic stimulation, increased sympathetic tone, increased release of catecholamines and other "stress" hormones, and decreased secretion of anabolic hormones. The postsurgical and trauma catabolic state can be worsened if the process continues.

Each separate part of the pain pathway (periphery, spinal cord, brain, and cerebral cortex) can be influenced so that the nociceptive signal is diminished or eliminated.

FORMULATION OF A TREATMENT PLAN

When designing a treatment plan it is important to understand the characteristics of the pathologic process responsible for the patient's pain.

The answer to the following questions is crucial in establishing the most effective therapeutic approach possible.

WHERE DOES IT HURT?

Is the location of pain appropriate for the injury sustained, the pathologic process, or for the surgery performed? Unrecognized injuries or pathology responsible for acute pain may be present. Sometimes pain may have nothing to do with the current acute problem in patients with underlying problems with chronic pain.

HOW MUCH DOES IT HURT?

Each patient should be asked to try to quantify his or her pain using visual, verbal, or numeric analog scales [27,28] (Fig. 23-1). With these measurements, each patient serves as his or her own control, and the response to treatment is best measured as change from the baseline value.

Pain in intubated and sedated patients can be assessed even if they are unable to communicate verbally. Various markers of sympathetic activity, such as restlessness, sweating, tachycardia,

lacrimation, pupillary dilation, and hypertension can be graded as signs of pain intensity, although any one of these is not an adequate measure of pain intensity by itself [29].

WHAT DOES IT FEEL LIKE?

Pain can be categorized as nociceptive and/or neuropathic. Nociceptive pain is transmitted through nonmyelinated C sensory fibers and small, myelinated A fibers [30] via the dorsal root ganglion and spinothalamic pathways in the spinal cord to the thalamus, periaqueductal grey, and other centers in the brain. Nociceptive pain encompasses somatic and visceral pain.

Somatic pain can be superficial, due to nociceptive input arising from skin, subcutaneous tissues, and mucous membranes; or it can be deep, arising from muscles, tendons, joints, or bones. It is usually described as sharp, pricking, well localized (superficial) or dull, aching, less well localized (deep).

Visceral pain is due to a disease process or abnormal function of an internal organ or its covering (parietal pleura, pericardium, peritoneum). It can be frequently associated with nausea, vomiting, sweating, and changes in heart rate and blood pressure.

Neuropathic pain is due to injury or dysfunction of the peripheral and/or central nervous system. Abnormal numbers and positioning of sodium channels in damaged neurons are responsible for the reduced response threshold and firing of action potentials even in the absence of a stimulus [31].

The N-methyl D-aspartate receptor is thought to be involved in the pathophysiology of neuropathic pain and other chronic pain states. In pathologic states, the N-methyl D-aspartate receptor is activated inappropriately, leading to a state of heightened excitability of pain pathways known as "wind-up" [32–34].

Neuropathic pain is usually described as burning, tingling, and numbing and can be associated with allodynia (pain caused by normally innocuous stimulus) and hyperalgesia.

Breakthrough pain refers to an episodic surge in pain against a background of well-controlled pain. It can be an increase in the patient's usual pain just before the next dose of regular analgesic.

Incident pain is a particular form of breakthrough pain, such as that brought on by movement or dressing changes.

MEDICAL MANAGEMENT

ICU patients commonly have pain and physical discomfort from many factors such as preexisting diseases, acutely painful medical conditions, invasive procedures, or trauma [35]. Pain and discomfort can also be caused by monitoring and therapeutic devices (catheters, drains, endotracheal tubes), routine nursing care (e.g., airway suctioning, physical therapy, dressing changes) and prolonged immobility [24,36]. Unrelieved pain may contribute to inadequate sleep, causing exhaustion and disorientation. Agitation in an ICU patient may also result from inadequate pain relief. Pain may also contribute to pulmonary dysfunction through localized guarding of muscles around the area of pain and a generalized muscle rigidity or spasm that restricts movement of the chest wall and diaphragm [37]. Effective analgesia tends to diminish pulmonary complications in postoperative patients [38].

Five-Point Global Scale	None A Little = 1 Some = 2 A Lot = 3 The Worst = 4
Verbal Quantitative Scale	0.......5.......10 None Worst imaginable
Visual Pain Analog Scale	No Worst .... Pain Pain Place a mark on the line

FIGURE 23-1. Several scales that can be useful for the evaluation of patient "self-reports" of pain before and after treatment. [From Stevens DS, Edwards WT: Management of pain in the critically ill. *J Intensive Care Med* 5:258, 1990, with permission.]

Several studies have demonstrated that the combined use of analgesics and sedatives ameliorates the stress response in critically ill patients [19,39–42].

NONPHARMACOLOGIC TREATMENTS

Nonpharmacologic interventions including attention to proper positioning of patients, stabilization of fractures, and elimination of irritating physical stimulation (e.g., proper positioning of ventilator tubing to avoid traction on the endotracheal tube) are important to maintain patient comfort. Studies have documented the successful use of transcutaneous electrical nerve stimulation in treating postoperative pain, pain associated with rib fractures, and burn pain [43–45]. One clinical investigation of burn patients shows that auricular acupuncture-like transcutaneous electrical nerve stimulation significantly reduces pain after dressing changes and wound debridement when compared to placebo [46].

Modifications of the ICU environment, such as creating units with single rooms [47], decreasing noise [48], and providing lighting that better reflects a day-night orientation [47], may help patients achieve normal sleep patterns and also improve pain control.

PHARMACOLOGIC TREATMENTS

Different classes of medications can be used to provide adequate analgesia in critically ill patients.

Nonsteroidal Antiinflammatory Drugs

Nonsteroidal antiinflammatory drugs (NSAIDs) interfere with the production of prostaglandins; they may diminish the inflammatory response to trauma and surgery and thereby decrease the nociceptive input; they also may augment analgesia when used in combination with opioids.

Ketorolac tromethamine (Toradol) has been shown to be effective in reducing opioid requirements after major surgery [49] without depressing the respiratory drive [50]; when used in combination with epidural blockade, it improves also chest and shoulder pain after thoracic surgery [51].

Ketorolac and other NSAIDs may cause nausea, peptic ulceration, and inhibition of platelet function [52,53]. Severe bronchospasm may occur in patients with asthma, nasal polyposis, and allergy to aspirin [54,55]; appropriate caution should be used when prescribing ketorolac in the unconscious patient. Ketorolac is contraindicated in the presence of acute or chronic renal failure as well as in the presence of hypovolemia and other conditions associated with decreased tissue perfusion; it should not be administered for more than 5 consecutive days and should always be used with appropriate monitoring of the renal function.

The role of the more selective COX-2 inhibitors in the critically ill patients remains unknown. Selective COX-2 inhibiting agents cause less gastrointestinal irritation with long-term use than traditional NSAIDs [56]. The slow onset of action of some agents may decrease their utility for acute pain management.

For patients in whom NSAIDs are contraindicated, acetaminophen may represent a good alternative. In combination with an opioid, acetaminophen produces a greater analgesic effect than higher doses of the opioid alone [57]. Care must be taken to avoid excessive and potentially hepatotoxic doses, especially in patients with a significant history of alcohol intake or a poor nutritional status [58].

Opioids

Opioids remain the main pharmacologic means for the treatment of acute pain in the ICU patient (Table 23-1).

Desirable attributes of a useful opioid include rapid onset of action, ease of titration, lack of accumulation of the parent drug or its metabolites, and low cost. Of the commonly used opioids, fentanyl has the most rapid onset and shortest duration of action; it causes only minor hemodynamic changes and does not affect the inotropic state of the heart. Virtually all hemodynamic variables including cardiac output and systemic and pulmonary vascular resistance, are unchanged after large doses of fentanyl [59]. Because fentanyl

TABLE 23-1.   Guidelines for Front-Loading Intravenous Analgesia

Drug	Total Front-Load Dose	Increments	Cautions
Morphine	0.08–0.12 mg/kg	0.03 mg/kg q 10 min	Hypotension (histamine) Nausea/vomiting Biliary colic Acute/chronic renal failure Elderly
Methadone	0.08–0.12 mg/kg	0.03 mg/kg q 15 min	Accumulation/sedation Elderly
Hydromorphone	0.02 mg/kg	25–50 μg/kg q 10 min	Same as morphine
Fentanyl	1–3 μg/kg	0.5–2.00 μg/kg/h	Accumulation/sedation Elderly Skeletal muscle rigidity
Remifentanil	0.25–1.00 μg/kg	0.05–2.00 μg/kg/min	Pain on discontinuation Skeletal muscle rigidity
Ketamine	0.2–0.5 mg/kg	0.5–2.00 mg/kg/h	Delirium Increased ICP High myocardial O_2 requirement Hypotension Decreased co

ICP, intracranial pressure; q, every.

is lipid-soluble, the duration of action with small doses (50 to 100 μg) is short as a result of redistribution from the brain to other tissues. Larger cumulative doses, including the doses delivered via a continuous infusion, become dependent on elimination as opposed to redistribution with possible drug accumulation and prolonged effects [60].

Morphine has a slower onset and longer duration of action; hypotension may result from vasodilation (secondary to release of histamine) and one of its active metabolites (morphine 6-glucuronide) may cause prolonged sedation in the presence of renal insufficiency.

Hydromorphone is a semisynthetic opioid that is 5- to 10-fold more potent than morphine, but with a similar duration of action; it has minimal hemodynamic effects and lacks a clinically significant active metabolite, and it causes minor to no histamine release [35,60].

Methadone is a synthetic opioid agent with properties similar to morphine that can be given enterally and parenterally [60]. It has a much longer duration of action than morphine but a similar receptor-associated adverse effect profile, although it is less sedating if the appropriate dose is carefully titrated. Although methadone is not the drug of choice for an acutely ill patient whose hospital course is rapidly changing, it is a good alternative for the patient who has a long recovery ahead and an anticipated prolonged ventilatory wean. Often when the patient's clinical conditions are stable, transitioning from fentanyl or morphine infusions to methadone intravenously (IV) or via a feeding tube can help simplify care regimens and decrease dependence on infusions [60].

Remifentanil has not been widely studied in ICU patients; it requires the use of a continuous infusion because of its very short duration of action. Furthermore, the rapid offset of analgesia with remifentanil may result in a greater incidence of pain at the time of the discontinuation of the infusion, especially when compared with other longer acting opioids [61]. The short duration of action could be beneficial in selected patients requiring interruptions of analgesia medications administration to allow neurologic examinations [62].

OPIOIDS SIDE EFFECTS. Adverse effects of opioid analgesics are common and may occur frequently, especially in ICU patients. These effects may aggravate the patient's illness and prolong the clinical course [63].

Respiratory depression is a concern in spontaneously breathing patients or those receiving partial ventilatory support. Hypotension is usually the result of the combination of sympatholysis, vagally mediated bradycardia, and histamine release (when using morphine) [64,65]; particular care should be taken in patients with hemodynamic instability [66]. Gastric retention and ileus are common in critically ill patients, and intestinal hypomotility is enhanced by opioids [67,68]; routine prophylactic use of a stimulant laxative may minimize constipation. Opioids may increase intracranial pressure with traumatic brain injury, although the data are inconsistent and the clinical significance is unknown [69–71]. Withdrawal phenomena after opioid use in critically ill adult patients have been reported in rare cases only [72]. Addiction in adult patients receiving opioids also seems to be unusual; in a large series of 11,882 patients treated with various opioids, only 4 were reported to have become addicted [73]. Methadone in high doses has also been associated with prolongation of the QTc interval in the electrocardiogram as well as the risk of development of torsade de pointes [74–76].

OPIOIDS ADMINISTRATION TECHNIQUES. Opioid analgesics should be administered on a continuous or scheduled intermittent basis, with supplemental bolus doses as required [77]. When analgesics are administered only on an "as needed" basis, it is almost impossible to achieve a minimal effective analgesic plasma concentration with subsequent poor overall pain control [78].

When a continuous infusion is used, a protocol incorporating daily awakening from analgesia and sedation (sedation vacation) may allow more effective analgesic titration with a lower total dose of opioid; daily awakening may also be associated with a shorter duration of ventilation and ICU stay [79]. For patients in whom a long recovery and a prolonged ventilatory wean are anticipated, the use of a long-acting opioid (e.g., methadone) for background pain control in association with supplemental bolus doses of a short-acting opioid is indicated.

In patients who are not critically ill, patient-controlled analgesia (PCA), has been reported to result in stable drug concentrations, a good quality of analgesia, less sedation, less opioid consumption, and potentially fewer side effects, including respiratory depression [40,80]. In addition, a basal rate or continuous infusion mode can be used for consistent analgesia during sleep. Patient selection is important when PCA is used, and particular attention should be paid to the patient's cognition, hemodynamic reserve, and previous opioid exposure in order to achieve optimal treatment and minimize the possibility of adverse events. PCA devices can also be used for nurse-controlled analgesia.

Transdermal fentanyl represents a different treatment approach, which could be used in patients who are hemodynamically stable and with more chronic analgesic needs. The patch provides consistent drug delivery, but the extent of absorption varies depending on the permeability, temperature, perfusion, and thickness of the skin. Fentanyl patches are usually not a recommended modality for acute analgesia because of their 12- to 24-hour delay to peak effect [81], and similar lag time to complete offset once the patch is removed.

Ketamine

Ketamine is an intravenous anesthetic that has analgesic properties. It works by blocking the *N*-methyl D-aspartate receptor as well as activating the mu receptor [30,60,82]. Ketamine is usually metabolized in the liver, and its major metabolite is norketamine [83]. Norketamine is one-third to one-fifth as potent as ketamine as an anesthetic but it has been demonstrated to have analgesic properties [84,85]. Ketamine also has a rapid onset and short duration of action [86].

Blood pressure and spontaneous respiration are maintained under ketamine anesthesia/analgesia [87]; also, ketamine has an important neuroprotective role and hinders the progression of cerebral ischemia [88], even though it has been reported that ketamine may increase intracranial pressure and cerebral blood flow in man [89]. Schwedler et al. [90] have shown that intracranial pressure, cerebral blood flow, and perfusion pressure are unchanged during ketamine anesthesia; in addition, when ketamine is administered, either in animals or humans, during controlled ventilation, only minimal if any increase in intracranial pressure can be observed [91,92].

Subhypnotic doses of ketamine administered as infusions have been used for critically ill ICU patients who are very difficult to sedate with opioid and benzodiazepine infusions [93]. These low-dose ketamine infusions (less than 5 μg per kg per minute) do not seem to be associated with the usual adverse effects of ketamine such as hypertension, tachycardia, increased intracranial pressure, excessive secretions, and vivid dreams and hallucinations [94]. Because of its potential adverse effects, ketamine is not recommended for routine sedation and analgesia of the critically ill patient, but it can be useful for more difficult situations and/or when short surgical procedures with intense pain, such as placement of chest tubes, dressing changes, and/or wound debridement in burn patients are necessary [60,94].

Other Drugs

Other medications such as anticonvulsants, antidepressants, sodium-channel blockers, and muscle relaxants (e.g., baclofen) have a minimal role in the management of acute pain in the critically ill patient, although they may become part of a strategy aimed at treating the patient's pain problem beyond the time of his or her stay in the ICU.

Topical anesthetics can be used in association with short-acting opioids and/or ketamine for dressing changes in burn patients or in patients with large, open wounds (e.g., patients with necrotizing fasciitis). Particular attention has to be paid to the amount of medication used in order to avoid dangerous side effects/complications secondary to local anesthetic accumulation and toxicity.

Benzodiazepines, barbiturates, propofol, phenothiazines, butyrophenones are usually given in combination with opioids [95]. They are used for anxiolysis, sedation, and production of amnesia, but not for analgesia, because they have no analgesic properties.

REGIONAL ANALGESIA TECHNIQUES

Recent studies suggest that advances in perioperative anesthesia and analgesia improve pain relief and patient satisfaction and can affect outcome in surgical and trauma patients. Neuraxial anesthesia and analgesia and peripheral nerve blockade have the potential to reduce or eliminate the physiologic stress response to surgery and trauma, decreasing the possibility of surgical complications and improving outcome [96–99].

Used alone or in combination with other treatment modalities, regional analgesia techniques are an invaluable tool to address pain-related problems in critically ill patients, but the indications for their use must be established correctly; postsurgical and trauma ICU patients are at risk for numerous complications and the use of an inappropriate regional analgesia technique can cause a deterioration of the patient's clinical status, affecting a potentially favorable outcome.

The purpose of this section is to discuss risk and benefits of neuraxial and peripheral nerve blockade for the management of pain in the critically ill patient.

GENERAL CONSIDERATIONS

There are several general considerations [100] related to regional analgesia:

- In general, given the lack of cooperation and communication in many critically ill patients, those undergoing regional analgesia with continuous catheters in ICUs require a higher level of vigilance than do ward patients. Blocks and catheters ideally should be placed and managed by intensivists trained in anesthesia or pain medicine; otherwise, close cooperation between the intensive care team and the acute pain service of the hospital is required.

- Because of the frequently large and confusing numbers of catheters in critically ill patients, the risk of drug errors and wrong administration of drugs through continuous regional analgesia catheters may be higher. Well-trained and highly qualified personnel are the best safeguard against these complications, as well as eye-catching labels, standardized care protocols, and specially designed connectors for those catheters.

- Comprehensive diagnostic approaches should be undertaken (e.g., computed tomography/magnetic resonance imaging scans) whenever there are clinical signs of possible bleeding complications (e.g., suspected epidural or retroperitoneal hematoma).

- Frequent observation for infectious complications and careful adherence to aseptic technique during placement and tunneling of the catheters should always be followed. Catheters do not need to be removed routinely after certain time intervals, but only when clinical signs of infection appear. If a catheter gets disconnected, the decision to reconnect or remove the catheter must be based on the individual patient's clinical situation. Cuvillon et al. [101] have reported a high overall incidence of colonization (57%) of femoral catheters without septic complications when disconnected catheters were reconnected after a thorough disinfection of the outer surface.

- The overall risk of permanent neurologic damage or death from regional anesthesia and analgesia seems to be low in the perioperative settings [102–104]. Although these studies include critically ill patients, there are no specific subgroup data available.

INTERCOSTAL NERVE BLOCKS

Single and continuous intercostal nerve blocks are used to provide analgesia in patients with thoracic injuries, such as rib fractures, as well as for treating postoperative pain. Immediate pain relief after intercostal nerve block as well as improvement in pulmonary mechanics have been demonstrated in several reports [105–107].

This technique provides analgesia without widespread sympathetic blockade or weakness of major muscle groups, disadvantages that may be seen with epidural local anesthetics. Also, studies have shown that injection into one intercostal groove blocks not only the intercostal nerve of that groove, but also the one above and below because of subpleural tracking [108,109].

Intercostal nerve blocks are associated with the risk of pneumothorax (0.073% to 19%) [110] and the possibility of systemic toxic reactions to the local anesthetics if excessive amounts are used. The patient's coagulation status must always be checked before performing an intercostal nerve block because of the risk of bleeding and hematoma formation subsequent to the laceration of an intercostal vessel [111].

Although not frequently used, intercostal nerve blocks can be extremely useful in the ICU patient, especially when used as a single injection for painful procedures (e.g., placement of chest tubes), or when the patient's hemodynamic conditions are compromised enough to discourage the use of thoracic epidural analgesia.

PARAVERTEBRAL BLOCK

Paravertebral nerve blocks provide analgesia for thoracic and upper abdominal pain. Paravertebral nerve blockade can be performed with a single injection of local anesthetic or a continuous catheter technique [112]. Injection into a paravertebral catheter causes flow laterally into an intercostal space as well as up and down the ipsilateral paravertebral space [113,114]. Several intercostal nerves are thus bathed with local anesthetic, providing analgesia over several dermatomal levels.

The advantages of paravertebral block are similar to those of the intercostal technique. Analgesia can be obtained without widespread cardiovascular effects because only unilateral sympathetic blockade is produced.

Because the site of injection is medial to the scapula, this block is easier to perform at high thoracic levels than are intercostal blocks. In contrast to routine intercostal blocks, the posterior primary ramus of the intercostal nerve is covered by this block, providing analgesia of the posterior spinal muscles and the costovertebral ligaments.

Risks of this technique include pneumothorax, epidural blockade, and inaccurate catheter placement [115].

INTERPLEURAL ANALGESIA

With this technique a conventional epidural catheter is placed into the interpleural space, between the parietal and visceral pleurae, using a Tuohy or Crawford stylet needle [116]. The usual point of injection is at the angle of the rib, approximately 8 to 10 cm lateral to the posterior midline. The technique is similar to that used to perform a thoracentesis (i.e., the needle is "walked off" the superior border of the rib), with the bevel of the needle directed cephalad. Entry into the interpleural space is detected by a "hanging drop" technique, in which the "negative pressure" on entry into the interpleural space is recognized when a drop of preservative-free normal saline placed on the hub of the needle is sucked inward [117]. An epidural catheter is then advanced 5 to 10 cm into the interpleural space. Once the catheter is in place, intermittent injections or a continuous infusion of local anesthetic may be used. Care must be exercised with the use of a continuous infusion to avoid accumulation of a toxic dose of local anesthetic. If a posterior approach is not possible, an anterior approach may also be used. The catheter also may be positioned in the interpleural space under direct vision during surgery [118].

It is uncertain how interpleural analgesia works. Possibilities include diffusion of local anesthetic through the parietal pleura, superficially, to block the intercostal nerves, or posteromedially to reach the paravertebral area to block nerve roots and sympathetic ganglia [118,119]. Intercostal nerves are anesthetized [120], but to a lesser extent than with standard percutaneous intercostal techniques [119]. Sympathetic blockade also has been reported, which may account for the relief of visceral pain seen with this technique [121–124]. The block tends to be denser in dependent areas, which may require patients to be in the lateral position when each "top up" dose is given [116,120,123].

Bupivacaine is absorbed very rapidly from the interpleural space, and it is unclear whether epinephrine slows this absorption [125,126].

Inadequate analgesia may occur with interpleural blockade in the presence of a thoracostomy tube because drainage may remove a large amount of the anesthetic agent from the interpleural space [127]. Interpleural analgesia is probably best used only if one side of the thorax or upper abdomen is involved [128]. Because of concerns about local anesthetic toxicity and bilateral thoracic sympathetic blockade, other methods of analgesia are preferable in patients with bilateral pain, and bilateral interpleural catheters are not recommended. Also, the possibility of ipsilateral phrenic nerve blockade with interpleural blockade contributes to the hazards associated with bilateral interpleural blockade [129–131].

Contraindications to the use of interpleural analgesia include (a) fibrosis of the pleura, which may make it difficult to identify the pleural space; (b) blood or fluid within the pleural space; and (c) recent thoracic infection, which may cause rapid absorption of the local anesthetic, leading to toxicity.

PERIPHERAL NERVE BLOCKS FOR THE UPPER EXTREMITIES

Severe trauma to the shoulders or arms is often part of multiple injuries secondary to traffic or workplace accidents. These injuries may be associated with blunt chest trauma requiring mechanical ventilation, and can contribute to severe pain, especially during positioning [100]. If the orthopaedic injury is part of a complex trauma including brain injury, in which the mental status of the patient may be altered and opioid-based analgesia regimens might mask the neurologic condition, adequate analgesia can be provided for the shoulder or upper limb with continuous interscalene [132–134], continuous cervical paravertebral [134–137], or infraclavicular [138] approaches to the brachial plexus.

There are concerns regarding the placement of regional blocks in ICU patients with impaired mental status due to neurologic injury or therapeutic sedation. Benumof [139] has reported several serious complications, including spinal cord injury, related to the interscalene approach that might have been associated with sedation or general anesthesia. In sedated critically ill patients, a combination of ultrasound and nerve stimulation for the placement of interscalene catheters and a technique with a less medial needle direction, such as the approach described by Meier et al. [140,141], should help to minimize the risk of complications [142]. Blocking of the phrenic nerve with the consequent loss of hemidiaphragmatic function [143] should always be considered when planning an interscalene approach to the brachial plexus. Although phrenic nerve blockade may have negligible effects in mechanically ventilated patients, it may impair weaning from mechanical ventilation in high-risk patients.

The continuous infraclavicular [134–138,144–146], and axillary [134,147–149] approaches provide good analgesia for the arm, elbow, and hand. The small risk of pneumothorax must be considered against the slightly higher success rate and easier catheter maintenance of the infraclavicular approach versus the axillary approach, but can be neglected if a chest tube is already in place. A more lateral approach [150–152] might help to reduce the pneumothorax risk further.

PERIPHERAL NERVE BLOCKS FOR THE LOWER EXTREMITIES

Femoral nerve blocks and catheters are helpful in the management of acute pain from femoral fractures in the period between the injury and shortly after surgical stabilization [153,154]. Ultrasonographic guidance [155] may limit the pain with nerve stimulation, which could be treated with small doses of IV remifentanil or ketamine. A fascia iliaca compartment block [156,157] might be a valid alternative.

Continuous femoral nerve catheters provide excellent pain relief for the whole leg when used in combination with a sciatic nerve block [158]. Whether an anterior [159], posterior mid-gluteal [160], subgluteal [161], or classic Labat approach with one or two injections [162] to the sciatic nerve is chosen depends on the skills of the operator and the ability to place the patient in the appropriate position for the procedure. If a combination of catheter techniques is indicated, as often is the case for the lower extremity, the total daily dose of local anesthetic must be adjusted based on catheter location, mixtures with epinephrine, drug interactions, and disease states [163].

EPIDURAL ANALGESIA

Epidural analgesia is the regional analgesia technique most frequently used in the ICU [164].

Indications for the use of epidural analgesia in the ICU include penetrating and blunt chest trauma with or without rib fractures [165–168], thoracic [169,170], and abdominal surgery [171–173], major vascular surgery [174,175], major orthopaedic surgery [176], acute pancreatitis [177], paralytic ileus [178–181], cardiac surgery [182,183], and intractable angina pain [184,185].

Because high-risk patients seem to profit most from epidural analgesia [186,187] and the current available literature does not address the specific problem of the critically ill patient with multiple comorbidities and organ failure, an individual approach is always necessary [188].

Although the issues of consent, possible coagulopathy, and infection can be addressed easily in elective conditions, they become a major problem in patients with multiple trauma or extremely painful conditions (e.g., acute pancreatitis). Regarding the patient's coagulation status, the current recommendations of the American Society of Regional Anesthesia, and the German Society of Anesthesia and Intensive Care should be followed [189–191]. Adequate safety intervals during the administration of anticoagulant drugs are equally important for the placement and removal of epidural catheters and should always be respected [192].

There is also controversy about the safety of placing epidural catheters in sedated patients [193–195]; also, confirmation of a good catheter position can be difficult in the critically ill patient if sensory level testing is not reliable. Even though an awake and cooperative patient usually facilitates the placement of an epidural catheter, minimizing the possibility of disastrous complications, literature data document the small frequency of serious neurologic adverse events associated with epidural catheter placement in anesthetized and/or heavily sedated patients [195].

Positioning the patient for the procedure may also represent a challenge depending on the underlying injury and the number and position of tubes, catheters, or external fixation devices present. Maximum barrier precaution similar to the placement of central lines should always be considered when placing epidural catheters in the critically ill patient. Tunneling the catheter should also be considered to prevent dislocation and reduce possible catheter site infections [196].

To confirm the correct position of the epidural catheter, electrical stimulation during placement (Tsui test) or a postplacement radiograph with a small amount of contrast medium may be helpful [197,198].

Bolus injections of long-acting local anesthetics such as bupivacaine and ropivacaine or the discontinuation of continuous infusions every morning can help neurologic assessment.

The most common side effects of epidural blocks are bradycardia and hypotension related to sympathetic block; this can be more pronounced with intermittent bolus dosing in patients with hypovolemia or reduced venous return secondary to high positive end-expiratory pressure ventilation. Continuous low-rate local anesthetic and/or opioid (morphine) infusions can be safely used in this particular clinical setting. If the clinical conditions do not permit the placement of an epidural catheter but the patient really could benefit from it (e.g., flail chest and acute respiratory distress syndrome secondary to severe blunt chest trauma), it would be appropriate to wait for an improvement of the patient's clinical conditions before proceeding with the placement of the epidural catheter.

Current sepsis and bacteremia are considered contraindications to neuraxial blockade; however, many ICU patients present with a clinical picture of systemic inflammatory response syndrome. Fever and increased white blood cell counts alone in the absence of positive blood cultures do not provide a reliable diagnosis of bacteremia. The combination of the serum markers C-reactive protein, procalcitonin, and interleukin-6, have been shown to indicate bacterial sepsis with a high degree of sensitivity and specificity [199–202] and can guide the decision as to whether to place an epidural catheter.

INFLUENCE OF ADEQUATE PAIN MANAGEMENT ON COMPLICATIONS, OUTCOME, AND LENGTH OF HOSPITAL STAY

PULMONARY FUNCTION AND PULMONARY COMPLICATIONS

The prevention of pulmonary complications is one of the major goals of providing analgesia in postsurgical and trauma patients.

Adequate pain control can reduce the incidence of postoperative atelectasis, pneumonia, and hypoxemia by directly influencing these variables as well as by affecting the reduction in functional residual capacity that follows major abdominal and thoracic surgery [203,204].

A meta-analysis of randomized controlled clinical trials, published in 1998, has assessed improvements in pulmonary outcomes comparing systemic and epidural opioids, and epidural local anesthetics. Use of epidural opioids (morphine) is associated with significantly less atelectasis and a reduced incidence of pulmonary complications when compared with systemic opioids. However, epidural local anesthetics significantly reduce the incidence of pulmonary complications, atelectasis, and pneumonia more than epidural opioids, and raise the postoperative partial pressure of oxygen even more [204]. A meta-analysis of 141 randomized trials has found an overall 39% reduction in pneumonia and a 59% reduction in respiratory depression in patients treated with thoracic epidural analgesia/anesthesia, compared with patients treated with general anesthesia and PCA [187]. Furthermore, a recently published randomized controlled trial has demonstrated that, when feasible, epidural analgesia improves the outcome in patients with traumatic chest wall pain associated with multiple rib fractures by decreasing the rate of nosocomial pneumonia and the duration of mechanical ventilation [168].

We believe that the available literature data support the conclusion that adequate pain control, and particularly a correct use of epidural analgesia, can improve pulmonary outcomes by attenuating the physiologic response to surgery, controlling postoperative and trauma pain, permitting earlier extubation, and reducing length of ICU stay.

GASTROINTESTINAL FUNCTION

Gastrointestinal ileus dramatically affects morbidity and length of hospital stay after major surgery and trauma [178]. Blockage of afferent pain signals and efferent sympathetic reflex arcs by using intraoperative and postoperative epidural anesthesia/analgesia techniques abolish the stress response and minimize the effect of surgery and trauma on bowel function. In addition, the anatomy of the autonomic nervous system permits the use of epidural anesthesia and analgesia to block the inhibitory sympathetic efferents to the gut while preserving the stimulatory parasympathetic efferents [97,205].

COAGULATION

The clinical merits of epidural analgesia's effects on coagulation have been addressed in two meta-analyses of randomized clinical trials. Rodgers et al. [187] have observed a 44% reduction in deep venous thrombosis and a subsequent 55% reduction in pulmonary embolism when epidural analgesia and anesthesia techniques were used in comparison to general anesthesia. Another analysis of 22 randomized studies in patients undergoing lower abdominal and lower extremity orthopaedic surgery found a significant reduction in thromboembolic complications when general epidural anesthesia and analgesia was compared to general anesthesia and systemic analgesia (28% to 62%, respectively) [206].

Overall, epidural analgesia reduces the risk of postsurgical and trauma embolic complications by improving venous blood flow, attenuating the sympathetic response to surgery, and through the anticoagulant properties of local anesthetics.

ENDOCRINE AND METABOLIC STRESS RESPONSE

The stress response to surgery and trauma initiates a cascade of physiologic and metabolic events with the release of neuroendocrine mediators and cytokines (interleukin-1, interleukin-6, tumor necrosis factor-α), which produce the clinical sequelae of tachycardia, hypertension, fever, immunosuppression, and

protein catabolism, which is related to increased morbidity and mortality [17,19,207,208]. The magnitude of the stress response correlates with cardiac, vascular, and infectious morbidity; the attenuation of the response usually decreases these morbidities [206]. Two studies have demonstrated the superiority of epidural analgesia over other analgesics in blunting the stress response. Kehlet and Holte [42] evaluated the effects of IV PCA, NSAIDs, and epidural analgesia on attenuating the stress response in an effort to reduce morbidity and mortality. Only epidural analgesia significantly reduced the magnitude of the stress response. As further support, a study by Moller et al. [209] found that IV PCA provided effective postoperative analgesia without altering the magnitude of the stress response after surgery.

The decline in serum catecholamines and their subsequent effect of reduced tachycardia, hypertension, and reduced myocardial oxygen consumption may explain the observed reduced cardiac morbidity when epidural analgesic techniques are used [19]. A similar study [210] has demonstrated a reduction in graft occlusions and lower plasma catecholamine levels in a series of patients with epidurals undergoing lower extremity vascular surgery. Additionally, sympathetic activation increases metabolism, resulting in hyperglycemia and protein catabolism, both of which have been implicated in infectious complications and impaired wound healing [211].

OVERALL MORTALITY/COST/LENGTH OF STAY

As reviewed previously, epidural analgesia affects positively several important outcome measures (e.g., vascular graft patency, deep venous thrombosis, intestinal ileus). There are, however, good data that suggest that epidural anesthesia and analgesia result in improved postsurgical and trauma mortality, cost of care, or hospital length of stay [212,213]. Retrospective studies have concluded that effective epidural analgesia does affect length of stay. A large retrospective study of 462 consecutive cancer patients undergoing surgery reported that both ICU days (1.3 days vs. 2.8 days) and hospital length of stay (11 days vs. 17 days) were decreased in patients treated with perioperative epidural anesthesia and analgesia techniques compared with those treated with general anesthesia and IV PCA [214]. Also, a recent randomized trial in patients undergoing colonic surgery reported not only a positive impact on bowel function and intake of food, but also long-lasting effects on exercise capacity and health-related quality of life [215].

CONCLUSIONS

- Pain control in critically ill patients is of paramount importance. Achieving adequate levels of analgesia in these patients decreases the stress response to surgery and trauma and improves morbidity and mortality.
- Lack of education, fear of possible side effects, and inappropriate use of medications contribute to the ineffective treatment of pain in critically ill ICU patients. The expertise of pain management specialists and anesthesiologists is often necessary for the management of complex situations
- Choosing the treatment plan that best fits the patient's clinical conditions is mandatory. A potentially favorable

outcome can be altered if inappropriate pain modalities are chosen and used.

- A rational multimodal approach including the use of nonpharmacologic, pharmacologic, and regional analgesia techniques is desirable and often needed. The continued use of these techniques extended into the postoperative period may shorten recovery time and speed discharge.
- Always assess and monitor the effects of a treatment modality on the patient's pain and clinical conditions as well. Be prepared to make changes in therapy as needed.
- Regional analgesia techniques (epidural, peripheral nerve blockade), although proven safe and effective, are underused in the management of pain in critically ill patients. They allow a decrease in the overall use of opioid analgesics and sedatives and reduce the possibility of developing potentially dangerous side effects. A correct indication as well as an appropriate timing for their use is required in order to increase their beneficial effects.
- The availability of new technologies (e.g., ultrasonography) may improve the quality of upper and lower extremity peripheral nerve blocks. Even though no data are available yet, it is reasonable to predict that the complication rate associated with performing peripheral nerve blocks in heavily sedated patients will significantly decrease with the routine use of ultrasound devices.

REFERENCES

1. Whipple JK, Lewis KS, Quebberman EJ, et al: Analysis of pain management in critically ill patients. *Pharmacotherapy* 15:592, 1995.
2. Cohen S, Christo P, Moroz L: Pain management in trauma patients. *Am J Phys Med Rehabil* 83(2):142, 2004.
3. Hewitt PB: Subjective follow-up of patients from a surgical intensive therapy ward. *BMJ (Clin Res)* 4:669, 1970.
4. Marks RM, Sachar EJ: Undertreatment of medical inpatients with narcotic analgesics. *Ann Intern Med* 78:173, 1973.
5. Jones J, Hoggart B, Withey J, et al: What the patients say: a study of reactions to an intensive care unit. *Intensive Care Med* 5:89, 1979.
6. Ferrante FM, Oray EJ, Rocco AG, et al: A statistical model for pain in patient-controlled analgesia and conventional intramuscular opioid regimens. *Anesth Analg* 67:457, 1988.
7. Jacob E, Puntillo K: Variability of analgesic practices for hospitalized children on different pediatric specialty units. *J Pain Symptom Manage* 20:59, 2000.
8. Edwards WT: Optimizing opioid treatment of postoperative pain. *J Pain Symptom Manage* 5:S24, 1990.
9. Oden RV: Acute postoperative pain: incidence, severity, and etiology of inadequate treatment. *Anesthesiol Clin North Am* 7:1, 1989.
10. Fields HC: Sources of variability in the sensation of pain. *Pain* 33:195, 1988.
11. Austin KL, Stapleton JV, Mather LV: Multiple intramuscular injections: a major source of variability in analgesic response to meperidine. *Pain* 8:47, 1980.
12. Bates MS: Ethnicity and pain, a biocultural model. *Soc Sci Med* 24:47, 1987.
13. Bates MS, Edwards WT, Anderson KO: Ethnocultural influences on variation in chronic pain perception. *Pain* 52:101, 1993.
14. Lavies N, Hart L, Rounsefell B, et al: Identification of patient, medical and nursing staff attitudes to postoperative opioid analgesia: stage 1 of a longitudinal study of postoperative analgesia. *Pain* 49:313, 1992.
15. Zalon ML: Nurses' assessment of postoperative patients' pain. *Pain* 54:329, 1993.
16. Woolf CJ, Salter MW: Neuronal plasticity: increasing the gain in pain. *Science* 288:1765, 2000.
17. Hedderich R, Ness TJ: Analgesia for trauma and burns. *Crit Care Clin* 15:167, 1999.
18. Anand KJ, Hickey PR: Halothane-morphine combined with high dose sufentanil for anesthesia and postoperative analgesia in neonatal cardiac surgery. *N Engl J Med* 326:1, 1992.
19. Yeager MP, Glass DD, Neff RK, et al: Epidural anesthesia and analgesia in high-risk surgical patients. *Anesthesiology* 66:729, 1987.
20. Schreiber S, Galai-Gat T: Uncontrolled pain following physical injury as the core-trauma in posttraumatic stress disorder. *Pain* 54:107, 1993.
21. Pembrook L: JCAHO has new pain management standards. *Anesthesiology News* 1:52, 1999.
22. *Pain Management: Understanding JCAHO Requirements and Patient Implications. Briefings on JCAHO.* Marblehead, MA, The Greeley Company, 2000.
23. de Rond MEJ, de Wit R, van Dam FSAM, et al: A pain monitoring program for nurses: effect on the administration of analgesics. *Pain* 89:25, 2000.
24. Desbiens NA, Wu AW, Broste SK, et al: Pain and satisfaction with pain control in seriously ill hospitalized adults: findings from the SUPPORT research investigators. *Crit Care Med* 246:1953, 1996.
25. Woolf CJ, Chong MS: Preemptive analgesia: treating postoperative pain by preventing the establishment of central sensitization. *Anesth Analg* 77:362, 1993.
26. Kehlet H: The stress response to anaesthesia and surgery: release mechanism and modifying factors. *Clin Anaesth* 2:15, 1984.
27. Huskisson EC: Visual analog scales, in Melzack R (ed): *Pain Measurement and Assessment.* New York, Raven, 1983; p 33.
28. Stevens DS, Edwards WT: Management of pain in the critically ill. *J Intensive Care Med* 5:258, 1990.
29. Rawal N, Tandon B: Epidural and intrathecal morphine in intensive care units. *Intensive Care Med* 11:129, 1985.
30. De Pinto M, Dunbar P, Edwards WT: Pain Management. *Anesthesiol Clin North Am* 24:19, 2006.
31. Banning A, Sjogren P, Henriken H: Pain causes in 200 patients referred to a multidisciplinary cancer pain clinic. *Pain* 45:45, 1991.
32. Stucky CL, Gold MS, Zhang X: Mechanisms of pain. *Proc Natl Acad Sci USA* 98:11845, 2001.
33. Dickenson AH: Spinal pharmacology of pain. *Br J Anaesth* 75:193, 1995.
34. Elliott K, Minami N, Kolesnikov Y, et al: The NMDA receptor antagonists, LY274614 and MK-801, and the nitric oxide synthase inhibitor, NG-nitro-L-arginine, attenuate analgesic tolerance to the mu opioid morphine but not to the kappa opioids. *Pain* 56:69, 1994.
35. Jacobi J, Fraser, GL, Coursin D, et al: Clinical practice guidelines for the sustained use of sedatives and analgesics in the critically adult. *Crit Care Med* 30(1):119, 2002.
36. Novaes MA, Knobel E, Bork AM, et al: Stressors in the ICU. perception of the patient, relatives, and healthcare team. *Intensive Care Med* 25:1421, 1999.
37. Desai PM: Pain management and pulmonary dysfunction. *Crit Care Clin* 15:151, 1999.
38. Gust R, Pecher S, Gust A: Effect of patient controlled analgesia on pulmonary complications after coronary artery by-pass grafting. *Crit Care Clin* 27:2218, 1999.
39. Mangano DT, Silician D, Hollenberg M, et al: Postoperative myocardial ischemia: therapeutic trials using intensive analgesia following surgery. *Anesthesiology* 76:342, 1992.
40. Parker SD, Breslow MJ, Frank SM, et al: Catecholamines and cortisol responses to lower extremity revascularization: correlation with outcome variables. *Crit Care Med* 23:1954, 1995.
41. Ford G, Whitelaw W, Rosenal T, et al: Diaphragm function after upper abdominal surgery in humans. *Am Rev Respir Dis* 127:431, 1987.
42. Kehlet H, Holte K: Effect of postoperative analgesia on surgical outcome. *Br J Anaesth* 87:62, 2001.
43. Hamza MA, White PF, Ahmed HE, et al: Effect of the frequency of transcutaneous electrical nerve stimulation on the postoperative opioid analgesic requirement and recovery profile. *Anesthesiology* 91:1232, 1999.
44. Kimball KL, Drews JE, Walker S, et al: Use of TENS for pain reduction in burn patients receiving Travase. *J Burn Care Rehabil* 81:28, 1987.
45. Oncel M, Sencan S, Yildiz H, et al: Transcutaneous electrical nerve stimulation for pain management in patients with uncomplicated minor rib fractures. *Eur J Cardiothorac Surg* 22:13, 2002.
46. Lewis SM, Clelland JM, Knowles CJ, et al: Effects of auricular acupuncture-like transcutaneous electrical nerve stimulation on pain levels following wound care in patients with burns: a pilot study. *J Burn Care Rehabil* 11:322, 1990.
47. Horsburgh CR: Healing by design. *N Engl J Med* 333:735, 1995.
48. Wallace CJ, Robins J, Alvord LS, et al: The effect of earplugs on sleep measures during exposure to simulated intensive care unit noise. *Am J Crit Care* 8:210, 1999.
49. O'Hara DA, Fragen RJ, Kinzer M, et al: Ketorolac tromethamine as compared with morphine sulphate for treatment of postoperative pain. *Clin Pharmacol Ther* 41:556, 1987.
50. Bravo LJCB, Mattie H, Spierdik, et al. The effects on ventilation of ketorolac in comparison with morphine. *Eur J Clin Pharmacol* 35:491, 1988.
51. Burgess FW, Anderson DM, Colonna D, et al: Ipsilateral shoulder pain following thoracic surgery. *Anesthesiology* 78:365, 1993.
52. Strom BL, Berlin JA, Kinman JL, et al: Parenteral ketorolac and risk of gastrointestinal and operative site bleeding. *JAMA* 275:376, 1996.
53. Thwaites BK, Nigus DB, Bouska GW, et al: Intravenous ketorolac tromethamine worsens platelet function during knee arthroscopy under spinal anesthesia. *Anesth Analg* 82:1176, 1996.
54. Zikowski D, Hord AH, Haddox D, et al: Ketorolac-induced bronchospasm *Anesth Analg* 76:417, 1993.
55. Haddow GR, Riley E, Isaacs R, et al: Ketorolac, nasal polyposys, and bronchial asthma: a cause for concern. *Anesth Analg* 76:420, 1993.
56. Bombardier C, Laine L, Reicin A, et al: Comparison of upper gastrointestinal toxicity of rofecoxib and naproxen in patients with rheumatoid arthritis. *N Engl J Med* 343:1520, 2000.
57. Peduta VA, Ballabio M, Stefanini S: Efficacy of propacetamol in the treatment of postoperative pain: Morphine sparing effects in orthopedic surgery. Italian Collaborative Group on Propacetamol. *Acta Anesthesiol Scand* 42:293, 1998.
58. Zimmerman HJ, Maddrey W: Acetaminophen hepatotoxicity with regular intake of alcohol; analysis of instances of therapeutic misadventures. *Hepatology* 22:767, 1995.
59. Stanley T, Webster L: Anesthetic requirements and cardiovascular effects of fentanyl-oxygen and fentanyl-diazepam-oxygen anesthesia in man. *Anesth Analg* 57:411, 1978.
60. Liu L, Gropper MA: Postoperative analgesia and sedation in the adult intensive care unit. A guide to drug selection. *Drugs* 63(8):755, 2003.
61. Muellejans B, Lopez A, Cross MH, et al: Remifentanil versus fentanyl for analgesia based

sedation in the intensive care unit: a randomized double-blind controlled trial. *Crit Care* 2(8):R1, 2004.

62. Tipps, LB, Coplin WM, Murry KR, et al: Safety and feasibility of continuous infusion of remifentanil in the neurosurgical intensive care unit. *Neurosurgery* 46:596, 2000.

63. Prielipp RC, Coursin DB, Wood KE, et al: Complications associated with sedative and neuromuscular blocking agents in critically ill patients. *Crit Care Clin* 11:983, 1995.

64. Grossman M, Abiose A, Tangphao O, et al: Morphine-induced venodilation in humans. *Clin Pharmacol Ther* 60:554, 1996.

65. Flacke JW, Flacke WE, Bloor BC, et al: Histamine release by four narcotics: a double-blind study in humans. *Anesth Analg* 66:723, 1987.

66. McArdle P: Intravenous analgesia. *Crit Care Clin* 15:89, 1999.

67. Yuan C, Foss JF, O'Connor MF, et al: Effects of low-dose morphine on gastric emptying in healthy volunteers. *J Clin Pharmacol* 38:1017, 1998.

68. Heyland DK, Tougas G, King D, et al: Impaired gastric emptying in mechanically ventilated, critically ill patients. *Intensive Care Med* 22:1339, 1996.

69. Albanese J, Viviand X, Potie F, et al: Sufentanil, fentanyl, and alfentanil in head trauma patients. A study on cerebral hemodynamics. *Crit Care Med* 27:407, 1999.

70. Sperry RJ, Bailey PL, Reichman MV, et al: Fentanyl and sufentanil increase intracranial pressure in head trauma patients. *Anesthesiology* 77:416, 1992.

71. DeNaal M, Munar F, Poca MA, et al: Cerebral hemodynamic effects of morphine and fentanyl in patients with severe head injury. *Anesthesiology* 92:11, 2000.

72. Walder B, Tramer, MR: Analgesia and sedation in critically ill patients. *Swiss Med Wkly* 134:333, 2004.

73. Porter J, Jick H: Addiction rare in patients treated with narcotics. *N Engl J Med* 302:123, 1980.

74. Kornick CA, Kilburn MJ, Santiago-Palma J, et al: QTc interval prolongation associated with intravenous methadone. *Pain* 105(3):499, 2003.

75. Walker PW, Klein D, Kasza L: High dose methadone and ventricular arrhythmias; a report of three cases. *Pain* 103(3):321, 2003.

76. Cruciani RA, Sekine R, Homel P, et al: Measurement of QTc in patients receiving chronic methadone therapy. *J Pain Symptom Manage* 29(4):385, 2005.

77. Acute Pain Management Guidelines Panel: *Acute Pain Management: Operative or Medical Procedures and Trauma. Clinical Practice Guidelines.* Rockville, MD, Agency for Health Care Policy and Research, 1992; AHCPR publication no. 92-0032.

78. Dasta JF, Fuhrman TF, McCandles C: Patterns of prescribing and administering drugs for agitation and pain in patients in a surgical intensive care unit. *Crit Care Med* 22:974, 1994.

79. Kress JP, Pohlman AS, O'Connor MF, et al: Daily interruptions of sedative infusions in critically ill patients undergoing mechanical ventilation. *N Engl J Med* 342:1472, 2000.

80. Boldt J, Thaler E, Lehmann A, et al: Pain management in cardiac surgery patients: comparison between standard therapy and patient-controlled analgesia regimen. *J Cardiothorac Vasc Anesth* 12:654, 1998.

81. Lehmann KA, Zech L: Transdermal fentanyl: clinical pharmacology *J Pain Symptom Manage* 7:58, 1992.

82. Irifune M, Shimizu T, Nomoto M, et al: Ketamine-induced anesthesia involves the N-methyl-D aspartate receptor channel complex in mice. *Brain Res* 596(1-2):1, 1992.

83. Cohen ML, Chan SL, Way WL, et al: Distribution in brain and metabolism of ketamine in the rat after intravenous administration. *Anesthesiology* 39:370, 1973.

84. Grant IS, Nimmo WS, Clements JA: Pharmacokinetics and analgesic effects of IM and oral ketamine. *Br J Anesth* 53:805, 1981.

85. Shimoyama M, Shimoyama N, Gorman AL, et al: Oral ketamine is antinociceptive in the rat formalin test: role of metabolite norketamine. *Pain* 81:85, 1999.

86. Hijazi Y, Bodonian C, Bolon M, et al: Pharmacokinetics and haemodynamics of ketamine in intensive care patients with brain or spinal cord injury. *Br J Anesth* 90(2):155, 2003.

87. White PF, Way WL, Trevor AJ: Ketamine—its pharmacology and therapeutic uses. *Anesthesiology* 56:119, 1982.

88. Marcoux FX, Goodrich JE, Dominick MA: Ketamine prevents ischemic neuronal injury. *Brain Res* 452:329, 1988.

89. Takeshit a H, Okuda Y, Sari A: The effects of ketamine on cerebral circulation and metabolism in man. *Anesthesiology* 36:69, 1972.

90. Schwedler M, Miletich DJ, Albrecht RF: Cerebral blood flow and metabolism following ketamine administration. *Can Anaesth Soc J* 29:222, 1982.

91. Pfenninger E, Grunert A, Bowdler I, et al: The effect of ketamine on intracranial pressure during hemorrhagic shock under conditions of both spontaneous breathing and controlled ventilation. *Acta Neurochir* 78:113, 1985.

92. Mayberg TS, Lam AM, Domino KB, et al: Cerebral blood flow velocity and ADVO2 response to ketamine in neurosurgical patients. *Anesthesiology* 79:A204, 1993.

93. Joachimsson PO, Heldstrand U, Eklund A: Low dose ketamine infusion for analgesia during postoperative ventilator treatment. *Acta Anesthesiol Scand* 30(8):697, 1986.

94. Edrich T, Friedrich AD, Eltzschig HK, et al: Ketamine for long term sedation and analgesia of a burn patient. *Anesth Analg* 99(3):893, 2004.

95. Mather LE, Phillips GD: Opioids and adjuvants: principles of use, in Cousins MJ, Phillips GD (eds): *Acute Pain Management*, New York, Churchill Livingstone, 1986; p 77.

96. Moraca RJ, Sheldon DG, Thirlby RC: The role of epidural anesthesia and analgesia in surgical practice. *Ann Surg* 238(5):663, 2003.

97. Liu S, Carpenter RL, Neal JM, et al: Epidural anesthesia and analgesia. *Anesthesiology* 82:1474, 1995.

98. Grass JA: The role of epidural anesthesia and analgesia in postoperative outcome. *Anesthesiol Clin North Am* 18:407, 2000.

99. Groban L, Zvara DA, Deal DD, et al: Effect of epidural anesthesia and analgesia on perioperative outcome. *Ann Surg* 234:560, 2001.

100. Schultz-Stubner S, Boezaart A, Hata SJ: Regional analgesia in the critically ill. *Crit Care Med* 33(66):1400, 2005.

101. Cuvillon P, Ripart J, Lalourcey L, et al. The continuous femoral nerve block catheter for postoperative analgesia: bacterial colonization, infectious rate, and adverse effects. *Anesth Analg* 93:1045, 2001.

102. Auroy Y, Benhamou D, Bargues L, et al: Major complications of regional anesthesia in France: the SOS regional Anesthesia Hotline Service. *Anesthesiology* 97:1274, 2002.

103. Auroy Y, Narchi P, Messiah A, et al: Serious complications related to regional anesthesia: results of a prospective survey in France. *Anesthesiology* 87:479, 1997.

104. Moen V, Dahlgren N, Irestedt L: Severe neurologic complications after central neuraxial blockade in Sweden 1990–1999. *Anesthesiology* 101:950, 2004.

105. Osinowo OA, Zahrani M, Softah Abdullateef: Effect of intercostal nerve block with 0. 5% bupivacaine on peak expiratory flow rate and arterial oxygen saturation in rib fractures. *J Trauma* 56(2):345, 2004.

106. Pedersen WM, Schulze S, Hoier-Madsen K, et al: Air-flow meter assessment of the effect of intercostal nerve blockade on respiratory function in rib fractures. *Acta Chir Scand 1* 49:119, 1983.

107. Watson DS, Panian S, Kendall V, et al: Pain control after thoracotomy; bupivacaine versus lidocaine in continuous intercostal nerve blockade. *Ann Thorac Surg* 67:825, 1999.

108. Moore DC: Intercostal nerve block: spread of India ink injected to the rib's costal groove. *Br J Anaesth* 53:325, 1981.

109. Murphy DF: Continuous intercostal nerve blockade: an anatomical study to elucidate its mode of action. *Br J Anaesth* 56:627, 1984.

110. Moore DC: Intercostal nerve blockade for postoperative somatic pain following surgery of thorax and upper abdomen *Br J Anaesth* 47:284, 1975.

111. Nielsen CH: Bleeding after intercostal nerve block in a patient anticoagulated with heparin. *Anesthesiology* 71:162, 1989.

112. Eason NJ, Wyatt R: Paravertebral thoracic block: a reappraisal. *Anesthesia* 34:638, 1979.

113. Conacher ID, Kokri M: Postoperative paravertebral blocks for thoracic surgery. *Br J Anaesth* 59:155, 1987.

114. Karmakar MK, Chui PT, Joyny GM, et al: Thoracic paravertebral block for management of pain associated with multiple fractured ribs in patients with concomitant lumbar spinal trauma. *Reg Anesth Pain Med* 26:169, 2001.

115. Purcell-Jones G, Pither CE, Justins DM: Paravertebral somatic nerve blockade: a clinical, radiographic, and computed tomographic study in chronic pain patients. *Anesth Analg* 68:32, 1989.

116. Reiestad F, Stromskag KE: Interpleural catheter in the management of postoperative pain; a preliminary report. *Reg Anesth* 11:89, 1986.

117. Squier RC, Morrow JS, Roman R: Hanging-drop for intrapleural analgesia. *Anesthesiology* 70:882, 1989.

118. Kambam JR, Hammond J, Parris WCW, et al: Intrapleural analgesia for post-thoracotomy pain and blood levels following bupivacaine intrapleural injection. *Can J Anaesth* 36:106, 1989.

119. Covino BG: Interpleural regional anesthesia. *Anesth Analg* 67:427, 1988.

120. Riegler FX, Pelligrino DA, VaBoncoeur TR: An animal model of intrapleural analgesia. *Anesthesiology* 69:A365, 1988.

121. Sihota MK, Ikuta PT, Holmblad BR, et al: Successful pain management of chronic pancreatitis and post-herpetic neuralgia with intrapleural technique. *Reg Anesth* 13[Suppl 2]:40, 1988.

122. Sihota MK, Holmblad BR" Horner's syndrome after intrapleural anesthesia with bupivacaine for post-herpetic neuralgia. *Acta Anesthesiol Scand* 32:593, 1988.

123. Reiestad F, McIlvaine WB, Kvalheim L, et al: Interpleural analgesia in treatment of upper extremity reflex sympathetic dystrophy. *Anesth Analg* 69:671, 1988.

124. Durrani Z, Winnie AP, Ikuta P: Interpleural catheter analgesia for pancreatic pain. *Anesth Analg* 67:479, 1988.

125. Kambam JR, Handte RE, Flanagan J, et al: Intrapleural anesthesia for post-thoracotomy pain relief. *Anesth Analg* 66:S90, 1987.

126. Denson D, Sehlhorst CS, Schulz REG, et al: Pharmacokinetics of intrapleural bupivacaine: effects of epinephrine. *Reg Anesth* 13[Suppl 1]:47, 1988.

127. Chan VWS, Arthur GR, Ferrante FM: Intrapleural bupivacaine administration for pain relief following thoracotomy. *Reg Anesth* 13[Suppl 2]:70, 1988.

128. Raj P: Intrapleural anesthesia applications and contraindications. *Anesthesiol Alert* 1:1, 1988.

129. Aguilar JL, Montero A, Vidal LF, et al: Intrapleural analgesia and phrenic nerve palsy. *Reg Anesth* 15:45, 1990.

130. Kowalski SE, Bradley BD, Greengrass RA, et al: Effects of interpleural bupivacaine (0.5%) on canine diaphragmatic function. *Anesth Analg* 75:400, 1992.

131. Lauder GR: Interpleural analgesia and phrenic nerve paralysis. *Anesthesia* 48:315, 1993.

132. Boezaart AP, de Beer JF, du Toit C, et al: A new technique of continuous interscalene nerve block. *Can J Anaesth* 46:275, 1999.

133. Brown DL: Brachial plexus anesthesia: an analysis of options. *Yale J Biol Med* 66:415, 1993.

134. Schultz-Stubner S: Brachial plexus. *Anesth Analg* 52:643, 2003.

135. Boezaart AP, de Beer JF, Nell MF: Early experience with continuous cervical paravertebral block using a stimulating catheter. *Reg Anesth Pain Med* 28:406, 2003.

136. Boezaart AP, Koorn R, Borene S, et al: Continuous brachial plexus block using the posterior approach. *Reg Anesth Pain Med* 28:70, 2003.

137. Boezaart AP, Koorn R, Rosenquist RW: Paravertebral approach to the brachial plexus: an anatomic improvement in technique. *Reg Anesth Pain Med* 28:241, 2003.

138. Ilfeld BM, Enneking FK: Brachial plexus infraclavicular block success rate and appropriate endpoints. *Anesth Analg* 95:784, 2002.

139. Benumof JL: Permanent loss of cervical spinal cord function associated with interscalene block performed under general anesthesia. *Anesthesiology* 93:1541, 2000.

140. Meier G, Bauereis C, Maurer H, et al: Interscalene plexus block. Anatomic requirements—anesthesiologic and operative aspects. *Anaesthetist* 50:333, 2001.

141. Meier G, Bauereis C, Heinrich C, et al: Interscalene brachial plexus catheter for anesthesia and postoperative pain therapy. Experience with a modified technique. *Anaesthetist* 46:715, 1997.

142. Marhofer P, Greher M, Kapral S: Ultrasound guidance in regional anesthesia. *Br J Anaesth* 94(1):7, 2005.

143. Sala-Clanch X, Lazaro JR, Correa J, et al: Phrenic nerve block caused by interscalene brachial plexus block: effects of digital pressure and a low volume of local anesthetic. *Reg Anesth Pain Med* 24:231, 1999.

144. Neuberger M, Kaiser H, Rembold-Schuster I, et al: Vertical infraclavicular brachial plexus blockade. A clinical study of reliability of a new method for plexus anesthesia of the upper extremity. *Anaesthetist* 47:595, 1998.

145. Borene SC, Edwards JN, Boezaart AP: At the cords, the pinkie towards: interpreting infraclavicular motor responses to neurostimulation. *Reg Anesth Pain Med* 29:125, 2004.

146. Sandhu NS, Capan LM: Ultrasound-guided infraclavicular brachial plexus block. *Br J Anaesth* 89:254, 2002.

147. Ang ET, Lassale B, Goldfarb G: Continuous axillary brachial plexus block. A clinical and anatomical study. *Anesth Analg* 63:680, 1984.

148. Sia S, Lepri A, Campolo MC, et al: Four injection brachial plexus block using a peripheral nerve stimulator: a comparison between axillary and humeral approaches. *Anesth Analg* 95:1075, 2002.

149. Retzl G, Kapral S, Greher M, et al: Ultrasonographic findings of the axillary part of the brachial plexus. *Anesth Analg* 92:1271, 2001.

150. Kapral S, Jandrasits O, Schabernig C, et al: Lateral infraclavicular plexus block vs axillary block for hand and forearm surgery. *Acta Anaesthesiol Scand* 43:1047, 1999.

151. Greher M, Retzl G, Niel P, et al: Ultrasonographic assessment of topographic anatomy in volunteers suggests a modification of the infraclavicular vertical brachial plexus block. *Br J Anaesth* 88:632, 2002.

152. Jandard C, Gentili ME, Girar DF, et al: Infraclavicular block with lateral approach and nerve stimulation: extent of anesthesia and adverse effects. *Reg Anesth Pain Med* 27:37, 2002.

153. Finlayson BJ, Underhill TJ: Femoral nerve block for analgesia in fractures of the femoral neck. *Arch Emerg Med* 5:173, 1988.

154. Tan TT, Coleman MM: Femoral blockade for fractured neck of femur in the emergency department. *Ann Emerg Med* 42:596, 2003.

155. Marhofer P, Schrogendorfer K, Koinig H, et al: Ultrasonographic guidance improves sensory block and onset time of three-in-one blocks. *Anesth Analg* 85:854, 1997.

156. Lopez S, Gros T, Bernard N, et al: Fascia iliaca compartment block for femoral bone fractures in prehospital care. *Reg Anesth Pain Med* 28:203, 2003.

157. Cuignet O, Pirson J, Boughrough J, et al: The efficacy of continuous fascia iliaca compartment block for pain management in burn patients undergoing skin grafting procedures. *Anesth Analg* 98:1077, 2004.

158. Kaden V, Wolfel H, Kirsch W: Experiences with a combined sciatic and femoral block in surgery of injuries of the lower leg. *Anesthesiol Reanim* 14:299, 1989.

159. Barbero C, Fuzier R, Samii K: Anterior approach to the sciatic nerve block: adaptation to the patient's height. *Anesth Analg* 98:1785, 2004.

160. Franco CD: Posterior approach to the sciatic nerve in adults: is Euclidean geometry still necessary? *Anesthesiology* 98:723, 2003.

161. Di Benedetto P, Casati A, Bertini L, et al: Posterior subgluteal approach to block the sciatic nerve: description of the technique and initial clinical experience. *Eur J Anaesthesiol* 19:682, 2002.

162. Bailey SL, Parkinson SK, Little WL, et al: Sciatic nerve block. A comparison of single versus double injection technique. *Reg Anesth Pain Med* 19:9, 1994.

163. Rosenberg PH, Veering BT, Urmey WF: Maximum recommended doses of local anesthetics: a multifactorial concept. *Reg Anesth Pain Med* 29:564, 2004.

164. Naber L, Jones G, Halm M: Epidural analgesia for effective pain control. *Crit Care Nurs* 14:69, 1994.

165. Holcomb JB, McMullin NR, Kozar RA, et al: Morbidity from rib fractures increase after age 45. *J Am Coll Surg* 196:549, 2003.

166. Flagel BT, Luchette FA, Reed L: Half-a-dozen ribs: the breakpoint for mortality. *Surgery* 138(4):718, 2005.

167. Karmakar MK, Ho AM: Acute pain management of patients with multiple fractured ribs. *J Trauma* 54:615, 2003.

168. Bulger EM, Edwards WT, Klotz P, et al: Epidural analgesia improves outcome after multiple rib fractures. *Surgery* 136(2):426, 2004.

169. Asantila R, Rosenberg PH, Scheinin B: Comparison of different methods of postoperative analgesia after thoracotomy. *Acta Anaesthesiol Scand* 30:421, 1986.

170. Licker M, Spiliopoulos A, Frey JG, et al: Risk factors for early mortality and major complications following pneumonectomy for non-small cell carcinoma of the lung. *Chest;* 121:1890, 2002.

171. Peyton PJ, Myles PS, Silbert BS, et al: Perioperative epidural analgesia and outcome after major abdominal surgery in high-risk patients. *Anesth Analg* 96:548, 2003.

172. Carli F, Trudel JL, Belliveau P: The effect of intraoperative thoracic epidural anesthesia and postoperative analgesia on bowel function after colorectal surgery: a prospective randomized trial. *Dis Colon Rectum* 44:1083, 2001.

173. Jorgensen H, Wettersley J, Moiniche S, et al: Epidural local anesthetics versus opioid-based analgesic regimens on postoperative gastrointestinal paralysis, PONV, and pain after abdominal surgery. *Cochrane Database Syst Rev* ;CD001893, 2000.

174. Albani A, Renghi A, Gramaglia L, et al: Regional anesthesia in vascular surgery: a multidisciplinary approach to accelerate recovery and postoperative discharge. *Minerva Anestesiol* 67:151, 2001.

175. Bush RL, Lin PH, Reddy PP, et al: Epidural analgesia in patients with chronic obstructive pulmonary disease undergoing transperitoneal abdominal aortic aneurysmorraphy: a multi-institutional analysis. *Cardiovasc Surg* 11:179, 2003.

176. Wu CL, Anderson GF, Herber R, et al: Effect of postoperative epidural analgesia on morbidity and mortality after total hip replacement surgery in Medicare patients. *Reg Anesth Pain Med* 28:271, 2003.

177. Niesel HC, Klimpel L, Kaiser H, et al: Epidural blockade for analgesia and treatment of acute pancreatitis. *Reg Anesth* 14:97, 1991.

178. Baig MK, Wexner SD: Postoperative ileus: a review. *Dis Colon Rectum* 47:516, 2004.

179. Kreis ME, Kasparek MS, Becker HD, et al: Postoperative ileus: Part II—clinical therapy. *Zentralbl Chir* 128:320, 2003.

180. Holte K, Kehlet H: Postoperative ileus: progress towards effective management. *Drugs* 62:2603, 2002.

181. Kehelt H, Holte K: Review of postoperative ileus. *Am J Surg* 182:3S, 2001.

182. Peterson KL, DeCampli WM, Pike NA, et al: A report of two-hundred-twenty cases of regional anesthesia in pediatric cardiac surgery. *Anesth Analg* 90:1014, 2000.

183. Aybek T, Kessler P, Dogan S, et al: Awake coronary artery by-pass grafting: utopia or reality? *Ann Thorac Surg* 75:1165, 2003.

184. Sworkdal N: Pro: Anesthesiologists' role in treating refractory angina: spinal cord stimulators, thoracic epidurals, therapeutic angiogenesis, and other emerging options. *J Cardiothorac Vasc Anesth* 17:536, 2003.

185. Marchertiene I: Regional anesthesia for patients with cardiac disease. *Medicina (Kaunas)* 39:721, 2003.

186. Thompson JS: The role of epidural analgesia and anesthesia in surgical outcomes. *Adv Surg* 36:297, 2002.

187. Rodgers A, Walker N, Schug S, et al: Reduction of postoperative mortality and morbidity with epidural or spinal anesthesia: results from overview of randomized trials. *BMJ* 321:1493, 2000.

188. Burton AW, Eappen S: Regional anesthesia techniques for pain control in the intensive care unit. *Crit Care Clin* 15:77, 1999.

189. Kaplan R: ASRA consensus statements for anticoagulated patients. American Society of Regional Anesthesia. *Reg Anesth Pain Med* 24:477, 1999.

190. Horlocker TT, Wedel DJ, Benzon H, et al: Regional anesthesia in the anticoagulated patient: defining the risks (the second ASRA Consensus Conference on Neuraxial Anesthesia and Anticoagulation). *Reg Anesth Pain Med* 28:172, 2003.

191. Gogarten W, Van Aken H, Buttner J, et al: Regional anesthesia and thromboembolism prophylaxis/anticoagulation. Revised guidelines of the German Society of Anesthesiology and Intensive Care Medicine. *Anaesth Intensivemed* 44:218, 2003.

192. Vandermeulen E, Gogarten W, Van Aken H: Risks and complications following peridural anesthesia. *Anaesthetist* 46[Suppl 3]:S179, 1997.

193. Bromage PR, Benumof JL: Paraplegia following intracord injection during attempted epidural anesthesia under general anesthesia. *Reg Anesth Pain Med* 23:104, 1998.

194. Krane EJ, Dalens BJ, Murat I, et al: The safety of epidurals placed during general anesthesia. *Reg Anesth Pain Med* 23:433, 1998.

195. Horlocker TT, Abel MD, Messick JM, et al: Small risk of serious neurologic complications related to lumbar epidural catheter placement in anesthetized patients. *Anesth Analg* 96:1547, 2003.

196. Herwaldt LA, Coffin SA, Schulz-Stubner S: Nosocomial infections associated with anesthesia, in Mayhall CG (ed): *Hospital Epidemiology and Infection Control*, 3rd ed. Philadelphia, Lippincott, Williams & Wilkins, 2004; p 1073.

197. Tsui BC, Gupta S, Finucane B: Confirmation of epidural catheter placement using nerve stimulation. *Can J Anaesth* 45:640, 1998.

198. Tsui BC, Guenther C, Emery D, et al: Determining epidural catheter location using nerve stimulation with radiological confirmation. *Reg Anesth Pain Med* 25:306, 2000.

199. Bell K, Wattie M, Byth K, et al: Procalcitonin: a marker of bacteremia in SIRS. *Anaesth Intensive Care* 31:629, 2003.

200. Bu B, Pan J, Chen D, et al: Serum procalcitonin and interleukin-6 levels may help to differentiate systemic inflammatory response of infectious and non-infectious origin. *Chin Med J (Engl)* 116:538, 2003.

201. Luzzani A, Polati E, Dorizzi R, et al: Comparison of procalcitonin and C-reactive protein as markers of sepsis. *Crit Care Med* 31:1737, 2003.

202. Delevaux I, Andre M, Colombier M; et al: Can procalcitonin measurement help in differentiating between bacterial infection and other kinds of inflammatory processes? *Ann Rheum Dis* 62:337, 2003.

203. Fratacc MD: Diaphragmatic shortening after thoracic surgery in humans. Effects of mechanical ventilation and thoracic epidural anesthesia. *Anesthesiology* 79:654, 1993.

204. Ballantyne JC, Carr DB, deFerranti S, et al: The comparative effects of postoperative analgesic therapies on pulmonary outcome: cumulative meta-analyses of randomized, controlled trials. *Anesth Analg* 86:598, 1998.

205. Carpenter RL: Gastrointestinal benefits of regional anesthesia/analgesia. *Reg Anesth* 21:13, 1996.

206. Hosoda R, Hattori M, Shimada Y: Favorable effects of epidural analgesia on hemodynamics, oxygenation, and metabolic variables in the immediate post-anesthetic period. *Acta Anesthesiol Scand* 37:469, 1993.

207. Carli F, Webster J, Pearson M, et al: Protein metabolism after abdominal surgery: effects of 24-h extradural block with local anesthetic. *Br J Anaesth* 67:729, 1991.

208. Udelsman R: Endocrine and molecular responses to surgical stress. *Curr Probl Surg* 8:663, 1991.

209. Moller IW, Dinesen K, Sondergard S, et al: Effect of patient-controlled analgesia on plasma catecholamine, cortisol and glucose concentrations after cholecystectomy. *Br J Anaesth* 61:160, 1988.

210. Christopherson R, Beattie C, Frank SM, et al: The perioperative ischemia randomized anesthesia trial study group: perioperative morbidity in patients randomized to epidural or general anesthesia for lower extremity surgery. *Anesthesiology* 79:422, 1993.

211. Kehlet H: The surgical stress response: should it be prevented? *Can J Surg* 34:565, 1991.

212. Carli F, Phil M, Mayo N, et al: Epidural analgesia enhances functional exercise capacity and health-related quality of life after colonic surgery. *Anesthesiology* 97:540, 2002.

213. Riff JR, Jaromzik N, Myles PS: Epidural anesthesia and analgesia and outcome of major surgery: a randomized trial. *Lancet* 359:1276, 2002.

214. Jayr C, Mollie A, Bourgain JL, et al: Postoperative pulmonary complications: general anesthesia with postoperative parenteral morphine compared with epidural analgesia. *Surgery* 104:57, 1987.

215. Park WY, Thompson JS, Lee KK: Department of Veterans Affairs Cooperative Study #345 Study Group. Effect of epidural anesthesia and analgesia on perioperative outcome. A randomized controlled Veteran Affairs Cooperative Study. *Ann Surg* 234:560, 2001.

J. Matthias Walz
Raimis Matulionis
Khaldoun Faris

CHAPTER **24**

Therapeutic Paralysis

Despite the routine use of neuromuscular blocking agents (NMBA) in the intensive care unit (ICU), limited data are currently available to guide the clinician with respect to appropriate indications, choice of agents, and the depth of neuromuscular blockade necessary to achieve a desired therapeutic effect.

The most common indications for the use of NMBAs in the ICU include emergency or elective intubations, optimization of patient-ventilator synchrony, the management of increased intracranial pressure, reduction of oxygen consumption and the treatment of muscle spasms associated with tetanus. According to the American College of Critical Care Medicine and the Society of Critical Care Medicine clinical practice guidelines for sustained neuromuscular blockade in the adult critically ill patient, they should be used only when all other means of optimizing a patient's condition have been used. This recommendation is based on concern that the administration of NMBAs may worsen patient outcome when administered during a course of critical illness, particularly if the patient is receiving systemic steroids at the same time [1–4]. In a recent international multicenter trial, 13% of patients on mechanical ventilation received NMBAs for at least 1 day, which was associated with longer duration of mechanical ventilation, longer weaning time and stay in the ICU, and higher mortality [5].

In addition to the pharmacology of the most commonly administered agents, we will briefly review the biology of the neuromuscular junction (NMJ), its alterations during the course of critical illness, and the resulting implications for the use of depolarizing and nondepolarizing NMBAs. Recommendations for administration of NMBAs to ICU patients based on available evidence will be provided.

PHARMACOLOGY OF NMBAs

The NMJ consists of the motor nerve terminus, acetylcholine (ACh), and the muscle end-plate. In response to neuronal action potentials, ACh is released from presynaptic axonal storage vesicles into the synapse of the NMJ. Both the presynaptic membrane and postsynaptic end-plate contain specialized nicotinic ACh receptors (nAChRs). The chemical signal is converted into an electrical signal by binding of two ACh molecules to the receptor, causing a transient influx of sodium and calcium, and efflux of potassium from muscle cells. This depolarization propagates an action potential that results in a muscle contraction. Unbound ACh is quickly hydrolyzed in the synapse by the enzyme acetylcholinesterase to acetic acid and choline,

thus effectively controlling the duration of receptor activation. A repolarization of the motor end-plate and muscle fiber then occurs.

THE NICOTINIC ACETYLCHOLINE RECEPTOR

The nAChR is built of five subunit proteins forming an ion channel. This ionic channel mediates neurotransmission at the NMJ, autonomic ganglia, spinal cord, and the brain. During early development, differentiation and maturation of the NMJ and transformation of the nAChR takes place: Fetal nAChRs gradually disappear with a rise of new, functionally distinct, mature nAChRs.

These mature nAChRs (also termed *adult, innervated, ε-containing*) have a subunit composition of $\alpha 2\beta\epsilon\delta$ in the synaptic muscle membrane. The only structural difference from the fetal nAChR is in substitution of the γ for the ϵ subunit, although functional, pharmacologic, and metabolic characteristics are quite distinct. Mature nAChRs have a shorter burst duration and a higher conductance to Na+, K+, and Ca²+ and are metabolically stable with a half-life averaging about 2 weeks. The 2 α, β, δ, and ϵ/γ subunits interact to form a channel and an extracellular binding site for ACh and other mediators as well. As mentioned previously, simultaneous binding of two ACh molecules to $\alpha\delta$ and $\alpha\epsilon$ subunits of a nAChR initiates opening of the channel and a flow of cations down their electrochemical gradient. In the absence of ACh or other mediators, the stable closed state (a major function of ϵ and γ subunits) normally precludes channel opening [6].

Adult skeletal muscle retains the ability to synthesize not only adult, but also fetal (often called *immature* or *extrajunctional*) type nAChRs. The synthesis of fetal nAChRs might be triggered in response to altered neuronal input such as loss of nerve function or prolonged immobility, or in the presence of certain disease states. The major differences between fetal and adult type of nAChRs is that fetal receptors migrate across the entire membrane surface and adult ones are mostly confined to the muscle end-plate. Secondly, these fetal nAChRs have much shorter half-life and are more ionically active with prolonged open channel time that exaggerates the K+ efflux. Lastly, these receptors are much more sensitive to depolarizing agents such as succinylcholine and resistant to nondepolarizing neuromuscular blockers.

The functional difference between depolarizing and nondepolarizing neuromuscular blockers lies in their interaction with AChRs. Depolarizing neuromuscular blockers are structurally similar to ACh and bind to and activate AChRs. Nondepolarizing neuromuscular blockers are competitive antagonists. There is emerging evidence pointing to yet another variant nAChR subunit (α7 acetylcholine receptors [α7nAChRs]), recently described to be expressed in muscle also [7]. These receptors not only bind ACh and succinylcholine, but also agonists such as choline and nicotine, as well as antagonists such as pancuronium, cobra toxin, and α-bungarotoxin [8].

DEPOLARIZING NEUROMUSCULAR BLOCKERS

Succinylcholine is the only depolarizing neuromuscular blocker in clinical use. Its use is limited to facilitating rapid-sequence intubation in the emergency setting. Succinylcholine mimics the effects of ACh by binding to the ACh receptor and inducing a persistent depolarization of the muscle fiber. Muscle contraction remains inhibited until succinylcholine diffuses away from the motor end-plate and is metabolized by serum (pseudo-) cholinesterase [9]. The clinical effect of succinylcholine is a brief excitatory period, with muscular fasciculations followed by neuromuscular blockade and flaccid paralysis. The intravenous dose of succinylcholine is 1 to 1.5 mg per kg and offers the most rapid onset of action (60 to 90 seconds) of the NMBAs. Recovery to 90% muscle strength after an intravenous dose of 1 mg per kg takes from 9 to 13 minutes [10]. Succinylcholine is also suitable for intramuscular administration; however, there are several limitations. Firstly, the required dose is higher (4 mg per kg) and time to maximum twitch depression is significantly longer (approximately 4 minutes). Secondly, the duration of action of succinylcholine after intramuscular injection is prolonged. It should be noted that the most frequent indication for intramuscular succinylcholine is for the treatment of laryngospasm in pediatric patients without intravenous access; however, the dose range listed here has also been verified in the adult population [11,12].

Potential adverse drug events associated with succinylcholine include hypertension, arrhythmias, increased intracranial and intraocular pressure, hyperkalemia, malignant hyperthermia, myalgias, and prolonged paralysis [13]. Neuromuscular blockade can persist for hours in patients with genetic variants of pseudocholinesterase isoenzymes [14]. Contraindications to succinylcholine use include major thermal burns, significant crush injuries, spinal cord transection, malignant hyperthermia, and upper or lower motor neuron lesions. Caution is also advised in patients with open globe injuries, renal failure, serious infections, and near-drowning victims [15].

NONDEPOLARIZING NMBAs

Nondepolarizing NMBAs function as competitive antagonists and inhibit ACh binding to postsynaptic nAChRs on the motor end-plate. They are categorized on the basis of chemical structure into two classes: benzylisoquiniliniums and aminosteroids. Within each of these classes, the therapeutic agents may further be categorized as short-acting, intermediate-acting, or long-acting agents. The benzylisoquinolinium agents commonly used in the critical care setting include mivacurium, atracurium, cisatracurium, and doxacurium, whereas the aminosteroid agents include vecuronium, rocuronium, pancuronium, and pipecuronium.

The nondepolarizing NMBAs are administered by the intravenous route and have volumes of distribution (V_ds) ranging from 0.2 to 0.3 L per kg in adults.

A clinical relationship exists between the time to onset of paralysis and neuromuscular blocker dosing, drug distribution, and ACh-receptor sensitivity. An important factor to consider is V_d, which may change as a result of disease processes. Cirrhotic liver disease and chronic renal failure often result in an increased V_d and decreased plasma concentration for a given dose of water-soluble drugs. However, drugs dependent on renal or hepatic excretion may have prolonged clinical effect. Therefore, a larger initial dose but smaller maintenance dose may be appropriate.

Alterations in V_d affect both peak neuromuscular blocker serum concentrations and time to paralysis. The pharmacokinetic and pharmacodynamic principles of commonly used NMBAs are summarized in Table 24-1.

MIVACURIUM

Mivacurium is a short acting, nondepolarizing NMBA that is structurally related to atracurium. The time of onset is 2 to 4 minutes, with a clinical duration of 12 to 18 minutes. It is eliminated through hydrolysis by plasma cholinesterases and can be administered by bolus dose or continuous infusion [9,16].

ATRACURIUM

Atracurium is an intermediate-acting nondepolarizing agent. Neuromuscular paralysis typically occurs between 3 and 5 minutes and lasts for 25 to 35 minutes after an initial bolus dose. Atracurium undergoes ester hydrolysis as well as Hofmann degradation, a nonenzymatic breakdown process that occurs at physiologic pH and body temperature, independent of renal or hepatic function [17]. Renal and hepatic dysfunction should not affect the duration of neuromuscular paralysis. The neuroexcitatory metabolite laudanosine is renally excreted. Laudanosine is epileptogenic in animals and may induce CNS excitation in patients with renal failure who are receiving prolonged atracurium infusions. Atracurium may induce histamine release after rapid administration.

CISATRACURIUM

Cisatracurium and atracurium are similar intermediate-acting nondepolarizing agents. A bolus dose of 0.2 mg per kg of cisatracurium usually results in neuromuscular paralysis within 1.5 to 2.5 minutes and lasts 45 to 60 minutes. When compared with atracurium, cisatracurium is 3 times as potent and has a more desirable adverse drug event profile, including lack of histamine release, minimal cardiovascular effects, and less interaction with autonomic ganglia. Cisatracurium also undergoes ester hydrolysis as well as Hofmann degradation. However, plasma laudanosine concentrations after cisatracurium administration

TABLE 24-1.   Pharmacokinetic and Pharmacodynamic Principles of Nondepolarizing Neuromuscular Blockers[a]

	Benzylisoquinolinium Agents		
	Cisatracurium (Nimbex)	Atracurium (Tracrium)	Doxacurium (Nuromax)
Introduced	1996	1983	1991
95% Effective dose (mg/kg)	0.05	0.25	0.025–0.030
Initial dose (mg/kg)	0.1–0.2	0.4–0.5	Up to 0.1
Onset (min)	2–3	3–5	5–10
Duration (min)	45–60	25–35	120–150
Half-life (min)	22–31	20	70–100
Infusion dose (μg/kg/min)	2.5–3.0	4–12	0.3–0.5
Recovery (min)	90	40–60	120–180
% Renal excretion	Hofmann elimination	5–10 (Hofmann elimination)	70
Renal failure	No change	No change	↑ Effect
% Biliary excretion	Hofmann elimination	Minimal	Unclear
Hepatic failure	Minimal to no change	Minimal to no change	?
Active metabolites	None but laudanosine	None but laudanosine	?
Histamine hypotension	No	Dose-dependent	No
Vagal block tachycardia	No	No	No
Ganglionic block hypotension	No	Minimal to none	No
Prolonged block reported	Rare	Rare	Yes

	Aminosteroidal Agents			
	Pancuronium (Pavulon)	Vecuronium (Norcuron)	Pipecuronium (Arduan)	Rocuronium (Zemuron)
Introduced	1972	1984	1991	1994
95% Effective dose (mg/kg)	0.07	0.05	0.05	0.30
Initial dose (mg/kg)	0.1	0.1	0.085–0.100	0.6–1.0
Onset (min)	2–3	3–4	5	1–2
Duration (min)	90–100	35–45	90–100	30
Half-life (min)	120	30–80	100	—
Infusion dose (μg/kg/min)	1–2	1–2	0.5–2.0	10–12
Recovery (min)	120–180	45–60	55–160	20–30
% Renal excretion	45–70	50	50+	33
Renal failure	↑ Effect	↑ Effect	↑ Duration	Minimal
% Biliary excretion	10–15	35–50	Minimal	<75
Hepatic failure	Mild ↑ effect	Mild ↑ effect	Minimal	Moderate
Active metabolites	3-OH and 17-OH pancuronium	3-desacetylvecuronium	None	None
Histamine hypotension	No	No	No	No
Vagal block tachycardia	Modest to marked	No	No	At high doses
Ganglionic block hypotension	No	No	No	No
Prolonged ICU block	Yes	Yes	No	No

↑, increased; ICU, intensive care unit.
[a]Modified from Grenvik A, Ayres SM, Holbrook PR, et al: *Textbook of Critical Care.* 4th ed. Philadelphia, WB Saunders, 2000; and Watling SM, Dasta JF: Prolonged paralysis in intensive care unit patients after the use of neuromuscular blocking agents: a review of the literature. *Crit Care Med* 22(5):884, 1994.

are 5 to 10 times lower than those detected after administration of atracurium [18,19].

ROCURONIUM

Rocuronium is the fastest onset, shortest-acting aminosteroidal NMBA. A bolus dose of 0.6 mg per kg usually results in neuromuscular paralysis within 60 to 90 seconds. It may be considered an alternative to succinylcholine for rapid-sequence intubation (0.8 to 1.2 mg per kg), although, even with large doses, the onset of action is slower as compared to succinylcholine [20]. Rocuronium is primarily eliminated in the liver and bile. Hepatic or renal dysfunction may reduce drug clearance and prolong recovery time.

VECURONIUM

An initial intravenous bolus dose of 0.1 mg per kg of vecuronium typically results in neuromuscular paralysis within 3 to 4 minutes and lasts 35 to 45 minutes. Vecuronium lacks vagal effects such as tachycardia and hypertension and produces negligible histamine release. Hepatic metabolism produces three active metabolites, the most significant being 3-desacetylvecuronium, with 50% to 70% the activity of the parent drug. Both vecuronium and its active metabolites are renally excreted. There is the potential for prolonged neuromuscular paralysis in patients with renal dysfunction receiving vecuronium by continuous infusion [21].

PANCURONIUM

Pancuronium is a long-acting nondepolarizing agent that is structurally similar to vecuronium. Unique features of pancuronium are its vagolytic and sympathomimetic activities and potential to induce tachycardia, hypertension, and increased cardiac output. Pancuronium is primarily excreted unchanged (60% to 70%) in the urine and bile, whereas the remaining 30% to 40% is hydroxylated by the liver to 3-hydroxypancuronium. It has 50% the activity of the parent drug and is renally eliminated. Renal dysfunction may result in the accumulation of pancuronium and its metabolites [22].

DOXACURIUM

Doxacurium is the most potent nondepolarizing agent available, but it has the slowest onset (as long as 10 minutes). Doxacurium is practically devoid of histaminergic, vagolytic, or sympathomimetic effects. Doxacurium undergoes minimal hepatic metabolism, and excretion occurs unchanged in both the urine and bile, with significantly prolonged effects seen in patients with renal dysfunction and, to a lesser extent, hepatic disease [23,24].

PIPECURONIUM

Pipecuronium is structurally related to pancuronium and its duration of action is 90 to 100 minutes, making it the longest-acting NMBA. Pipecuronium is metabolized to 3-desacetylpipecuronium by the liver, and both the parent compound and metabolite are renally excreted. When compared with pancuronium, pipecuronium has a longer duration of action, less histamine release, and minimal cardiovascular effects [25].

REVERSAL AGENTS

The clinical effects of nondepolarizing neuromuscular blockers can be reversed by acetylcholinesterase inhibitors (anticholinesterases). These agents increase the synaptic concentration of ACh by preventing its synaptic degradation and allow it to competitively displace nondepolarizing MBAs from postsynaptic nAChRs on the motor end-plate. Because anticholinesterase drugs (e.g., neostigmine, edrophonium, pyridostigmine) also inhibit acetylcholinesterase at muscarinic receptor sites, they are used in combination with the antimuscarinic agents (e.g., atropine or glycopyrrolate) to minimize adverse muscarinic effects (e.g., bradycardia, excessive secretions, and bronchospasm) while maximizing nicotinic effects. Typical combinations include neostigmine and glycopyrrolate (slower-acting agents) and edrophonium and atropine (faster-acting agents). The depth of neuromuscular blockade determines how rapidly neuromuscular activity returns [26].

DRUG INTERACTIONS

A substantial number of medications commonly used in clinical practice have the potential for interaction with NMBAs. These interactions typically influence the degree and duration of clinical effects through either potentiation of or resistance to neuromuscular blockade. The most clinically relevant drug interactions with NMBA are discussed here and summarized in Table 24-2.

Aminoglycosides and other antibiotics (e.g., tetracyclines, clindamycin, vancomycin) have the ability to potentiate neuromuscular blockade and prolong the action of nondepolarizing agents through mechanisms including the inhibition of presynaptic ACh release, reduction of postsynaptic receptor sensitivity to ACh, blockade of cholinergic receptors, and impairment of ion channels. Penicillin and cephalosporin antibiotics do not interact with NMBAs and thus do not influence the degree of neuromuscular blockade.

Local, inhalational, and intravenous anesthetic and sedative agents may potentiate neuromuscular blockade. Local anesthetics reduce ACh release and decrease muscle contractions through direct membrane effects, whereas inhalational anesthetics desensitize the postsynaptic membrane and also depress muscle contractility.

Cardiovascular drugs such as furosemide, procainamide, quinidine, beta-blockers, and calcium channel blockers have the ability to potentiate neuromuscular blocking effects. The role of the calcium ion in the release of ACh from vesicles into

TABLE 24-2.   Drug Interactions with Neuromuscular Blocking Agents[a]

Therapeutic Agent	Potential Interaction
Antibiotics	
Aminoglycosides	Potentiate blockade; decreased acetylcholine release
Tetracyclines	Potentiate blockade
Clindamycin, lincomycin	Potentiate blockade
Vancomycin	Potentiate blockade
Sedative/anesthetics	Potentiate blockade
Cardiovascular agents	
Furosemide	Low doses: Potentiate blockade; high doses: Antagonize blockade
Beta-blockers	Potentiate blockade
Procainamide	Potentiate blockade
Quinidine	Potentiate blockade
Calcium channel blockers	Potentiate blockade
Methylxanthines	Antagonize blockade
Antiepileptic drugs	
Phenytoin	Acute: Potentiate blockade; chronic: Resistance to blockade
Carbamazepine	Resistance to blockade
Ranitidine	Antagonize blockade
Lithium	Potentiate blockade
Immunosuppressive agents	
Azathioprine	Mild antagonism; phosphodiesterase inhibition
Cyclosporin	Potentiate blockade
Corticosteroids	Potentiate steroid myopathy
Local anesthetics	Potentiate blockade

[a]Adapted from Buck ML, Reed MD: Use of nondepolarizing neuromuscular blocking agents in mechanically ventilated patients. *Clin Pharm* 10(1):32, 1991.

the synapse has been well established, although the exact interaction between calcium channel blockers and NMBAs remains to be determined. Verapamil, a calcium channel blocker, has local analgesic effects and direct skeletal muscle effects, but its significance in drug interaction with NMBAs remains to be defined.

Chronic antiepileptic therapy, specifically phenytoin and carbamazepine, can increase the resistance to neuromuscular blocking effects, whereas the acute administration of phenytoin potentiates neuromuscular blockade. Chronic phenytoin therapy appears to induce an upregulation of ACh receptors, resulting in increased postsynaptic sensitivity. Carbamazepine has been shown to induce resistance and shorten recovery times in combination with both pancuronium and vecuronium, possibly resulting from competition at the NMJ [9,27].

MONOTORING OF NMBAs

Current guidelines recommend the routine monitoring of depth of neuromuscular blockade in critically ill patients [1]. It is important to remember that NMBAs have no analgesic and sedative effect. Careful clinical monitoring of the patient for signs consistent with inadequate sedation—such as tachycardia, hypertension, salivation. and lacrimation—while receiving NMBAs is important. A recommendation to use monitors such as the Bispectral Index or the Patient State Index to ensure adequate depth of sedation while receiving MBAs seems plausible; however, more studies are needed to determine whether these monitors are reliable and cost-effective in the critical care setting, and whether they contribute to improved outcomes [28–30]. The modality of choice to monitor the depth of nondepolarizing neuromuscular blockade at present is train-of-four (TOF) monitoring. To determine the depth of blockade, four supramaximal stimuli are applied to a peripheral nerve (ideally, the ulnar nerve to assess an evoked response of the adductor pollicis muscle) every 0.5 seconds (2 Hz). Each stimulus in the train causes the muscle to contract, and "fade" in the response provides the basis for evaluation. To obtain the TOF ratio, the amplitude of the fourth response is divided by the amplitude of the first response. Before administration of a nondepolarizing muscle relaxant, all four responses are ideally the same: The TOF ratio is 1 to 1. During a partial nondepolarizing block, the ratio decreases (fades) and is inversely proportional to the degree of blockade [31].

Three prospective clinical trials have examined the question whether the routine use of TOF monitoring in the ICU will increase cost-effectiveness and decrease the incidence of prolonged neuromuscular weakness. TOF monitoring for vecuronium appears to improve outcome and decrease the cost of therapy. However, these outcomes could not be demonstrated for the benzylisoquinolinium agents, atracurium, and cisatracurium [32–34].

ADVERSE EFFECTS OF DEPOLARIZING AND NONDEPOLARIZING NMBAs IN CRITICALLY ILL PATIENTS

Significant progress has been made in the recent past in our understanding of the changes in regulation and distribution of ACh receptors during a course of critical illness. The majority of patients hospitalized in an ICU will undergo postsynaptic upreg-

ulation of nAChRs due to immobility, upper and/or lower motor neuron lesions, and/or pharmacologic denervation (such as NMBAs, aminoglycoside antibiotics). As previously outlined, immature receptors are not confined to the NMJ proper, but can be found over the entire surface of skeletal muscle (Fig. 24-1). This will lead to increased sensitivity to depolarizing NMBAs and decreased sensitivity to nondepolarizing NMBAs. Furthermore, these changes in receptor distribution and physiology put the patient at a heightened risk for succinylcholine-induced hyperkalemia. This is based on the fact that immature (fetal) and $\alpha 7nAChRs$ are low conductance channels with prolonged opening times and significantly higher potassium efflux into the systemic circulation as compared to mature (adult) nAChRs. Furthermore, succinylcholine is metabolized more slowly as compared to ACh, thus prolonging the "open" state of the immature receptors. Upregulation of receptors during periods of immobilization have been described as early as 6 to 12 hours into the disease process. Therefore, it seems advisable to avoid succinylcholine in critically ill patients beyond 48 to 72 hours of immobilization and/or denervation. In contrast, a reduction in the number of postsynaptic nAChRs will result in resistance to depolarizing and increased sensitivity to nondepolarizing NMBAs. For conditions associated with the potential for ACh receptor upregulation see Table 24-3.

ACQUIRED NEUROMUSCULAR DISORDERS OF CRITICAL ILLNESS

Two distinct neuromuscular disease entities have been described in the recent past, critical illness polyneuropathy (CIP) and critical illness myopathy (CIM). These conditions occur in up to 50% to 70% of patients meeting diagnostic criteria for the systemic inflammatory response syndrome as well as in patients immobilized and on mechanical ventilation for more than a week [35]. They manifest as limb weakness and difficulty in weaning from the mechanical ventilator. Nondepolarizing muscle relaxants of both classes, aminosteroids and benzylisoquiniliniums, have been associated with the development of these neuromuscular disorders [36–39]; however, the etiology appears to be multifactorial and includes alterations in microvascular blood flow in conditions of sepsis/systemic inflammatory response syndrome, and the concomitant administration of corticosteroids [35]. There is evidence suggesting that high-dose corticosteroids have direct physiologic effects on muscle fibers, resulting in a typical myopathy with loss of thick-filament proteins. Atrophy and weakness are observed primarily in muscles of trunk and extremities, and functional denervation of muscle with NMBAs in conjunction with corticosteroid therapy seems to heighten the risk of myopathy [38,40]. Furthermore, methylprednisolone and hydrocortisone both antagonize nAChRs, possibly potentiating the effects of NMBAs [41]. A differential diagnosis of weakness in ICU patients is presented in Table 24-4.

CRITICAL ILLNESS POLYNEUROPATHY

Electrophysiologic findings of CIP are consistent with a primary, axonal degeneration, resulting in reduction in amplitudes of the compound muscle action potential and sensory nerve action potential. Although several case reports have suggested that NMBAs are causative agents in the etiology of this disorder [37,42–45], prospective studies of CIP have not confirmed a

FIGURE 24-1. Schematic of the succinylcholine (SCh)-induced potassium release in an innervated (*top*) and denervated (*bottom*) muscle. In the innervated muscle, the systemically administered succinylcholine reaches all of the muscle membrane but depolarizes only the junctional ($\alpha1$, $\beta1$, δ, ε) receptors because acetylcholine receptors (AChRs) are located only in this area. With denervation, the muscle (nuclei) expresses not only extrajunctional ($\alpha1$, $\beta1$, δ, γ) AChRs but also $\alpha7$AChRs throughout the muscle membrane. Systemic succinylcholine, in contrast to acetylcholine released locally, can depolarize all of the upregulated AChRs, leading to massive efflux of intracellular potassium into the circulation, resulting in hyperkalemia. The metabolite of succinylcholine, choline, and possibly succinylmonocholine can maintain this depolarization via $\alpha7$AChRs, enhancing the potassium release and maintaining the hyperkalemia. [From Martyn JA, Richtsfeld M: Succinylcholine-induced hyperkalemia in acquired pathologic states: etiologic factors and molecular mechanisms. *Anesthesiology* 104:158, 2006, with permission.]

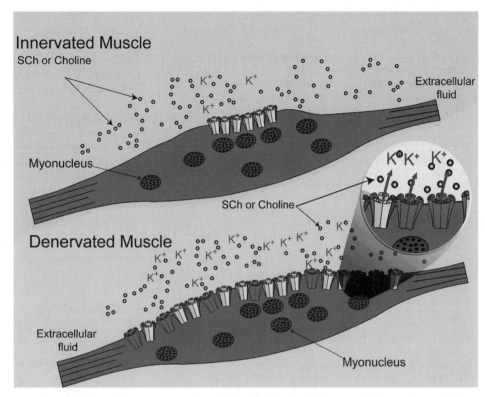

correlation between the use of NMBAs, steroids, and CIP [46,47]. It seems plausible, however, that NMBAs contribute to nerve and muscle damage during a course of critical illness. Their use should be avoided whenever possible until more prospective data demonstrating their safety in critically ill patients are available [46,48].

CRITICAL ILLNESS MYOPATHY

CIM can occur in association with, or independently from, CIP. A group of several myopathies of critical illness are now thought to be part of the same syndrome; those include acute quadriplegic myopathy, critical care myopathy, acute corticosteroid myopathy, acute hydrocortisone myopathy, acute myopathy in severe asthma, and acute corticosteroid and pancuronium-associated myopathy [49]. The major feature of this syndrome is flaccid, diffuse weakness involving all limb muscles and the neck flexors, and often the facial muscles and the diaphragm. As with CIP, this can result in difficulty to wean from the mechanical ventilator. The syndrome is more difficult to diagnose than CIP, and

TABLE 24-3. Conditions Associated with the Potential for Nicotinic Acetylcholine Receptor Upregulation

Severe infection/SIRS

Muscle atrophy associated with prolonged immobility

Thermal injury

Upper and/or lower motor neuron defect

Prolonged pharmacologic or chemical denervation (e.g., NMBAs, magnesium, aminoglycoside antibiotics, clostridial toxins)

NMBAs, neuromuscular blocking agents; SIRS, systemic inflammatory response syndrome.

diagnostic evaluations include electrophysiologic studies and muscle biopsy and laboratory evaluations (plasma creatine kinase levels). Again, there is no definitive evidence suggesting that NMBAs are causative agents for this syndrome, but rather a component in a multifactorial etiology. However, the incidence of CIP and CIM appears to be higher in ICUs where these agents are more frequently used [50,51].

TABLE 24-4. Weakness in Intensive Care Unit Patients: Etiologies and Syndromes[a]

Prolonged recovery from neuromuscular blocking agents (secondary to parent drug, drug metabolite, or drug-drug interaction)

Myasthenia gravis

Eaton-Lambert syndrome

Muscular dystrophy

Guillain-Barré syndrome

Central nervous system injury or lesion

Spinal cord injury

Steroid myopathy

Mitochondrial myopathy

Human immunodeficiency virus-related myopathy

Critical illness myopathy

Disuse atrophy

Critical illness polyneuropathy

Severe electrolyte toxicity (e.g., hypermagnesemia)

Severe electrolyte deficiency (e.g., hypophosphatemia)

[a]Adapted from Murray MJ, Cowen J, DeBlock H, et al: Clinical practice guidelines for sustained neuromuscular blockade in the adult critically ill patient. *Crit Care Med* 30(1):142, 2002, with permission.

TABLE 24-5. Recommendations for Administration of Neuromuscular Blocking Agents (NMBAs) to ICU Patients[a]

1. Develop, use, and document a standardized approach for administering and monitoring NMBA.
2. Use NMBA only after optimizing ventilator settings and sedative and analgesic medication administration.
3. Establish the indications and clinical goals of neuromuscular blockade, and evaluate at least daily.
4. Select the best NMBA based on patient characteristics:
   A. Use intermittent NMBA therapy with pancuronium, doxacurium, or other suitable agent if clinical goals can be met.
   B. If continuous infusion is required and renal or hepatic dysfunction is present, select atracurium or cisatracurium, and avoid vecuronium.
5. Use the lowest effective dose for the shortest possible time (<48 h if possible), particularly if corticosteroids are concomitantly administered.
6. Administer adequate analgesic and/or sedative medication during neuromuscular blockade, and monitor clinically and by bispectral array EEG if available.
7. Systematically anticipate and prevent complications, including provision of eye care, careful positioning, physical therapy, and DVT prophylaxis.
8. Avoid the use of medications that affect NMBA actions. Promptly recognize and manage conditions that affect NMBA actions.
9. Adjust NMBA dosage to achieve clinical goals (i.e., patient-ventilator synchrony, apnea, or complete paralysis).
10. Periodically (i.e., at least once or twice daily) perform NMBA dosage reduction, and preferably cessation (drug holiday) if clinically tolerated, to determine whether neuromuscular blockade is still needed, and to perform physical and neurologic examination.
11. Periodically perform and document a clinical assessment in which spontaneous respiration as well as limb movement and/or the presence of DTRs are observed during steady-state infusion and/or during dosage reduction/cessation. With deep blockade, muscle activity may be present only during dosage reduction/cessation.
12. Perform and document scheduled (i.e., every 4–8 h) TOF testing for patients receiving vecuronium NMBA and/or undergoing deep neuromuscular blockade (i.e., apnea or complete paralysis), and adjust dosage to achieve one-fourth or more twitches. If clinical goals cannot be met when one-fourth or more twitches are present during steady-state infusion, demonstrate one-fourth or more twitches during dosage reduction/cessation. Consider TOF testing in all patients

DTR, deep tendon reflexes; DVT, deep venous thrombosis; EEG, electroencephalogram; TOF, train of four.
[a]Modified from Gehr LC, Sessler CN: Neuromuscular blockade in the intensive care unit. *Semin Respir Crit Care Med* 22:175, 2001, with permission.

The question whether CIP and CIM increase hospital mortality was recently addressed by Latronico et al. [52]. Although only limited data are available suggesting that CIP increases ICU and hospital mortality in critically ill patients, CIP and CIM appear to be important causes of increased morbidity during and after acute care hospital stay [52].

SUMMARY AND RECOMMENDATIONS

Although there is currently insufficient evidence to demonstrate an unequivocal link between the use of NMBAs and an increase in morbidity and mortality in critically ill patients, it seems pru-

dent to perform a careful risk-benefit analysis prior to the administration of this class of drugs in the ICU setting. More prospective data are needed to identify proper indications, selection of agents, and doses in the ICU setting. Concomitant use of drugs predisposing patients for the development of CIM-like steroids and aminoglycoside antibiotics should alert the clinician for the increased risk of CIP/CIM in this setting. Succinylcholine can subject patients who are immobilized with upper and lower motor neuron lesions or with burns to a markedly increased risk for succinylcholine-induced hyperkalemia, and should be avoided in the ICU whenever possible. For recommendations for the administration of NMBAs to ICU patients, please see Table 24-5.

Acknowledgements

We would like to thank Drs. Jerry D. Thomas and Greg A. Bauer for their significant contributions to previous revisions of this chapter.

REFERENCES

1. Murray MJ, Cowen J, DeBlock H, et al: Clinical practice guidelines for sustained neuromuscular blockade in the adult critically ill patient. *Crit Care Med* 30:142, 2002.
2. Rudis MI, Guslits BJ, Peterson EL, et al: Economic impact of prolonged motor weakness complicating neuromuscular blockade in the intensive care unit. *Crit Care Med* 24:1749, 1996.
3. Leatherman JW, Fluegel WL, David WS, et al: Muscle weakness in mechanically ventilated patients with severe asthma. *Am J Respir Crit Care Med* 153:1686, 1996.
4. Watling SM, Dasta JF: Prolonged paralysis in intensive care unit patients after the use of neuromuscular blocking agents: a review of the literature. *Crit Care Med* 22:884, 1994.
5. Arroliga A, Frutos-Vivar F, Hall J, et al: Use of sedatives and neuromuscular blockers in a cohort of patients receiving mechanical ventilation. *Chest* 128:496, 2005.
6. Naguib M, Flood P, McArdle JJ, et al: Advances in neurobiology of the neuromuscular junction: implications for the anesthesiologist. *Anesthesiology* 96:202, 2002.
7. Fischer U, Reinhardt S, Albuquerque EX, et al: Expression of functional alpha7 nicotinic acetylcholine receptor during mammalian muscle development and denervation. *Eur J Neurosci* 11:2856, 1999.
8. Tsuneki H, Salas R, Dani JA: Mouse muscle denervation increases expression of an alpha7 nicotinic receptor with unusual pharmacology. *J Physiol* 547:169, 2003.
9. Taylor P. *Agents Acting at the Neuromuscular Junction and Autonomic Ganglia.* 10th ed. New York, McGraw Hill, 2001.
10. Viby-Mogensen J: Correlation of succinylcholine duration of action with plasma cholinesterase activity in subjects with the genotypically normal enzyme. *Anesthesiology* 53:517, 1980.
11. Schuh FT: The neuromuscular blocking action of suxamethonium following intravenous and intramuscular administration. *Int J Clin Pharmacol Ther Toxicol* 20:399, 1982.
12. Sutherland GA, Bevan JC, Bevan DR: Neuromuscular blockade in infants following intramuscular succinylcholine in two or five per cent concentration. *Can Anaesth Soc J* 30:342, 1983.
13. Durant NN, Katz RL: Suxamethonium. *Br J Anaesth* 54:195, 1982.
14. Pantuck EJ: Plasma cholinesterase: gene and variations. *Anesth Analg* 77:380, 1993.
15. Wadbrook PS: Advances in airway pharmacology. Emerging trends and evolving controversy. *Emerg Med Clin North Am* 18:767, 2000.
16. Frampton JE, McTavish D: Mivacurium. A review of its pharmacology and therapeutic potential in general anaesthesia. *Drugs* 45:1066, 1993.
17. Fisher DM, Canfell PC, Fahey MR, et al: Elimination of atracurium in humans: contribution of Hofmann elimination and ester hydrolysis versus organ-based elimination. *Anesthesiology* 65:6, 1986.
18. Eastwood NB, Boyd AH, Parker CJ, et al: Pharmacokinetics of 1R-cis 1'R-cis atracurium besylate (51W89) and plasma laudanosine concentrations in health and chronic renal failure. *Br J Anaesth* 75:431, 1995.
19. Newman PJ, Quinn AC, Grounds RM, et al: A comparison of cisatracurium (51W89) and atracurium by infusion in critically ill patients. *Crit Care Med* 25:1139, 1997.
20. Wright PM, Caldwell JE, Miller RD: Onset and duration of rocuronium and succinylcholine at the adductor pollicis and laryngeal adductor muscles in anesthetized humans. *Anesthesiology* 81:1110, 1994.
21. Conway EE Jr: Persistent paralysis after vecuronium administration. *N Engl J Med* 327:1882, 1992.
22. Reeves ST, Turcasso NM. Nondepolarizing neuromuscular blocking drugs in the intensive care unit: a clinical review. *South Med J* 90:769, 1997.
23. Basta SJ, Savarese JJ, Ali HH, et al: Clinical pharmacology of doxacurium chloride. A new long-acting nondepolarizing muscle relaxant. *Anesthesiology* 69:478, 1988.
24. Fisher DM, Reynolds KS, Schmith VD, et al: The influence of renal function on the pharmacokinetics and pharmacodynamics and simulated time course of doxacurium. *Anesth Analg* 89:786, 1999.

25. Atherton DP, Hunter JM: Clinical pharmacokinetics of the newer neuromuscular blocking drugs. *Clin Pharmacokinet* 36:169, 1999.

26. McManus MC: Neuromuscular blockers in surgery and intensive care, Part 2. *Am J Health Syst Pharm* 58:2381, 2001.

27. Booij LH: Neuromuscular transmission and its pharmacological blockade. Part 2: Pharmacology of neuromuscular blocking agents. *Pharm World Sci* 19:13, 1997.

28. Nasraway SS Jr., Wu EC, Kelleher RM, et al. How reliable is the Bispectral Index in critically ill patients? A prospective, comparative, single-blinded observer study. *Crit Care Med* 30:1483, 2002.

29. Schneider G, Heglmeier S, Schneider J, et al: Patient State Index (PSI) measures depth of sedation in intensive care patients. *Intensive Care Med* 30:213, 2004.

30. Vivien B, Di Maria S, Ouattara A, et al: Overestimation of Bispectral Index in sedated intensive care unit patients revealed by administration of muscle relaxant. *Anesthesiology* 99:9, 2003.

31. Naguib M, Lien CA: Pharmacology of muscle relaxants and their antagonists, in *Miller's Anesthesia.* 6th ed. New York, Churchill Livingstone, 2005.

32. Baumann MH, McAlpin BW, Brown K, et al: A prospective randomized comparison of train-of-four monitoring and clinical assessment during continuous ICU cisatracurium paralysis. *Chest* 126:1267, 2004.

33. Rudis MI, Sikora CA, Angus E, et al: A prospective, randomized, controlled evaluation of peripheral nerve stimulation versus standard clinical dosing of neuromuscular blocking agents in critically ill patients. *Crit Care Med* 25:575, 1997.

34. Strange C, Vaughan L, Franklin C, et al: Comparison of train-of-four and best clinical assessment during continuous paralysis. *Am J Respir Crit Care Med* 156:1556, 1997.

35. Bolton CF: Neuromuscular manifestations of critical illness. *Muscle Nerve* 32:140, 2005.

36. Davis NA, Rodgers JE, Gonzalez ER, et al: Prolonged weakness after cisatracurium infusion: a case report. *Crit Care Med* 26:1290, 1998.

37. Giostra E, Magistris MR, Pizzolato G, et al: Neuromuscular disorder in intensive care unit patients treated with pancuronium bromide. Occurrence in a cluster group of seven patients and two sporadic cases, with electrophysiologic and histologic examination. *Chest* 106:210, 1994.

38. Larsson L, Li X, Edstrom L, et al: Acute quadriplegia and loss of muscle myosin in patients treated with nondepolarizing neuromuscular blocking agents and corticosteroids: mechanisms at the cellular and molecular levels. *Crit Care Med* 28:34, 2000.

39. Marik PE: Doxacurium-corticosteroid acute myopathy: another piece to the puzzle. *Crit Care Med* 24:1266, 1996.

40. Behbehani NA, Al-Mane F, D'Yachkova Y, et al: Myopathy following mechanical ventilation for acute severe asthma: the role of muscle relaxants and corticosteroids. *Chest* 115:1627, 1999.

41. Kindler CH, Verotta D, Gray AT, et al: Additive inhibition of nicotinic acetylcholine receptors by corticosteroids and the neuromuscular blocking drug vecuronium. *Anesthesiology* 92:821, 2000.

42. Faragher MW, Day BJ, Dennett X: Critical care myopathy: an electrophysiological and histological study. *Muscle Nerve* 19:516, 1996.

43. Gooch JL, Suchyta MR, Balbierz JM, et al: Prolonged paralysis after treatment with neuromuscular junction blocking agents. *Crit Care Med* 19:1125, 1991.

44. Hirano M, Ott BR, Raps EC, et al: Acute quadriplegic myopathy: a complication of treatment with steroids, nondepolarizing blocking agents, or both. *Neurology* 42:2082, 1992.

45. Rossiter A, Souney PF, McGowan S, et al: Pancuronium-induced prolonged neuromuscular blockade. *Crit Care Med* 19:1583, 1991.

46. Berek K, Margreiter J, Willeit J, et al: Polyneuropathies in critically ill patients: a prospective evaluation. *Intensive Care Med* 22:849, 1996.

47. Leijten FS, de Weerd AW: Critical illness polyneuropathy. A review of the literature, definition and pathophysiology. *Clin Neurol Neurosurg* 96:10, 1994.

48. Latronico N, Fenzi F, Recupero D, et al: Critical illness myopathy and neuropathy. *Lancet* 347:1579, 1996.

49. Lacomis D, Zochodne DW, Bird SJ: Critical illness myopathy. *Muscle Nerve* 23:1785, 2000.

50. Lacomis D, Petrella JT, Giuliani MJ: Causes of neuromuscular weakness in the intensive care unit: a study of ninety-two patients. *Muscle Nerve* 21:610, 1998.

51. Zifko UA, Zipko HT, Bolton CF: Clinical and electrophysiological findings in critical illness polyneuropathy. *J Neurol Sci* 159:186, 1998.

52. Latronico N, Shehu I, Seghelini E: Neuromuscular sequelae of critical illness. *Curr Opin Crit Care* 11:381, 2005.

Arif Showkat
Sergio R. Acchiardo
William F. Owen, Jr.

CHAPTER **25**

Dialysis Therapy in the Intensive Care Setting

OVERVIEW OF DIALYSIS MODALITIES

Bones can break, muscles can atrophy, glands can loaf, even the brains can go to sleep, without immediately endangering our survival; but should the kidneys fail neither bone, muscle, gland, nor brain could carry on.

Homer W. Smith (1895–1962)

In 1839, Addison [1] reported that stupor, coma, and convulsions were consequences of diseased kidneys, which was referred to as Bright's disease for much of that century [2]. Almost 50 years later, Tyson [3] noted that uremic symptoms depend on retention of urea and allied substances in the blood, which, when they have accumulated to a sufficient quantity, act on the nervous system producing delirium and convulsions or coma.

These rudimentary observations relevant to the pathobiology of symptomatic renal failure suggested that therapy should be directed at mitigating the retention of nitrogenous products of metabolism. In September 1945, Kolff [4] dialyzed a 67-year-old woman with acute oliguric renal failure. Although this was a successful effort, dialysis remained an experimental tool until Teschan [5] described its use in treating Korean War casualties with posttraumatic renal failure in 1955. In 1960, Scribner et al. [6] devised an exteriorized arteriovenous access for long-term hemodialysis and initiated a 39-year-old man with end-stage renal disease (ESRD) on regular dialysis treatments. By the mid-1960s, hemodialysis was becoming conventional therapy for acute renal failure (ARF) and its application was expanding to patients with ESRD.

Conceptually, peritoneal dialysis is an older technique than hemodialysis, but its practical application was delayed by numerous unsuccessful attempts to treat both acute and end-stage renal disease patients [7]. Results were poor because of technical problems with catheters, peritonitis, and dialysate fluid composition. The subsequent development of commercially prepared dialysate and the introduction of the silicon-cuffed catheter by Tenckhoff and Schechter [8] in 1968 heralded the modern era of peritoneal dialysis. Despite those improvements, peritoneal dialysis was still a somewhat unsatisfactory technique until 1976, when Popovich et al. [9] advocated "portable equilibration" from which continuous ambulatory peritoneal dialysis is modeled.

Because ARF is potentially reversible, an aggressive pursuit should be undertaken to identify and correct the cause. Within the intensive care unit (ICU) setting, although elements of chronicity may or may not be present, most cases of renal failure that require dialytic support are acute in nature. Therefore, most of the subsequent discussion focuses on patients with ARF as well as those with advanced chronic renal failure within the ICU. Unless specifically noted, all subsequent discussions are applicable to both.

Dialysis fulfills two biophysical goals: the addition or removal ("clearance") of solute and the elimination of excess fluid from the patient ("ultrafiltration"). These two processes can be performed simultaneously or at different times. The dialysis procedures in common use are hemodialysis, hemofiltration, a combination of these, and peritoneal dialysis (Table 25-1).

HEMODIALYSIS

Hemodialysis is a diffusion-driven, size-discriminatory process for the clearance of relatively small solutes such as electrolytes and urea [less than 300 daltons (Da)]. Larger solutes are typically cleared far less readily. During hemodialysis, ultrafiltration is engendered by the generation of negative hydraulic pressure on the dialysate side of the dialyzer. The major components of the hemodialysis system are the artificial kidney or dialyzer; the respective mechanical devices that pump the patient's blood and the dialysate through the dialyzer; and the dialysate, which is a fluid having a specified chemical composition used for solute clearance. During the performance of "conventional" intermittent hemodialysis, the patient's blood and dialysate are pumped continuously through the dialyzer in opposite (countercurrent) directions at flow rates averaging 300 and 500 mL per minute, respectively. The dialysate passes through the dialyzer only once (single-pass system) and is discarded after interaction with the blood across the semipermeable membrane of the dialyzer. The efficiency of hemodialysis can be augmented by the use of dialyzers that are more porous to water and solutes. Those kidneys with enhanced performance characteristics are described as high-efficiency or high-flux dialyzers, depending on their ultrafiltration capacity and ability to remove larger molecular weight solutes such as β_2-microglobulin. High-efficiency hemodialysis uses a high-porosity dialyzer that has an ultrafiltration coefficient greater than 10 and less than 20 mL per mm Hg per hour. High-flux hemodialysis uses an even more porous dialyzer with an ultrafiltration coefficient greater than

TABLE 25-1.   Dialysis Modalities

Technique	Dialyzer	Physical Principle
Hemodialysis		
Conventional	Hemodialyzer	Concurrent diffusive clearance and UF
Sequential UF/ clearance	Hemodialyzer	UF followed by diffusive clearance
UF	Hemodialyzer	UF alone
Hemofiltration		
SCUF	Hemofilter	Arteriovenous UF without a blood pump
CAVH	Hemofilter	Arteriovenous convective transport without a blood pump
CAVHD	Hemofilter	Arteriovenous hemodialysis without a blood pump
CAVHDF	Hemofilter	Arteriovenous hemofiltration and hemodialysis without a blood pump
CVVH	Hemofilter	Venovenous convective transport with a blood pump
CVVHD	Hemofilter	Venovenous hemodialysis with a blood pump
CVVHDF	Hemofilter	Venovenous hemofiltration and hemodialysis with a blood pump
Peritoneal dialysis		
Intermittent	None	Exchanges performed for 10–12 h every 2–3 d
CAPD	None	Manual exchanges performed daily during waking hours
CCPD	None	Automated cycling device performs exchanges nightly

CAPD, continuous ambulatory peritoneal dialysis; CAVH, continuous arteriovenous hemofiltration; CAVHD, continuous arteriovenous hemodialysis; CAVHDF, continuous arteriovenous hemodiafiltration; CCPD, continuous cycling peritoneal dialysis; CVVH, continuous venovenous hemofiltration; CVVHD, continuous venovenous hemodialysis; CVVHDF, continuous venovenous hemodiafiltration; SCUF, slow continuous ultrafiltration; UF, ultrafiltration.

20 mL per mm Hg per hour and greater clearances of solutes greater than 300 Da.

Variables of the hemodialysis procedure that may be manipulated by the dialysis care team are the type of dialyzer (determines the solute clearance and ultrafiltration capacity of the dialysis treatment), the dialysate composition (influences solute clearance and loading), the blood and dialysate flow (influences solute clearance), the hydraulic pressure that drives ultrafiltration, and the duration of dialysis.

These dialytic parameters should be prescribed so as to afford patients the optimal "dose" of dialysis [10]. Dialysis dose can be determined either by measuring the fractional reduction of blood urea nitrogen with each dialysis or by measurement of the total amount of urea removed in each dialysis. Fractional reduction of urea can be measured by volume-adjusted fractional clearance of urea, Kt/V_{urea}, where K is the dialyzer's urea clearance, t is the time on dialysis, and V is the volume of distribution of urea. It can also be expressed as the percentage reduction in urea during a single hemodialysis treatment (urea reduction ratio or URR) [11], which is defined mathematically as

$$[1 - (\text{postdialysis blood urea nitrogen concentration} \div \text{predialysis blood urea nitrogen concentration})] \times 100$$

In ARF patients, fractional urea reduction (Kt/V) is found to overestimate the actual amount of urea removed [12]. In a steady state, the urea distribution volume approximates total body water because urea is freely permeable across cell membranes and equilibrates rapidly among different body spaces.

The relationship of urea kinetics and dialysis dose is more complex in ARF patients, however, possibly due to their unstable hemodynamics. Volume of urea distribution has been found to exceed total body water in patients with ARF by approximately 20% [13,14]. In addition, ARF is usually characterized by hypercatabolism and negative nitrogen balance. Taking into account these different limitations, a method for calculating equilibrated Kt/V has been proposed for dialysis dose measurement in ARF [15].

HEMOFILTRATION AND HEMODIAFILTRATION

In contrast to the diffusion-driven solute clearance of hemodialysis, hemofiltration depends principally on convective transport. The patient's blood is conveyed through an extremely high-porosity dialyzer (hemofilter), resulting in the formation of a protein-free hemofiltrate that resembles plasma water in composition. In the case of arteriovenous hemofiltration, the major determinant of perfusion of the hemofilter is the patient's mean arterial pressure, whereas the hydrostatic pressure gradient between the blood and hemofiltrate compartments provides the driving force for the formation of the filtrate. For effective hemofiltration, the mean arterial pressure should be maintained at more than 70 mm Hg.

If a hemofiltrate is formed but is not replaced by a replacement fluid, the process is called *slow continuous ultrafiltration*. Little solute clearance occurs during slow continuous ultrafiltration. An alternative technique that enhances solute clearance is to replace the lost volume continuously with a physiologic solution lacking the solute to be removed. If an arteriovenous blood path is used, the process is called *continuous arteriovenous hemofiltration* (CAVH). A venovenous circuit may be used with blood flow driven by a blood pump, and this procedure is referred to as *continuous venovenous hemofiltration* (CVVH). Optimal solute clearance is achieved by combining diffusive clearance and convective transport. This is accomplished by circulating dialysate through the hemofilter with or without high ultrafiltration rates (continuous arteriovenous hemodiafiltration [CAVHDF] and continuous arteriovenous hemodialysis [CAVHD], respectively). Alternatively, these procedures may be performed using venovenous access with a blood pump to generate adequate flow rates (continuous venovenous hemodiafiltration [CVVHDF] and continuous venovenous hemodialysis [CVVHD], respectively). Hemodiafiltration combines high ultrafiltration rate (requiring replacement fluid) and dialysate flow for clearance. Collectively, all these modalities are termed *continuous renal replacement therapies* (CRRT). Due to the availability of reliable blood pumps, precise ultrafiltration controllers, and the desire to avoid the morbidity of arterial cannulation, venovenous therapies have greatly diminished the use of arteriovenous modes of CRRT.

PERITONEAL DIALYSIS

Solute clearance in peritoneal dialysis is gradient-driven, whereas ultrafiltration during peritoneal dialysis depends on the osmolality of the dialysis solution. In stable ESRD patients, maintenance peritoneal dialysis is performed daily, either by manual instillation and drainage of the dialysate during waking hours (continuous ambulatory peritoneal dialysis) or while sleeping using an automated dialysate cycling device (continuous cycling peritoneal dialysis). The dialysate is allowed to dwell in the peritoneal cavity for variable intervals depending on the clearance and ultrafiltration goals (described as an "exchange"). The dialysate volume is usually 1.5 to 2.0 L per instillation, but can be as great as 3 L for the overnight dwell while the patient is recumbent.

In the acute setting, after the placement of a peritoneal dialysis catheter, peritoneal dialysis is easily initiated and discontinued with limited personnel and equipment. As in ambulatory ESRD patients, peritoneal dialysis for ARF may be performed manually or using an automated cycler. If it is performed acutely using an uncuffed dialysis catheter, rather than the conventional Dacron-cuffed catheters used for ESRD patients, 60 to 80 L of dialysate are exchanged during 48 to 72 hours, and the catheter is removed. The risk of peritonitis increases significantly thereafter without a cuffed catheter. A soft Dacron-cuff catheter is preferred if extended periods of peritoneal dialysis are expected.

A major disadvantage of peritoneal dialysis is its relative inefficiency for solute clearance, which may be problematic for patients in the ICU, who are often hypercatabolic and require high clearance of nitrogenous wastes. The advantages of peritoneal dialysis are that it obviates the use of anticoagulation, uses a biologic membrane (the peritoneum) for dialysis, and demands much less nursing time if automated cycling is used. Careful attention has to be paid to the patient's nitrogen balance because substantial losses of protein and amino acid may occur through the peritoneum [16].

INDICATIONS FOR DIALYSIS IN RENAL FAILURE

Whereas in chronic renal failure the therapeutic objective is for dialysis to substitute for absent renal function indefinitely, in patients with ARF, the goal of dialytic therapy is to support the patient while awaiting the recovery of adequate renal function to sustain life. In patients with ARF who have had insufficient time to establish compensatory or adaptive physiologic alterations, it is mandatory that dialysis be initiated promptly. Absolute indications for the initiation of dialysis are uremic serositis, uremic encephalopathy, hyperkalemia resistant to conservative therapy, hypervolemia unresponsive to high doses of diuretics, and acidosis that is not adequately corrected with alkali. In addition, there are selected conditions that typically are not life-threatening and that can be managed by more conservative means. These conditions are relative indications for the initiation of dialysis. Examples include azotemia in the absence of uremia, hypercalcemia, hyperuricemia, hypermagnesemia, and bleeding exacerbated by uremia.

ABSOLUTE DIALYSIS INDICATIONS

Uremic Encephalopathy and Serositis

Of the complications of uremia, few respond as dramatically to dialysis as those involving the central nervous system (CNS). Tremor, asterixis, diminished cognitive function, neuromuscular irritability, seizures, somnolence, and coma are all reversible manifestations of uremia that merit the provision of dialysis [17]. Reversible cardiopulmonary complications of uremia, such as uremic pericarditis and uremic lung, respond to the initiation of an adequate dialysis regimen, but clinical resolution is more protracted than for the CNS manifestations of uremia [18,19]. Uremic pericarditis is characterized by the presence of noninfectious inflammation of both layers of the pericardium. It is accompanied by pericardial neovascularization and the development of a serofibrinous exudative effusion. Injudicious use of systemic anticoagulation for hemodialysis or other indications may induce intrapericardial hemorrhage and cardiac tamponade, although these complications may also occur spontaneously. Development of uremic cardiac tamponade has been reported to be associated with prolonged ARF and inadequate renal replacement therapy [20]. Uremic pericarditis may also be associated with systolic dysfunction of the left ventricle and serosal inflammation with pleural hemorrhage. Uremic lung is a poorly understood late pulmonary complication of uremia demonstrating a roentgenographic pattern of atypical pulmonary edema that is not necessarily associated with elevated pulmonary capillary wedge pressures. It is also treated by dialysis.

There is a poor correlation between the blood urea nitrogen (BUN) and the development of uremic signs and symptoms. The BUN reflects not merely the degree of renal insufficiency but also the dietary protein intake, hepatocellular function, and protein catabolic rate. It is thus not surprising that uremic manifestations may arise with a BUN less than 100 mg per dL. In addition to the absolute level, the temporal rate of increase of the BUN seems to influence the development of uremia. Patients with a precipitous decline in renal function, such as those with ARF, typically manifest uremic symptoms at lesser degrees of azotemia than do patients whose renal function declines more gradually, such as those with chronic progressive kidney disease. Finally, selected patient populations, such as children, the elderly, and individuals with diabetes mellitus, appear to have a lower threshold for manifesting uremic symptoms.

Hyperkalemia

During the course of progressive renal insufficiency, the capacity to excrete potassium is compromised and the adaptive cellular uptake declines [17]. The need for emergent treatment of hyperkalemia is based on the degree of hyperkalemia, rate of rise, symptoms, and presence of electrocardiographic changes. Patients with chronic renal failure develop adaptive mechanisms to excrete potassium [18,21]. In contrast, hyperkalemia in the setting of ARF is usually poorly tolerated. In the absence of indications for urgent treatment, conservative measures will suffice. These interventions include limiting daily intake of potassium (oral or parenteral), discontinuing incriminating medications, augmenting potassium excretion in the urine or stool (if oliguric), and implementing strategies to minimize cardiotoxicity [22–24]. Hemodialysis can reduce serum potassium by 1 to 1.5 mmol per L per hour [25]. Peritoneal dialysis and CRRT are not as effective as intermittent hemodialysis in lowering serum potassium in acute, severe hyperkalemia. The decision to start emergency hemodialysis should not preclude treatment with nondialytic measures.

Hypervolemia

Hypervolemia is a common complication of renal insufficiency, in both the inpatient and outpatient setting. The obligatory volume of fluids, medications, and food administered to hospitalized patients often exceeds their excretory capacity, even if nonoliguric.

Integral to the prevention and treatment of hypervolemia is the administration of diuretics. Even patients with advanced renal insufficiency (glomerular filtration rate [GFR] less than 15 mL per minute) may respond to aggressive doses of loop diuretics. The absence of an adequate diuretic response (diuresis that is inadequate to meet the volume challenge from obligatory fluids) is an absolute indication for dialysis. Fluid removal can be accomplished by hemodialysis, hemofiltration, or peritoneal dialysis (ultrafiltration). Ultrafiltration rates of more than 3 L per hour can be achieved during hemodialysis, 1 to 3 L per hour during hemofiltration, and usually less than 1 L per hour during peritoneal dialysis.

Acidosis

As renal function declines, endogenously generated organic acids and exogenously ingested acids are retained, and the capacity to generate and reclaim bicarbonate becomes increasingly compromised. In patients who are not hypercatabolic or receiving an acid load, acid generation occurs at a rate of approximately 1 mEq per kg per day, resulting in an uncorrected decline in serum bicarbonate concentration to as low as 12 mEq per L [26]. Therefore, in patients with renal failure, metabolic acidosis is the typical acid-base disturbance.

Severe acidosis in the context of ARF can result in changes in mental state leading to coma and can provoke hypotension by depressing myocardial contractility and causing vasodilatation. The correction of acidosis is thus a major concern, especially in the intensive care setting. Less severe acidosis may be corrected by administration of exogenous oral alkali therapy.

Because both bicarbonate and citrate are administered as sodium salts, volume overload is a risk. Excessive correction of severe metabolic acidosis (plasma bicarbonate less than 10 mEq per L) may have adverse consequences, including paradoxical acidification of the cerebrospinal fluid and increased tissue lactic acid production. An initial partial correction to 15 to 20 mEq per L is quite appropriate.

With these concerns in mind, if progressively larger doses of alkali therapy are required to control acidosis in renal failure, dialysis is indicated. Hemodialysis is also useful in treating acidosis accompanying salicylate, methanol, and ethylene glycol poisonings [27–30], offering the added benefit of clearing the parent compounds and their toxic metabolites (methanol [formic acid] and ethylene glycol [glycolic acid, oxalate]).

RELATIVE DIALYSIS INDICATIONS

Non–life-threatening indications for dialysis can typically be managed with more conservative interventions. Multiple relatively mild manifestations of ARF may provoke consideration of dialysis when present simultaneously. For example, a hypercatabolic trauma patient with ARF manifested by a gradually increasing serum potassium concentration, declining serum bicarbonate concentration, falling urine output, and a mildly diminished sensorium does not fulfill any of the absolute criteria for the initiation of dialysis. However, in such a case, the need for dialysis is almost inevitable, and the patient's care is not improved by withholding dialysis until a life-threatening complication of renal failure develops.

Other subcritical chemical abnormalities may be approached with hemodialysis. Hypercalcemia and hyperuricemia associated with ARF are common in patients with malignancies and tumor lysis syndrome, respectively [31,32]. Hypermagnesemia in renal failure is usually the result of the injudicious use of magnesium containing cathartics or antacids [33]. These metabolic disorders are readily corrected by deletion of the excessive electrolyte from the dialysate. For example, hypercalcemia that is unresponsive to conventional conservative interventions may be corrected by hemodialysis with a reduced calcium dialysate (less than 2.5 mEq per L).

Bleeding from the skin and gastrointestinal tract are common manifestations of platelet dysfunction in renal insufficiency. The hemostatic defect of renal insufficiency, an impairment of platelet aggregation and adherence, is reflected in the typical threefold prolongation of the bleeding time [33–36]. Although either peritoneal or hemodialysis can correct the platelet defect [37], more conservative therapies are available [38–42].

PROPHYLACTIC DIALYSIS AND RESIDUAL RENAL FUNCTION

The presence of definitive indications such as severe hyperkalemia and overt uremia prompts the decision to initiate dialysis without further delay. However, in the absence of such emergent indications, the timing of the initiation of dialysis is more a matter of judgment. Prevailing opinion dictates that dialysis should be initiated prophylactically in ARF when life-threatening events appear imminent, understanding that it may be difficult to predict imminent events in so volatile a context.

Several small trials of prophylactic renal replacement therapy revealed conflicting results. Forty-four coronary artery bypass graft patients with chronic kidney disease (serum creatinine more than 2.5 mg per dL) were studied with prophylactic hemodialysis [43]. Patients who were prophylactically dialyzed before surgery had a lower rate of acute renal failure, in-hospital mortality, and shorter hospital stay than those who were not. In the second trial of chronic renal failure patients (creatinine clearance less than 50 ml per minute) needing elective cardiac catheterization, periprocedural CVVHF helped to decrease the risk of development of ARF, and improve in-hospital and long-term outcome [44]. In contrast, three trials of prophylactic hemodialysis given to chronic renal failure patients during [45] or immediately after [46,47] exposure to radiocontrast material failed to show any benefit compared to the nonhemodialysis group treated with intravenous fluid.

An additional consideration in the timing of dialysis is its influence on residual renal function and length of recovery from ARF. Numerous observations suggested an important and possibly deleterious effect of dialysis on residual renal function. Several investigators have observed that in posttraumatic ARF treated with hemodialysis, there were pathologically demonstrable fresh, focal areas of tubular necrosis 3 to 4 weeks after the initial renal injury [48,49]. The only culpable hemodynamic insults experienced during this period were short-lived episodes of intradialytic hypotension. Furthermore, the initiation of dialysis is frequently associated with an acute decline in urine output [50]. It has been observed that in patients with advanced renal failure, the institution of hemodialysis results in progressive deterioration in GFR over several months [51]. The fact that peritoneal dialysis does not provoke a similar relentless decline in residual renal function [52] suggests that this may be a consequence of combined hemodialysis-induced hypotension with abnormal vascular compensation and complement-mediated injury resulting from immunogenic dialyzer membrane materials [53,54]. Preserving residual renal function must be a high priority in managing patients with severe renal insufficiency [55]. Even modest preservation of GFR may ease fluid management in patients with ARF. A residual GFR of approximately 15 mL per minute is equivalent to 5 hours of hemodialysis with a dialyzer, having a urea clearance of 160 mL per minute. The clearance of middle-molecular-weight solutes is especially enhanced with endogenous function compared with hemodialysis.

Relatively few studies have examined the issue of the timing of dialysis initiation, and most are reports from the early days of dialytic therapy. In 1960, Teschan et al. [56] described their success with the initiation of hemodialysis before the onset of frank uremia. Using this protocol, dialysis was continued on a daily basis to maintain the BUN less than 150 mg per dL until recovery occurred. Compared with historical control subjects who were dialyzed for severe uremia alone, patient survival was greatly improved. In later years, two relevant randomized prospective studies were performed. In one study, 18 posttraumatic ARF patients were randomized to initiate hemodialysis at low (predialysis BUN and creatinine levels less than 70 mg per dL and 5 mg per dL, respectively) or high BUN threshold treatment groups (predialysis BUN approximately 150 mg per dL or overt uremia as an indication for dialysis). Continued hemodialysis was performed only when these thresholds were reached. The study reported 64% survival in the low BUN group compared with 20% in the high BUN group [57]. Sepsis and hemorrhage were frequent complications in the high BUN group. As intriguing

as these observations are, none of these studies was sufficiently optimally designed as to allow definitive conclusions.

In a prospective randomized trial of 106 ARF patients, Bouman et al. [58] compared the effect of early (within 12 hours of meeting the criteria for ARF) and late (meeting traditional criteria) initiation of CVVH. The mean serum urea nitrogen at the start of renal replacement therapy was 47 mg per dL in the groups with early initiation of dialysis compared to 105 mg per dL in the group with late initiation. No significant difference was found between the groups regarding patient survival and recovery of renal function. Overall patient survival in the study was 72.6%, which is significantly higher than most studies with ARF, and might indicate enrollment of less-sick patients in the study. Recognition of early ARF and early initiation of CVVHDF in a group of patients with cardiac surgery yielded more positive results [59]. Sixty-one patients with cardiac surgery were treated with CVVHDF for early ARF (decrease in urine output to less than 100 mL within 8 hours, with no response to 50 mg of furosemide) versus late ARF (serum creatinine above 5 mg per dL or serum potassium above 5.5 mEq per L). Patients who received early CVVHDF had significantly lower ICU and overall hospital mortality compared with patients treated with late CVVHDF. Positive clinical outcome was also seen in acute liver failure patients with ARF who received early renal replacement therapy (BUN 117.3 $\pm$ 32.8 mg per dL) compared with late (BUN 44.64 $\pm$ 19.5 mg per dL) [59].

In summary, although dialytic therapy is an essential tool in the management of ARF, its use or abuse may have detrimental effects on patient outcome. The physician must avoid the temptation to intervene in the course of ARF based purely on the patient's reaching a threshold blood urea or creatinine level. Proper consideration of the patient's overall condition, expected course of renal failure, fluid and nutritional requirements, and the presence of comorbid conditions is a wiser approach.

PRACTICAL APPLICATION OF ENGINEERING PRINCIPLES

HEMODIALYSIS AND HEMOFILTRATION

Clearance

The most fundamental biophysical principle of dialysis is solute movement across a semipermeable membrane by diffusion. Diffusional movement of a solute from a region of higher concentration to that of a lower concentration is governed by Fick's law:

$$J = -DA \times (dc/dx)$$

where J is the solute flux, D its diffusivity, A is the area available for diffusion, and dc is the change in the concentration of the solute over the intercompartmental distance, dx. For a particular model of dialyzers, dx and A are constant, and for an individual solute, D is constant. It is clear that solute flux is influenced by the surface area and the physical structure of the membrane, the variables that define the clearance characteristic of a given dialyzer.

In clinical practice, the clearance of a solute not only depends on the dialyzer but also the blood and dialysate flow rates, expressed by the following equation:

$$K = [Q_{Bi} \times (C_{Bi} - C_{B0})] \div C_{Bi}$$

In this expression, K is the diffusive clearance of the solute from the blood, Q_{Bi} is the rate at which blood containing the solute flows into the dialyzer, C_{Bi} is the concentration of the solute in the blood entering the dialyzer (arterial end), and C_{B0} is the concentration of the remaining solute at the egress side of the blood compartment (venous end). This mathematical description is accurate for the situation in which the solute is not initially present in the dialysate ($C_{Di} = 0$). Usually, the dialysate passes through the dialyzer only once (single-pass dialysis system), and there is minimal convective transport of the solute during its clearance. Thus, the clearance of a solute during dialysis may be functionally defined as the volumetric removal of the solute from the patient's blood. Within the practical application of this formulation, the clearance of a solute can be modified by altering the patient's blood flow into the dialyzer (Q_{Bi}).

A similar relationship exists for the dialysate and the diffusive clearance of a solute from the blood:

$$K = [Q_{Di} \times (C_{D0} - C_{Di})] \div C_{Bi}$$

where Q_{Di} is the flow rate of the dialysate into the dialyzer, and C_{D0} and C_{Di} are the concentrations of solute at the dialysate outlet and inlet ends of the hemodialyzer, respectively. Thus, an additional means of augmenting the diffusive clearance of a solute from the blood into the dialysate, or vice versa, is to increase the dialysate flow rate. Increases in blood, dialysate flow, or both do not improve the clearance linearly. As blood and dialysate flow rates are increased, resistance and turbulence within the dialyzer occur, resulting in a decline in clearance per unit flow of blood or dialysate. For conventional dialyzers, this limitation occurs above 300 and 500 mL per minute, respectively, for blood and dialysate flows. Limitations for high-flux dialyzers are observed at above 400 and 800 mL per minute for blood and dialysate flow rates.

The clearance characteristics of dialyzers, as provided by their manufacturers, are determined in vitro; the influence of plasma proteins on solute clearance is not accounted for, and the actual in vivo diffusivity is usually lower [61]. The clearance of a solute by a given dialyzer is a unique property of that solute. Molecules larger than 300 Da, such as vitamin B_{12} or β_2-microglobulin, typically have lower K values compared with smaller solutes, such as urea and potassium. The clearance of these larger solutes from blood depends to a greater extent on ultrafiltration and the passive movement of solute (convective transport). The summary interaction between the diffusive clearance and convective transport of a solute is expressed as

$$J = (K \times [1 - Q_f/Q_{Bi}] + Q_f) \times C_{Bi} = KC_{Bi}$$

where Q_f is the ultrafiltration rate, and K is the sum of the convective and diffuse clearances. If the diffusive clearance (K) is large, as is true for urea, the influence of the ultrafiltration rate is not great. As the diffusive clearance for a solute declines because of increasing molecular weight (value of K approaches Q_f), the proportionate contribution of convective transport to solute movement increases greatly. The practical application of convective transport of solutes alone is observed during pure hemofiltration (CAVH, CVVH) because no dialysate is passed through the hemofilter (preventing diffusive clearance).

Ultrafiltration

An equally important operational variable in the dialysis procedure is the ultrafiltration coefficient (K_f), defined by

$$K_f = Q_f \div (P_B - P_D)$$

where Q_f is the ultrafiltration rate, and P_B and P_D are the mean pressures in the blood and dialysate compartments, respectively. Analogous to the information derived for the clearance of a particular solute for a specific dialyzer, each dialyzer also has an ultrafiltration coefficient. Because these values are typically derived in vitro, similar limitations exist for their application to the in vivo situation. It is not unusual for an individual dialyzer's in vitro and in vivo ultrafiltration coefficients to vary by 10% to 20% in either direction.

The ultrafiltration coefficient for a dialyzer operationally defines the volume of ultrafiltrate formed per unit time in response to a given pressure differential (P_B minus P_D) across the dialysis membrane, and is expressed in *milliliters per millimeters of mercury per hour*. It is therefore possible to use the ultrafiltration coefficient to calculate the quantity of pressure that must be exerted across the dialysis membrane (transmembrane pressure [TMP]) to achieve a given volume of ultrafiltration during a dialysis session. To make this calculation, it is first necessary to quantitate the pressure that is exerted across the dialysis membrane from the blood to the dialysate compartment. During ultrafiltration, the serum oncotic pressure increases in the dialyzer's blood compartment from the arterial to the venous end, but this is usually a relatively negligible biophysical factor. The net pressure across the dialysis membrane that arises from the flow of blood and dialysate is defined by the following equation:

$$P_{net} = [(P_{Bi} - P_{B0}) \div 2] - [(P_{Di} + P_{D0}) \div 2]$$

where P_{Bi}, P_{B0}, P_{D0}, and P_{Di} are the pressures measured at the inflow and outflow ports of the blood and dialysate compartments, respectively. If the P_{net} is too low to provide for adequate ultrafiltration during a dialysis session ($P_{net} \times$ ultrafiltration coefficient $\times$ dialysis time < target ultrafiltrate volume), additional pressure can be generated across the dialysis membrane by creating negative pressure in the dialysate compartment. The effective pressure, or TMP, required can be derived from TMP = desired weight loss $\div$ (ultrafiltration coefficient $\times$ dialysis time).

The performance of ultrafiltration during hemodialysis has been greatly simplified by the development of dialysis machines that possess volumetric control systems ("ultrafiltration controllers"). Ultrafiltration with these devices is remarkably precise, and weight loss can be affected in a linear manner per unit of time. Such exact volumetric control is a prerequisite for high-flux hemodialysis in which high-porosity dialyzers are used.

During most hemodialysis treatments, ultrafiltration and solute clearance are performed simultaneously. However, it is possible to segregate the two procedures temporally by a modification of the hemodialysis procedure described as sequential ultrafiltration clearance [62]. This modification of the conventional hemodialysis procedure is accomplished by first ultrafiltering the patient to a desired volume and then conducting diffusive clearance without ultrafiltration. During the initial ultrafiltration phase, diffusive clearance is prevented by not pumping dialysate through the dialyzer. During the second phase, no negative pressure is instituted, and the small fluid losses secondary to P_{net} are balanced by the infusion of saline. Sequential ultrafiltration clearance has distinct hemodynamic advantages over conventional hemodialysis, making it a particularly useful technique for aggressive fluid removal within a short interval. When ultrafiltration is performed concurrently with diffusive solute clearance, intravascular volume losses may exceed the rate of translocation of fluid from the interstitium. If these losses are not counterbalanced by an appropriate increase in the peripheral vascular resistance and venous refilling, hypotension occurs [63]. With sequential ultrafiltration clearance, these hemodynamic abnormalities are attenuated, and up to 4 L per hour may be removed without causing hypotension. However, unless the total time allotted to dialysis is increased during sequential ultrafiltration clearance, solute clearance is compromised and inadequate dialysis may occur.

During CRRT, ultrafiltration is governed by physical principles different from those for hemodialysis. Because the driving force for blood flow during CAVH is the mean arterial pressure, and the resistance in the blood path that arises from the hemofilter and lines is low, the hydraulic pressure in the blood compartment of the hemofilter is also low. Therefore, during CAVH, the *principle* driving force for the formation of an ultrafiltrate is the negative hydrostatic pressure within the ultrafiltrate compartment of the hemofilter. This effective negative pressure (P_h) is generated by the weight of the column within the ultrafiltration collection line and is calculated by P_h = height difference (cm) between the hemofilter and collection bag × 0.74. Therefore, to increase or decrease the rate of fluid formation during hemofiltration, the collection bag is either lowered below or raised to the level of the hemofilter. In contrast to hemodialysis, the increase in oncotic pressure at the venous end of the hemofilter is of sufficient magnitude that little ultrafiltration occurs at this end. Because significant convective solute clearance occurs with hemofiltration, little clearance occurs at the venous end of the hemofilter. This situation is most likely to occur when the amount of ultrafiltrate formed is maximal and when the blood flow rate through the hemofilter is low. It is therefore undesirable to have the net ultrafiltration rate greater than 25% of the blood flow rate [64]. Excessively large amounts of ultrafiltrate can result from a kinked or thrombosed venous return line because increased resistance will translate into increased hydraulic pressure in the blood compartment.

The ultrafiltrate formed during hemofiltration is free of protein and has a solute composition that closely resembles that of the aqueous component of plasma. The quantity of a selected solute that is removed is determined by the volume of ultrafiltrate formed, by its concentration in the blood (and therefore in the ultrafiltrate), and by the composition of the replacement solution. For example, if hemofiltration results in the formation of 0.5 L ultrafiltrate per hour and the ultrafiltrate and the replacement solution contain 5 and 0 mEq per L of potassium, respectively, 30 mEq of potassium will be cleared in 12 hours.

As mentioned previously, hemofiltration usually necessitates replacement fluid because of the inherently high rate of associated ultrafiltration. The replacement solution can be administered immediately before (predilutional hemofiltration) or after the hemofilter (postdilutional hemofiltration), simultaneously into both locations (pre- and postdilution hemofiltration), or into the peripheral venous circulation [65]. Predilution hemofiltration offers the advantage of diluting plasma proteins, effectively lowering the thrombogenicity of the hemofilter and increasing the ultrafiltration rate for a given hydrostatic pres-

sure. However, this technique also reduces the concentration of solutes in the blood entering the hemofilter and therefore may compromise their clearance. Alternatively, the replacement solution can be administered incompletely before the hemofilter, with the balance being infused immediately after the hemofilter. This offers the advantages of predilutional hemofiltration and avoids the clearance disadvantages.

SOLUTE CLEARANCE AND FLUID MANAGEMENT IN CONTINUOUS RENAL REPLACEMENT THERAPY

Solute clearance and fluid management in CRRT is closely related. Fluid status in CRRT can be managed by two strategies [66]. Most commonly, CRRT is started with a fixed rate of replacement fluid, and the ultrafiltration rate is adjusted according to patient's fluid status. When the patient requires negative fluid balance and significant ultrafiltration, this helps to achieve adequate solute clearance. On the other hand, zero or positive fluid balance will require reduction in ultafiltration and thereby impairment in solute clearance. An alternate option is to start CRRT at a fixed ultrafiltration rate that will provide adequate solute clearance. Positive, negative, and zero fluid balance in this strategy is achieved by adjusting the replacement fluid rate.

PERITONEAL DIALYSIS

Clearance

The simplest kinetic model of solute transport in peritoneal dialysis is that of two compartments separated by a membrane, with the two pools representing blood in the mesenteric vasculature and dialysate in the peritoneal cavity. Solutes passing from the blood into the dialysate compartment encounter three structures of resistance: the capillary endothelium, the interstitial tissues, and the mesothelial cell layer of the peritoneum. Solute clearance occurs both by diffusion and convective transport in peritoneal dialysis. As within the context of hemodialysis, diffusion (according to Fick's law) can be expressed as $J = -DA \times dc/dx$, where J is the solute flux, D is the diffusion coefficient of that solute, A is the functional surface area of the membrane, dx is the diffusion distance, and dc is the concentration gradient. DA/dx is known as the *mass transfer area coefficient* (MTAC), and the *concentration gradient* is the difference between the plasma (CP) and dialysate (CD) concentrations. Hence,

$$J = \text{MTAC} \times (\text{CP} - \text{CD})$$

As is evident from these principles of solute transfer, the diffusive clearance can clearly be influenced by the concentration gradient; the diffusion coefficient, which is solute size-dependent; and the characteristics of the peritoneal membrane. As the concentrations approximate each other (CP − CD nears zero), diffusive clearance declines. Thus, to increase clearance, the concentration gradient must be maintained with frequent change of dialysate (increase the number of exchanges with shorter dwell times). The benefit of increasing dialysate exchange rate (above 3.5 L per hour) is limited by the fact that this decreases the effective time available for contact between the dialysate and the peritoneum. A successful alternative to aid clearance is to increase the volume of dialysate per exchange from 2.0 to 3.0 L. These volumes are usually well tolerated by adults, especially when recumbent. The larger volume of dialysate allows more contact with the peritoneum, facilitating clearance. Increments in the dialysate volume have been shown to augment mass transfer area coefficient [67,68].

Because ultrafiltration and clearance occur concurrently during peritoneal dialysis, the use of hyperosmolal dialysates augments the clearance of solutes. In this situation, convective transport is added to diffusive clearance. The use of the most osmotically active dialysate (4.25% dextrose) can increase urea clearance by approximately 50% [69]. If the peritoneal vascular surface area is adequate, urea clearance and ultrafiltration are not limited by peritoneal blood flow [70–73]. For example, in patients in shock, the clearance of urea is depressed only by approximately 30%; intraperitoneal vasodilators augment small solute clearance by only 20%.

Ultrafiltration

In peritoneal dialysis, the net pressure generated favors movement of water from the dialysate into the capillaries. Therefore, an active osmotic solute (typically dextrose) is used to facilitate ultrafiltration. As is the situation for solute clearance, ultrafiltration is maximal at the beginning of an exchange and declines as the osmolality gradient declines during equilibration. Hyperglycemia, by decreasing the osmolal gradient, also impairs ultrafiltration. Even with optimal exchange frequency and volume, ultrafiltration rates during peritoneal dialysis are usually at least 700 mL per hour. The ultrafiltrate formed is hypoosmolal to serum, so hypernatremia is a common complication of excessive ultrafiltration.

COMPONENTS OF THE DIALYSIS PROCESS

HEMODIALYSIS AND HEMOFILTRATION

Dialyzers and Hemofilters

Virtually all commercially available hemodialyzers are configured as large cylinders packed with hollow fibers through which the blood flows (hollow-fiber dialyzer). The dialysate flows through the dialyzer, bathing these fibers, usually in a countercurrent direction. The membrane for these dialyzers is composed of a variety of modified biologic or synthetic materials such as regenerated cellulose, cuprophan, hemophan, cellulose acetate, polysulfone, polymethylmethacrylate, and polyacrylonitrile [74]. The surface area available for solute transport and the filling volume of the blood and dialysate compartments vary significantly among different dialyzers and are a function of the membrane material. These materials vary in their characteristics for solute transport and ultrafiltration, the degree to which they are tolerated by the patient's immune system ("biocompatibility"), costs, and capacity to be reused. The choice of dialysis membrane materials has been suggested to influence the outcome of patients with ARF, but these findings are inconsistent [75,76].

The impetus to develop more efficient dialyzers stems from the desire to decrease hemodialysis treatment time through faster solute clearance. A secondary goal is to improve clearance of larger solutes that may be toxic, such as β_2-microglobulin. A putative disadvantage of these efficient larger-pore dialyzers is that they may more readily permit the transmembrane backflux of bacterial-derived lipopolysaccharides from the dialysate into the dialyzer blood compartment (backfiltration) [77]. The resultant patient exposure to the pyrogen results in an acute nonbacteremic, febrile illness described as a pyrogen reaction. The use of bicarbonate-buffered dialysates, which permit the growth of Gram-negative bacteria, and ultrafiltration controllers that limit the rate of ultrafiltration may also contribute to the occurrence of pyrogen reactions.

Use of polyacrylonitrile membrane (specifically, AN-69, Hospal Corp, Lyon, France) in patients receiving angiotensin-converting enzyme inhibitors can result in anaphylactoid reaction [78]. Increased production of bradykinin by the contact of blood with the membrane and impaired degradation of bradykinin by the angiotensin-converting enzyme inhibitors appears to be the mechanism behind the hypotension.

The characteristic requirements of a dialyzer or hemofilter used in CRRT must be considered from a different perspective. Because the driving force for hemofiltration is the mean arterial pressure of a low-speed venous pump and clearance is disproportionately dependent on convection of low resistance, a high K_{uf} hemofilter is required. Hemofilters are usually composed of polysulfone, polymethylmethacrylate, or polyacrylonitrile because cuprophan does not have sufficient hydraulic permeability at TMP of 30 to 70 mm Hg. Hemofilters are available in two geometric configurations: the hollow-fiber or the parallel-plate configuration (blood and dialysate separated by a flat, semipermeable membrane).

In continuous hemodialysis techniques (CAVHD, CVVHD), solute transport is limited by the dialysate flow rate, unlike conventional intermittent hemodialysis. The blood flow rate is usually 100 to 150 mL per minute, and dialysate flow rate is generally 16 to 30 mL per minute. The rapidity of solute equilibration across the dialysis membrane, which is a function of the hemofilter, determines the type of hemofilter that can be used.

Dialysates for Hemodialysis

The composition of the dialysate is the other key variable of the dialysis process that determines the outcome of this procedure (Table 25-2). Although sodium and potassium are typically the only components of the dialysate that are adjusted to meet the demands of specific clinical situations, the other constituents are equally critical. The dialysate is stored as a liquid or powdered concentrate that is diluted in a fixed ratio to yield the final solute concentration.

TABLE 25-2. Dialysate Formulation for Peritoneal Dialysis and Conventional Hemodialysis

Solute	Range (Usual Concentration)
Peritoneal dialysis	
Na^+	132 mEq/L
K^+	0
Cl^-	96 mEq/L
Lactate	35 mEq/L
Ca^+	2.5 or 3.5 mEq/L
Mg^+	0.5 or 1.5 mEq/L
Glucose	1.5%, 2.5%, or 4.25% g/dL
Conventional hemodialysis	
Na^+	138–145 mEq/L (140)
K^+	0–4 mEq/L (2)
Cl^-	100–110 mEq/L (106)
HCO_3^-	35–45 mEq/L (38)
Ca^+	1.0–3.5 mEq/L (2.5)
Mg^+	1.5 mEq/L (1.5)
Dextrose	1.0–2.5 mEq/L (2)

GLUCOSE. Before hydraulic-driven ultrafiltration became available, the dialysate glucose concentration was maintained at above 1.8 g per L to generate an osmotic gradient between the blood and the dialysate [79]. Although this was effective for inducing ultrafiltration, some patients developed morbidity from hyperosmolality. Currently, dialysates are glucose-free, normoglycemic (0.00% to 0.25%), or modestly hyperglycemic (more than 0.25%). Hemodialysis with a glucose-free dialysate results in a net glucose loss of approximately 30 g and stimulates ketogenesis and gluconeogenesis [80]. Such alterations in intermediary metabolism may be particularly deleterious in chronically or acutely ill hemodialysis patients who are malnourished or on a medication such as propranolol that may induce hypoglycemia [81,82]. These effects are ameliorated by the use of a normoglycemic dialysate. Additional metabolic consequences occurring from the use of a glucose-free dialysate include an accelerated loss of free amino acids into the dialysate [83], a decline in serum amino acids [84], and enhanced potassium clearance stemming from relative hypoinsulinemia [80]. Therefore, the dialysate glucose concentration should be maintained at normoglycemic concentrations.

SODIUM. Historically, the dialysate sodium concentration was maintained on the low side (more than 135 mEq per L) to prevent interdialytic hypertension, exaggerated thirst, and excessive weight gains. However, hyponatremic dialysates increase the likelihood of loss of sodium by diffusion with two consequent possible side effects [85]. First, loss of intravascular sodium can cause osmotic shift of fluid from extracellular to intracellular compartment leading to intracellular overhydration. This will lead to CNS symptoms of dialysis disequilibrium syndrome. The second effect of loss of intravascular volume is intradialytic hypotension and associated symptoms of cramps, headache, nausea, and vomiting. Use of hypernatremic dialysate helps to prevent net sodium loss and adverse effects of low dialysate sodium. This also permits enhanced ability to ultrafiltrate these patients. However hypernatremic dialysate carries the risk of inadequate sodium removal, polydipsia, and refractory hypertension. The hemodynamic alterations are minimized in the setting of equal dialysate and serum sodium concentrations. Thus, there has been an appropriate increase in the dialysate sodium to 140 to 145 mEq per L.

The newer dialysate delivery systems permit real-time modification of dialysate sodium concentrations during hemodialysis by the use of variable-dilution proportioning systems. The technique of sodium "profiling" to fit a patient's hemodynamic needs has been espoused as a means of accomplishing optimal blood pressure support without increased thirst at the completion of the treatment. The modulation of dialysate sodium concentration can be executed in several patterns [86]. Sodium profiling may reduce the frequency of hypotension during ultrafiltration without decreasing the dialysis time committed to diffusive clearance, as is the case with sequential ultrafiltration clearance [87]. However, it is unclear if this technique offers any advantage over a fixed dialysate sodium of 140 to 145 mEq per L [88–90]. Furthermore, interdialytic weight gains appear unaffected by sodium modeling. Combining dialysate sodium concentration with ultrafiltration profiling reduces intradialytic symptoms compared with standard dialysis with constant dialysate sodium and ultrafiltration [91].

POTASSIUM. Unlike urea, which usually behaves as a solute distributed in a single pool with a variable volume of distribution, only 1% to 2% of the total body store of 3,000 to 3,500 mEq of potassium are present in the extracellular space. The flux of potassium from the intracellular compartment to the extracellular space, and subsequently across the dialysis membrane to the dialysate compartment, is unequal. Therefore, the efficacy of potassium removal in hemodialysis is highly variable, difficult to predict, and influenced by dialysis-specific and patient-specific factors [92].

During hemodialysis, approximately 70% of the potassium removed is derived from the intracellular compartment. Because 50 to 80 mEq of potassium are removed in a single dialysis session and only 15 to 20 mEq of potassium are present in the plasma, life-threatening hypokalemia would be the consequence of hemodialysis if this was not the case [92]. However, the volume of distribution of potassium is not constant; the greater the total-body potassium, the lower its volume of distribution [93]. As a result, the fractional decline in plasma potassium during a single dialysis session is greater if the prehemodialysis level is higher. Optimal potassium elimination by hemodialysis is accomplished by daily short hemodialysis treatments instead of protracted sessions every other day. The transfer of potassium from intracellular to extracellular compartment usually occurs more slowly than the transfer from the plasma across the dialysis membrane [93,94], making it difficult to predict the quantity of potassium that will be removed during hemodialysis. A practical consequence of the discordant transfer rates is that the plasma potassium measured immediately after the completion of hemodialysis is approximately 30% less than the steady-state value measured after 5 hours. Therefore, hypokalemia based on blood measurements obtained immediately after the completion of hemodialysis should not be treated with potassium supplements.

The transcellular distribution of potassium is influenced by several variables, including the blood insulin concentration (insulin promotes potassium uptake by cells, lowering its intradialytic clearance), catecholamine activity (β-agonists promote cellular uptake of potassium and a-agonists stimulate the cellular egress of potassium, attenuating and increasing the intradialytic clearance of potassium, respectively) [95], sodium-potassium adenosine triphosphatase activity (pharmacologic inhibition diminishes potassium uptake into cells, which may enhance intradialytic clearance), and systemic pH (alkalemia augments transcellular potassium uptake, which may diminish dialytic clearance of potassium) [95]. Modification of dialysate that can enhance reduction in serum potassium includes use of lower dialysate potassium, glucose-free dialysate, and increased dialysate bicarbonate [96]. Use of higher concentration of HCO_3 dialysate (39 mmol per L vs. 35 mmol per L and 27 mmol per L) can result in a more rapid decrease in serum potassium concentration, although the reduction in serum potassium is thought to be due to transfer of potassium from extracellular to intracellular fluid compartment, and not due to removal by dialysis [97]. Paradoxically, it has been observed that, as the gradient for potassium clearance from blood into the dialysate is increased by decreasing the dialysate potassium concentration, the uptake of bicarbonate from the dialysate declines. This interaction between buffer base and potassium in the dialysate is significant: a 1-mEq increase in the potassium gradient results in a decline in bicarbonate loading of 50 mEq.

This interaction should not be overlooked in planning the dialysate prescription for patients being dialyzed for severe acidosis [98]. Use of lower dialysate potassium (1 mEq per L vs. 3 mEq per L) can increase postdialysis blood pressure possibly through increasing peripheral resistance [99]. However, dialysis efficiency seems unaffected.

Because the selection of the dialysate potassium concentration is empirical, most patients are dialyzed against a potassium concentration of 1 to 3 mEq per L. For stable patients who do not have significant cardiac disease or who are not taking cardiac glycosides, a dialysate potassium concentration of 2 to 3 mEq per L is appropriate. In a patient with a history of cardiac disease, especially with arrhythmias and cardiac glycoside usage, the dialysate potassium should be increased to 3 to 4 mEq per L [100]. Such patients are at the greatest risk for the development of dysrhythmias associated with intradialytic potassium flux.

Most cardiac morbidity attributable to the dialysate potassium concentration occurs during the first half of the dialysis session because of the rapid decline in serum potassium concentration associated with large blood-to-dialysate potassium gradient. The sudden fall in serum potassium concentration during the initial phase of hemodialysis can prolong the QTc interval even in patients without cardiac disease [101,102]. The rapidity of the fall in the plasma potassium concentration, rather than the absolute plasma concentration, appears to determine the risk of cardiac arrhythmias. The effect of dialysate potassium modeling on this initial rapid decline in serum potassium and cardiac arrhythmias was studied in a prospective randomized trial [103]. Hemodialysis patients were randomized to either a fixed dialysate potassium (2.5 mEq/L) or to an exponentially declining dialysate potassium (3.9 to 2.5 mEq/L) that maintains a constant blood-to-dialysate potassium concentration gradient (1.5 mEq/L). Even though the total decreases in serum potassium concentration were similar in both groups, patients with variable dialysate potassium had fewer premature ventricular contractions, particularly in the first hour of dialysis. If a patient has a significant deficit in total body potassium, postdialysis hypokalemia can occur, even if the dialysate potassium concentration is greater than the serum potassium concentration. This seemingly contradictory situation arises because of the potential for a delayed conductance of potassium from the dialysate into the patient, compared with its movement from the extracellular space into the intracellular compartment.

BASES. Although bicarbonate was used as the original base used in dialysate in the early 1960s, it was superseded by acetate, which is more stable in aqueous solution at neutral pH in the presence of divalent cations. It was found that vascular instability is much more problematic with predominantly acetate-containing dialysates than bicarbonate-containing dialysates [104–107]. The hemodynamic instability associated with acetate is worsened by hyponatremic dialysates and is lessened with a normonatremic dialysate [105,108,109].

Hemodialysis using bicarbonate-buffered dialysate prevents these complications. The transient anion gap metabolic acidosis associated with acetate dialysis is avoided with bicarbonate-based dialysis. A supraphysiologic bicarbonate concentration in the dialysate not only attenuates the diffusive gradient from blood to dialysate but generally allows the patient to achieve a net positive bicarbonate balance. Additionally, dialysis-induced hypoxemia is attenuated by a bicarbonate dialysate.

Bicarbonate is now used routinely as the buffer in hemodialysis solutions. Bicarbonate dialysis is now feasible because of the widespread availability of proportioning systems that permit mixing of the separate concentrates containing bicarbonate and divalent cations close to the final entry point of the dialysate into the dialyzer. Unlike the more acidic and hyperosmolal acetate-based dialysate, liquid bicarbonate concentrates and reconstituted bicarbonate dialysates support the growth of Gram-negative bacteria such as *Pseudomonas, Acinetobacter, Flavobacterium,* and *Achromobacter;* filamentous fungi; and yeast. Because of the propensity of the dialysate to support bacterial growth, and the morbidity associated with the presence of such growth in the dialysate, strict limits are placed on bacterial growth and presence of lipopolysaccharide in the dialysate, and frequency of dialyzer reuse [110].

A bicarbonate-based dialysate of 30 to 35 mEq per L is conventionally used. Bicarbonate concentrations above 35 mEq per L may result in the development of a metabolic alkalosis with secondary hypoventilation, hypercapnia, and hypoxemia. Use of higher dialysate bicarbonate to correct metabolic acidosis might have a beneficial effect on patient's nutritional status. In maintenance hemodialysis patients, use of higher dialysate bicarbonate (40 mEq per L) to keep predialysis total CO_2 concentration above 23 mmol per L is associated with significant decrease in protein degradation. If a bicarbonate dialysate is unavailable, acetate at an equivalent concentration is suitable, but large-surface-area dialyzers or dialyzers with high-efficiency or high-flux transport characteristics cannot be used.

CALCIUM. Patients with renal failure are prone to develop hypocalcemia, hyperphosphatemia, hypovitaminosis D, and hyperparathyroidism. Positive calcium balance is thus useful as an adjunct during hemodialysis for controlling metabolic bone disease [111–113]. In patients with renal failure requiring dialysis, more than 60% of the calcium is not bound to plasma proteins and is in a diffusible equilibrium during hemodialysis [114]. During hemodialysis, serum ionized calcium level is directly related to the dialysate calcium concentration and it varies in a time-dependent manner [115]. Assuming free conductance of calcium across the dialysis membrane secondary to diffusive clearance and an additional contribution secondary to convective losses, a dialysate calcium concentration of roughly 3.5 mEq per L (7.0 mg per dL) is necessary to prevent intradialytic calcium losses [116]. Various complications such as vascular calcification, calciphylaxis, and adynamic bone disease have been attributed to increased calcium load over the years in chronic hemodialysis patients. To avoid the risks of these complications and to allow the use of vitamin D and calcium-containing phosphate binders, it has been recommended that 2.5 mEq per L dialysate calcium be used in maintenance hemodialysis patients [117].

A reduction in the dialysate calcium may exacerbate vascular instability during hemodialysis. Dialysate calcium of 2.5 mEq per L, compared to 3.5 mEq per L, is associated with a significant decrease in intradialytic blood pressure in both healthy as well as cardiac-compromised hemodialysis patients [117,118]. Low dialysate calcium is also reported to be associated with increased QTc intervals during hemodialysis [119]. Intradialytic increases in serum ionized calcium concentration augment left ventricular performance without an accompanying alteration in the peripheral vascular resistance [117]. Several modifications in dialysate compositions have been tried to ameliorate the cardiovascular adverse effects associated with low calcium dialysate. Use of higher magnesium dialysate (1.5 mEq per L) along with dialysate calcium of 2.5 mEq per L was also found to prevent both symptomatic and asymptomatic intradialytic hypotension [120].

MAGNESIUM. The serum magnesium concentration, like that of potassium, is a poor indicator of total body magnesium stores. Only about 1% of the total body magnesium is present in the extracellular fluid, and only 60% of this amount (approximately 25 mEq) is free and diffusible [121]. Because of scant extrarenal clearance, removal during hemodialysis is the primary route of elimination for magnesium in patients with renal failure.

Because the ideal serum magnesium concentration in patients with ESRD is debatable, the appropriate dialysate magnesium concentration is unresolved. Many centers use a 1.0-mEq per L dialysate magnesium concentration.

CHLORIDE. Chloride is the major anion in the dialysate. Because of the constraint of maintaining electrical neutrality in the dialysate, chloride concentration is determined by the concentration of cations.

Dialysates and Replacement Fluid for Continuous Renal Replacement Therapy

Typical dialysate flow rates for continuous hemodialysis or hemodiafiltration are 800 to 1,000 mL per hour (vs. 500 to 800 mL per minute for conventional hemodialysis), and the dialysate is usually delivered into the dialyzer by a continuous infusion pump. The principal mechanism for solute clearance in techniques using hemofiltration convection. To achieve adequate solute clearance, the ultrafiltration volume is large (12 to 24 L per day), making fluid replacement obligatory for CAVH, CVVH, CAVHDF, and CVVHDF. Because the composition of the ultrafiltrate is similar to that of the aqueous phase of plasma, the ideal replacement solution should approximate the normal plasma composition minus the solutes that need removal. Standard peritoneal dialysis solutions have been used in many centers as dialysate or replacement solution for CRRT. Because of the risk of hyperglycemia, it has been recommended that solutions based on supraphysiologic concentrations of glucose should be avoided [122]. Various standard commercial fluids are available now for use as dialysates or replacement fluids in CRRT. Some are lactate-based (Hemofiltration solution, Baxter Healthcare Corporation, IL, U.S.A.; Hemosol, Hospal, Lyon, France) while others are bicarbonate-based (Prismasate, Gambro Renal Products, Lakewood, CO, U.S.A.; Accusol, Baxter Healthcare Corporation, IL, U.S.A.; Normocarb, Dialysis Solution Inc., Richmond, OH, U.S.A.). Compared to bicarbonate-based buffer, lactate buffer is associated with more hemodynamic instability [123]. Bicarbonate buffer is also preferred in patients with lactic acidosis, hepatic failure, and in patients who needs high-volume hemofiltration. Even with the availability of various commercial solutions with different compositions, customized dialysates and replacement fluid is required in some situations. Trisodium citrate used in regional citrate anticoagulation requires the replacement fluid or dialysate to have little or no alkali supplement. Consequently, custom replacement

fluid is prepared with trisodium citrate as the source for base [124].

On-site replacement solutions can be made by the addition of various solutes to standard intravenous dextrose 5% water or saline. The single-bag approach is easiest, in which bicarbonate is mixed with calcium and magnesium. Because of the potential for solute precipitation, single bags have limited use. Alternately, bicarbonate can be prepared separately from the calcium- and magnesium-containing solutions, and the two bags of replacement solutions can be infused sequentially or concurrently through different infusion ports.

Anticoagulation for Intermittent Hemodialysis

Despite the impaired capacity of platelets to aggregate and adhere in most patients with advanced renal failure, the interaction of plasma with the dialysis membrane results in activation of the clotting cascade, thrombosis in the extracorporeal circuit, and the resultant dysfunction of the dialyzer [125]. Dialyzer thrombogenicity is determined by its composition, surface charge, surface area, and configuration [126]. In addition, the propensity for intradialytic clotting is influenced by the blood flow through the dialyzer; the extent of blood recirculation in the extracorporeal circuit (newly dialyzed blood reentering the dialyzer); the amount of ultrafiltration; and the length, diameter, and composition of the lines between the patient and the dialyzer. Patient-specific variables that influence thrombogenicity and determine the requirements for anticoagulants include the presence of congestive heart failure, malnutrition, neoplasia, blood transfusions, and comorbid coagulopathies such as disseminated intravascular coagulation, warfarin therapy, or hepatic synthetic dysfunction.

Because of its low cost, ready availability, ease of administration, simplicity of monitoring, and relatively short biologic half-life, unfractionated heparin is the most widely used anticoagulant for dialysis. The time constraints of hemodialysis are such that the partial thromboplastin time cannot be used to monitor the effectiveness of anticoagulation. Instead, an activated clotting time (ACT) is often used. In this assay, whole blood is mixed with an activator of the extrinsic clotting cascade, such as kaolin, diatomaceous earth, or ground glass, and the time necessary for the blood to first congeal is monitored. The normal range is 90 to 140 seconds.

The precise method of heparin administration is influenced by the patient's comorbid illness and varies among dialysis providers. The simplest method of heparin administration is systemic administration, in which 2,000 to 5,000 U of heparin are administered at the initiation of dialysis followed by a constant infusion of 1,000 U per hour. The target ACT is approximately 50% above baseline. Another method of systemic anticoagulation is to administer repeated boluses of heparin (100 U per kg of dry weight at the start) when the ACT falls below target.

Use of low-molecular-weight heparin (LMWH) as a source of anticoagulation has become quite widespread. Several forms of LMWH have been used as anticoagulant in hemodialysis. Elimination of LMWH is impaired in renal failure. Pharmacokinetic studies of several LMWH in hemodialysis patients revealed that a single dose of dalteparin, enoxaparin, and danaparoid provided adequate anticoagulation during the duration of hemodialysis without any significant adverse effects [127]. Mean doses of LMWH in the study are dalteparin, 39 U per kg; enoxaparin, 0.70 mg per kg; and danaparoid, 35 U per kg. These doses are significantly less than the recommended doses used in patients with normal renal function. In a prospective, randomized, crossover trial, single-dose enoxaparin sodium is found to be an effective, convenient, albeit costly, alternative to unfractionated heparin in intermittent hemodialysis patients [128].

Because the degree of anticoagulation during systemic anticoagulation is relatively intensive, it is appropriate only for stable patients who are at no risk for bleeding. Therefore, in the ICU, systemic anticoagulation is rarely used. Less intensive anticoagulation is achieved with fractional heparinization, in which the target ACT is maintained at 15% ("tight fractional") or 25% ("fractional") greater than the baseline value. Five hundred to 3,000 U of heparin are administered at the initiation of dialysis, followed by a continuous heparin infusion at an initial rate of 500 to 1,000 U per hour.

Heparin exposure may be minimized with "regional" heparinization. By this method, the extracorporeal circuit alone is anticoagulated with heparin and the effect is reversed before the extracorporeal blood is returned to the patient [129]. Problems associated with this method of anticoagulation include complexity of balancing the infusion rate, bleeding from rebound anticoagulation because of the dissociation of the heparin–protamine complex [130], and side effects of protamine (flushing, bradycardia, dyspnea, and hypotension). Alternatively, regional anticoagulation may be achieved with sodium citrate as the anticoagulant [131]. Citrate binds to calcium and forms a dialyzable salt, thereby depleting the extrinsic and intrinsic clotting cascades of the obligatory cofactor, calcium. A 4% solution of trisodium citrate is initially infused into the arterial line at 200 mL per hour, and the infusion rate is adjusted after 20 minutes to maintain the ACT of the machine at 25% over baseline. This process is reversed on the venous side distal to the filter by infusion of 10% calcium chloride at 30 mL per hour. Although very effective [131,132], the principal disadvantages of this technique are the requirements for additional infusions and close monitoring of the patient's calcium and acid-base status (as citrate is metabolized to generate bicarbonate, increasing the risk of alkalemia). Imbalance of ionized calcium associated with citrate anticoagulation can lead to cardiac arrest and death in extreme cases [133]. The dialysate used in citrate regional anticoagulation must be calcium-free with lower sodium and bicarbonate concentration.

Regional anticoagulation can be associated with significant and relatively frequent side effects [134]. In high-risk situations in which regional anticoagulation may be contraindicated (e.g., heparin-induced thrombocytopenia, allergy to protamine, unfamiliarity of personnel with technique), dialysis may be performed without heparin [134–137]. In this technique, the hemodialyzer is first rinsed with 1 L of 0.45% saline containing 3,000 to 5,000 U of heparin. Hemodialysis is immediately initiated using the maximum blood flow tolerated, and the dialyzer is flushed every 15 to 30 minutes with 50 mL of saline. Although not feasible with large-volume ultrafiltration, compromised blood flow, or the intradialytic administration of blood products, heparin-free dialysis may be the safest choice for any ICU patient at risk of bleeding. Intermittent hemodialysis without heparin in ICU patients does not appear to affect the solute clearance.

Anticoagulation must be individualized based on the patient's risk of hemorrhage. Clearly, the risk of thrombosis of the dialytic circuit is a secondary consideration. Guidelines for anticoagulation based on comorbid conditions are as follows:

- Patients who are bleeding, or at significant risk of bleeding, have a baseline major thrombostatic defect, are within 7 days of a major operative procedure or within 14 days of intracranial surgery should be dialyzed without heparin or by regional anticoagulation.
- Patients who are within 72 hours of a needle or forceps biopsy of a visceral organ should be dialyzed without heparin or by regional anticoagulation.
- Patients who are beyond the temporal limits established for the first two items can be dialyzed with fractional heparinization. If they have previously received fractional heparinization without incurring morbidity, they can now be considered for systemic anticoagulation.
- Patients with pericarditis should be dialyzed without heparin or by regional anticoagulation.
- Patients who have undergone minor surgical procedures within the previous 72 hours should be dialyzed under fractional anticoagulation.
- Patients anticipated to receive a major surgical procedure within 8 hours of hemodialysis should be dialyzed without heparin or by regional anticoagulation. If they are within 8 hours of a minor procedure, fractional anticoagulation is appropriate.
- Dialysis patients who developed heparin-induced antibody can be treated with direct thrombin inhibitors such as argatroban or danaparoid for intradialytic anticoagulation [136,137].

ANTICOAGULATION FOR CONTINUOUS RENAL REPLACEMENT THERAPY

The need for anticoagulation in CRRT is driven by its relatively low blood flow rate (100 to 150 mL per minute) and prolonged continuous exposure of blood to the dialyzer membrane. Thus, even by modifying the procedure to minimize thrombogenicity (using relatively short arterial and venous lines, changing to a parallel-plate configuration for the hemofilter, performing predilutional hemofiltration), heparin is usually required [138]. Predictably, aggressive ultrafiltration that results in hemoconcentration, reduced blood flows, and blood passage through long venous lines creates a very thrombogenic environment within the hemofilter and venous side of the blood circuit. In CRRT, the required intensity of anticoagulation usually is similar to that associated with systemic heparinization for hemodialysis. After a systemic loading dose of heparin, an initial maintenance infusion of approximately 10 U per kg per hour is administered and titrated to maintain the partial thromboplastin time in the arterial line 50% greater than control. Obviously, such concentrated heparinization compromises the use of this technique for patients at risk for bleeding.

Alternatives to the standard systemic heparinization technique described here have been proposed for patients at high risk of bleeding. These include citrate regional anticoagulation [139,140] and use of heparin with protamine [141]. Two prospective randomized trials compared regional citrate anticoagulation to systemic heparin anticoagulation in CRRT patients [142,143]. Both trials demonstrated the superiority of citrate anticoagulation over heparin in terms of filter survival time and prevention of bleeding. As in intermittent hemodialysis, in patients with CVVH, dalteparin, a LMWH is found to be effective, safe but more costly alternative to unfractionated heparin [144].

CRRT modalities can be performed without anticoagulation, although this usually compromises the performance of the hemofilter, necessitating that it be replaced frequently. This technique involves rinsing the kidney and lines with heparinized saline in the method described for heparin-free hemodialysis [145].

Thrombosis within the hemofilter is easy to recognize by the characteristic striped clotting of the usually white fibers within the hollow-fiber dialyzer. However, the parallel-plate configuration is assembled in such a manner that the interior of the hemofilter cannot be visualized. In this circumstance, clotting of the hemofilter can be defined inferentially by the decline in the ultrafiltration rate, decrease in dialysate urea nitrogen-to-BUN ratio (less than 0.6 is significant), or both [146].

Hemodialysis Angioaccess

An adequately functioning angioaccess is a prerequisite for any extracorporeal blood-purification technique. There are two categories of access-related issues in the intensive care setting: ESRD patients with established permanent access and patients with ARF requiring temporary angioaccess for hemodialysis or CRRT.

The vascular access of choice for maintenance hemodialysis patients is the endogenous arteriovenous native vein fistula. This is because of its ease of construction, long-term survival, and lower incidence of infection compared with other modalities of vascular access [147]. Many patients with ESRD, particularly older and diabetic patients, do not have adequate arterial or venous anatomy to allow the creation of a native fistula. Many patients with ESRD do not have adequate arterial or venous anatomy; in these patients, a prosthetic arteriovenous fistula or arteriovenous graft is implanted. Relevant to care within the ICU, it should be appreciated that acute thrombosis of either a native vein or graft fistula may occur from intravascular volume depletion secondary to overzealous ultrafiltration, systemic hypotension from a comorbid condition like sepsis, or excessive local pressure for hemostasis after removal of the hemodialysis needles. Judicious care must be taken to preserve patency of these fistulas, especially prohibiting their use for routine cannulation or phlebotomy, measurement of blood pressure, or subjection to constricting dressings or tourniquets.

The type of angioaccess needed for dialysis in the setting of ARF in the ICU is determined by the chosen modality of dialytic therapy. If hemodialysis is adopted, a venous catheter will suffice. If CRRT is preferred, there is the option of using arteriovenous or venovenous methods. The latter is currently favored because it allows direct regulation of blood flow and, consequently, higher blood flows can be achieved relatively independent of the mean arterial pressure [148]. Higher blood flows also permit less intense anticoagulation because they minimize clotting of the extracorporeal circuit. Acute angioaccess for hemodialysis or venovenous CRRT may be achieved with vascular catheters. Vascular complications such as aneurysm, bleeding, and limb ischemia are less likely to occur with a venous access [149,150]. The oldest and safest means of establishing angioaccess for hemodialysis is to place a single- or double-lumen coaxial catheter in the femoral vein by the Seldinger technique [151]. The incidence of serious complication from femoral vein dialysis catheters is only 0.2% [152]. Femoral vein catheters are available in a number of lengths and diameters. To prevent blood recirculation, the 24-cm length is preferable so that the tip of the catheter is in the inferior vena cava.

Alternative sites for catheter-based angioaccess are the subclavian or internal jugular veins. Right internal jugular catheters provide superior blood flow compared to left ones. Because of higher rates of stenosis, subclavian vein catheters should be avoided if possible, especially in patients who might require permanent arteriovenous dialysis access in the future. Compared with the femoral vein, internal jugular vein catheters have the advantages of fewer local infections, longer local positioning, enhanced patient mobility [152], and less catheter malfunction [153]. Early catheter complications such as local bleeding, hemothorax, pneumothorax, hemopericardium [154], arrhythmia [155], and hemomediastinum are usually related to catheter insertion. Internal jugular catheters are best placed under ultrasound guidance to minimize insertion-related complications [156]. Even though anatomical variations of the femoral veins are rare, in certain circumstances (e.g., very obese patients or those without a palpable femoral artery or who have had previous femoral catheterization or surgery) sonographic localization should be considered for catheter insertion [157]. Late-occurring complications such as arteriovenous fistula formation, local catheter infection or sepsis [158], central vein thrombosis or stenosis [159], and catheter malfunction are particularly vexing. Infectious complications are a function of the duration of catheter usage. The risk of infection is found to increase exponentially for femoral catheters between the first and second weeks, and for internal jugular catheter between the third and fourth weeks. Femoral catheters should thus be removed or changed after 1 week and internal jugular catheters after 3 weeks [160]. The typical pathogenesis of catheter infections involves migration of bacteria down the catheter sheath to colonize the skin adjacent to the catheter entry site [161]. This may be discouraged by the use of topical antibiotics like mupirocin [156]. When an infection occurs, the usual therapy is 10 to 14 days of systemic antibiotics and removal of the dialysis catheter. Suppurative thrombophlebitis and endocarditis require prompt discontinuation of the catheter and 4 to 6 weeks of bactericidal antibiotics. Central venous thrombosis (which occurs more commonly with subclavian vein catheters) necessitates immediate removal of the catheter [162]. Use of povidone and mupirocin in dry-gauze dressings in patients with acute dialysis catheter have been shown to decrease the risk of bacteremia.

Inadequate or absent blood flow results in catheter malfunction. It is most often secondary to intraluminal thrombosis or catheter malposition. Thrombolytics such as tissue plasminogen activator have been used successfully for restoration of blood flow in thrombosed dialysis catheters [163,164]. If thrombolytic therapy fails to restore flow, the catheter may be malpositioned. The catheter can be threaded with a guidewire, removed, and a replacement catheter repositioned.

Site-specific instructions for placing venous catheters via the Seldinger technique can be found in Chapter 2.

Hemofiltration Angioaccess

The techniques used to establish venous access for CVVH or CVVHD are exactly as described previously. The principal advantage of an arteriovenous access for CRRT (CAVH) is that it allows the use of a very simple extracorporeal circuit without a blood pump or an air embolus monitor. On the other hand, arteriovenous circuits require the placement of an additional catheter for arterial access. There are only two forms of arteriovenous access: wide-bore single-lumen femoral artery and vein catheters and, much less commonly, the Scribner shunt (an external plastic arteriovenous fistula). Scribner shunts should not be placed in patients with peripheral vascular disease who may develop digital ischemia. The proper technique for femoral artery cannulation is described in Chapter 3.

PERITONEAL DIALYSIS

Dialysates

Compared with the dialysates used for hemodialysis or hemofiltration, the composition of the dialysates used for peritoneal dialysis is relatively constant (see Table 25-2). Hypokalemia in patients on maintenance peritoneal dialysis is usually managed by increasing the dietary potassium intake. If oral therapy is ineffective or unfeasible, potassium can be added to the dialysate to attenuate the diffusive gradient. A typical potassium concentration in the dialysate is 1 to 4 mEq per L. The dialysate calcium concentration varies from 2.5 to 3.5 mEq per L; the choice of dialysate calcium depends on the patient's propensity to develop hypercalcemia. The other electrolyte present in the dialysate is chloride, the concentration of which is determined solely by the requirements to achieve electrical neutrality.

Ultrafiltration during peritoneal dialysis is achieved by the infusion of a hyperosmolal dialysate. Dextrose in concentrations of 1.5%, 2.5%, or 4.25% is used to induce ultrafiltration. Because the osmotic gradient is less with a 1.5% dextrose-containing dialysate than with a 4.25% dialysate, the fall-off in ultrafiltration develops relatively sooner using the 1.5% dextrose solution. Likewise, if the osmotic gradient is attenuated by the development of hyperglycemia, ultrafiltration will decline. Therefore, in peritoneal dialysis patients with glucose intolerance, ultrafiltration with dialysates containing high levels of glucose may be compromised if glycemic control is not maintained. A glucose polymer, icodextrin, is being used in peritoneal dialysis solutions for chronic peritoneal dialysis patients with ultrafiltration difficulties [165]. Icodextrin has a molecular weight of 17,000 Da and acts as a colloid osmotic agent. Because of slower absorption of icodextrin, it is able to maintain the osmotic gradient for longer period of time than dextrose containing dialysate. So far, its effectiveness in ARF patients has not been evaluated.

Access to the Peritoneal Cavity

Immediate access for peritoneal dialysis may be provided in the acute setting by the percutaneous placement of a stylet-guided, rigid, uncuffed catheter connected to a closed-gravity, manual instillation drainage system or to an automated dialysate cycler.

The procedure for placement of a temporary peritoneal dialysis catheter is as follows:

1. The urinary bladder is emptied to prevent inadvertent perforation.
2. The abdomen is prepared with povidone-iodine solution and draped, as it would be for an abdominal paracentesis.
3. A point one third of the distance between the umbilicus and symphysis pubis is infiltrated with local anesthetic to the peritoneum.

4. To distend the peritoneum, 1 to 2 L of 1.5% dextrose peritoneal dialysate is introduced into the peritoneal cavity via a 16-gauge spinal needle or Angiocath (Becton, Dickinson and Company, Franklin Lakes, NJ).
5. A small puncture is made at the same site with a scalpel blade.
6. The stylet-guided catheter is inserted into the skin puncture site and passed through the skin, underlying fascia, and linea alba. Entry of the catheter tip into the peritoneum is evident by a sudden reduction in resistance and by appearance of dialysis fluid in the transparent catheter.
7. If cloudy or feculent fluid is withdrawn, the bowel has been punctured [166], and the dialysis catheter should be left in place until a decision is made regarding the need for a diagnostic procedure (e.g., contrast computed tomography). Intravenous antibiotics to cover bowel bacteria (e.g., gentamicin and metronidazole or ampicillin-sulbactam) should be started. If peritoneal dialysis is to be continued, another access site should be chosen, and the process repeated. If the peritoneal drainage is clear, the stylet is withdrawn until the obturator point meets the catheter tip. The catheter is then advanced into the posteroinferior area of the peritoneal cavity and connected to a closed-gravity manual instillation drainage system or to an automatic cycler.
8. The catheter may finally be secured to the skin with a superficial purse-string suture.

Although simple to insert and position in the peritoneal cavity, patients must remain supine, and the risk of infection is so great that the uncuffed catheters must be removed after 48 to 72 hours [167]. If dialysis is required for more than 72 hours, a new site should be selected and the original catheter removed.

An alternative means of establishing access into the peritoneal cavity with much greater permanency, and one that permits patient ambulation, is to install a flexible Silastic catheter with one or two Dacron cuffs. The most frequently used dual-cuffed catheter is the Tenckhoff catheter, which has an open end and multiple holes in the distal 15 cm of the catheter. The catheter cuffs minimize bacterial migration down the catheter tract. Such catheters are not only highly desirable for ESRD patients on continuous peritoneal dialysis but also in the ARF population, if the expected duration of dialytic support by peritoneal dialysis is more than 2 weeks.

Placement of stylet-guided temporary catheters can be difficult and dangerous in patients who have intraabdominal adhesions, which usually result from prior abdominal surgery. Adhesions may cause compartmentalization of dialysate in the peritoneal cavity, greatly impeding inflow and outflow of dialysate, even with a properly positioned catheter. Adhesions also decrease the membrane surface area available for solute clearance and ultrafiltration. For this reason, peritoneal dialysis is not generally offered to patients with renal failure who have had previous major abdominal surgery and likely have intraabdominal adhesions.

Catheter malfunction, manifested by slow dialysate instillation, drainage, or both, may be caused by catheter malpositioning (catheter tip migration, entrapment in adhesions, or kinking) or luminal obstruction (blood clot, fibrin, or incarcerated omentum). An initial approach to this problem is to obtain an abdominal plain radiograph to determine the position of the catheter tip. If appropriately positioned, a thrombolytic may be instilled into the catheter [168]. After the liquid is aspirated, an exchange may be attempted. If catheter dysfunction continues, it should be replaced. Catheter exit site infection, as evident by local redness and drainage, needs to have antibiotic treatment and usually does not mandate a change of catheter to a new exit location. More extensive infections, such as tunnel infection with or without peritonitis, obligate removal of the catheter and transient substitution of peritoneal dialysis with another dialytic modality.

Effectiveness of Peritoneal Dialysis in Acute Renal Failure

Advantages of peritoneal dialysis in ARF include easy and quick implementation, nonreliance on vascular access and systemic anticoagulation, and avoidance of hemodynamic instability. Considering that a 24 L per day exchange of 1.5% dextrose-containing dialysate typically results in a urea clearance of approximately 17 mL per minute, peritoneal dialysis is a low-efficiency procedure. Therefore, it is not surprising that this technique may be inappropriate for management of hyper-catabolic patients with ARF. As a result, despite the theoretical advantages, use of peritoneal dialysis for ARF is becoming less frequent in developed countries [169]. But it remains an important modality of dialysis in developing countries [170]. The spectrum of ARF cases in developed countries has changed over the years. Increasingly, ICUs are faced with patients with ARF in the setting of sepsis, multiorgan dysfunction syndrome, and complicated underlying diseases and hypercatabolic state. These patients require significant volume and solute removal beyond the capability of low-efficiency peritoneal dialysis. Different peritoneal dialysis regimens with automated machine have been tried to improve its efficiency. In a crossover trial of 87 mild-to-moderate hypercatabolic patients with ARF, high-flow tidal peritoneal dialysis was able to provide adequate solute clearance [170].

To achieve negative fluid balance with peritoneal dialysis in hypercatabolic patients, exchanges with high dextrose-containing dialysate are often required. Absorption of high-dextrose dialysate will result in hyperglycemia and increased CO_2 production with worsening of respiratory failure. In-creased abdominal pressure-associated peritoneal dialysis can also compromise pulmonary function, especially in patients who already have respiratory failure. A prospective study of patients with ARF associated with systemic infection showed superiority of CVVHDF over peritoneal dialysis in terms of patient survival and correction of azotemia and acidosis [171].

For many adults on maintenance peritoneal dialysis, the contribution of residual renal function to solute clearance is critical for achieving adequate peritoneal dialysis. In a peritoneal dialysis patient, the loss of residual renal function due to a severe comorbid illness or nephrotoxic medication such as an aminoglycosides may render a previously satisfactory dialysis regimen inadequate. Such patients should have their daily number of exchanges increased empirically or they should be switched to hemodialysis.

SELECTED ISSUES IN DIALYTIC THERAPY FOR ACUTE RENAL FAILURE

MEMBRANE BIOCOMPATIBILITY IN HEMODIALYSIS

The development of a wide array of dialyzers allows an easier selection to fulfill the dialytic solute and ultrafiltration needs of the patient. However, with the advent of these newer membranes, an added criterion for selection of membranes in the management of ARF and the ESRD population is its *biocompatibility* [172]. The interaction of both soluble and cellular components of the blood with the dialysis membrane may influence the length of recovery from acute ischemic renal failure [173]; incidence of dialysis-associated symptoms and signs such as fever, hypotension, and hypoxemia [174–177]; and immunologic dysfunction and infectious susceptibility [178–180].

A plethora of alterations in cellular functions and physiologic responses has been described in association with hemodialysis using cellulosic-based membranes. These findings are listed in Table 25-3. Membranes without these proinflammatory effects are described as *biocompatible*. Another aspect of biocompatibility is the ability of the membrane to adsorb activated proinflammatory substances from the blood. Highly adsorptive membranes can efficiently reduce levels of factor D (an essential enzyme of the alternative pathway activation) [192], bradykinin, and

TABLE 25-3. Evidence of Bioincompatibility (Proinflammatory) Effects of Conventional Dialysis Membranes

Proinflammatory Reactant or Function	Finding	Reference
C3a and C5a	Increased intradialytic generation in vivo	181
Leukocyte adhesion molecules	Induction of increased expression in vivo	182,183
Reactive oxygen species	Increased production by granulocytes in vivo	184
Coagulation pathway	Increased activation in vitro	185
Kallikrein-kinin system	Increased activity in vitro	186
Cytokines, including IL-1, IL-6, tumor necrosis factor	Increased production by monocytes in vitro and in vivo	187–189
IL-2 receptor	Altered expression in vivo	190
Monocyte function	Altered phagocytic activity in vitro	191
Natural killer cell function	Altered in vitro	191

IL, interleukin.

pyrogenic cytokines such as interleukin (IL)-1 and tumor necrosis factor.

Dialyzer membranes composed of bioincompatible materials are typically derived from cellulose, whereas biocompatible membrane dialyzers are usually synthetic materials, such as polysulfone, polymethylmethacrylate, polyamide, or polyacrylonitrile. Many adverse pathobiologic consequences of hemodialysis that arise from membrane interactions are thought to be attenuated by using biocompatible membranes. This has led to an increased preference for these membrane materials for dialyzers in maintenance hemodialysis. Because of the high ultrafiltration requirement for CRRT, and the inability of cellulosic dialyzers to fulfill this requirement, CRRT is always performed with highly porous biocompatible dialyzers.

Several reviews have examined the impact of dialysis membrane type on outcome in patients with ARF [193–198]. Based on in vitro models of ischemic ARF [199] and several in vivo interventional trials, the use of biocompatible membranes has been espoused to enhance patient survival, expedite recovery from ARF, and diminish the need for dialytic support [200,201]. However, those reports are not uniform; more recent studies failed to show any superiority of biocompatible membrane [202–205]. Study addressing patient symptoms such as hypotensive episodes, angina, and bronchospasm during hemodialysis have not demonstrated any difference between membrane types [206]. Although catabolic effects were demonstrated in experimental single hemodialysis sessions with bioincompatible membranes, a long-term study found an increase in serum albumin in both groups of patients treated with biocompatible and bioincompatible membranes [207]. In the same study, flux characteristics of the membranes were not found to have a significant effect on nutritional parameters. Because of the inconsistent nature of the available evidence, it is not justifiable to exclude bioincompatible membrane dialyzers categorically in the treatment of patients with ARF [208,209]. However, with the reduction in cost differential between bioincompatible and biocompatible dialyzers, there are less persuasive economic reasons to use bioincompatible membranes in ARF [210].

DOSE OF DIALYSIS

As is true for maintenance peritoneal and hemodialysis, the amount of solute clearance provided during ARF likely affects outcomes [211]. As previously described, using urea as a surrogate uremic toxin, the amount of urea removed can be quantitated by various methods such as Kt/V, URR and SRI (the actual amount of urea removed). For maintenance hemodialysis patients, a URR of less than 60% to 65% and Kt/V less than 1.2 is associated with an increased odds risk of death [212,213]. A similar dose-response relationship for ARF patients on dialysis has not been validated.

In an outcome analysis of patient survival with ARF, the mean delivered Kt/V was significantly higher among survivors (0.90 ± 0.04 vs. 0.76 ± 0.05) [214]. However, it was observed that the quantity of hemodialysis exerted no influence for the highest and lowest patient disease severity quartiles but did have an impact on the survival of patients with moderate severity scores. It is not surprising that the amount of dialysis would have no discernible influence when extreme disease severity and comorbidity are the competing risks. Similarly, in a retrospective review of 844 ARF patients requiring hemodialysis during a period of 7 years, dialysis dose did not affect survival in patients with very low and high severity of disease [215]. However, dialysis dose did correlate with survival in patients with intermediate severity of disease. A mean Kt/V greater than 1.0 and time-averaged BUN clearance (TAC$_{UREA}$) less than 45 mg per dL was associated with improved survival. In a randomized controlled trial of ARF patients treated with CRRT, higher intensity CVVH (filtration rate of 35 mL per kg per hour and 45 mL per kg per hour) was associated with improved survival compared to lower intensity CVVH (filtration rate of 20 mL per kg per hour) [216]. Another randomized controlled trial of high and low doses of CVVH failed to replicate these results [66]. Three CRRT modalities were used in the study in 106 severely ill ARF patients, early initiation of high-volume CVVH (72 to 96 L per 24 hours), early initiation of low-volume CVVH (24 to 36 L per 24 hours) and late initiation of low-volume CVVH (24 to 36 L per 24 hours). No difference was found among the groups regarding course or outcome. The study was underpowered and raised questions about patient selection criteria.

In the first prospective study of dialysis dose in ARF patients treated with intermittent hemodialysis, higher dialysis dose with daily intermittent hemodialysis improved survival compared to alternative-day intermittent hemodialysis [217]. Patients with daily intermittent hemodialysis received significantly higher weekly delivered dialysis dose (Kt/V 5.8 ± 0.4) compared to patients with alternate-day intermittent hemodialysis (Kt/V 3.0 ± 0.6). Although several questions have been raised about the study (patient recruitment, power, dosing level comparisons), this was the first study to prospectively help recognize a potential relationship between dialysis dose and patient outcome in intermittent hemodialysis patients with ARF. Results of these trials are being more rigorously tested in an ongoing, multicenter, randomized control trial, the Veterans Affairs/National Institutes of Health Acute Renal Failure Trial Network Study [218]. Higher dialysis dose in the study is delivered with 6-times-a-week intermittent hemodialysis in hemodynamically stable patients, and CVHDF rate of 35 mL per kg per hour or 6 times a week slow low-efficiency dialysis in hemodynamically, unstable patients. Lower dialysis dose is delivered with similar modalities, but intermittent hemodialysis and slow low-efficiency dialysis are provided 3 times week, and CVVHDF is provided with rate of 20 mL per kg per hour. There is inadequate information to recommend a *minimum* or optimal delivered dose of hemodialysis in ARF. However, there is no reason to anticipate that the delivered hemodialysis dose should be less than a Kt/V of 1.2 or URR of 65%, as recommended for maintenance hemodialysis patients.

CONTINUOUS VERSUS INTERMITTENT DIALYTIC THERAPY

Advocates of CRRT espouse several putative advantages of CRRT over intermittent hemodialysis. Fluid removal is a common reason for initiating dialysis in ARF, and this can easily be achieved by either CRRT or hemodialysis. However, because of its intermittent nature, significant volume expansion can occur between hemodialysis treatments, especially if the patient is receiving parenteral nutrition. In contrast, CRRT allows precise hourly adjustments of the ultrafiltration rate that readily permits the removal of more than 10 L per day. Because ultrafiltration with CRRT is gradual, hemodynamic stability may be more readily maintained. Therefore, a principal advantage of CRRT is that it permits the allocation of nutrition with less concern for volume overload [219]. Similarly, the continuous dynamic nature of CRRT may allow better correction of azotemia and acidemia [220]. Seven hours of daily intermittent hemodialysis are necessary to achieve similar levels of urea clearance as CRRT [221]. In a comparison between CVVH and hemodialysis in patients with ARF, CRRT provided better control of azotemia for equal amounts of therapy [222].

Sepsis syndrome and multiorgan failure in association with ARF augur a poor outcome, perhaps related to the activity of proinflammatory substances such as activated complement fragments, platelet-activating factor, arachidonic acid metabolites, kinins, selected cytokines, and proteases [223,224]. It has been speculated that CRRT may improve patient outcomes by removing these inflammatory mediators in sepsis and multiorgan failure syndrome with renal failure. Several human studies demonstrated that hemofiltration removes inflammatory mediators like tumor necrosis factor, IL-1β, IL-6, platelet-activating factor, and complement fragments from circulation [225,226]. The mechanism of removal is through convective clearance or by the adsorption to the hemofilter membrane. Clinical studies in patients with ARF have revealed that higher doses of convective clearance (45 mL per kg per hour) enhanced survival of patients with sepsis compared to lower doses (20 mL per kg per hour) [227].

Despite these advantages, CRRT has not been demonstrated to be of added benefit over conventional dialysis in improving patients' outcomes. Several prospective randomized trials tried to demonstrate differences in clinical outcomes. In a multicenter, randomized, controlled trial of 166 patients with ARF, treatment by intermittent hemodialysis resulted in lower mortality (41.5%) compared with CVVHDF (59.5%) [227]. However, patients randomized to CVVHDF had more severe disease. After statistical adjustment for this difference, both groups had similar mortality. A single-center prospective study of CVVH versus intermittent hemodialysis was done with 80 ARF patients [228]. Patients in the two groups had similar severity of illness score and received same dialysis dose (goal Kt/V, 3.6 per week). Even though patients treated with CVVH achieved greater volume control and hemodynamic stability, there was no benefit in terms of survival or renal recovery compared to that of intermittent hemodialysis. A similar study of ARF patients treated with CVVHDF and intermittent hemodialysis found no difference in ICU and hospital mortality [229].

Most of the trials comparing CRRT and intermittent hemodialysis have had problems with either improper randomization, inadequate number of subjects, or inability to blind the trials. Open design of the trials also could contribute to the bias, as hemodynamically unstable patients are more likely to be treated by CRRT rather than conventional hemodialysis. Therefore, the inability to demonstrate a favorable effect on mortality for CRRT may be a consequence of patient selection bias (i.e., treatment by indication), which biases toward the null. The possibility also exists that CRRT may have deleterious consequences, and thus contribute to competing risks. For example, adverse effects may be produced by eliminating beneficial cytokines such as, IL-1 receptor antagonist, IL-10 (peptides with antagonistic effects against IL-1), and tumor necrosis factor [230].

There are operational drawbacks in the use of CRRT. These include the greater need for anticoagulation, increased frequency of access-related problems due to its continuous use, intensive nursing support requirements, lack of mobility for the patient (not a consideration if the patient is ventilated), slower onset of removal of electrolytes in emergent cases, and cost, which is estimated to be 2.5 times that of conventional hemodialysis.

A hybrid technique known as extended daily dialysis uses the advantages of two forms of renal replacement therapies [231]. The process involves longer duration (8 to 12 hours) of daily hemodialysis using low blood and dialysate flow rates, and low ultrafiltration using a conventional hemodialysis machine. In a prospective randomized trial of 39 critically ill patients with oliguric ARF, extended daily dialysis provided similar solute clearance, correction of acidosis, and hemodynamic stability as CVVH [232].

NUTRITION

The importance of adequate nutrition in patients with ESRD and chronic kidney disease has been strongly stated [233–235]. Critically ill patients with ARF are at high risk for malnutrition, in part because of reduced nutritional intake and also hypercatabolic processes, such as sepsis, glucocorticoid therapy, surgical trauma, and especially multiple organ failure [236]. Dialysis itself may adversely affect nutritional status; amino acids and water-soluble vitamins are readily removed with dialysis. CRRT has been shown to affect amino acid loss with risk of negative nitrogen balance [237]. Both CVVHDF and CVVHD have been imputed. One specific effect of CRRT on amino acid pool is the disproportionate loss of the amino acid, glutamine [238,239]. Glutamine is needed for protein production and is the major intracellular amino acid-regulating signal trafficking of proteins. Peritoneal dialysis also causes substantial protein losses, far more so than conventional hemodialysis or CRRT. Apart from protein removal from the body, the process of hemodialysis causes catabolism, leading to a net loss of protein stores [240]. This is found to be true irrespective of the membranes used in hemodialysis.

In past years, protein intake was severely restricted in patients with ARF in an effort to reduce uremic symptoms. However, institution of adequate nutritional support has appropriately become standard practice. In a prospective randomized trial of 50 ARF patients on CRRT, protein intake of 2.5 g per kg per day increased the likelihood of achieving positive nitrogen balance and improving the patient's survival [241]. This and other prospective trials found no risk from this high level of protein delivery [242]. As stated earlier, dialysis should be initiated relatively early for ARF to permit adequate nutritional support, especially in catabolic patients. Dialysis should be prescribed as needed to control azotemia without compromising nutrition, even if treatments are prolonged (5 to 6 hours) or more frequent (four to six per week). Current recommendations for nutrition in patients with ARF include enteral and parenteral administration of 25 to 30 kcal per kg day of energy and 1.2 to 1.5 g of protein per kg per day [243].

DISCONTINUING DIALYSIS

Recovery from ARF usually occurs within 4 weeks, but may take 6 to 8 weeks if a severe insult has occurred or if preexisting renal insufficiency was present. It is imperative to periodically examine factors that may be associated with functional recovery. Generally, a urine output of less than 0.75 L per day is insufficient to provide clearance of obligate solute. However, the urine output alone cannot be used to gauge the safety of discontinuing dialysis, particularly in critically ill patients. This aspect of care must be individualized, balancing the risks of holding renal replacement therapy against the benefit and risks of continued dialysis, which includes the reduced chance for recovery of renal function with continued therapy.

Several laboratory parameters may provide clues that renal function is returning. A urine osmolality dissimilar to that of plasma or a specific gravity of greater than 1.020 or less than 1.010 indicates the ability of the kidney to concentrate or dilute the urine, a capacity lost when renal tubular function is severely impaired. Paradoxically, the BUN concentration may increase during recovery because of improved tubular reabsorptive capacity. As renal function improves, the serum creatinine concentration typically plateaus or slowly decreases. If the interdialytic rate of rise of the serum creatinine concentration is progressively less, renal function may be improving. If the serum creatinine concentration decreases between dialysis treatments and the patient is not threatened by volume overload or metabolic complications, dialysis should be withheld and the patient followed carefully.

Discontinuing dialysis because of a patient's relentlessly declining overall condition is far more challenging because of the frequent uncertainty in defining the patient's prognosis [244]. In most critically ill patients who develop ARF, the extent of comorbid disease (e.g., sepsis, cardiac failure, and surgical trauma) determines the clinical outcome. Withdrawing dialysis may be appropriate when further aggressive care is ineffective but will almost certainly hasten death. In one study of severe ARF patients requiring renal replacement therapy, renal replacement therapy was withdrawn in more than 70% of patients who subsequently died. Like most ethical dilemmas encountered by ICU staff, the care of the dying patient must be individualized to reflect the wishes of the patient or his or her designated advocate [244]. It is imperative to fully inform the patient or his or her health care proxy, or both, of the potential risks and benefits of dialysis before it is begun. In cases in which the patient, his or her health proxy, and the proximate caregivers are ambivalent because of an uncertain outcome, it may be helpful to recommend a trial of dialysis for a defined period. After this time, the patient's clinical condition can be reassessed and the decision to proceed with additional dialysis treatments readdressed. The institution of dialysis does not mandate that this intervention be continued indefinitely. Many patients agree to short-term dialysis therapy but elect a priori to decline chronic dialysis if it is later deemed necessary, based on quality of life considerations. A thoughtful, realistic, and compassionate approach to the patient with ARF should allow the patient, his or her family, and physicians to share in decision-making.

MATCHING THE DIALYSIS MODALITY TO THE PATIENT

There is no consensus as to the definitive dialysis modality for a particular clinical situation [245,246]. We offer these guidelines based on our experiences and our assessment of the available evidence (Table 25-4):

- If a large volume of fluid removal is required, hemodialysis or CRRT is the preferred treatment. In situations in which

TABLE 25-4. Considerations Relevant to the Selection of a Dialysis Modality

Patient-specific	*Dialysis-specific*
Residual renal function	Membrane composition
Cardiovascular status	Membrane surface area
Pulmonary status	Ultrafiltration coefficient
Volume status	Dialysate composition
Volume load	Sodium
Medications	Potassium
Comorbid conditions	Base
Surgery	Calcium
Myocardial or coronary disease	Dextrose
Coagulopathy	Magnesium
Hemorrhage	Blood and dialysate flow
Sepsis	Dialysis duration and frequency
Arrhythmias	Dialysate volume[a]
Malnutrition	Angioaccess
Diabetes mellitus	Peritoneal access[a]
Burns	Anticoagulation
Vasculopathy	

[a]Applicable to peritoneal dialysis only.

the expected ultrafiltration volume is more than 10% of the body weight, CRRT should take precedence.
- If solute clearance is the main consideration, hemodialysis or CRRT is the choice. Note that CAVHDF and CVVHDF achieve the greatest solute clearance with time.
- If rapid fluid or solute correction is needed (such as for hyperkalemia), hemodialysis is the most efficient in the shortest amount of time.
- If anticoagulation is contraindicated, heparin-free hemodialysis (for those with high demands for clearance) or peritoneal dialysis (for those with lower demands for clearance) would be appropriate.
- If the patient is hemodynamically unstable, peritoneal dialysis is the safest option. CRRT may be considered as an alternative.
- If vascular access cannot be established, peritoneal dialysis is the only option.
- Because of its restrictions on mobility, CRRT may present more of a problem for conscious patients.
- In neurosurgical patients or patients with hepatic coma and cerebral edema, CRRT and peritoneal dialysis are less likely to increase intracerebral pressure further by inducing osmotic dysequilibrium [247,248].
- In hypercatabolic patients who require large fluid volumes for nutritional support, CRRT is advantageous.
- If dialysis nursing support is not available, peritoneal dialysis is the simplest to manage.
- Hemodialysis is most efficient for rapid removal of drug or toxin

Regardless of the dialysis modality selected, it is vital that the full range of dialysis techniques is available. The selection of one form of therapy does not preclude change to another when the dynamics of the clinical condition alter.

TABLE 25-5.   Dialysis Complications

Hemodialysis	Hemofiltration
Hypotension	Bleeding
Cramps	Thrombosis of hemofilter
Bleeding	Technical mishaps
Leukopenia	Incorrect dialysate mixture,
Arrhythmias	incorrect replacement
Infections	solution, contaminated
Hypoxemia	dialysate, air embolism
Pyrogen reactions	Hemolysis
Dialysis dysequilibrium	Angioaccess dysfunction
syndrome	Hypotension
Angioaccess dysfunction	Congestive heart failure
Technical mishaps	Peritoneal dialysis
Incorrect dialysate	Peritonitis
mixture, contaminated	Catheter infections
dialysate, air embolism,	Catheter dysfunction
spallation	Abdominal pain
	Visceral perforation
	Pleural effusion
	Respiratory failure
	Technical mishaps
	Inappropriate dialysate
	composition, contaminated
	dialysate

SELECTED COMPLICATIONS OF DIALYSIS

CONVENTIONAL HEMODIALYSIS

Complications from hemodialysis may arise from ultrafiltration, solute clearance, or technical variances (Table 25-5).

Cardiovascular Complications

Hypotension during hemodialysis is a common complication. There are many factors that may play a role in the pathophysiology of intradialytic hypotension [249]. These complications are listed in Table 25-6. Intradialytic hypotension is typically ascribed to excessive ultrafiltration (frank intravascular volume depletion resulting in diminished left ventricular filling pressure) or to an excessive rate of ultrafiltration (volume removal from the intravascular space at a rate that exceeds the capacity of interstitial fluid to migrate into this compartment). Common additional

TABLE 25-6.   Pathophysiology of Hypotension during Hemodialysis

Contributing Factors	*Probable Mechanism(s)*
Hypovolemia	Excessive fluid removal or ultrafiltration at a rate exceeding that at which interstitial fluid moves to intravascular space; hemorrhage
Reduced cardiac output	Systolic or diastolic left ventricular dysfunction due to drugs or comorbid conditions; pericardial disease
Autonomic dysfunction	Associated with uremia, comorbid states (e.g., diabetes mellitus), certain medications (e.g., beta-blockers)
Reduced vascular tone	Associated with certain medications (e.g., narcotic analgesics) and with comorbid states such as sepsis
Response to dialysis system	Acetate, low calcium, low sodium in dialysate; bioincompatible dialyzer membranes

contributory factors include left ventricular dysfunction (systolic or diastolic secondary to comorbid illness or medications), autonomic dysfunction (secondary to disease processes or medications), lack of pressor hormone stimulation, inappropriate vasodilatation (secondary to sepsis, medications), disease of the pericardium or the pericardial space, and bleeding. It is important to appreciate that other critical components of the dialysis procedure may contribute to the development of hypotension. These include the choice of dialysate (buffer, sodium, and calcium concentration), dialyzer membrane composition, and porosity. Specific provocative issues are the (a) vasodilatory and cardiodepressant effects of acetate; (b) impairment of vasoconstriction, exacerbation of autonomic dysfunction, and declining serum osmolality with a hyponatremic dialysate; (c) vasodilatory and cardiodepressant effects of a lowered calcium dialysate; (d) cellulosic membrane-induced complement activation; (e) cellulosic membrane-induced or acetate-induced hypoxemia; (f) complement or pyrogen-induced production of proinflammatory cytokines; and (g) immediate hypersensitivity of dialysis membrane mediated by kallikrein/bradykinin activation.

Preemptive strategies should be taken to prevent hypotension in the setting of hemodialysis [250]. In intermittent hemodialysis, real-time changes in dialysate sodium with sodium balance-neutral sodium profiles in combination with ultrafiltration profiles help to prevent intradialytic hypotension-related discomforts as well as less sodium and weight gain [251]. Hemodialysis in acute setting should have higher calcium dialysate (3.5 mEq per L) to prevent hemodynamic instability [252]. Use of isothermic (adjusting dialysis temperature to keep body temperature unchanged) or hypothermic dialysis helps to prevent the risk of symptomatic hypotension during hemodialysis [253]. Cooler dialysate results in increased myocardial contractility [254] and peripheral vasoconstriction [255]. The ultrafiltration rate (as calculated to achieve the estimated dry weight) should be closely regulated, and a volumetric-controlled machine is preferable. The time on dialysis can be increased if large-volume ultrafiltration is desired (decreased rate of ultrafiltration) and sequential ultrafiltration clearance can be instituted to give better cardiovascular tolerance. The use of a biocompatible dialyzer membrane may provide additional benefit, as discussed earlier. Antihypertensive medications should be withheld before each treatment in patients prone to hypotension during dialysis. Hypotension is managed acutely by intravenous infusion of saline [256], hypertonic saline, dextran [257], or albumin. Ultrafiltration rate should be transiently reduced with continuation of hemodialysis. In hemodynamically unstable patients, inotropic agents and supplemental oxygen may be required. Other potential causes of low blood pressure during hemodialysis should be considered, such as myocardial ischemia with left ventricular dysfunction, arrhythmias, and pericardial tamponade from hemorrhage and bleeding.

Dialysis-associated arrhythmias occur most often in patients with comorbid cardiovascular disease, cardiac glycoside administration, a concurrent rapid decline in plasma potassium concentration, or a combination of these factors [258]. In high-risk patients, the dialysate potassium concentration should be increased to 3 to 4 mEq per L. Interdialytic hyperkalemia can be managed by more frequent dialysis treatments or the supplemental administration of Kayexalate, if not contraindicated because of gastrointestinal dysfunction. Myocardial ischemia and hypoxemia must be ruled out and treated if present.

Dialysis Dysequilibrium

The *dialysis dysequilibrium syndrome* is an admixture of neurologic symptoms and signs associated with the excessive removal of solute that occurs with the initiation of hemodialysis or in the setting of a dramatic increase in the amount of hemodialysis delivered to a chronically poorly dialyzed patient. The precise pathobiology of this disorder is undefined but seems to center about an increase in intracerebral pressure [259], which has been attributed to a combination of reduced expression of urea transporter and increased expression of aquaporin in brain cells [260]. During rapid solute clearance with hemodialysis, urea departure from the cerebrospinal fluid is delayed. The brain becomes relatively hyperosmolal, and water shifts into the brain [261]. The intracerebral accumulation of organic osmolytes, such as inositol, glutamine, and glutamate in the brain [262], is an adaptation to the hyperosmolality in chronic azotemia. These osmolytes further contribute to the discrepancy in osmolality during rapid hemodialysis. These alterations result in paradoxic intracerebral swelling. Because such adaptation occurs less in ARF, dialysis dysequilibrium is uncommon in this setting. The clinical manifestations may range from mere headache and nausea to disorientation, seizures, coma, and even death, when especially severe [263].

The simplest way to prevent dialysis dysequilibrium is to slow solute clearance during hemodialysis by using a smaller surface area dialyzer, decreasing blood and dialysate flows, circulating the blood and dialysate in a concurrent direction, and decreasing the duration of dialysis. Alternatively, dialysis can also be initiated using peritoneal dialysis or CVVH with less solute clearance. Additional preventive strategies include the intradialytic administration of mannitol or dextrose or the use of a high sodium- or urea-containing dialysate [264]. The use of a high-sodium dialysate appears to be the most effective strategy. The intent is to minimize the decline in serum osmolality by using urea or substituting another osmolyte for urea. Finally, in high-risk patients who require aggressive solute clearance, the patient should receive a loading dose of phenytoin before the initiation of hemodialysis, and a maintenance dose should be continued during the subsequent 72 hours as a full dialysis schedule is achieved. Once dialysis dysequilibrium has developed, therapy consists of administration of anticonvulsants and reducing cerebral edema by inducing hyperventilation and administering mannitol. Neurosurgical patients with stable ESRD treated by hemodialysis may exhibit a similar propensity to develop cerebral edema, and caution should be undertaken in performing hemodialysis in this group of patients [265].

Hypoxemia

In some hemodialysis patients, a 5- to 35-mm Hg decline in arterial oxygen tension is observed. For most patients, this decline in arterial oxygen tension is usually of no clinical significance. However, in critically ill, nonventilated patients with preexisting respiratory and cardiac compromise, this decline in O_2 tension can result in overt respiratory failure, CNS hypoxemia, cardiac arrhythmias, hypotension, or a combination of these. Dialysis-associated hypoxemia appears to result from the interaction of the dialysate, dialysis membrane, lungs, and respiratory control center. As discussed earlier in this chapter, with acetate-based dialysates, CO_2 is cleared from the blood into the dialysate.

The dialysance of CO_2 results in hypocapnia, which causes compensatory hypoventilation and hypoxemia (normocapnic hypoventilation) [266]. Less contributory to the development of dialysis-associated hypoxemia is the interaction between blood complement and selected dialysis membrane materials. Cellulosic membrane materials activate complement by the alternate pathway, giving rise to anaphylatoxins that alter pulmonary regional ventilatory and perfusion patterns [267]. In addition, leukocyte interactions with the dialysis membrane enhance cell membrane expression of selected leukocyte adhesion molecules, causing leukocyte pulmonary sequestration [268]. Modifications of the hemodialysis procedure that minimize this complication include the use of a bicarbonate-based dialysate containing 30 to 35 mEq per L and use of a biocompatible dialysis membrane material. Patients at high risk should have their inspired oxygen concentration empirically increased during the hemodialysis treatment.

Technical Errors

Because intradialytic treatment monitoring techniques have improved, technical mishaps that compromise patient safety (such as air emboli, hemolysis, and misformulated dialysate) are now remarkably uncommon. As discussed earlier, pyrogen reactions are a persistent and vexing problem that result from the development of high-porosity dialysis membranes and ultrafiltration controllers, combined with the greatly increased utility of bicarbonate-based dialysates. Arguably, strict adherence to prescribed guidelines for water and dialysate purity can minimize this occurrence [269]. In the case of a suspected pyrogen reaction, blood cultures should be performed, and the patient should be treated with systemic antibiotics until the possibility of septicemia has been eliminated.

CONTINUOUS RENAL REPLACEMENT THERAPY

Technical evolution and increased experience have made CRRT a well-tolerated therapy with low complication rates. The most frequent complications are those related to vascular access and the need for intensive anticoagulation. Less frequently, problems arise from balancing ultrafiltration and clearance needs. Complications from establishing and maintaining angioaccess have been previously discussed.

Bleeding is the most vexing problem encountered with CRRT techniques. Its risk is increased by the continuous need for anticoagulation during CRRT. Bleeding may be internal (gastrointestinal, intracerebral, or both) or localized to the catheter insertion site. Although not typically life-threatening, infection of a hematoma or distortion and compression of vascular anatomy can be problematic if protracted dialysis is needed. An infected hematoma may lead to sepsis in a critically ill patient.

Because automated safeguards are fewer with CRRT and replacement solutions are often needed, the potential for error is greater than with intermittent hemodialysis. A vigilant and experienced staff is mandatory. A host of metabolic abnormalities may develop as a consequence of variances in the replacement solution or the dialysate. For example, if CAVH is performed in the absence of a bicarbonate-containing replacement solution, severe hyperchloremic metabolic acidosis can develop. Excessive solute replacement can result in hypernatremia, metabolic alkalosis, hyperkalemia, hypercalcemia, and hypermagnesemia. Inadequate solute replacement may cause hyponatremia, hyperchloremic metabolic acidosis, hypokalemia, hypocalcemia, and hypomagnesemia. The removal of phosphate is usually substantial in CRRT and may necessitate replacement.

Techniques like CRRT, which depend on convective clearance, obligate the formation of large volumes of ultrafiltrate and require the administration of a replacement fluid. This must be done with precision because errors can result in gross fluid imbalances of both extremes. Changes in key hemodynamic parameters (central venous pressure, mean arterial pressure, pulmonary artery wedge pressure) should prompt reassessment and changes to the prescriptions. Adequate patient and techni-

cal surveillance can prevent this problem. A meticulously maintained flow chart, recording the progress of the procedure and displaying an ongoing ledger of the patient's fluid balance, is absolutely essential.

PERITONEAL DIALYSIS

The most common complication of peritoneal dialysis is peritonitis, which is reviewed in detail elsewhere [270]. Although peritonitis may occur as a consequence of bacteremia, it usually results from introduction of bacteria through the catheter

TABLE 25-7. Summary of Evidence-Based Conclusions in Dialysis Therapy

Topic	Finding	Reference
Does prophylactic RRT reduce risk of ARF?	In a small randomized trial, preoperative HD given to CKD patients undergoing CABG surgery was associated with fewer cases of postoperative ARF, less mortality, shorter hospital stay than without HD.	43
	In another trial, patients with CKD experienced reduced incidence of ARF from CVVH given around time of radiocontrast exposure.	44
	In three other studies, patients receiving HD during or after radiocontrast exposure had no reduction of incidence of ARF.	45–47
Does timing of initiation of RRT influence outcomes in ARF?	In a small ($n = 18$), prospective, randomized trial with trauma patients, early HD (at BUN <70 mg/dL) associated with better survival than later treatment.	57
	In a similar but larger ($n = 106$) study in patients, no difference in mortality or recovery from ARF seen between early vs. late treated patients.	58
	In studies of early vs. late institution of CVVHD in the settings of cardiac surgery or liver failure, earlier treatment led to better outcomes.	59
Does adjustment of dialysate potassium concentration influence morbidity in ARF patients being dialyzed?	In a randomized, prospective trial, less ventricular ectopic activity occurred in patients receiving modeled potassium concentration during HD treatments than in patients receiving treatment with dialysate containing a fixed concentration of potassium.	103
Are "biocompatible" dialyzer membranes better tolerated or associated with better outcomes in ARF than conventional membranes?	Results of randomized, controlled trials have been inconclusive. Some trials have shown better outcomes with biocompatible than with cellulosic membranes.	200–201
	Other trials have failed to demonstrate any difference in outcomes or tolerability between membrane types.	202–207
Does intensity of RRT affect outcome in ARF?	*CRRT*	
	In a randomized, controlled trial, ARF patients undergoing CVVH received either a high or lower intensity ultrafiltration protocol. Survival was better in the more aggressively treated group.	216
	A second similar study failed to find any difference, but raised methodologic questions.	66
	IHD	
	In a prospective trial, ARF patients treated with daily HD had better survival rates than alternate-day IHD. Further corroboration of this study is being sought in a larger study in progress.	217
Does continuous RRT offer an advantage over IHD?	In a multicenter, randomized trial involving 166 ARF patients, no difference was found in survival between patients treated with IHD and patients treated with CVVHD when group data were adjusted for case severity.	227
	In a separate single-center, prospective study ($n = 80$), no difference was found in outcome of patients receiving CVVH vs. IHD.	228
	A similar study comparing CVVHD with IHD also yielded no significant difference in survival rates.	229
Should protein intake be adjusted in ARF?	In a randomized trial in 50 patients undergoing CRRT for ARF, a higher protein intake (2.5 g/kg/d) offered significant metabolic and survival benefits.	241

ARF, acute renal failure; BUN, blood urea nitrogen; CABG, coronary artery bypass graft; CKD, chronic kidney disease; CRRT, continuous renal replacement therapy; CVVD, continuous venovenous hemofiltration; CVVHD, continuous venovenous hemodiafiltration; HD, hemodialysis; IHD, intermittent HD; RRT, renal replacement therapy.

during an exchange or from bacterial migration along the catheter tunnel. The incidence of peritonitis has declined, predominantly because of equipment advances [271]. The diagnosis of bacterial peritonitis is not difficult. Symptoms and signs of fever, abdominal pain and tenderness, and cloudy dialysate effluent are noted within 6 to 24 hours of the provoking event. In acute peritoneal dialysis, with its typically rapid cycling and short dwell times, dialysate turbidity may be less apparent. The peritoneal fluid white blood cell count of more than 100 cells per μL with at least 50% polymorphonuclear leukocytes indicates presence of infection in peritoneal dialysis patients. Routine sentinel cell counts and cultures of dialysate fluid may help detect early infections. Antibiotics should be initiated while awaiting definitive culture results. *Staphylococcus aureus* and *Staphylococcus epidermidis* account for more than 50% of the cases of bacterial peritonitis, although polymicrobial [272] and fungal infections should not be discounted in the ICU. Appropriate antibiotics may be administered intraperitoneally [270]. Initial coverage for Gram-positive and Gram-negative organisms is recommended, to be modified pending culture results. A popular regimen consists of vancomycin, 2 g intraperitoneally, repeated every 7 days for duration of treatment or until culture results dictate otherwise, along with levofloxacin, 250 mg orally or intravenously. Daily peritoneal fluid white blood cell count with differential should be done to follow the response to therapy. Resistant or recurrent peritonitis may necessitate removal of the catheter for the duration of treatment [273]. In some severe cases of peritonitis, discontinuation of peritoneal dialysis should be considered.

Common metabolic abnormalities associated with peritoneal dialysis are hyperglycemia, hyper- and hyponatremia, hypokalemia, and hypercalcemia. Insulin may be required for adequate glycemic control, and hypokalemia can be corrected with addition of potassium into the dialysate.

Less common, but with devastating ramifications, is hydrothorax, which may occur in approximately 5% of patients [274] and results from tracking of dialysate through a rent in the diaphragm and into the pleural space. The diagnosis is straightforward with thoracocentesis; the pleural fluid has a high glucose and urea content. At the very least, hydrothorax should prompt a reduction in dwell volume. Placing the patient in reverse Trendelenburg position may reduce the tendency of dialysate to leak into the chest cavity. If these measures fail to control the problem, changing to another dialytic modality is recommended.

BIOARTIFICIAL KIDNEY

A novel device based on tissue engineering in a continuous hemofiltration modality is under study in ARF patients [275]. A renal tubule-assist device (RAD) is incorporated in a CVVHF circuit in addition to the usual hemofiltration dialyzer. A RAD comprises a commercial hemofiltration unit, in which human renal tubule cells have been grown to confluence along the inner surface of the hollow fibers. Early clinical trials with RAD and CVVHF in humans with ARF demonstrated an additional effect of reduction in inflammatory cytokines as well as a survival benefit [276].

Advances in dialysis therapy, based on randomized, controlled trials or metaanalyses of such trials, are summarized in Table 25-7.

REFERENCES

1. Addison T: On the disorders of the brain connected with diseased kidneys. *Guys Hosp Rep* 4:1, 1839.
2. Bright R: Cases and observations illustrative of renal disease 77 accompanied with the secretion of albuminous urine. *Guys Hosp Rep* 1:338, 1836.
3. Tyson J: Acute parenchymatous nephritis. *Boston Med Surg J* 111:193, 1884.
4. Kolff WJ: *The Artificial Kidney* [dissertation]. Groningen, The Netherlands, University of Groningen, 1946.
5. Teschan PE: Hemodialysis in military casualties. *Trans Am Soc Artif Int Organs* 2:52, 1955.
6. Scribner BH, Buri R, Caner JEZ, et al: The treatment of chronic uremia by means of intermittent dialysis: a preliminary report. *Trans Am Soc Artif Int Organs* 6:114, 1960.
7. Odel HM, Ferns DO, Power H: Peritoneal lavage is an effective means of extra renal excretion. *Am J Med* 9:63, 1950.
8. Tenckhoff H, Schechter H: A bacteriologically safe peritoneal access device. *Trans Am Soc Artif Intern Organs* 14:181, 1968.
9. Popovich RP, Moncrief JW, Decherd JB, et al: The definition of a novel portable/wearable equilibrium dialysis technique [abstract]. *Trans Am Soc Artif Intern Organs* 5:64, 1976.
10. Evanson JA, Himmelfarb J, Wingard R, et al: Prescribed versus delivered dialysis in acute renal failure patients. *Am J Kidney Dis* 32:832, 1998.
11. Lowrie E, Lew N: The urea reduction ratio (URR): a simple method for evaluating hemodialysis treatment. *Contemp Dial Nephrol* 12:11, 1991.
12. Evanson JA, Ikizler TA, Hakim RH: Measurement of the delivery of dialysis in acute renal failure. *Kidney Int* 55:1501, 1999.
13. Himmelfarb J, Evanson E, Hakim RH, et al: Urea volume of distribution exceeds total body water in patients with acute renal failure. *Kidney Int* 61:317, 2002.
14. Ikizler TA, Sezer MT, Flakoll PJ, et al, for the PICARD study group: Urea space and total body water measurements by stable isotopes in patients with acute renal failure. *Kidney Int* 65:725, 2004.
15. Kanagasundaram NS, Greene T, Larive AB, et al, on behalf of the PICARD study group: Prescribing an equilibrated intermittent hemodialysis dose in intensive care unit acute renal failure. *Kidney Int* 64:2298, 2003.
16. Dulaney JT, Hatch FE: Peritoneal dialysis and loss of proteins: a review. *Kidney Int* 26:253, 1984.
17. Brouns R, De Deyn PP: Neurological complications in renal failure: a review. *Clin Neruol Neurosurg* 107:1, 2004.
18. Locke S, Merrill JP, Tyler HR: Neurologic complications of acute uremia. *N Engl J Med* 108:75, 1961.
19. Drueke T, Le Pailleur C, Zingraff J, Jungers P: Uremic cardiomyopathy and pericarditis. *Adv Nephrol* 9:33, 1980.
20. Zakynthinos E, Theodorakopoulou M, Zakynthinos S, et al: Hemorrhagic cardiac tamponade in critically ill patients with acute renal failure. *Heart Lung* 33:55, 2004.
21. Allon M: Hyperkalemia in end stage renal disease: mechanisms and management. *J Am Soc Nephrol* 6:1134, 1995.
22. Bastl C, Hayslett JP, Binder HJ: Increased large intestinal secretion of potassium in renal insufficiency. *Kidney Int* 12:9, 1977.
23. Kunis CL, Lowenstein J: The emergency treatment of hyperkalemia. *Med Clin North Am* 65:165, 1981.
24. Allon M, Shanklin N: Effect of bicarbonate administration on plasma potassium in dialysis patients: interactions with insulin and albuterol. *Am J Kidney Dis* 28:508, 1996.
25. Weiner DI, Wingo CS: Hyperkalemia: a potential killer. *J Am Soc Nephrol.* 9:1535, 1998.
26. Van Ypersele de Strihou C, Frans A: The pattern of respiratory compensation in chronic uremic acidosis. *Nephron* 7:37, 1970.
27. Garella S: Extracorporeal techniques in the treatment of exogenous intoxication. *Kidney Int* 33:735, 1988.
28. Mbane B, Borron SW, Baud FJ: Current recommendations for treatment of severe toxic alcohol poisonings. *Intensive Care Med* 31:189, 2005.
29. Gonda A, Gault H, Churchill D, et al: Hemodialysis for methanol intoxication. *Am J Med* 64:749, 1978.
30. Peterson CD, Collins AJ, Himes JM, et al: Ethylene glycol poisoning: pharmacokinetics during therapy with ethanol and hemodialysis. *N Engl J Med* 304:21, 1981.
31. Davidson MB, Thakkar S, Schreiber MJ, et al: Pathophysiology, clinical consequences, and treatment of tumor lysis syndrome. *Am J Med* 116:546, 2004.
32. Kjellstrand CM, Campbell DC, von Hartitzch B, et al: Hyperuricemic acute renal failure. *Arch Intern Med* 133:349, 1974.
33. Randall RE, Cohen MD, Spray CC: Hypermagnesemia in renal failure. *Ann Intern Med* 61:73, 1964.
34. Remuzzi G: Bleeding in renal failure. *Lancet* 1:1205, 1988.
35. Livio M, Gotti E, Marchesi D, et al: Uremic bleeding: role of anemia and beneficial effect of red cell transfusion. *Lancet* 2:1013, 1982.
36. Escolar G, Cases A, Bastida E, et al: Uremic platelets have a functional defect affecting the interaction of von Willebrand factor with glycoprotein IIb–IIIa. *Blood* 76:1336, 1990.
37. Nenci G, Berrittini M, Agnelli G, et al: The effect of peritoneal dialysis, hemodialysis, and kidney transplantation on blood platelet function. Platelet aggregation to ADP and epinephrine. *Nephron* 23:287, 1979.
38. Janson PA, Jubeliere SJ, Weinstein MJ, et al: Treatment of the bleeding tendency in uremia with cryoprecipitate. *N Engl J Med* 308:8, 1980.
39. Mannucci PM, Remuzzi G, Pusineri F, et al: Deamino-8-D-arginine vasopressin shortens the bleeding time in uremia. *N Engl J Med* 308:8, 1983.
40. Moia M, Vizzotto L, Cattaneo M, et al: Improvement of the hemostatic defect of uraemia after treatment with recombinant human erythropoietin. *Lancet* 2:1227, 1987.
41. Livio M, Mannucchi PM, Bignano G, et al: Conjugated estrogens for the management of bleeding associated with renal failure. *N Engl J Med* 315:731, 1986.

42. Lohr JW, Schwab SJ: Minimizing hemorrhagic complications in dialysis patients. *J Am Soc Nephrol* 2:961, 1991.

43. Durmaz I, Yagdi T, Engin C: Prophylactic dialysis in patients with renal dysfunction undergoing on-pump coronary artery bypass surgery. *Ann Thorac Surg* 75:859, 2003.

44. Marenzi G, Marana I, Bartorelli A, et al: The prevention of radiocontrast-agent-induced nephropathy by hemofiltration. *N Eng J Med* 349:1333, 2003.

45. Frank H, Werner D, Ludwig J: Simultaneous hemodialysis during coronary angiography fails to prevent radiocontrast induced nephropathy in chronic renal failure. *Clin Nephrol* 60:176, 2003.

46. Vogt B, Ferrari P, Schönholzer C, et al: Prophylactic hemodialysis after radiocontrst media in patients with renal insufficiency is potentially harmful. *Am J Med* 111:692, 2001.

47. Hsieh YC, Ting CT, Liu TJ, et al: Short- and long-term renal outcomes of immediate prophylactic hemodialysis after cardiovascular catheterizations in patients with severe renal insufficiency. *Int J Cardiol* 101:407, 2005.

48. Conger JD: Does hemodialysis delay recovery from acute renal failure? *Semin Dial* 3:146, 1990.

49. Solez L, Morel-Maroger L, Sraer J: The morphology of acute tubular necrosis in man: analysis of 57 renal biopsies and comparison with the glycerol model. *Medicine* 58:362, 1979.

50. Yeh BPY, Tomki DJ, Stacy WK, et al: Factors influencing sodium and water excretion in uremic man. *Kidney Int* 7:103, 1975.

51. Ogata K: Clinicopathological study of kidneys from patients on chronic dialysis. *Kidney Int* 37:1333, 1990.

52. Rottermbourg J: Residual renal function and recovery of renal function in patients treated by CAPD. *Kidney Int* 43[Suppl 40]:S106, 1993.

53. Conger JD, Robinette JB, Schrier RW: Smooth muscle calcium and endothelial-derived relaxing factor in abnormal vascular responses of acute renal failure. *J Clin Invest* 82:532, 1988.

54. Hakim RM: Clinical implications of hemodialysis membrane biocompatibility. *Kidney Int* 44:484, 1993.

55. Lynn RI, Feinfeld DA: Importance of residual renal function in end-stage renal disease. *Semin Dial* 2:1, 1989.

56. Teschan PE, Baxter CR, O'Brien TF, et al: Prophylactic hemodialysis in the treatment of acute renal failure. *Ann Intern Med* 53:992, 1960.

57. Conger JD: A controlled evaluation of prophylactic dialysis in post-traumatic acute renal failure. *J Trauma* 15:1056, 1975.

58. Bouman CSC, Oudemans-van Straaten HM, Tijssen JGP, et al: Effects of early high-volume continuous venovenous hemofiltration on survival and recovery of renal function in intensive care patients with acute renal failure: a prospective, randomized trial. *Crit Care Med* 30:2205, 2002.

59. Demirkiliç U, Kuralay E, Yenicesu M, et al: Timing of replacement therapy for acute renal failure after cardiac surgery. *J Card Surg* 19:17, 2004.

60. Tsai HB, Wu VC, Yang MT, et al: Outcome in the acute liver failure patients treated with renal replacement therapy for acute renal failure: comparison between early or late dialysis [abstract]. *J Am Soc Nephrol* 16:540A, 2005.

61. Babb AL, Farrell P, Uvelli DA, et al: Hemodialyzer evaluation by examination of solute molecular spectra. *Trans Am Soc Artif Int Organs* 18:98, 1972.

62. Asaba H, Bergstrom J, Furst P, et al: Sequential ultrafiltration and diffusion as alternatives to conventional hemodialysis. *Proc Clin Dial Transplant Forum* 6:29, 1976.

63. Bradley JR, Evans DB, Cowley AJ: Comparison of vascular tone during haemodialysis with ultrafiltration and during ultrafiltration followed by haemodialysis: a possible mechanism for dialysis hypotension. *BMJ* 19:300, 1990.

64. Forni LG, Hilton PJ: Continuous hemofiltration in the treatment of acute renal failure. *N Engl J Med* 336:1303, 1997.

65. Geronemus R, von Albertini B, Glabman S, et al: Enhanced molecular clearance in hemofiltration. *Proc Clin Dial Transplant Forum* 8:47, 1985.

66. Mehta RL: Continuous renal replacement therapy in the critically ill patient. *Kidney Int* 67:781, 2005.

67. Brandes J, Emerson P, Campbell D, et al: The relationship between body size, fill volume and mass transfer area coefficient in PD [abstract]. *Am Soc Nephrol* 3:407, 1992.

68. Schonfeld P, Diaz-Buxo JA, Keen M, et al: The effect of body position, surface area (BSA), and intraperitoneal exchange volume (Vip) on the peritoneal transport constant [abstract]. *Am Soc Nephrol* 4:416, 1993.

69. Henderson LW: Peritoneal ultrafiltration dialysis. Enhanced urea transfer using hypertonic peritoneal dialysis fluid. *J Clin Invest* 45:950, 1966.

70. Nolph KD, Ghods AJ, Van Stone JC: The effects of intraperitoneal vasodilators on peritoneal clearances. *Trans Am Soc Artif Int Organs* 22:586, 1976.

71. Nolph KD, Ghods AJ, Brown PA: Effects of intraperitoneal nitroprusside on peritoneal clearances with variations in dose, frequency of administration, and dwell times. *Nephron* 24:4, 1979.

72. Miller FN, Nolph KD, Harris PD: Microvascular and clinical effects of altered peritoneal solutions. *Kidney Int* 15:630, 1979.

73. Grzegorzewska AE, Moore HL, Nolph KD, et al: Ultrafiltration and effective peritoneal blood flow during peritoneal dialysis in the rat. *Kidney Int* 39:608, 1991.

74. Clark WR, Gao D: Properties of membranes used for hemodialysis therapy. *Semin Dial* 15:191, 2002.

75. Schiffl H, Lang SM, Konig A, et al: Biocompatible membranes in acute renal failure: prospective case controlled study. *Lancet* 344:570, 1994.

76. Himmelfarb J, Rubin NT, Chandran P, et al: A multicenter comparison of dialysis membranes in the treatment of acute renal failure requiring dialysis. *J Am Soc Nephrol* 9:257, 1998.

77. Mion CM, Canaud B, Francesqui MP, et al: Bicarbonate concentrate: a hidden source of microbial contamination of dialysis fluid. *Blood Purif* 7:32, 1987.

78. Tielemans C, Madhoun P, Lenaers P, et al: Anaphylactoid reactions during hemodialysis on AN69 membranes in patients receiving ACE inhibitors. *Kidney Int* 38:982, 1990.

79. Mendelssohn S, Swartz CD, Yudis M, et al: High glucose concentration dialysate in chronic hemodialysis. *Trans Am Soc Artif Int Organs* 13:249, 1967.

80. Ward RA, Walthen RL, Williams TE, et al: Hemodialysate composition and intradialytic metabolic, acid-base, and potassium changes. *Kidney Int* 32:129, 1987.

81. Arem R: Hypoglycemia. *Endocrinol Metab Clin North Am* 18:103, 1989.

82. Grajower MM, Walter L, Albin J: Hypoglycemia in chronic hemodialysis patients: association with propranolol use. *Nephron* 26:126, 1980.

83. Kopple JD, Swendseid ME, Shinaberger JH, et al: The free and bound amino acids removed by hemodialysis. *Trans Am Soc Artif Int Organs* 19:309, 1973.

84. Ganda OP, Aoki TT, Soeldner JS, et al: Hormone-fuel concentrations in anephric subjects: effects of hemodialysis (with special references to amino acids). *J Clin Invest* 57:1403, 1976.

85. Locatelli F, Covic A, Yaqoob M, et al: Optimal composition of the dialysate, with emphasis on its influence on blood pressure. *Nephrol Dial Transplant* 19:785, 2004.

86. Stiller S, Bonnie-Scorn E, Mann H, et al: A critical review of sodium profiling for hemodialysis. *Semin Dial* 14:337, 2001.

87. Raja RM: Sodium profiling in the elderly hemodialysis patients. *Nephrol Dial Transplant* 11[Suppl 8]:42, 1996.

88. Palmer BF: The effect of dialysate composition on systemic hemodynamics. *Semin Dial* 5:54, 1992.

89. Raja R, Kramer M, Barber K, et al: Sequential changes in dialysate sodium during hemodialysis. *Trans Am Soc Artif Int Organs* 29:649, 1983.

90. Paganini EP, Sandy D, Moreno L, et al: The effect of sodium and ultrafiltration modelling on plasma volume changes and hemodynamic stability in intensive care patients receiving hemodialysis for acute renal failure: a prospective, stratified, randomized, cross-over study. *Nephrol Dial Transplant* 11[Suppl 8]:32, 1996.

91. Oliver ML, Edwards LJ, Churchill DN: Impact of sodium and ultrafiltration profiling on hemodialysis-related symptoms. *J Am Soc Nephrol* 12:151, 2001.

92. Ketchersid TL, Van Stone JC: Dialysate potassium. *Semin Dial* 4:46, 1991.

93. Feig PU, Shook A, Sterns RH: Effect of potassium removal during hemodialysis on the plasma potassium concentration. *Nephron* 27:25, 1981.

94. Hou S, McElroy PA, Nootes S, et al: Safety and efficacy of low potassium dialysate. *Am J Kidney Dis* 13:137, 1989.

95. Ozuer M, Aksoy, Dortlemez O, et al: Effects of cardioselective (β1) and nonselective (both β1 and β2) adrenergic blockade on serum potassium in patients with chronic renal failure undergoing hemodialysis. *Kidney Int* 26:584, 1984.

96. Zehnder C, Gutzwiller JP, Schneditz D, et al: Low-potassium and glucose-free dialysis mainitains urea but enhances potassium removal. *Nephrol Dial Transplant* 16:78, 2001.

97. Heguilén RM, Sciurano C, Bellusci AD, et al: The faster potassium-lowering effect of high dialysate bicarbonate concentrations in chronic hemodialysis patients. *Nephrol Dial Transplant* 20:591, 2005.

98. Redaelli B, Sforzini B, Bonoldi L, et al: Potassium removal as a factor limiting the correction of acidosis during dialysis. *Proc EDTA-ERA* 19:366, 1982.

99. Dolson GM, Ellis KJ, Bernardo MV et al: Acute decrease in serum potassium augment blood pressure. *Am J Kidney Dis* 26:321, 1995.

100. Morrison G, Michelson EL, Brown S, et al: Mechanism and prevention of cardiac arrhythmias in chronic hemodialysis patients. *Kidney Int* 17:811, 1980.

101. Cupisti A, Galetta F, Caprioli R, et al: Potassium removal increases the QTc interval dispersion during hemodialysis. *Nepron* 82:122, 1999.

102. Lorincz I, Matyus J, Zilahi Z, et al: QT dispersion in patients with end-stage renal failure and during hemodialysis. *J Am Soc Nephrol* 10:1297, 1999.

103. Redaelli B, Locatelli F, Limido D, et al: Effect of a new model of hemodialysis potassium removal to the control of ventricular arrhythmias. *Kidney Int* 50:609, 1996.

104. Mastrangelo F, Rizzelli S, Corliano C: Benefits of bicarbonate dialysis. *Kidney Int* 28[Suppl 17]:S188, 1985.

105. Henrich WL: Hemodynamic instability during hemodialysis. *Kidney Int* 30:605, 1986.

106. Wolff J, Pendersen T, Rossen M, et al: Effects of acetate and bicarbonate dialysis on cardiac performance, transmural myocardial perfusion and acid-base balance. *Int J Artif Organs* 9:105, 1986.

107. Daugirdas JT: Dialysis hypotension: a hemodynamic analysis. *Kidney Int* 39:233, 1991.

108. Wehle B, Asaba H, Castenfors J, et al: The influence of dialysis fluid composition on the blood pressure response during dialysis. *Clin Nephrol* 10:62, 1978.

109. Borges HF, Fryd DS, Rosa AA, et al: Hypotension during acetate and bicarbonate dialysis in patients with acute renal failure. *Am J Nephrol* 1:24, 1981.

110. Ward RA, Luehmann DA, Klein E: Are current standards for the microbiological purity of hemodialysate adequate? *Semin Dial* 2:69, 1989.

111. Sherman RA: On lowering dialysate calcium. *Semin Dial* 1:78, 1988.

112. Goodman WG, Coburn JW: The use of 1,25-dihydroxyvitamin D3 in early renal failure. *Annu Rev Med* 43:27, 1992.

113. Sutton RA, Cameron EC: Renal osteodystrophy: pathophysiology. *Semin Nephrol* 12:91, 1992.

114. Wing AJ: Optimum calcium concentration of dialysis fluid for hemodialysis. *BMJ* 4:145, 1968.

115. Kyriazis J, Glotos J, Gerimani I, et al: Dialysate calcium profiling during hemodialysis: use and clinical implications. *Kidney Int* 61:276, 2002.

116. Raman A, Chong YK, Sreenevasan GA: Effects of varying dialysate calcium concentrations on the plasma calcium fractions in patients on dialysis. *Nephron* 16:181, 1976.

117. Eknoyan G, Levin A, Levin NW: 2003 KDOQI guidelines: bone metabolism and disease in chronic kidney disease. *Am J Kidney Dis* 42[Suppl 4]:1, 2003.

118. Van Dar Sande FM, Cheriex EC, Van Kuuk WHM, et al: Effect of dialysate calcium concentration on intradialytic blood pressure course in cardiac compromised patients. *Am J Kidney Dis* 32:125, 1998.

119. Ni SE, Virtanen VK, Pasternack AI, et al: QTc dispersion increases during hemodialysis with low-calcium dialysate. *Kidney Int* 57:2117, 2000.
120. Kyriazis J, Kalogeropoulou K, Bilirakis L: Dialysate magnesium level and blood pressure. *Kidney Int* 66:1221, 2004.
121. Vaporean ML, Van Stone JC: Dialysate magnesium. *Semin Dial* 6:46, 1993.
122. Kellum JA, Mehta RL, Angus DC, et al: The first international consensus conference on continuous renal replacement therapy. *Kidney Int* 62:1855, 2002.
123. Barenbrock M, Hausberg M, Matzkies F, et al: Effects of bicarbonate- and lactate-buffered replacement fluids on cardiovascular outcome in CVVH patients. *Kidney Int* 58:1751, 2000.
124. Bihorac A, Ross E: Continuous venovenous hemofiltration with citrate-based replacement fluid: efficacy, safety, and impact on nutrition. *Am J Kidney Dis* 46:908, 2005.
125. Cazenave JP, Mulvihill J: Interaction of blood with surfaces: hemocompatibility and thromboresistance of biomaterials. *Contrib Nephrol* 62:188, 1988.
126. Grant ME, Lovell HB, Wiegmann TB: Current use of anticoagulation in hemodialysis. *Semin Dial* 4:168, 1991.
127. Polkinghorne KR, McMahon LP, Becker GJ: Pharmacokinetic studies of dalteparin (Fragmin), enoxaparin (Celexane), and danaproid sodium (Orgaran) in stable chronic hemodialysis patients. *Am J Kidney Dis* 40:990, 2002.
128. Saltissi D, Morgan C, Westhuyzen J, et al: Comparison of low-molecular-weight heparin (enoxaparin sodium) and standard unfractionated heparin for hemodialysis anticoagulation. *Nephrol Dial Transplant* 14:2698, 1999.
129. Gordon LA, Simon ER, Richards JM: Studies in regional heparinization. II. Artificial kidney hemodialysis without systemic heparinization—preliminary report of a method using simultaneous infusion of heparin and protamine. *N Engl J Med* 255:1063, 1956.
130. Swartz R, Port F: Preventing hemorrhage in high risk hemodialysis: regional versus low-dose heparin. *Kidney Int* 16:513, 1979.
131. Flanigan MJ, Pillsbury L, Sadewasser G, et al: Regional hemodialysis anticoagulation: hypertonic tri-sodium citrate or anticoagulant citrate dextrose-A. *Am J Kidney Dis* 27:519, 1996.
132. Apsner R, Buchmayer H, Gruber D, et al: Citrate for long-term hemodialysis: prospective study of 1,009 consecutive high-flux treatments in 59 patients. *Am J Kidney Dis* 45:557, 2005.
133. Charney DI, Salmond R: Cardiac arrest after hypertonic citrate anticoagulation for chronic hemodialysis. *ASAIO Trans* 36:M217, 1990.
134. Schwab S, Onorato J, Shara L, et al: Hemodialysis without anticoagulation: 1 year prospective trial in hospitalized patients at risk for bleeding. *Am J Med* 83:405, 1987.
135. McGill RL, Blas A, Bialkin S, et al: Clinical consequences of heparin-free hemodialysis. *Hemodial Int* 9:393, 2005.
136. Tang IY, Cox DS, Murry PT, et al: Argatroban and renal replacement therapy in patients Heparin-induced thrombocytopenia. *Ann Pharmacother* 39:231, 2004.
137. O'Shea SI, Ortel TL, Kovalik EC: Alternative methods of anticoagulation for dialysis-dependent patients with heparin-induced thrombocytopenia. *Semin in Dialysis* 16:61, 2003.
138. Ronco C, Brendolan A, Gragantini L, et al: Continuous arteriovenous hemofiltration. *Contrib Nephrol* 48:70, 1985.
139. Palsson R, Niles JL: Regional citrate anticoagulation in continuous venovenous hemofiltration in critically ill patients with high risk of bleeding. *Kidney Int* 55:1991, 1999.
140. Tolwani AJ, Campbell RC, Schenk MB, et al: Simplified citrate anticoagulation of continuous renal replacement therapy. *Kidney Int* 60:370, 2001.
141. Kaplan AA, Petrillo R: Regional heparinization for continuous arteriovenous hemofiltration. *Trans Am Soc Artif Int Organs* 33:312, 1987.
142. Monchi M, Berghmans M, Ledoux D, et al: Citrate vs. heparin for anticoagulation in continuous venovenous hemofiltration: a prospective randomized study. *Intensive Care Med* 30:260, 2004.
143. Kutsogiannis D, Gibney RTN, Stollery D, et al: Regional citrate versus systemic heparin anticoagulation for continuous renal replacement in critically ill patients. *Kidney Int* 67:2361, 2005.
144. Reeves JH, Cumming AR, Gallagher L, et al: A controlled trial of low-molecular-weight heparin (dalteparin) versus unfractionated heparin as anticoagulant during continuous venovenous hemodialysis with filtration. *Crit Care Med* 27:2224, 1999.
145. Smith D, Paganini EP, Suhoza K, et al. Non-heparin continuous renal replacement therapy is possible, in Nose J, Kjellstrand CM, Ivanovich P (eds): *Progress in Artificial Internal Organs.* Cleveland, OH, ISAO Press, 1985, p 32.
146. Mehta R: Anticoagulation strategies for continuous renal replacement therapies: what works? *Am J Kidney Dis* 28[Suppl 3]:S-8, 1996.
147. Fan PY, Schwab SJ: Vascular access: concepts for the 1990s. *J Am Soc Nephrol* 3:1, 1992.
148. Storck M, Hartl WH, Zimmerer E, et al: Comparison of pump-driven and spontaneous continuous hemofiltration in postoperative ARF. *Lancet* 337:452, 1991.
149. Bellomo R, Parkin G, Love J, et al: A prospective comparative study of CAVHDF and CVVHDF in critically ill patients. *Am J Kidney Dis* 21:400, 1993.
150. Tominaga G, Ingegno M, Ceraldi C, et al: Vascular complications of CAVH in trauma patients. *J Trauma* 35:285, 1993.
151. Nidus B, Matalon R, Katz C: Hemodialysis using femoral vein cannulation. *Nephron* 13:416, 1974.
152. Besarab A, Al-Ejel F: Creating and maintaining acute access for hemodialysis. *Semin Dial* [Suppl 1]:S-2, 1996.
153. Hryszko T, Brzosko S, Mazerska M, et al: Risk factors of nontunneled noncuffed hemodialysis catheter malfunction. A prospective study. *Nephron Clin Pract* 96:c43, 2004.
154. Edwards H, King TC: Cardiac tamponade from central venous catheters. *Arch Surg* 117:965, 1982.
155. Fiaccadori E, Gonzi G, Zambrelli P, et al: Cardiac arrhythmias during central venous catheter procedure in ARF. a prospective study. *J Am Soc Nephrol* 7:1079, 1996.
156. NKF-K/DOQI Clinical Practice Guidelines for Vascular Access: Update 2000. *Am J Kidney Dis* 37[Suppl 1]:S137, 2001.
157. Seyahi N, Kahveci A, Erek E, et al. Ultrasound imaging findings of femoral veins in patients with renal failure and its impact on vascular access. *Nephrol Dial Trnsplant* 20:1864, 2005.
158. Naumovic RT, Jovanovic DB, Djukanovic LJD: Temporary vascular catheters for hemodialysis: a 3-year prospective study. *Int J Artif Organs* 27:848, 2004.
159. Schwab SJ, Quarles LD, Middleton JP, et al: Hemodialysis-associated subclavian vein stenosis. *Kidney Int* 33:1156, 1988.
160. Oliver MJ: Risk of bacteremia from temporary hemodialysis catheter by site of insertion and duration of use: a prospective study. *Kidney Int* 58:2543, 2000.
161. Goldstein MB: Prevention of sepsis from central vein dialysis catheters. *Semin Dial* 5:106, 1992.
162. Cimochowski G, Sartan J, Worley E, et al: Clear superiority of internal jugular access route over the subclavian vein for temporary access: an angiographic study in 52 patients with 102 venograms. *Kidney Int* 31:230, 1987.
163. Daeihagh P, Jordon J, Rocco M, et al: Efficacy of tissue plasminogen activator administration on patency of hemodialysis access catheters. *Am J Kidney Dis* 36:77, 2000.
164. Nguyen TV, Dikun M: Establishing an alteplase dosing protocol for hemodialysis-catheter thrombosis. *Am J Health Syst Pharm* 61:1922, 2004.
165. Moberly JB, Mujais S, Gehr T, et al: Review of clinical trial experience with icodextrin. *Kidney Int* 62[Suppl 81]:S46, 2002.
166. Ash S, Daugirdas J: Peritoneal access devices, in Daugirda J, Black P, Ing T (eds): *Handbook of Dialysis.* 3rd ed. Philadelphia, Lippincott Williams & Wilkins, 2001, p 309.
167. Passadakis P, Oreopoulos D: Peritoneal dialysis in acute renal failure. *Int J Artif Organ* 26:265, 2003.
168. Strippoli P, Pilolli D, Dimgrone G, et al: A hemostasis study in CAPD patients during fibrinolytic intraperitoneal therapy with urokinase (UK). *Adv Perit Dial* 5:97, 1989.
169. Hyman A, Mendelssohn DC: Current Canadian approaches to dialysis for acute renal failure in the ICU. *Am J Nephrol* 22:29, 2002.
170. Chitalia VC, Almeida AF, Khanna R, et al: Is peritoneal dialysis adequate for hypercatabolic acute renal failure in developing countries? *Kidney Int* 61:747, 2002.
171. Phu NH, Hien TT, Mai NTH, et al: Hemofiltration and peritoneal dialysis in infection-associated acute renal failure in Vietnam. *N Engl J Med* 347:895, 2002.
172. Lazarus JM, Owen WF: Role of biocompatibility in dialysis morbidity and mortality. *Am J Kidney Dis* 24:1019, 1994.
173. Hakim R, Wingrad RL, Parker RA: Effect of dialysis membrane in the treatment of patients with ARF. *N Engl J Med* 331:1336, 1994.
174. Henderson LW, Koch KM, Dinarello CA, et al: Hemodialysis hypotension: the interleukin hypothesis. *Blood Purif* 1:3, 1983.
175. Dinarello CA, Koch KM, Shaldon S: Interleukin-1 and its relevance to patients treated with hemodialysis. *Kidney Int* 33[Suppl 24]:S21, 1988.
176. Tetta C, David S, Biancone L, et al: Role of platelet activating factor in hemodialysis. *Kidney Int* 43[Suppl 39]:S154, 1993.
177. Ing TS, Wong FK, Cheng YL, et al: The first-use syndrome revisited: a dialysis center's perspective. *Nephrol Dial Transplant* 10[Suppl 10]:39, 1995.
178. Roccatello D, Mazzucco G, Coppo R, et al: Functional changes of monocytes due to dialysis membranes. *Kidney Int* 32:84, 1989.
179. Vanholder R, Ringoir S, Dhondt A, et al: Phagocytosis in uremic and hemodialysis patients: a prospective and cross sectional study. *Kidney Int* 39:320, 1991.
180. Vanholder R, Ringoir S: Polymorphonuclear cell function and infection in dialysis. *Kidney Int* 42[Suppl 38]:S91, 1992.
181. Hakim RM: Recent advances in the biocompatibility of hemodialysis membranes. *Nephrol Dial Transplant* 10[Suppl 10]:7, 1995.
182. Aranout A, Hakim RM, Todd R, et al: Increased expression of an adhesion-promoting surface glycoprotein in the granulocytopenia of hemodialysis. *N Engl J Med* 312:457, 1985.
183. Himmelfarb J, Zaoui P, Hakim R: Modulation of granulocyte LAM-1 and MAC-1 during dialysis. A prospective, randomized controlled trial. *Kidney Int* 41:388, 1992.
184. Himmelfarb J, Ault KA, Holbrook D, et al: Intradialytic granulocyte reactive oxygen species production: a prospective, cross-over trial. *J Am Soc Nephrol* 4:178, 1993.
185. Ward RA: Effects of hemodialysis on coagulation and platelets: are we measuring membrane biocompatibility? *Nephrol Dial Transplant* 10[Suppl 10]:12, 1995.
186. Schulman G, Hakim R, Arias R, et al: Bradykinin generation by dialysis membranes: possible role in anaphylactic reaction. *J Am Soc Nephrol* 3:1563, 1993.
187. Shaldon S, Lonnemann G, Koch KM: Cytokine relevance in biocompatibility. *Contrib Nephrol* 79:227, 1989.
188. Schindler R, Lonnemann G, Shaldon S, et al: Transcription, not synthesis, of interleukin-1 and tumor necrosis factor by complement. *Kidney Int* 37:85, 1990.
189. Pertosa G, Gesualdo L, Tarantino EA, et al: Influence of hemodialysis on interleukin-6 production and gene expression by peripheral blood mononuclear cells. *Kidney Int* 43[Suppl 39]:S149, 1993.
190. Zaoui P, Green W, Hakim RM: Hemodialysis with cuprophan membrane modulates interleukin-2 receptor expression. *Kidney Int* 39:1020, 1991.
191. Zaoui P, Hakim RM: Natural killer-cell function in hemodialysis patients: effect of the dialysis membrane. *Kidney Int* 43:1298, 1993.
192. Pascual M, Schifferli JA: Adsorption of complement factor D by polyacrylonitrile dialysis membranes. *Kidney Int* 43:903, 1993.
193. Modi GK, Pereira JG, Jaber BL: Hemodialysis in acute renal failure: does the membrane matter. *Semin Dial* 14:318, 2001.
194. Subramanian S, Venkataraman R, Kellum JA: Influence of dialysis membranes on outcomes in acute renal failure: a meta-analysis. *Kidney Int* 62:1819, 2002.
195. Jaber BL, Lau J, Schmid CH, et al: Effect of biocompatibility of hemodialysis membranes on mortality in acute renal failure: a meta-analysis. *Clin Nephrol* 57:274, 2002.
196. Locatelli F: Influence of membranes on mortality. *Nephrol Dial Transplant* 11[Suppl 2]:116, 1996.

197. Himmerfarb J, Hakim R: The use of biocompatible dialysis membranes in acute renal failure. *Adv Ren Replace Ther* 4[Suppl 1]:72, 1997.

198. Karsou SA, Jaber BL, Pereira BJG: Impact of intermittent hemodialysis variables on clinical outcomes in acute renal failure. *Am J Kidney Dis* 35:980, 2000.

199. Schulman G, Fogo A, Gung A, et al: Complement activation retards resolution of acute ischaemic renal failure in the rat. *Kidney Int* 40:1069, 1991.

200. Schiffl LA, Lang SM, Konig A, et al: Biocompatible membrane in ARF. prospective case control study. *Lancet* 344:570, 1994.

201. Alkhunaizi A, Schrier R: Management of acute renal failure: new perspectives. *Am J Kidney Dis* 28:315, 1996.

202. Liano F, Pascual J: Epidemiology of acute renal failure: a prospective, multicenter, community-based study. Madrid Acute Renal Failure Study Group. *Kidney Int* 50:811, 1996.

203. Gastaldello K, Melot C, Kahn R-J, et al: Comparison of cellulose diacetate and polysulfone membranes in the outcome of acute renal failure: a prospective randomized study. *Nephrol Dial Transplant* 15:224, 2000.

204. Albright RC, Smelser JM, McCarthy JT, et al: Patient survival and renal recovery in acute renal failure: randomized comparison of cellulose acetate and polysulfone membrane dialyzers. *Mayo Clin Proc* 75:1141, 2000.

205. Jorres A, Gahl GM, Dobis C, et al: Hemodialysis-membrane biocompatibility and mortality of patients with dialysis-dependent acute renal failure: a prospective randomised multicenter trial. *Lancet* 354:1337, 1999.

206. Bergamo Collaborative Dialysis Study Group: Acute intradialytic well-being: results of a clinical trial comparing polysulfone and cuprophane. *Kidney Int* 40:714, 1991.

207. Parker TF, Wingard RL, Husni L, et al. Effect of the membrane biocompatibility on nutritional parameters in chronic hemodialysis patients. *Kidney Int* 49:551, 1996.

208. Krazlin B, Reuss A, Gretz N, et al: Recovery from ischaemic renal failure: independence from dialysis membrane type. *Nephron* 73:644, 1996.

209. Jacobs C: Membrane biocompatibilty in the treatment of acute renal failure: what is the evidence in 1996? *Nephrol Dial Transplant* 12:38, 1997.

210. Mehta R, McDonald B, Gabbai F, et al: Effect of biocompatible membranes on outcomes from acute renal failure in the ICU. *J Am Soc Nephrol* 7:1457, 1996.

211. Hakim RM, Breyer J, Ismail N, et al: Effects of dose of dialysis on morbidity and mortality. *Am J Kidney Dis* 23:661, 1994.

212. Owen WF, Lew NL, Liu YL, et al: The urea reduction ratio and serum albumin concentration as predictors of mortality in patients undergoing hemodialysis. *N Engl J Med* 329:1001, 1993.

213. Hemodialysis Adequacy Work Group: NKF-KDOQI clinical practice guidelines for hemodialysis: an update, in *Kidney Dialysis Outcomes Quality Initiative*. Philadelphia, National Kidney Foundation, 2001.

214. Bellomo R, Ronco C: Nutritional management of ARF in the critically ill patients. *Am J Kidney Dis* 28[Suppl 3]:S58, 1996.

215. Paganini EP, Taployai M, Goormastic M, et al: Establishing a dialysis/patient outcome link in intensive care unit acute dialysis for patients with acute renal failure. *Am J Kidney Dis* 28[Suppl 3]:S81, 1996.

216. Ronco C, Bellomo R, Homel P, et al: Effects of different doses in continuous veno-venous hemofiltration on outcomes of acute renal failure: a prospective randomized trial. *Lancet* 356:26, 2000.

217. Schffl H, Lang HM, Fisher R: Daily hemodialysis and the outcome of acute renal failure. *N Eng J Med* 346:305, 2002.

218. Palevsky PM, O'Connor T, Smith MW, et al: Design of the VA/NIH Acute Renal Failure Trial Network (ATN) study: intensive versus conventional renal support in acute renal failure. *Clinical Trials* 2:423, 2005.

219. Bellomo R, Ronco C: ARF in the intensive care unit: adequacy of dialysis and the case for continuous therapies. *Nephrol Dial Transplant* 11:424, 1996.

220. Paganini EP, Taployai M, Goormastic M, et al: Establishing a dialysis/patient outcome link in intensive care unit acute dialysis for patients with acute renal failure. *Am J Kidney Dis* 28[Suppl 3]:S81, 1996.

221. Frankenfeld DC, Reynolds HN, Wiles CE, et al: Urea removal during continuous hemofiltration of conventional dialytic therapy and acute continuous hemodialfiltration in the management of ARF in the critically ill. *Renal Fail* 15:595, 1993.

222. Clark WR, Mueller BA, Alaka KJ, et al: A comparison of metabolic control by continuous and intermittent therapies in ARF. *J Am Soc Nephrol* 4:1413, 1994.

223. Billiau A, Vandekerckhove F: Cytokines and their interactions with other inflammatory mediators in the pathogenesis of sepsis and septic shock. *Eur J Clin Invest* 21:559, 1991.

224. Parillo JE: Pathogenetic mechanisms of septic shock. *N Engl J Med* 328:1471, 1993.

225. Bellomo R, Tipping P, Boyce N: CVVH with dialysis removes cytokines from the circulation of septic patients. *Crit Care Med* 21:522, 1993.

226. Ronco C, Tetta C, Lupi H, et al: Removal of platelet activating factors in experimental CAVH. *Crit Care Med* 23:99, 1995.

227. Mehta RL, McDonald B, Pahl M, et al: Continuous versus intermittent dialysis for acute renal failure in the ICU. results from a randomized multicenter trial. *J Am Soc Nephrol* 7:1456, 1996.

228. Augustine JJ, Sandy D, Paganini EP, et al: A randomized controlled trial comparing intermittent with continuous dialysis in patients with ARF. *Am J Kidney Dis* 44:1000, 2004.

229. Uehlinger DE, Jakob SM, Frey FJ, et al: Comparison of continuous and intermittent renal replacement therapy for acute renal failure. *Nephrol Dial Transplant* 20:1630, 2005.

230. Journois D, Silvester W: Continuous hemofiltration in patients with sepsis or multiorgan failure. *Semin Dial* 9:175, 1996.

231. Kumar VA, Yeuin JY, Don BR: Extended daily dialysis vs. continuous hemodialysis for ICU patients with acute renal failure: a two-year single center report. *Int J Artif Organs* 27:371, 2004.

232. Kielstein JT, Kretschmer U, Fliser D, et al: Efficacy and cardiovascular tolerability of extended dialysis in critically ill patients: a randomized controlled study. *Am J Kidney Dis* 43:342, 2004.

233. Lowrie EG, Lew NL: Death risk in hemodialysis patients: the predictive value of commonly measured variables and an evaluation of death risk differences between facilities. *Am J Kidney Dis* 15:458, 1990.

234. NKF-K/DQOI. *Clinical Practice Guidelines for Nutrition in Chronic Renal Failure*. New York, National Kidney Foundation, 2001.

235. Chertow G, Bullard A, Lazarus JM: Nutrition and dialysis prescription. *Am J Nephrol* 16:79, 1996.

236. Chima CS, Meyer L, Hummell AC, et al: Protein catabolic rate in patients with acute renal failure on continuous arteriovenous hemofiltration and total parenteral nutrition. *J Am Soc Nephrol* 3:1516, 1993.

237. Mokrzycki MH, Kaplan AA: Protein losses in continuous renal replacement therapies. *J Am Soc Nephrol* 7:2259, 1996.

238. Maxvold NJ, Smoyer WE, Custer JR, et al: Amino acid loss and nitrogen balance in critically ill children with acute renal failure: a prospective comparison between classic hemofiltration and hemofiltration with dialysis. *Crit Care Med* 28:1161, 2000.

239. Novak I, Sramek V, Pittrova H, et al: Glutamine and other amino acid losses during continuous venovenous hemodiafiltration. *Artif Organs* 22:359, 1997.

240. Ikizler TA, Pupim LB, Brouillette JR, et al: Hemodialysis stimulates muscle and whole body protein loss and alters substrate oxidation. *Am J Physiol Endocrinol Metab* 282:E107, 2002.

241. Scheinkestel CD, Kar L, Marshall K, et al: Prospective randomized trial to assess caloric and protein needs of critically ill, anuric, ventilated patients requiring continuous renal replacement therapy. *Nutrition* 19:909, 2003.

242. Bellomo R, Tan HK, Bhonagiri S, et al: High protein intake during continuous hemodiafiltration: impact on amino acids and nitrogen balance. *Int J Artif Organs* 25:263, 2002.

243. Druml W: Nutritional management of acute renal failure. *Am J Kidney Dis* 37[Suppl S]:S89, 2001.

244. Renal Physicians Association and American Society of Nephrology: *Shared Decision Making in the Appropriate Initiation and Withdrawal from Dialysis. Clinical Practice Guideline Number 2.* Rockville, MD, Renal Physicians Association, 2000.

245. Mehta RL: Renal replacement therapy for acute renal failure: matching the method to the patient. *Semin Dial* 6:253, 1993.

246. Lazarus JM: Which dialytic therapy is best for the patient with an unstable cardiovascular system? Hemodialysis is the optimal therapy. *Semin Dial* 5:208, 1992.

247. Yoshida S, Tajika T, Yamasaki N, et al: Dialysis dysequilibrium syndrome in neurosurgical patients. *Neurosurgery* 20:716, 1987.

248. Krane NK: Intracranial pressure measurement in a patient undergoing hemodialysis and peritoneal dialysis. *Am J Kidney Dis* 13:336, 1989.

249. Daugirdas JT: Pathophysiology of dialysis hypotension: an update. *Am J Kidney Dis* 38[Suppl 4]:S11, 2001.

250. Leunissen KM, Kooman JP, van Kuijk W, et al: Preventing hemodynamic instability in patients at risk for intradialytic hypotension. *Nephrol Dial Transplant* 11[Suppl 2]:11, 1996.

251. Song JH, Park GH, Kim MJ, et al: Effect of sodium balance and the combination of ultrafiltration profile during sodium profiling hemodialysis on the maintenance of the quality of dialysis and sodium and fluid balances. *J Am Soc Nephrol* 16:237, 2005.

252. Daugirdas JT, Ross EA, Nissenson AR: Acute hemodialysis prescription, in Daugirdas JT, Blake PG, Ing TS (eds): *Handbook of Dialysis.* 3rd ed. Philadelphia, Lippincott Williams & Wilkins, 2001, p 110.

253. Maggiore Q: Isothermic dialysis for hypotension-prone patients. *Semin Dial* 15:187, 2002.

254. Levy FL, Grayburn PA, Henrich WL, et al: Improved left ventricular contractility with cool temperature hemodialysis. *Kidney Int* 41:961, 1992.

255. Agarwal R, Jost C, Henrich WL, et al: Thirty five degree Celsius dialysis increases periphery resistance and improves hemodynamic stability of patients. *J Am Soc Nephrol* 3:351, 1992.

256. Knoll GA, Grabowski JA, O'Rouke K, et al: A randomized, controlled trial of albumin versus saline for intradialytic hypotension. *J Am Soc Nephrol* 15:487, 2004.

257. Gong R, Lindberg J, Abrams J, et al: Comparison of hypertonic saline solutions and dextran in dialysis-induced hypotension. *J Am Soc Nephrol* 3:1808, 1993.

258. Rombola G, Colussi G, De FM, et al: Cardiac arrhythmias and electrolyte changes during hemodialysis. *Nephrol Dial Transplant* 7:318, 1992.

259. Silver SM, Sterns RH, Halperin ML: Brain swelling after dialysis: old urea or new osmoles? *Am J Kidney Dis* 28:1, 1996.

260. Trinh-Trang-Tan MM, Cartron JP, Bankir L: Molecular basis for the dialysis disequilibrium syndrom3: altered aquaporin and urea transporter expression in the brain. *Nephrol Dial Transplant* 20:1984, 2005.

261. Silver SM, DeSimone JA Jr, Smith DA, et al: Dialysis dysequilibrium syndrome in the rat: role of the reverse urea effect. *Kidney Int* 42:161, 1992.

262. Gullans SR, Verbalis JG: Control of brain volume during hyper- and hypoosmolar conditions. *Annu Rev Med* 44:289, 1993.

263. Arieff AI: Dialysis dysequilibrium syndrome: current concepts on pathogenesis. *Controv Nephrol* 4:367, 1982.

264. Doorenbos CJ, Bosma RJ, Lamberts PNJ: Use of urea containing dialysate to avoid disequilibrium syndrome, enabling intensive dialysis treatment in a diabetic patient with renal failure and severe metformin induced lactic acidosis. *Nephrol Dial Trnsplant* 16:1303, 2001.

265. Davenport A: Renal replacement therapy in the patient with acute brain injury. *Am J Kidney Dis* 37:457, 2001.

266. Aurigemma NM, Feldman NT, Gottlieb M, et al: Arterial oxygenation during hemodialysis. *N Engl J Med* 297:871, 1977.

267. De Broe ME: Hemodialysis-induced hypoxemia. *Nephrol Dial Transplant* 9[Suppl 2]:173, 1994.

268. Arnout MA, Hakim RM, Todd RF, et al: Increased expression of an adhesion promoting surface glycoprotein in the granulocytopenia of hemodialysis. *N Engl J Med* 312:457, 1985.

269. Bland LA, Favero MS, Arduino MJ: Should hemodialysis fluid be sterile? *Semin Dial* 6:34, 1993.

270. Piraino B, Bailie GR, Bernardini J, et al: ISPD Guidelines/Recommendations. Peritoneal dialysis-related infections. Recommendations: 2005 update. *Perit Dial Int*, 25:107, 2005.

271. Port FK, Held PJ, Nolph KD, et al: Risk of peritonitis and technique failure by CAPD connection technique: a national study. *Kidney Int* 42:967, 1992.

272. Holley JL, Bernardini J, Piraino B: Polymicrobial peritonitis on continuous peritoneal dialysis. *Am J Kidney Dis* 19:162, 1992.

273. Choi P, Nemati E, Banerjee A, et al: Peritoneal dialysis catheter removal for acute peritonitis:a retrospective analysis of factors associated with catheter removal and prolonged postoperative hospitalization. *Am J Kidney Dis* 43:103, 2004.

274. Nomoto Y, Suga T, Nakajima K, et al: Acute hydrothorax in CAPD—a collaborative study of 161 centers. *Am J Nephrol* 9:363, 1989.

275. Humes HD, Mackay SA, Funke AJ, et al: The bioartificial renal tubule assist device to enhance CRRT in acute renal failure. *Am J Kidney Dis* 30[Suppl 4]:S28, 1997.

276. Tumlin J, Wali R, Brennan K, et al: Effect of the renal assist device (RAD) on mortality of dialysis-dependent acute renal failure: a randomized, open-labeled, multicenter, phase II trial [abstract]. *J Am Soc Nephrol* 16:46A, 2005.

Theresa Nester
Michael Linenberger

CHAPTER **26**

Therapeutic Apheresis: Technical Considerations and Indications in Critical Care

TECHNICAL RATIONALE AND INSTRUMENTS

Apheresis means *to remove*. Apheresis instruments are designed to separate whole blood into its component parts in order to selectively remove one component and return the remaining components to the patient. By processing one or more blood volumes, a significant amount of pathologic solutes or cells may be removed while the intravascular compartment remains relatively euvolemic. In an exchange procedure, replacement fluid or blood is given back to the patient in order to allow plasma or red cells to be removed. With any apheresis procedure, some type of anticoagulant is added to the circuit to ensure that blood flows freely.

Centrifugation apheresis instruments use either a continuous or a discontinuous flow method to deliver blood to the separation device where blood cells and plasma are differentially sedimented according to their specific gravity. Continuous flow methods draw blood into the extracorporeal circuit, separate blood into components in the centrifugation chamber, divert the unwanted component into a collection bag, and return nonpathologic components to the patient without interruption (Fig. 26-1). Dual venous/catheter access is required for these procedures. Discontinuous, or intermittent, flow methods accomplish the same steps but draw, process, and return a discrete amount of blood extracorporeally before another discrete volume of blood is removed. Discontinuous procedures take a longer time than continuous procedures but require only single vein/catheter access [1,2].

Some apheresis instruments, predominantly used in Asia and Europe, use a membrane filtration technique to isolate plasma. The extracorporeal membrane consists either of a flat plate or a hollow fiber with a pore size that excludes cellular components from the filtrate. The plasma that is separated in the instrument is diverted for disposal or treatment, while the other blood components are returned to the patient [3].

Specialized columns and instruments have been developed to treat separated plasma, with the goal of selectively removing pathogenic proteins or other solutes. One example is the staphylococcal protein A–silica column, also known as the Prosorba column [4]. This device is Food and Drug Administration–approved for patients with moderate to severe arthritis and im-

mune thrombocytopenic purpura whose disease is refractory to other treatments. Plasma that is isolated by apheresis is passed through the column, where the protein A binds the Fc (fragment, crystallizable) portion of free immunoglobulin-G (IgG) and circulating immune complexes. Because the total amount of IgG removed by the column is relatively small, additional immunomodulatory mechanisms may be responsible for the therapeutic effect with this treatment. Two different columns are approved for patients with familial hypercholesterolemia who have failed combination drug therapy. The heparin extracorporeal LDL precipitation (HELP) system and Liposorber LA-15 system target the removal of low density lipoproteins (LDL) from separated plasma [5,6]. Additional columns and systems have been tested and used outside the United States. These include a dextran-sulfate column to remove anti-DNA and anticardiolipin antibodies and immobilized polymyxin B or other adsorbers to remove inflammatory cytokines and mediators of sepsis [7–9].

PHYSIOLOGIC PRINCIPLES

The effectiveness of an apheresis procedure in reducing a plasma molecule or cellular component depends on two factors: (a) the distribution of that component between the intravascular and extravascular space; and (b) the rate of regeneration of the component [10,11]. For solutes that move freely between intravascular and extravascular compartments, complete reequilibration between the compartments occurs at approximately 48 hours after a plasma exchange. Circulating blood cells also traffic between sites of vascular margination and/or splenic sequestration and this, in turn, can affect the efficiency of a therapeutic cytapheresis procedure.

The rate of intravascular regeneration of a pathologic solute or blood cell population after apheresis also depends on the rates of synthesis or production and decay or cell death. Plasma exchange typically removes large molecules at a rate that greatly exceeds their natural synthetic rate, thus a simple one-compartment mathematical model is used to predict the depletion of soluble plasma substances. Assumptions of the model are that the plasma removed is replaced with a fluid devoid of the target substance, and that complete mixing of the replacement fluid with the remaining intravascular plasma volume occurs [10]. Figure 26-2 depicts the kinetics of removal and

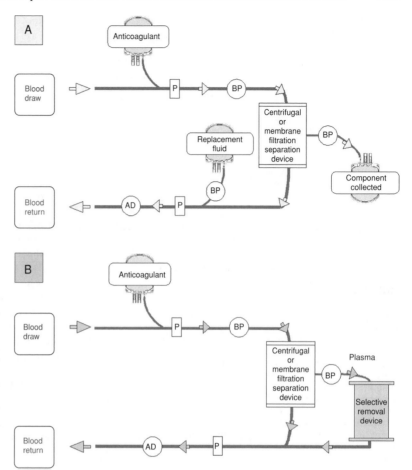

FIGURE 26-1.   A: Basic circuitry and instrumentation of component removal in a therapeutic apheresis procedure. Anticoagulant is added to the patient's blood as it is drawn and pumped to the separation device. The component to be collected is pumped from the device to a collection bag, and the remainder of the blood is returned, along with appropriate replacement fluid, to the patient. **B:** Circuitry and instrumentation for selective removal of pathogenic substance from the patient's plasma. The patient's anticoagulated blood is pumped to the separation device, and separated plasma is then delivered to the selective removal device. The purified plasma is then combined with the cellular portion of the patient's blood and returned to the patient. AD, air detector; BP, blood pump; P, pressure monitor.

regeneration of plasma IgG and IgM after therapeutic plasma exchange. The reliability of the one-compartment model to predict removal of soluble substances may be limited by conditions that cause an expanded plasma volume, such as paraproteinemia, molecules with rapid synthetic rates, and situations where rebound IgG production occurs, such as in the setting of humoral solid organ rejection due to a preformed antibody [12].

The efficiency of cell depletion by cytapheresis is less predictable than soluble substance removal by plasma exchange. Factors that may hinder the prediction include a rapid rate of cell production, such as occurs with untreated acute leukemia, the propensity of the spleen to sequester abnormal circulating cells or platelets, and miscalculation of the plasma volume of the patient. In general, a cytapheresis procedure in which 1.5 to 2.0 blood volumes are processed can be expected to remove approximately 35% to 85% of the target cells [13].

ANTICOAGULATION AND FLUID REPLACEMENT

Citrate is the most commonly used anticoagulant for plasma exchange and cytapheresis procedures. Heparin is often used with specialized column extraction systems and plasma membrane filtration. Current apheresis instruments limit both the anticoagulant (citrate or heparin) dose and rate of blood return based on the patient's total blood volume. The operator

can also adjust the ratio of anticoagulant to whole blood being processed.

The acid-citrate-dextrose (ACD) solution effectively chelates free or ionized plasma calcium, thereby preventing coagulation of blood and plasma in the apheresis circuit. The precise decrease in ionized calcium in vivo during an apheresis procedure is difficult to predict, as this depends on dilution, metabolism, redistribution, and excretion of infused citrate [14]. Fluid replacement with fresh frozen plasma (FFP) or albumin may decrease the ionized calcium further because of citrate in the FFP or calcium binding by albumin. Ionized calcium may typically decrease by 23% to 33%, as measured during donor apheresis procedures [15,16].

Citrate does not produce an anticoagulant effect in vivo. The half-life in patients with normal renal and hepatic function is approximately 30 minutes. In a patient with severe liver disease, where citrate will not be as quickly metabolized, the operator should reduce the amount and/or rate of ACD used during an exchange. In critically ill patients needing plasma exchange, it is advised that ionized calcium be monitored and intravenous calcium replacement be provided as needed. Some apheresis services use protocols for the infusion of intravenous calcium gluconate or calcium chloride during all therapeutic plasma exchanges [17].

Continuous reinfusion of extracorporeal heparin during an apheresis procedure will affect the patient's hemostatic parameters. The effect is measurable until the drug is metabolized, usually within 30 to 60 minutes of finishing the procedure. For

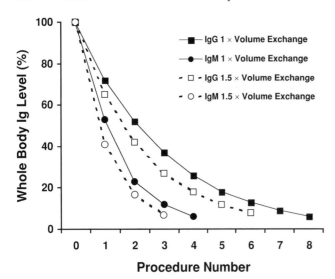

FIGURE 26-2. Hypothetical depletion of whole body immunoglobulin (Ig) levels by therapeutic plasma exchange. The 1-compartment model predicts that approximately 60% of the soluble substance will be removed from the plasma with a 1× plasma volume therapeutic exchange, and approximately 80% will be removed with a 1.5× volume exchange. Because roughly 50% of IgG distributes to the extravascular space, reequilibration between the intravascular and extravascular compartments occurs between sequential procedures, and 6 or 7 1× volume exchanges are needed to deplete whole body IgG to less than 10% of the pretreatment level. By comparison, IgM is predominantly intravascular, and therefore, only 3 or 4 1× volume exchanges are needed to deplete whole body IgM to less than 10%. By increasing the processing to 1.5× plasma volumes, the same therapeutic goal would require three procedures to deplete IgM and five procedures to deplete IgG.

patients already therapeutically anticoagulated with heparin, the anticoagulation normally used with apheresis may be reduced or eliminated. The primary providers of critically ill patients must communicate with the apheresis team all information regarding systemic anticoagulation, coagulopathy, and contraindications to anticoagulation, especially when heparin is planned for a therapeutic procedure. It is particularly important to document if the patient has known or suspected heparin-induced thrombocytopenia.

Replacement fluid used in plasma exchange may consist of FFP, albumin, or saline. The type of fluid depends on: (a) the patient's baseline hemostatic parameters, particularly fibrinogen; (b) the anticipated number and frequency of procedures; and (c) the condition being treated. For a patient with a neurologic illness, such as acute Guillain-Barré syndrome, 1 to 1.5 volume exchanges are typically performed every other day with 5% albumin as replacement fluid. This regimen and schedule allows the fibrinogen level to recover between procedures. Alternatively, if a condition requires that plasma exchange be performed daily, some FFP replacement will likely be needed to maintain the patient's fibrinogen at a hemostatic level. For conditions where a plasma component is felt to be an important part of the therapy, such as with thrombotic thrombocytopenic purpura, FFP should comprise at least half of the replacement fluid [18]. In such cases, fibrinogen and other coagulation factors will not be depleted.

An apheresis instrument that uses a centrifugation technique must deliver a specific volume of packed red cells to the separation chamber in order to maintain the cell/plasma density

gradient necessary for efficient selective extraction. The extracorporeal blood volume necessary for this purpose varies according to the specifications of the instrument and disposable tubing kit and the hematocrit of the patient. The American Association of Blood Banks (AABB) recommends that the extracorporeal blood volume (ECV) for a general procedure should not exceed 15% of a patient's total blood volume [19]. The implications for a therapeutic apheresis procedure can be illustrated by the following example. A 60 kg adult with a hematocrit of 40% has a total blood volume of: 60 kg × 70 mL/kg (the standard conversion factor for an adult male) = 4,200 mL; and a red cell volume of 4,200 mL × 40/100 = 1,680 mL. If the instrument requires 200 mL of extracorporeal red cell volume, then the ECV required to deliver that 200 mL will be 200/1,680 = 0.12, or 12% of the total blood volume. If, however, the same patient has a hematocrit of 20%, the red cell volume will be 4,200 mL × 20/100 = 840 mL; and the required ECV will be 200/840 = 0.24 or 24% of the total blood volume, which exceeds the AABB safety limit. Allogeneic red cells are required when the ECV exceeds 15%. These are either given to the patient as a transfusion prior to the procedure (to increase their pretreatment red cell volume), or used to "prime" the apheresis circuit at the beginning of the procedure (and returned to the patient as part of the return fluid).

VASCULAR ACCESS

The type of vascular access required for therapeutic apheresis depends on the status of the patient's peripheral veins, the condition being treated, and the anticipated treatment schedule. The vein or catheter must be able to withstand negative pressures associated with inlet rates ranging from 30 to 150 mL per minute for the draw line, and up to 150 mL per minute for blood being returned to the patient. For a patient needing only one exchange, it may be possible to use antecubital or forearm veins. A 16- to 18-gauge Teflon or silicone-coated steel, back-eye apheresis or dialysis-type needle is required for the draw line. The patient ideally will be able to help squeeze a ball during the exchange.

A large bore central venous catheter is often required for critically ill patients, especially those requiring daily procedures [20]. Temporary or long-term tunneled catheters for adults weighing more than 40 kg should be at least 10 French size. Smaller diameter short-term catheters are acceptable for smaller adults and pediatric patients (Table 26-1). Plastic central venous catheters such as those used for cardiac pressure monitoring are not adequate for the draw line because they collapse under the negative pressure generated from the high inlet flow rate. These catheters or a peripheral vein may be useful as return access under certain circumstances. Peripherally inserted central venous catheter (PICC) lines and port-a-catheters are also not options for venous access. Arteriovenous fistulas created for dialysis access can be used for therapeutic apheresis. The critical care team should consult with the apheresis team prior to placing venous access for the procedure.

LIMITATIONS AND POTENTIAL ADVERSE EVENTS

When considering therapeutic apheresis, two limitations should be remembered. First, apheresis is not the same as dialysis. It is not usually possible to end a procedure with a large net negative

TABLE 26-1.   Catheter Recommendations Based on Patient Weight

Patient Weight	Catheter Name	Manufacturer	Size/Gauge
Percutaneous (Non-tunneled) catheters for short-term apheresis			
5–15 kg	Hospal	Hemoaccess	8 Fr
	Soft-Line	Medcomp	7 Fr
15–35 kg	Quinton Mahurkar	Kendall	8 Fr–10 Fr
	Arrow DL	Arrow	8 Fr
35–70 kg	Quinton Mahurkar	Kendall	10 Fr–11.5 Fr
			12 Fr (triple lumen)
	Duo-Flow XTP	Medcomp	9 Fr
>70 kg	Quinton Mahurkar	Kendall	10 Fr–11.5 Fr
			12 Fr (triple lumen)
	Hemo-Cath	Medcomp	11.5 Fr
Tunneled catheters for long-term apheresis			
5–15 kg	Split cath	Medcomp	10 Fr
15–35 kg	Quinton Permcath	Kendall	10 Fr
35–70 kg	Quinton Permcath	Kendall	10 Fr
>70 kg	Hickman Dialysis	BARD	13.5 Fr
	Hickman TriFusion	BARD	12 Fr (Triple lumen)
	VasCath	BARD	
	Ash Split Cath	Medcomp	13 Fr
	Mahurkar Cuffed	Kendall	14 Fr
	TAL PALINDROME	Kendall	13.5 Fr
			14.5 Fr

Fr, French.

fluid balance (i.e., greater than 200 to 400 mL) because the deficit is colloid rather than crystalloid, and hypotension is likely to occur. A safe end fluid balance is plus or minus 10% to 15% of the total blood volume. Additionally, it is not recommended that red cells be transfused during the apheresis procedure (other than at the start as a blood "prime") because the cell separation gradient and cell/plasma interface in the separation chamber may be disturbed. The second limitation is that the procedure is almost always an adjunctive, rather than definitive, therapy for the condition being treated. Thus, while apheresis can be performed on very ill patients, one must carefully consider the risks that are associated with hemodynamic instability, hematologic abnormalities, the need for vascular access, and the priorities for more urgent primary treatments.

Possible adverse complications related to therapeutic apheresis are shown in Table 26-2. Central line complications include

TABLE 26-2.   Possible Adverse Effects of Therapeutic Apheresis

Central venous catheter-associated complications

Signs and symptoms of hypocalcemia and/or hypomagnesemia

Hypotension related to vasovagal reactions or fluid shifts

Transfusion reactions (i.e., when allogeneic red cells are used to "prime" the instrument or fresh-frozen plasma is used as part of the replacement fluid)

Altered hemostatic parameters (i.e., fibrinogen depletion with frequent plasma exchanges or thrombocytopenia with cytapheresis procedures)

Bradykinin reaction in patients on ACE inhibitors undergoing plasma exchange or plasma treatment

Removal of highly protein-bound drugs or immunoglobulins (with frequent plasma exchanges)

procedure-related events, infection, and bleeding [21]. Citrate toxicity occurs in approximately 0.8% to 1.2% of therapeutic procedures [22]. Higher risk is associated with larger process volumes, longer procedure duration, liver failure, alkalosis due to hyperventilation, and use of replacement fluid consisting of blood components that are collected and stored in ACD. Signs and symptoms include a metallic taste in the mouth, muscle or gastrointestinal cramps, perioral numbness, distal paresthesias, and chest tightness. In sedated or unconscious patients, severe citrate toxicity may manifest as tetany, muscle spasm including laryngospasm, a prolonged QTc interval and decreased myocardial contractility [23,24]. Hypomagnesemia and hypokalemia may also occur as the kidneys increase cation excretion into the urine to facilitate excretion of the citrate load. Although rare, fatal arrhythmias have occurred during therapeutic apheresis [25]. To avoid these complications, ionized calcium should be monitored and intravenous calcium infused, as indicated, either through the return line or as an additive with the albumin replacement fluid.

Hypotension or vasovagal reactions occur in roughly 0.5% to 1% of therapeutic apheresis procedures [24,26]. Patients with preexisting hemodynamic instability or diminished vascular tone, as seen in certain neurologic disorders, may be at particular risk. In such patients, a net negative end fluid balance must be avoided. Transfusion reactions may occur if blood components are part of the replacement fluid. Allergic reactions have been reported in some patients receiving albumin as the replacement fluid [27].

Hemostatic alterations and bleeding may occur in severely ill patients with baseline coagulopathy and/or severe thrombocytopenia. A typical 1.3-volume plasma exchange using albumin depletes most coagulation factors to approximately 25% to 45% of their preprocedure values [28]. Repletion time of these coagulation factors depends on their respective rates of synthesis, with most factors returning to baseline values by 24 hours. The exception is fibrinogen, which takes about 3 days to return to baseline values. Because fibrinogen levels are the most severely affected during the course of a series of plasma exchanges, preprocedure fibrinogen levels should be monitored, especially if the replacement fluid does not include at least 50% plasma. Therapeutic leukapheresis removes a portion of circulating platelets, and this decrement could be significant in a patient with preprocedure severe thrombocytopenia. The postprocedure platelet count and coagulation status should be monitored in a critically ill patient, particularly if an invasive procedure is needed shortly after apheresis.

In some patients undergoing plasma exchange with albumin as the replacement fluid, a severe reaction consisting of flushing, hypotension, bradycardia, and dyspnea has been linked to concomitant use of angiotensin-converting enzyme (ACE) inhibitors [29]. This reaction is mediated by bradykinin, which is thought to be generated by prekallikrein activating factor in the albumin preparation. These reports have led to the recommendation that ACE inhibitors be withheld for 24 to 48 hours (depending on the half-life of the specific drug) before plasma exchange using albumin [29]. If an emergency exchange is required in a patient on an ACE inhibitor, FFP should be used as the replacement fluid to avoid this reaction. Similar reactions involving ACE inhibitors have been seen in patients undergoing plasma treatment with specialized columns (e.g., the Prosorba column); thus, similar precautions must be followed [30].

An additional potential adverse effect of repeated plasma exchange is the removal of highly protein-bound therapeutic drugs and plasma immunoglobulins. The exact effects of exchange on individual drug levels have not been delineated. To avoid this complication, medications should be administered following a plasma exchange procedure whenever possible. Immunoglobulin levels should also be measured periodically in immunosuppressed patients undergoing a series of plasma exchanges, as these proteins will be nonselectively depleted from the circulation, and severe hypogammaglobulinemia could further predispose the patient to infections [31].

INDICATIONS IN CRITICAL CARE

Evidence-based guidelines for clinical applications are published by the American Society for Apheresis (ASFA) every few years [32]. Medical conditions are placed into categories from I to IV, with I indicating that therapeutic apheresis is known to be an effective primary or adjunct therapy based on randomized controlled clinical trials or broad noncontroversial experience, and category IV indicating no demonstrated efficacy of therapeutic apheresis for the condition. Examples of evidence-based indications for therapeutic apheresis are shown in Table 26-3.

In the intensive care unit, therapeutic plasma exchange (TPE) is likely to be the most frequent apheresis procedure used. Antibody-mediated conditions known to respond to plasma exchange include: idiopathic thrombotic thrombocytopenic purpura (TTP) [18,33–36]; demyelinating diseases including acute inflammatory demyelinating polyneuropathy/Guillain-Barré syndrome [37–39,66,67], severe, acute idiopathic inflammatory demyelinating diseases (Table 26-4), myasthenic crisis [40,41], demyelinating polyneuropathy with IgG and IgA [42,43]; antiglomerular basement membrane (Goodpasture's)

disease, and pulmonary hemorrhage associated with other forms of rapidly progressive glomerulonephritis (RPGN) [44–47]. Among patients with RPGN, the evidence supporting a potential benefit of plasma exchange derives from retrospective and case-control studies among more severely affected patients [69,70]; whereas randomized controlled trials have yielded supportive results in some studies [71] but not others [72,73] (see Table 26-4). With other disorders, such as Guillain-Barré syndrome and myasthenia gravis, plasma exchange is effective but not superior to or as tolerable as intravenous immunoglobulin infusion [66,67,74] (see Table 26-4).

Although sepsis has not yet been formally evaluated under ASFA evidence-based criteria, relatively recent data suggest that TPE might have a potential role in the setting of severe sepsis and multiorgan dysfunction. Two randomized controlled trials using either continuous plasma filtration versus supportive care [65] or plasma exchange versus standard care [48] have been published. No difference was observed in the 14-day mortality rates of 14 patients with sepsis syndrome receiving 34 hours of continuous plasma filtration and 16 untreated control patients (57% vs. 50%) [65] (see Table 26-4). By comparison, the 28-day mortality rate was 33.3% among 54 patients with sepsis and septic shock treated with one or two TPE treatments compared to 53.8% among 52 nontreated control patients ($p=0.05$) [48] (see Table 26-4). When differences between the control and experimental groups were considered using multiple logistic regression the significance of the treatment variable on mortality was $p=0.07$. A nonrandomized observational cohort study evaluated hemodynamic and mortality outcomes in critically ill surgical patients with sepsis treated with TPE and continuous venovenous hemofiltration (CVVHF) [49]. No overall difference in mortality was observed between treated patients and an untreated historical control group (42% vs. 46%); however, patients with organ failure limited to one or two systems appeared to benefit, with mortality rates of 10% among 10 treated patients and 38% among 16 untreated control patients [49]. Although encouraging, these data must be supported by results from additional well-designed randomized controlled trials before plasma exchange can be recommended as a noninvestigational therapy for this indication.

Use of red blood cell exchange may be warranted for patients with sickle cell disease who are experiencing stroke, acute chest syndrome, priapism, or multiple organ failure as a complication of their disease [50–53]. Exchange may reduce the chance of hyperviscosity complications compared to simple transfusion, as hemoglobin S-positive cells are removed and diluted to a target below 30% of the total red cell volume [54]. Of note, sufficient crossmatch compatible blood may be difficult to obtain for sickle cell patients who have been heavily transfused in the past and have multiple alloantibodies. Red cell exchange may also be used in patients with severe clinical manifestations of falciparum malaria or babesiosis [55,56]. Although a metaanalysis performed in 2002 showed no survival benefit of red cell exchange compared to antimalarials and aggressive supportive care alone [57], the Centers for Disease Control (CDC) recommends consideration of exchange as adjunctive therapy if *Plasmodium falciparum* parasitemia is greater than 10%, or if the patient has altered mental status, noncardiogenic pulmonary edema, or renal complications secondary to the infection. Quinidine administration should not be delayed and may be given concurrently with the exchange [58]. As in

TABLE 26-3. Evidence-Based Indication Categories for Therapeutic Apheresis for Disorders Potentially Affecting Critically Ill Patients

Disease	Apheresis Procedure	Indication Category
Renal		
Antiglomerular basement membrane antibody disease	Plasma exchange	I
Rapidly progressive glomerulonephritis	Plasma exchange	II
Acute renal failure with myeloma	Plasma exchange	II
Hemolytic uremic syndrome (HUS)	Plasma exchange	III
Allograft rejection	Plasma exchange	IV
Autoimmune and Rheumatologic		
Cryoglobulinemia	Plasma exchange	II
Idiopathic thrombocytopenic purpura (refractory)	Immunoadsorption	II
Systemic lupus erythematosus	Plasma exchange	III
Vasculitis	Plasma exchange	III
Catastrophic antiphospholipid syndrome	Plasma exchange	N/A
Hematologic		
Thrombotic thrombocytopenic purpura (TTP)	Plasma exchange	I
Hyperleukocytosis and leukostasis	Leukapheresis	I
Acute severe sickle cell disease	Red cell exchange	I
Thrombocytosis (myeloproliferative disorder)	Plateletpheresis	I
Posttransfusion purpura	Plasma exchange	I
Polycythemia vera or erythrocytosis	Erythrocytapheresis	II
Hyperviscosity (monoclonal IgM, IgA, IgG)	Plasma exchange	II
Coagulation factor inhibitors	Plasma exchange	II
Malaria or babesiosis	Red cell exhange	III
Neurologic		
Acute inflammatory demyelinating polyradiculopathy (Guillain-Barré syndrome)	Plasma exchange	I
Chronic inflammatory demyelinating polyradiculopathy	Plasma exchange	I
Myasthenia crisis	Plasma exchange	I
Demyelinating polyneuropathy with IgG and IgA	Plasma exchange	I
Demyelinating polyneuropathy with IgM	Plasma exchange	II
Lambert-Eaton myasthenia syndrome	Plasma exchange	II
Multiple sclerosis (acute, fulminant)	Plasma exchange	III
Other Disorders		
Drug overdose and poisoning	Plasma exchange	III
Acute hepatic failure	Plasma exchange	III
Toxic epidermal necrolysis	Plasma exchange	N/A
Severe sepsis and multiple-organ dysfunction syndrome (MODS)	Plasma exchange Plasma adsorption	N/A

Adapted from criteria endorsed by the American Association of Blood Banks (AABB): Smith JW, Weinstein R, for the AABB Hemapheresis Committee KL, et al: Therapeutic apheresis: a summary of current indication categories endorsed by the AABB and the American Society for Apheresis. *Transfusion* 43:820–822, 2003; and the American Society for Apheresis (ASFA): Mcleod BC: Introduction to the third issue: clinical applications of therapeutic apheresis. *J Clin Apheresis* 15:1–5, 2000.

Category I disease indications include those disorders for which therapeutic apheresis is standard and acceptable, either as primary treatment or as a first-line adjunct to other therapies, based on randomized controlled trials (RCT) or broad noncontroversial experience. Category II diseases are those for which the evidence is generally accepted as supportive or adjunctive based on RCT or case studies. Category III indications represent disorders for which apheresis is not clearly indicated because of unclear risk/benefit from controlled trials or lack of adequate data; however, apheresis may be reasonable as a salvage therapy when no other options exist. Category IV diseases include those for which no benefit or efficacy of therapeutic apheresis has been demonstrated, and application of this modality should be undertaken only in the context of an approved research protocol. N/A indicates that the disorder is not ranked by the AABB and ASFA criteria.

fulminant malaria, several case reports demonstrate that patients with overwhelming parasitemia from Babesia also quickly respond to red cell exchange [56]. Erythrocytapheresis (i.e., selective removal of red cells by apheresis) may be considered as an alternative to large volume phlebotomy in selected patients with uncontrolled erythrocytosis and polycythemia vera with acute thromboembolism, severe microvascular complications, or bleeding [59,60]. This method can quickly and more safely normalize the hematocrit in patients who are hemodynamically unstable.

Leukapheresis (i.e., selective removal of white blood cells) is commonly used in patients with acute myeloid leukemia (AML) experiencing symptoms of intravascular leukostasis. Signs and symptoms typically manifest as neurologic alterations or pulmonary compromise. Apheresis is indicated in a patient with AML and a circulating blast count greater than 50,000 per μL who is clearly demonstrating signs of intravascular leukostasis (i.e., not due to infection, bleeding or metabolic derangements) [59,61]. Leukapheresis may be warranted sooner in monocytic subtypes of AML, as signs of intravascular

TABLE 26-4. Randomized Controlled Trials and Systematic Reviews of Randomized Controlled Trials that Utilized Therapeutic Apheresis for Disorders in Critical Care Patients

Disease Category [Ref]	n	Intervention	Outcome
Severe sepsis and septic shock [48]	106	Plasma exchange (PE) vs. standard therapy	**28-day mortality** 18/54 (33%) PE 28/52 (54%) Control ($p = 0.05$)
Sepsis syndrome [65]	30	Plasmafiltration (PF) vs. standard therapy	**14-day mortality** 8/14 (57%) PF 8/16 (50%) Control ($p = 0.73$)
Acute inflammatory demyelinating polyradiculopathy/Guillain-Barré syndrome (systematic review of 6 trials) [66]	649	Plasma exchange (PE) vs. supportive care	**Mechanical ventilation at 4 wk** 85/315 (27%) Control 44/308 (14%) PE (RR 0.53; 95% CI 0.39 to 0.74, $p = 0.0001$) **Severe sequelae at 1 year** 55/328 (17%) Control 35/321 (11%) PE (RR 0.65; 95% CI 0.44 to 0.96, $p = 0.03$) **1-year mortality** 18/328 (5.5%) Control 15/321 (4.7%) PE (RR 0.85; 95% CI 0.42 to 1.45, $p = 0.70$)
Acute inflammatory demyelinating polyradiculopathy/Guillain-Barré syndrome (systematic review of five trials) [67]	582	Plasma exchange (PE) vs. intravenous immunoglobulin (IVIg)	**Median time to discontinuation of mechanical ventilation (2 studies)** 34 days ($n = 34$) PE vs. 27 d ($n = 29$) IVIg ($p =$ NS) 29 days ($n = 40$) PE vs. 26 d ($n = 44$) IVIg ($p =$ NS) **Mortality during follow-up** 9/286 (3.1%) PE 7/296 (2.4%) IVIg (RR 0.78; 95% CI 0.31 to 1.95, $p =$ NS)
Severe, acute idiopathic inflammatory demyelinating diseases of the central nervous system, including multiple sclerosis [68]	22	Active plasma exchange (PE) vs. sham PE (crossover allowed)	**≥ Moderate acute improvement** 8/19 (42%) Active PE therapy 1/17 (6%) Sham PE therapy
Rapidly progressive glomerulonephritis (RPGN), including antiglomerular basement membrane (anti-GBM) disease and antineutrophil cytoplasmic antibody (ANCA) associated disease [71]	44	Plasma exchange (PE) vs. immunoadsorption (IA)	**6-month median creatinine clearance** 49 mL/min PE 49 mL/min IA **6-month mortality** 1/23 (4.3%) PE 2/21 (9.5%) IA ($p =$ NS)
Rapidly progressive glomerulonephritis (RPGN), including antiglomerular basement membrane (anti-GBM) disease and antineutrophil cytoplasmic antibody (ANCA) associated disease [72]	33	Plasma exchange (PE) vs. standard therapy with immunosuppression	**Dialysis-free survival among patients with Type III RPGN** 42% PE ($n = 18$) 49% Control ($n = 15$; $p =$ NS)
Rapidly progressive glomerulonephritis (RPGN), including antiglomerular basement membrane (anti-GBM) disease and antineutrophil cytoplasmic antibody (ANCA) associated disease [73]	32	Plasma exchange (PE) vs. standard therapy with immunosuppression	**Patients on dialysis at study end** 3/16 (19%) PE 5/16 (31%) Control ($p =$ NS)
Thrombotic thrombocytopenic purpura [18]	102	Plasma exchange (PE) vs. plasma infusion (PI)	**6-month response rate** 40/51 (78%) PE 25/51 (49%) PI ($p = 0.002$) **6-month mortality** 11/51 (22%) PE 19/51 (37%) PI ($p = 0.036$)
Myasthenia gravis [74]	87	Plasma exchange (PE) vs. intravenous immunoglobulin (IVIg)	**Day 15 variation of myasthenic muscular score** +18 PE ($n = 41$) +15.5 IVIg ($n = 46$; $p = 0.65$)

CI, confidence interval; *n*, number; NS, not significant; RR, relative risk; vs., versus.

leukostasis may be seen at blast counts less than 50,000 per µL or after the start of chemotherapy. Prophylactic leukapheresis should be considered in AML with circulating blast counts greater than 100,000 per µL, particularly if the count is rapidly rising and definitive therapy with induction chemotherapy is delayed [59,62–64]. In comparison to AML, leukostasis complications are rare in patients with acute lymphoblastic leukemia (ALL) and circulating blast counts less than 400,000 per µL. Studies have shown that prophylactic leukapheresis for ALL with hyperleukocytosis does not offer additional benefit above aggressive supportive care and chemotherapy [61].

Plateletpheresis is indicated emergently in patients experiencing thrombosis or hemorrhage in the setting of uncontrolled thrombocytosis associated with a stem cell disorder. Such stem cell disorders include essential thrombocythemia, polycythemia vera, idiopathic myelofibrosis, or unclassified myeloproliferative disease. The goal of the plateletpheresis is to decrease the count below 1 million per μL, with a target closer to 500,000 per μL [59].

For any apheresis procedure, consultation with the apheresis team can be useful in assessing experience and available data for a given condition. The apheresis physician and team should be viewed as partners in determining the treatment plan. Initial discussion with the apheresis physician will include whether the indication is urgent or routine, the impact of apheresis on other treatment modalities, volume management, fluid replacement, and vascular access. Ongoing discussions should continue through the patient's course so that appropriate adjustments can be made to optimize the therapy.

REFERENCES

1. Burgstaler EA: Current instrumentation for apheresis, in McLeod BC, Price TH, Weinstein R (eds): *Apheresis: Principles and Practice*. 2nd ed. Bethesda, MD, AABB, 2003, pp 95–130.
2. Madore F: Plasmapheresis. Technical aspects and indications. *Crit Care Clin* 18:375–392, 2002.
3. Siami GA, Siami FS: Membrane plasmapheresis in the United States: a review over the last 20 years. *Ther Apher* 5:315–332, 2001.
4. Snyder HW Jr, Balint JP, Jones FR: Modulation of immunity in patients with autoimmune disease and cancer treated by extracorporeal immunoadsorption with Prosorba® column. *Semin Hematol* 26[Suppl 1]:31–41, 1989.
5. Mabuchi H, Koizumi J, Shimzu M, et al: Long-term efficacy of low-density lipoprotein apheresis on coronary heart disease in familial hypercholesterolemia. *Am J Cardiol* 82:1489–1495, 1998.
6. Armstrong VW, Schuff-Werner P, Eisenhauer T, et al: Heparin extracorporeal LDL precipitation (HELP): an effective apheresis procedure for lowering Lp(a) levels. *Chem Phys Lipids* 67-68:315–321, 1994.
7. Schneider M, Gaubitz M, Perniok A: Immunoadsorption in systemic connective tissue diseases and primary vasculitis. *Ther Apher* 2:117–120, 1997.
8. Kutsuki H, Takata S, Yamamoto K, et al: Therapeutic selective adsorption of anti-DNA antibody using dextran sulfate cellulose column (Selesorb) for the treatment of systemic lupus erythematosus. *Ther Apher* 2:18–24, 1998.
9. Kodama M, Tani T, Hanasawa H, et al: Treatment of sepsis by plasma endotoxin removal: Hemoperfusion using a polymyxin-B immobilized column. *J Emdotoxin Res* 4:293–297, 1997.
10. Weinstein R: Basic principles of therapeutic blood exchange, in McLeod BC, Price TH, Weinstein R (eds): *Apheresis: Principles and Practice*. 2nd ed. Bethesda, MD, AABB, 2003, pp 295–313.
11. Brecher ME: Plasma exchange: why we do what we do. *J Clin Apheresis* 17:207–211, 2002.
12. Kozaki K, Egawa H, Kasahara M, et al: Therapeutic strategy and the role of apheresis therapy for ABO incompatible living donor living transplantation. *Ther Apher* 9:285–291, 2005.
13. Hester J: Therapeutic cell depletion, in McLeod BC, Price TH, Weinstein R (eds): *Apheresis: Principles and Practice*. 2nd ed. Bethesda, MD, AABB, 2003, pp 283–294.
14. Crookston KP, Simon TL: Physiology of apheresis, in McLeod BC, Price TH, Weinstein R (eds): *Apheresis: Principles and Practice*. 2nd ed. Bethesda, MD, AABB, 2003, pp 71–79.
15. Bertholf MF, Mintz PD: Comparison of plateletpheresis using two cell separators and identical donors. *Transfusion* 29:521–523, 1989.
16. Bolan CD, Greer SE, Cecco SA, et al: Comprehensive analysis of citrate effects during plateletpheresis in normal donors. *Transfusion* 41:1165–1171, 2001.
17. Weinstein R: Prevention of citrate reactions during therapeutic plasma exchange by constant infusion of calcium gluconate with the return fluid. *J Clin Apheresis* 11:204–210, 1996.
18. Rock GA, Shumak KH, Buskard NA, et al: Comparison of plasma exchange with plasma infusion in the treatment of thrombotic thrombocytopenic purpura. The Canadian Apheresis Study Group. *N Engl J Med* 325:393–397, 1991.
19. Menitove J (ed): *Standards for Blood Banking and Transfusion Services*. 18th ed. Bethesda, MD, AABB, 1997, p 32.
20. Schonermarck U, Bosch T: Vascular access for apheresis in intensive care patients. *Therap Apher Dial* 7:215–220, 2003.
21. Sadler DJ, Saliken JC, So CB, et al: Apheresis: another indication for radiologically placed central venous catheters. *Can Assoc Radiol J* 50:177–181, 1999.
22. McLeod BC, Sniecinski I, Ciavarella D, et al: Frequency of immediate adverse effects associated with therapeutic apheresis. *Transfusion* 39:282–288, 1999.
23. Rock G, Buskard NA: Therapeutic plasmapheresis. *Curr Opin Hematol* 3:504–510, 1996.
24. Korach JM, Berger P, Giraud C, et al: Role of replacement fluids in the immediate complications of plasma exchange. French Registry Cooperative Group. *Intensive Care Med* 24:452–458, 1998.
25. Huestis DW: Risks and safety practices in hemapheresis procedures. *Arch Pathol Lab Med* 113:273–278, 1989.
26. Raphael JC, Chevret S, Gadjos P: Plasma exchange in neurological diseases. *Transfus Sci* 17:267–282, 1996.
27. Stafford CT, Lobel SA, Fruge BC, et al: Anaphylaxis to human serum albumin. *Ann Allergy* 61:85–88, 1988.
28. Chirnside A, Urbaniak SJ, Prowse CV, et al: Coagulation abnormalities following intensive plasma exchange on the cell separator, II: effects on factors I, II, V, VII, VIII, IX, X, and antithrombin III. *Br J Haematol* 48:627–634, 1981.
29. Owen HG, Brecher ME: Atypical reactions associated with use of angiotensin-converting enzyme inhibitors and apheresis. *Transfusion* 34:891–894, 1994.
30. Olbricht CJ, Schaumann D, Fischer D: Anaphylactoid reactions, LDL apheresis with dextran sulfate, and ACE inhibitors [letter]. *Lancet* 340:908–909, 1992.
31. Wing EJ, Bruns FJ, Fraley DS, et al: Infectious complications with plasmapheresis in rapidly progressive glomerulonephritis. *JAMA* 244:2423–2426, 1980.
32. Smith JW, Weinstein R, for the AHCKL, et al: Therapeutic apheresis: a summary of current indication categories endorsed by the AABB and the American Society for Apheresis. *Transfusion* 43:820–822, 2003.
33. Grima KM: Therapeutic apheresis in hematological and oncological diseases. *J Clin Apheresis* 15:28–52, 2000.
34. Lara PN Jr, Coe TL, Zhou H, et al: Improved survival with plasma exchange in patients with thrombotic thrombocytopenic purpura-hemolytic uremic syndrome. *Am J Med* 107:573–579, 1999.
35. George JN: How I treat patients with thrombotic thrombocytopenic purpura-hemolytic uremic syndrome. *Blood* 96:1223–1229, 2000.
36. Knobl P, Rintelen C, Kornek G, et al: Plasma exchange for treatment of thrombotic thrombocytopenic purpura in critically ill patients. *Intensive Care Med* 23:44–50, 1997.
37. Efficiency of plasma exchange in Guillain-Barré syndrome: role of replacement fluids. French Cooperative Group on Plasma Exchange in Guillain-Barré syndrome. *Ann Neurol* 22:753–761, 1987.
38. Vriesendorp FJ, Mayer RF, Koski CL: Kinetics of anti-peripheral nerve myelin antibody in patients with Guillain-Barré syndrome treated and not treated with plasmapheresis. *Arch Neurol* 48:858–861, 1991.
39. Van der Meche FG, Schmitz PI: A randomized trial comparing intravenous immune globulin and plasma exchange in Guillain-Barré syndrome. Dutch Guillain-Barré Study Group. *N Engl J Med* 326:1123–1129, 1992.
40. Kirmani JF, Yahia AM, Qureshi AI: Myasthenic crisis. *Curr Treat Options Neurol* 6:3–15, 2004.
41. Batocchi AP, Evoli A, Di Schino C, et al: Therapeutic apheresis in myasthenia gravis. *Ther Apher* 4:275–279, 2000.
42. Weinstein R: Therapeutic apheresis in neurological disorders. *J Clin Apheresis* 15:74–128, 2000.
43. Kiprov DD, Hofmann JC: Plasmapheresis in immunologically mediated polyneuropathies. *Therap Apher Dial* 7:189–196, 2003.
44. Winters JL, Pineda AA, McLeod BC, et al: Therapeutic apheresis in renal and metabolic diseases. *J Clin Apheresis* 15:53–73, 2000.
45. Madore F: Plasmapheresis. Technical aspects and indications. *Crit Care Clin* 18:375–392, 2002.
46. McCarthy LJ, Danielson CF, Rothenberger SS: Indications for emergency apheresis procedures. *Crit Rev Clin Lab Sci* 34:573–610, 1997.
47. Szczepiorkowski ZM: TPE in renal, rheumatic, and miscellaneous disorders, in McLeod BC, Price TH, Weinstein R (eds): *Apheresis: Principles and Practice*. 2nd ed. Bethesda, MD, AABB, 2003, pp 375–409.
48. Busund R, Koukline V, Utrobin U, et al: Plasmapheresis in severe sepsis and septic shock: a prospective, randomized, controlled trial. *Intensive Care Med* 28:1434–1439, 2002.
49. Schmidt J, Mann S, Mohr VD, et al: Plasmapheresis combined with continuous venovenous hemofiltration in surgical patients with sepsis. *Intensive Care Med* 26:532–537, 2000.
50. Uchida K, Rackoff WR, Ohene-Frempong K, et al: Effect of erythrocytapheresis on arterial oxygen saturation and hemoglobin oxygen affinity in patients with sickle cell disease. *Am J Hematol* 59:5–8, 1998.
51. Liem RI, O'Gorman MR, Brown DL: Effect of red cell exchange transfusion on plasma levels of inflammatory mediators in sickle cell patients with acute chest syndrome. *Am J Hematol* 76:19–25, 2004.
52. Lawson SE, Oakley S, Smith NA, et al: Red cell exchange in sickle cell disease. *Clin Lab Haematol* 21:99–102, 1999.
53. Wayne AS, Kevy SV, Nathan DG: Transfusion management of sickle cell disease. *Blood* 81:1109–1123, 1993.
54. Schmalzer EA, Lee JO, Brown AK, et al: Viscosity of mixtures of sickle and normal red cells at varying hematocrit levels. Implications for transfusion. *Transfusion* 27:228–233, 1987.
55. Tejura B, Sass DA, Fischer RA, et al: Transfusion-associated falciparum malaria successfully treated with red blood cell exchange transfusion. *Am J Med Sci* 320:337–341, 2000.
56. Evenson DA, Perry E, Kloster B, et al: Therapeutic apheresis for babesiosis. *J Clin Apheresis* 13:32–36, 1998.
57. Riddle MS, Jackson JL, Sanders JW, et al: Exchange transfusion as an adjunct therapy in severe plasmodium falciparum malaria: a meta-analysis . *Clin Infect Dis* 34:1192–1198, 2002.
58. Centers for Disease Control and Prevention: http://www.cdc.gov/malaria/facts.htm.
59. Zarkovic M, Kwaan HC: Correction of hyperviscosity by apheresis. *Semin Thromb Hemost* 29:535–542, 2003.
60. Valbonesi M, Bruni R: Clinical application of therapeutic erythrocytapheresis (TEA). *Transfus Sci* 22:183–194, 2000.
61. Porcu P, Farag S, Marcucci G, et al: Leukocytoreduction for acute leukemia. *Ther Apher* 6:15–23, 2002.

62. Lester TJ, Johnson JW, Cuttner J: Pulmonary leukostasis as the single worst prognostic factor in patients with acute myelocytic leukemia and hyperleukocytosis. *Am J Med* 79:43–48, 1985.

63. Dutcher JP, Schiffer CA, Wiernik PH: Hyperleukocytosis in adult acute nonlymphocytic leukemia: impact on remission rate and duration, and survival. *J Clin Oncol* 5:1364–1372, 1987.

64. Ventura GJ, Hester JP, Smith TL, et al: Acute myeloblastic leukemia with hyperleukocytosis: risk factors for early mortality in induction. *Am J Hematol* 27:34–37, 1988.

65. Reeves JH, Butt WW, Shann F, et al: Continuous plasmafiltration in sepsis syndrome. Plasmafiltration in Sepsis Study Group. *Crit Care Med* 27:2096–2104, 1999.

66. Raphael JC, Chevret S, Hughes RAC, et al: Plasma exchange for Guillain-Barré syndrome. *Cochrane Database Syst Rev* 2:CD001798, 2002.

67. Hughes RA, Raphael JC, Swan AV, et al: Intravenous immunoglobulin for Guillain-Barré syndrome. *Cochrane Database Syst Rev* 1:CD002063, 2006.

68. Weinshenker BG, O'Brien PC, Petterson TM, et al: A randomized trial of plasma exchange in acute central nervous system inflammatory demyelinating disease. *Ann Neurol* 46:878–886, 1999.

69. Klemmer PJ, Chalermskulrat W, Reif MS, et al: Plasmapheresis therapy for diffuse alveolar hemorrhage in patients with small-vessel vasculitis. *Am J Kidney Dis* 42:1149–1153, 2003.

70. Frasca GM, Soverini ML, Falaschini A, et al: Plasma exchange treatment improves prognosis of antineutrophil cytoplasmic antibody-associated crescentic glomerulonephritis; a case-control study in 26 patients from a single center. *Ther Apher Dial* 7:540–546, 2003.

71. Stegmayr BG, Almroth G, Berlin G, et al: Plasma exchange or immunoadsorption in patients with rapidly progressive crescentic glomerulonephritis. A Swedish multicenter study. *Int J Artif Organs* 22:81–87, 1999.

72. Zauner I, Bach D, Braun N, et al: Predictive value of initial histology and effect of plasmapheresis on long-term prognosis of rapidly progressive glomerulonephritis. *Am J Kidney Dis* 39:28–35, 2002.

73. Cole E, Cattran D, Magil A, et al: A prospective randomized trial of plasma exchange as additive therapy in idiopathic crescentic glomerulonephritis. The Canadian Apheresis Study Group. *Am J Kidney Dis* 20:261–269, 1992.

74. Gajdos P, Chevret S, Clair B, et al: Clinical trial of plasma exchange and high-dose intravenous immunoglobulin in myasthenia gravis. Myasthenia Gravis Clinical Study Group. *Ann Neurol* 41:789–796, 1997.

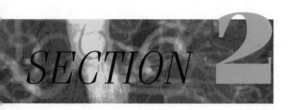

SECTION 2

MINIMALLY INVASIVE MONITORING

ALAN LISBON

Michael D. Howell
Frederick J. Curley
Nicholas A. Smyrnios

CHAPTER **27**

Routine Monitoring of Critically Ill Patients

The ability to intensively, continuously, and routinely monitor both usual vital signs and more specialized metrics forms one of the cornerstones of modern critical care. One of the key differences between intensive care units (ICUs) and other hospital units is the level of detail with which patients are routinely monitored. This careful monitoring alerts the health care team to changes in the patient's severity of illness—helping both to diagnose disease and assess prognosis. Careful monitoring also helps the health care team safely apply therapies such as volume resuscitation, vasoactive infusions, and mechanical ventilation.

This chapter deals with the routine and predominantly noninvasive monitoring that should be done for most patients in critical care units. It examines the indications for, the fundamental technology of, and the problems encountered in the routine monitoring of temperature, blood pressure, electrocardiographic (ECG) rhythm, ST segments, respiratory rate/pattern, and oxygen and carbon dioxide levels. In addition, it reviews noninvasive monitoring of tissue perfusion, with particular attention to gastric tonometry, sublingual capnometry, and transcutaneous oxygen and carbon dioxide monitoring.

TYPES OF MONITORING SYSTEMS

When ICUs came into being in the late 1950s, nurses monitored patients' vital signs intermittently. Continuous measurement was either unavailable or necessitated invasive procedures. The explosion in the use of technology during the past few decades has significantly changed critical care. All routine vital signs can now be monitored accurately, noninvasively, and continuously. As a result, today's patients are monitored more intensively and continuously in the ICU than in any other part of the hospital, with the possible exception of the operating room.

During the past decades, the trend in monitoring systems has been toward multipurpose systems that monitor a variety of parameters. Commercial systems now monitor multiple invasive and noninvasive blood pressures, core temperature, respiration, oxygenation, end-tidal carbon dioxide, central and mixed venous oxygen saturations, ECG rhythm, and ST segments. Multipurpose systems eliminate the need for multiple, freestanding devices, which also reduces clutter and improves workflow ergonomics at the bedside. They can coordinate the monitoring of different parameters and manage data from other sources such as a ventilator or infusion pump. These multipurpose monitoring systems also work in conjunction with commercially available critical care information systems to provide more efficient data management, quality assurance reports, and, in some cases, prospective data-driven alerts.

Monitoring systems for ICUs may be either configured or modular. Configured systems have all of their functions hardwired directly into the system. Modular systems have removable modules that interface with the monitor and contain information for each parameter to be monitored. Modular systems have gained popularity as the physiologic parameters being monitored have changed and expanded. Modular systems can be upgraded more easily than hardwired systems.

TEMPERATURE MONITORING

Temperature changes in the critically ill patient are associated with significant morbidity and mortality [1,2], making it clinically important to recognize an abnormal temperature. In one surgical ICU study, rectal temperatures on admission were normal in only 30% of patients, were above 37.6°C in 38%, and were below 36.8°C in 32% [3]. An abnormal temperature is frequently the earliest clinical sign of infection, inflammation, central nervous system dysfunction, or drug toxicity. Unfortunately, the type of thermometer and the site where the temperature is taken can affect the accuracy of this vital measurement. Clinicians should understand the impact of the thermometer type and the measurement site on obtaining an accurate and responsive estimation of the patient's core temperature.

TYPES OF THERMOMETERS

Mercury-in-Glass Thermometers

Although mercury-in-glass thermometers have historically been the most common type in clinical use, environmental and health concerns related to mercury have resulted in several state and local legislative efforts to phase out this type of thermometer [4,5]. Mercury and other liquid-expansion–based thermometers can give a falsely low measurement when the thermometer is left in place for less than 3 minutes; falsely high temperatures result from failure to shake the mercury down. Because of practical limitations in length, different models of mercury thermometers are used for the hypothermic temperature range.

Liquid Crystal Display Thermometers

Liquid crystal display (LCD) thermometers contain liquid crystals embedded in thin adhesive strips that are directly attached to the patient's skin. LCD thermometers can be applied to any area of the skin but are most commonly applied to the forehead for ease of use and steady perfusion. Like all skin temperature measurements, they may poorly reflect core temperature when the skin is hypoperfused or patients have vasomotor instability. Forehead skin temperature is typically lower than core temperatures by 2.2°C [6], and changes in LCD forehead temperature lag behind changes in core temperature by more than 12 minutes [7]. LCD skin thermometry is probably best used in patients with stable, normal hemodynamics who are not expected to experience major temperature shifts and in whom the trend of temperature change is more important than the accuracy of the measurement.

Standard Digital Thermometers: Thermocouples and Thermistors

Electric thermometers that convert the electrical temperature signal into digital displays frequently use thermocouples and thermistors as probes. Thermocouples and thermistors can be fashioned into thin wires and embedded in flexible probes that are suitable for placing in body cavities to measure deep temperature.

Thermocouples consist of a tight junction of two dissimilar metals. The voltage change across the junction can be precisely related to temperature. The measuring thermocouple must be calibrated against a second constant-temperature junction for absolute temperature measurements. The measured voltage changes are on the order of 50 μV per degree Celsius and must be amplified to generate a usable temperature display. In the range of 20°C to 50°C, thermocouples may have a linearity error of less than 0.1 [8].

Thermistors consist of semiconductor metal oxides in which the electrical resistance changes inversely with temperature. A linearity error of up to 4°C may occur over the temperature range of 20°C to 50°C, but this can be substantially reduced by making mathematical adjustments or placing a fixed resistance in parallel with the thermistor, which decreases its sensitivity and usable temperature range [8]. Thermistors are more sensitive, faster responding, and less linear than thermocouples or semiconductors [8,9]. Semiconductors measure temperature by taking advantage of the fact that the base-to-emitter voltage change is temperature-dependent, whereas the collector current of the silicon resistor is constant.

Tympanic Infrared Emission Detection Thermometers

Commonly used in a hospital setting, infrared emission-detection tympanic thermometers use a sensor that detects infrared energy emitted by the core temperature tissues behind the tympanic membrane [10]. The infrared emissions through the tympanic membrane vary linearly with temperature. The thermometer's sensor sends a signal to a microprocessor, which converts the signal into a digitally displayed temperature. Measurements are most accurate when the measuring probe blocks the entrance of ambient air into the ear canal and when the mid-posterior external ear is tugged posterosuperiorly so as to direct the probe to the anterior, inferior third of the tympanic membrane. Operator error due to improper calibration, setup, or poor probe positioning can significantly alter temperatures [11]. However, a study controlling for these factors still found that tympanic temperatures frequently disagree with pulmonary artery temperatures in critically ill patients. In this study, more than 25% of tympanic temperature measurements differed by more than 0.6°C.

TEMPORAL ARTERY INFRARED EMISSION DETECTION THERMOMETERS. More recently, infrared technology has also been used to noninvasively measure temperature over the temporal artery. Using these devices, a probe is passed over the forehead and searches for the highest temperature; some systems also scan the area behind the ear. An algorithm that estimates ambient heat loss and blood cooling then estimates the core temperature. The device is convenient, painless, and provides a rapid reading. One study of 57 critically ill adults found good correlation with pulmonary artery temperatures. However, patients in this study were normothermic and the authors concluded that these results should not be extrapolated to hypo- or hyperthermic patients [12]. In another study in patients with a broader temperature range, 89% of measurements differed from pulmonary artery temperatures by more than 0.5°C, the amount the authors had specified *a priori* as clinically significant [13]. Similar results have been found in febrile children [14]. Although comparatively few studies have assessed this method, it appears that temporal artery temperature measurements may differ significantly from measured core temperature in febrile or hypothermic critically ill patients.

MEASUREMENT SITES

The goal of temperature measurements is generally to estimate *core temperature*, the deep body temperature that is carefully regulated by the hypothalamus so as to be independent of transient small changes in ambient temperature. Core temperature exists more as a physiologic concept than as the temperature of an anatomic location. An ideal measurement site would be protected from heat loss, painless and convenient to use, and would not interfere with the patient's ability to move and communicate. No one location provides an accurate measurement of core temperature in all clinical circumstances.

Sublingual Temperature Measurements

Sublingual temperature measurements are convenient, but suffer numerous limitations. Although open- versus closed-mouth breathing [15] and use of nasogastric tubes do not alter temperature measurement [16], oral temperature is obviously altered if measured immediately after the patient has consumed hot or cold drinks. Falsely low oral temperatures may occur because of cooling from tachypnea [17]. Sixty percent of sublingual temperatures are more than 1°F lower than simultaneously measured rectal temperatures; 53% differ by 1°F to 2°F, and 6% differ by more than 2°F. Continuous sublingual measurement interferes with the patient's ability to eat and speak, and it is difficult to maintain a good probe position. Sublingual measurement is best suited for intermittent monitoring when some inaccuracy in measurement can be tolerated.

Axillary Temperature Measurements

Axillary temperatures have been used as an index of core temperature and can be taken with a mercury-in-glass thermometer, a flexible probe, or an LCD thermometer. Although some studies indicate close approximation of the axillary site with pulmonary artery temperatures [12], temperatures average 1.5°C to 1.9°C lower than tympanic temperatures [18]. Positioning the sensor over the axillary artery may improve accuracy. The accuracy and precision of axillary temperature measurements are less than at other sites [18], perhaps due in part to the difficulty of maintaining a good probe position.

Rectal Temperature Measurements

Rectal temperature is measured with a mercury-in-glass thermometer or a flexible temperature sensor. It is clearly the most widely accepted standard of measuring core temperature in clinical use. Before a rectal thermometer is inserted, a digital rectal examination should be performed because feces can blunt temperature measurement. Readings are more accurate when the sensor is passed more than 10 cm (4 inches) into the rectum [9]. Rectal temperature correlates well in most patients with distal esophageal, bladder, and tympanic temperatures [18,19]. Rectal temperatures typically responds to induced changes in temperature more slowly than other central measurement sites [20,21].

Esophageal Temperature Measurements

Esophageal temperature is usually measured with an electric, flexible temperature sensor. On average, esophageal temperatures are 0.6°C lower than rectal temperatures [22]. However, the measured temperature can vary greatly depending on the position of the sensor in the esophagus. In the proximal esophagus, temperature is influenced by ambient air [23]. During hypothermia, temperatures in different portions of the esophagus may differ by up to 6°C [23]. Stable, more accurate temperatures are reached when the sensor is 45 cm from the nose [23,24]. Because of the proximity of the distal esophagus to the great vessels and heart, the distal esophageal temperature responds rapidly to changes in core temperature [9]. Changes in esophageal temperature may inaccurately reflect changes in core temperature when induced temperature change occurs because of the inspiration of heated air, gastric lavage, or cardiac bypass or assist [9].

Tympanic Temperature Measurements

Health care providers must measure tympanic temperature with specifically designed thermometers that are commonly used in the ICU. However, several studies have questioned their reliability in estimating ICU patients' core temperatures [25–29]. Accuracy depends in part on operator experience; however, one study showed that even when trained and experienced ICU nurses use tympanic thermometers, the variability in repeated measurements was more than 0.5°F in 20% of patients [30]. Unlike temporal artery measurements, which are not known to have complications, tympanic temperature measurements come with some risk. Perforation of the tympanic membrane [31] and bleeding from the external canal due to trauma from the probe have been reported.

Temporal Artery Measurements

Temporal artery measurements are not known to have complications. Their accuracy is reviewed in a previous section.

Urinary Bladder Temperature Measurements

Providers can easily measure the urinary bladder temperature with a specially designed temperature probe embedded in a Foley catheter [18–21]. In patients undergoing induced hypothermia and rewarming, bladder temperatures correlate well with great vessel and rectal temperatures and less well with esophageal temperatures [19–21]. Bladder temperature under steady-state conditions is more reproducible than that taken at most other sites [19].

Central Circulation Temperature Measurements

ICU practitioners can measure the temperature of blood in the pulmonary artery using a thermistor-equipped pulmonary artery catheter. The temperature sensor is located at the distal tip and can record accurate great vessel temperatures once the catheter is in place in the pulmonary artery. Pulmonary artery temperatures are generally accepted as the gold standard for accurate measures of core temperature, although readings might be expected to differ from core temperature when heated air is breathed or warm or cold intravenous fluids are infused. Inserting a central venous thermistor specifically to monitor temperature is probably warranted only when other sites are believed to be unreliable, and when accurate, rapid, continuous temperature measurements are critical to the patient's management.

Selecting the Measurement Site

The site used to monitor temperature must be an individualized choice, but certain generalizations can be made. Bladder [19,32], esophageal, and rectal temperatures in general appear to be most accurate and reproducible [33], although rectal temperatures may lag behind other temperatures when the patient's status is changing quickly. Because esophageal, rectal, and bladder sites appear similar in performance, convenience may help dictate appropriate site selection. Routine measurement of esophageal temperatures would necessitate inserting an esophageal probe in patients. In addition, because small changes in position can affect the accuracy of the measurement, routine esophageal temperature measurement is probably of benefit only in patients undergoing treatment for hyperthermia or hypothermia. Meanwhile, rectal probes may be extruded and may be refused by patients. Reusable, electronic, sheath-covered rectal thermometers have been associated with the transmission of *Clostridium difficile* and vancomycin-resistant *Enterococcus* [34,35]. The third option, bladder temperature monitoring, is simplified by the fact that most critically ill patients have an indwelling Foley catheter. Monitoring the bladder temperature in these patients requires only a thermistor-equipped catheter. Patients with a thermistor-tipped pulmonary artery catheter already in place require no additional monitoring.

INDICATIONS FOR TEMPERATURE MONITORING

The Society of Critical Care Medicine's Task Force on Guidelines' recommendations for care in a critical care setting grades temperature monitoring as an essential service for all critical care units [36]. Critically ill patients are at high risk for temperature disorders because of debility, impaired control of temperature, frequent use of sedative drugs, and a high predisposition to infection. All critically ill patients should have core temperature measured at least intermittently. Patients with marked temperature abnormalities should be considered for continuous monitoring; patients undergoing active interventions to alter temperature, such as breathing heated air or using a cooling-warming blanket, should have continuous monitoring to prevent overtreatment or undertreatment of temperature disorders.

ARTERIAL BLOOD PRESSURE MONITORING

The first recorded blood pressure measurement occurred in 1733 and, somewhat surprisingly, was intraarterial pressure monitoring. The Reverend Stephen Hales placed a 9-foot brass tube in a horse's crural artery and found a blood pressure of about 8 feet 3 inches. This was obviously not clinically applicable. In the mid-1800s, Carl Ludwig recorded the first arterial pressure waveforms, but it was not until 1881 that the first noninvasive blood pressure recordings were made. In 1896, Riva-Rocci developed and popularized the mercury sphygmomanometer, which was then adopted and disseminated at least in part by Harvey Cushing. In 1905, Korotkoff developed techniques for detecting diastolic pressure by listening for what are now called Korotkoff sounds [37]. More clinical techniques of direct blood pressure measurement by intraarterial cannula were initially developed in the 1930s and popularized in the 1950s [38,39]. These measurements were soon accepted as representing true systolic and diastolic pressures.

Since that time, a variety of invasive and alternative indirect methods have been developed that equal and even surpass auscultation in reproducibility and ease of measurement. This section examines the advantages and disadvantages of various methods of arterial pressure monitoring and provides recommendations for their use in the ICU.

NONINVASIVE (INDIRECT) BLOOD PRESSURE MEASUREMENT

Providers can indirectly monitor blood pressure using a number of techniques, most of which describe the external pressure applied to block flow to an artery distal to the occlusion [40–44]. These methods therefore actually detect blood *flow*, not intraarterial pressure [40], although one method describes the pressure required to maintain a distal artery with a transmural pressure gradient of zero. These differences in what is actually measured are the major points of discrepancy between direct and indirect measurements.

Indirectly measured pressures vary depending on the size of the cuff used. Cuffs of inadequate width and length can provide falsely elevated readings. Bladder width should equal 40% and bladder length at least 60% of the circumference of the extremity measured [45]. Anyone who makes indirect pressure measurements must be aware of these factors and carefully select the cuff to be used.

MANUAL METHODS

Auscultatory (Riva-Rocci) Pressures

The traditional way to measure blood pressure involves inflating a sphygmomanometer cuff around an extremity and auscultating over an artery distal to the occlusion. Sounds from the vibrations of the artery under pressure (Korotkoff sounds) indicate systolic and diastolic pressures [43]. The level at which the sound first becomes audible is taken as the systolic pressure. The point at which there is an abrupt diminution in or disappearance of sounds is used as diastolic pressure [44]. This method, still commonly used in the ICU, yields an acceptable value in most situations. Its advantages include low cost, time-honored reliability, and simplicity. Disadvantages include operator variability, susceptibility to environmental noise, and the absence of Korotkoff sounds when pressures are very low. Auscultatory pressures also correlate poorly with directly measured pressures at the extremes of pressure [40,46]. Therefore, auscultatory pressures must be interpreted with full knowledge of their limitations in the critically ill.

Manual Oscillation Method

The oscillation method has served as the basis for the development of several automated blood pressure monitoring devices, but also continues to be used in manual blood pressure measurement. The first discontinuity in the needle movement of an aneroid manometer indicates the presence of blood flow in the distal artery and is taken as systolic pressure [40]. This oscillation is caused by vibration of the walls of the artery when blood begins to flow through it. The advantages of the oscillation method are its low cost and simplicity. The disadvantages include the inability to measure diastolic pressure, poor correlation with directly measured pressures [40], and lack of utility in situations in which Riva-Rocci measurements are also unobtainable. Aneroid manometers may also be inaccurate: in one study, 34% of all aneroid manometers in use in one large medical system gave inaccurate measurements, even when more lenient standards were used than those advocated by the National Bureau of Standards and the Association for the Advancement of Medical Instrumentation [47]. In the same survey, 36% of the devices were found to be mechanically defective, pointing out the need for regular maintenance. Although the manometers themselves can also be used for auscultatory measurements, oscillometric readings probably provide no advantage over auscultation in the ICU.

Palpation, Doppler, and Pulse-Oximetric Methods

Systolic pressures can be measured by any method that detects flow in a distal artery as the blood pressure cuff is slowly deflated. Palpation of the radial artery is the most commonly used technique; it is most useful in emergency situations in which Korotkoff sounds cannot be heard and an arterial line is not in place. The inability to measure diastolic pressure makes the palpation method less valuable for ongoing monitoring. In addition, palpation obtains no better correlation with direct measurements than the previously described techniques. In one study, variation from simultaneously obtained direct pressure measurements was as high as 60 mm Hg [46]. Like other indirect methods, palpation tends to underestimate actual values to greater degrees at higher levels of arterial pressure. Any method that detects blood flow distal to a sphygmomanometer cuff may be used in this fashion. Doppler machines are commonly used and may be particularly useful in situations where the pulse is not palpable or environmental noise precludes auscultation [48,49]. Pulse oximeters have been similarly used and correlate well with other methods; the point at which a plethysmographic trace appears is taken as the systolic pressure [50,51].

AUTOMATED METHODS

Automated indirect blood pressure devices measure the arterial blood pressure without manual inflation and deflation of the sphygmomanometer cuff. They operate on one of several principles: Doppler flow, infrasound, oscillometry, volume clamp, arterial tonometry, and pulse wave arrival time.

Doppler Flow

Systems that operate on the Doppler principle take advantage of the change in frequency of an echo signal when there is movement between two objects. Doppler devices emit brief pulses of sound at a high frequency that are reflected back to the transducer [52]. The compressed artery exhibits a large amount of wall motion when flow first appears in the vessel distal to the inflated cuff. This causes a change in frequency of the echo signal, known as a *Doppler shift*. The first appearance of flow in the distal artery represents systolic pressure. In an uncompressed artery, the small amount of motion does not cause a change in frequency of the reflected signal. Therefore, the disappearance of the Doppler shift in the echo signal represents diastolic pressure [53,54].

Infrasound

Infrasound devices use a microphone to detect low-frequency (20 to 30 Hz) sound waves associated with the oscillation of the arterial wall [42,55]. These sounds are processed by a minicomputer, and the processed signals are usually displayed in digital form [55].

Oscillometry

Oscillometric devices operate on the same principle as manual oscillometric measurements. The cuff senses pressure fluctuations caused by vessel wall oscillations in the presence of pulsatile blood flow [42,56]. Maximum oscillation is seen at mean pressure, whereas wall movement greatly decreases below diastolic pressure [57]. As with the other automated methods described, the signals produced by the system are processed electronically and displayed in numeric form.

Volume Clamp Technique

The volume clamp method avoids the use of an arm cuff. A finger cuff is applied to the proximal or middle phalanx to keep the artery at a constant size [58]. The pressure in the cuff is changed as necessary by a servocontrol unit strapped to the wrist. The feedback in this system is provided by a photoplethysmograph, which estimates arterial size. The pressure needed to keep the artery at its *unloaded volume* can be used to estimate the intraarterial pressure [59].

Arterial Tonometry

Arterial tonometry provides continuous noninvasive measurement of arterial pressure, including pressure waveforms. It slightly compresses the superficial wall of an artery (usually the radial). Pressure tracings obtained in this manner are similar to intraarterial tracings. A generalized transfer function can convert these tracings to an estimate of aortic pressure [60]. This method has not yet achieved widespread clinical use. One available system studied in ICU patients had approximately one-third of mean arterial pressure readings which differed by 10 mm Hg or more compared with intraarterial pressure measurements and was associated with significant drift during the course of the study [61]. Another recent system reported more accurate readings in patients undergoing anesthesia [62].

Pulse Wave Arrival Time

The time interval between the R wave of the ECG and the peripheral arrival of the plethysmographic pulse wave may reflect blood pressure change. This theory was tested in 15 critically ill infants and children. The relationship between systolic blood pressure and 1/pulse wave arrival time was not found to be close enough to be clinically useful [63]. However, researchers are actively investigating this area, have found good correlations between refinements of this method and standard measures of blood pressure, and are pursuing improvements of these systems [64,65]. At present, these systems are not routinely used clinically.

UTILITY OF NONINVASIVE BLOOD PRESSURE MEASUREMENTS

Only four of the methods described previously (infrasound, oscillometry, Doppler flow, and volume clamp) are associated with significant clinical experience. Of these, methods that use infrasound technology correlate least well with direct measures, with correlation coefficients of 0.58 to 0.84 compared with arterial lines [41,42,66]. Therefore, infrasound is rarely used in systems designed for critical care.

Although they have not been consistently accurate, automated methods have the potential to yield pressures as accurate as values derived by auscultation [67–69]. Commonly used oscillometric methods can correlate to within 1 mm Hg of the directly measured group average values [42,70,71] but may vary substantially from intraarterial pressures in individual subjects, particularly at the extremes of pressure. One study revealed as good a correlation with directly measured pressures as Riva-Rocci pressures have traditionally obtained [42]. Another study demonstrated that mean arterial pressures determined by auscultation were extremely close to those measured by automated devices [68].

When volume clamp methods using a finger cuff have been compared with standard methods in multiple studies [44,72–77], these devices have been found to respond rapidly to changes in blood pressure and give excellent correlation in group averages [78]. In one study looking at a large number of measurements, 95% of all measurements using this method were within 10 mm Hg of the directly measured values [67]. Studies by Aitken et al. [74] and Hirschl et al. [44] demonstrated acceptable correlation of volume clamp technique with systolic pressures measured directly. However, other studies have shown clinically significant differences between the volume clamp technique and invasively measured pressures in patients undergoing anesthesia [79–81].

One of the proposed advantages of automated noninvasive monitoring is patient safety [82]. Avoiding arterial lines eliminates the risk of vessel occlusion, hemorrhage, and infection. Automated methods have complications of their own, however. Ulnar nerve palsies have been reported with frequent inflation and deflation of a cuff [83]. Decreased venous return from the limb and eventually reduced perfusion to that extremity can also be seen when the cuff is set to inflate and deflate every minute [82–84].

In summary, automated noninvasive blood pressure monitoring forms a major component of modern critical care monitoring. Oscillometric and Doppler-based devices are adequate for frequent blood pressure checks in patients without hemodynamic instability, in patient-transport situations in which arterial lines cannot be easily used, and in the severely burned patient, in whom direct arterial pressure measurement may lead to an unacceptably high risk of infection [85]. Automated noninvasive blood pressure monitors have a role in following trends of pressure change [86] and when group averages, not individual measurements, are most important. In general, they have significant limitations in patients with rapidly fluctuating blood pressures and may diverge substantially from directly measured intraarterial pressures. Given these limitations, critical care practitioners should be wary of relying solely on these measurements in patients with rapidly changing hemodynamics or in whom very exact measurements of blood pressure are important.

DIRECT INVASIVE BLOOD PRESSURE MEASUREMENT

Direct blood pressure measurement is performed with an intraarterial catheter. Chapter 3 reviews insertion and maintenance of arterial catheters. Here we discuss the advantages and disadvantages of invasive monitoring compared with noninvasive means.

Arterial catheters contain a fluid column that transmits the pressure back through the tubing to a transducer. A low-compliance diaphragm in the transducer creates a reproducible volume change in response to the applied pressure change. The volume change alters the resistance of a Wheatstone bridge and is thus converted into an electrical signal. Most systems display the pressure in both wave and numeric forms.

Problems in Direct Pressure Monitoring

SYSTEM-RELATED PROBLEMS. Several technical problems can affect the measurement of arterial pressure with the arterial line. Transducers must be calibrated to zero at the level of the heart. Improper zeroing can lead to erroneous interpretation of essentially accurate measurements. Thrombus formation at the catheter tip can occlude the catheter, making accurate measurement impossible. This problem can be largely eliminated by using a 20-gauge polyurethane catheter, rather than a smaller one, with a slow, continuous heparin flush [87,88], although this may be associated with heparin-induced thrombocytopenia [89]. Because movement may interrupt the column of fluid and prevent accurate measurement, the patient's limb should be immobile during readings.

Direct pressure values are also affected by several factors specific to the measurement system itself. An effective design must take into account the transducer system's natural frequency, which is the frequency at which the system oscillates independent of changes in the measured variable. Signals with wavelengths that approach the natural frequency are amplified and may result in an exaggerated reported pressure [90]. This phenomenon is referred to as *overshoot*. Above the natural frequency, the signal is attenuated, which can cause the system to report an erroneously low pressure. Accurate recording systems require a natural frequency at least 5 times greater than the fundamental frequency (i.e., the range of expected heart rates) [91,92]. This is necessary to account for the multiple harmonic frequencies produced along with the main (fundamental) frequency.

The frequency response of the system is a phenomenon not only of transducer design but of the tubing and the fluid in it. The length, width, and compliance of the tubing all affect the system's response to change. Designs should use tubing shorter than 60 cm [93]. Small-bore catheters are preferable because they minimize the mass of fluid that can oscillate and amplify the pressure [92]. The compliance of the system (the change in volume of the tubing and the transducer for a given change in pressure) should be low [92]. In addition, bubbles in the tubing can affect measurements in two ways. Large amounts of air in the measurement system damp the system response and cause the system to underestimate the pressure [94]. This is usually easily detectable. Small air bubbles cause an increase in the compliance of the system and can significantly amplify the reported pressure [92–94].

SITE-RELATED PROBLEMS. Other problems arise in relation to the location of catheter placement. The radial artery is the most common site of arterial cannulation for pressure measurement. This site is accessible and can be easily immobilized to protect both the catheter and the patient. The major alternative site is the femoral artery. Both sites are relatively safe for insertion [87,95,96]. A systematic review of 19,617 radial, 3,899 femoral, and 1,989 axillary cannulations found that serious complications occurred infrequently (less than 1% of cannulations) and were similar between the sites [97]. In particular, and somewhat surprisingly, rates of infection appear similar between the femoral and radial sites [97,98]. The ulnar, brachial, dorsalis pedis, and axillary arteries are also used with some frequency [96,97,99,100]. Although there are a number of theoretical considerations about comparing blood pressures from one site to another, there are little data for critically ill patients. In 14 septic surgical patients on vasopressors, radial pressures were significantly lower than femoral arterial pressures. In 11 of the 14, vasopressor dose was reduced based on the femoral pressure without untoward consequences; after vasopressors were discontinued, radial and femoral pressures equalized. The authors concluded that clinical management based on radial artery pressures may lead to excessive vasopressor administration [101]. Similar significant differences in systolic pressures between the radial and femoral sites were found in the reperfusion phase of liver transplantation, although mean arterial pressures did not differ [102]. However, another larger observational study in critically ill patients [103], and one in hypotense anesthetized patients [104], found no clinically meaningful differences in blood pressures between the sites. Although data are sparse, mean arterial pressure readings between the radial and femoral sites are probably interchangeable.

Advantages

Despite technical problems, direct arterial pressure measurement offers several advantages. Arterial lines actually measure the end-on pressure propagated by the arterial pulse. In contrast, indirect methods report the external pressure necessary either to obstruct flow or to maintain a constant transmural vessel pressure. Arterial lines can also detect pressures at which Korotkoff sounds are either absent or inaccurate. Arterial lines provide a continuous measurement, with heartbeat-to-heartbeat blood pressures. In situations in which frequent blood drawing is necessary, indwelling arterial lines eliminate the need for multiple percutaneous punctures. Finally, analysis of the respiratory change in systolic or pulse pressure [105] may provide important information on cardiac preload and fluid responsiveness.

CONCLUSIONS

Indirect methods of measuring the blood pressure estimate the arterial pressure by reporting the external pressure necessary to either obstruct flow or maintain a constant transmural vessel pressure. Arterial lines measure the end-on pressure propagated by the arterial pulse. Direct arterial pressure measurement offers several advantages. Although an invasive line is required, the reported risk of complications is low [97]. Arterial lines provide a heartbeat-to-heartbeat measurement, can detect pressures at which Korotkoff sounds are either absent or inaccurate, and do not require repeated inflation and deflation of a cuff. Additionally, they provide easy access for phlebotomy and blood gas sampling, and they may provide additional information about cardiac status. Regardless of the method used, the mean arterial pressure should generally be the value used for decision-making in most critically ill patients.

ELECTROCARDIOGRAPHIC MONITORING

Almost all ICUs in the United States routinely perform continuous ECG monitoring. Continuous ECG monitoring combines the principles of ECG, which have been known since 1903, with the principles of biotelemetry, which were first put into practical application in 1921 [106,107]. Here we review the principles of arrhythmia monitoring, automated arrhythmia detection, and the role of automated ST segment analysis.

ECG monitoring in most ICUs is done over hard-wired apparatus. Skin electrodes detect cardiac impulses and transform them into an electrical signal, which is transmitted through wires directly to the signal converter and display unit. This removes the problems of interference and frequency restrictions seen in telemetry systems. Although this comes at the cost of reduced patient mobility, mobility is often not an immediate concern for this group of patients.

ARRHYTHMIA MONITORING IN THE INTENSIVE CARE UNIT

The American Heart Association's Practice Standards guideline considers continuous ECG monitoring a class I intervention for all patients with indications for intensive care, regardless of whether the patient's primary admitting diagnosis related to a cardiac problem [108]. Approximately 20% of ICU patients in a general ICU have significant arrhythmias, mostly atrial fibrillation or ventricular tachycardia [109], with a circadian variation in arrhythmia onset, peaking at about 2 PM for ventricular fibrillation [110]. There is also a substantial incidence of arrhythmia following major surgery [111–113]. Although no studies address whether monitoring for arrhythmias in a general ICU population alters outcomes, this monitoring is generally accepted and

considered standard care [108]. In postmyocardial infarction patients, on the other hand, the data are compelling. Arrhythmia monitoring was shown to improve the prognosis of patients admitted to the ICU for acute myocardial infarction many years ago [114–116]. It has been a standard of care in the United States since that time. Although ventricular tachycardia and fibrillation after myocardial infarction have declined in frequency over the years, they still occur in about 7.5% of patients [117]. Monitoring enables the rapid detection of these potentially lethal rhythms. Because thrombolytic therapy for acute myocardial infarction also leads to a slight increase in arrhythmias within 8 to 12 hours after successful reperfusion [118–120], the incidence of arrhythmias can be used as one indicator of successful reperfusion.

EVOLUTION OF ARRHYTHMIA MONITORING SYSTEMS FOR CLINICAL USE

After ICUs implemented continuous ECG monitoring, practitioners recognized some deficiencies with the systems. Initially, the responsibility for arrhythmia detection was assigned to specially trained coronary care nurses. Despite this, several studies documented that manual methods failed to identify arrhythmias, including salvos of ventricular tachycardia, in up to 77% of cases [121–123]. This failure was probably due to an inadequate number of staff nurses to watch the monitors, inadequate staff education, and faulty monitors [122]. Subsequently, monitors equipped with built-in rate alarms that sounded when a preset maximum or minimum rate was detected proved inadequate because some runs of ventricular tachycardia are too brief to exceed the rate limit for a given time interval [121,123]. Ultimately, computerized arrhythmia detection systems were incorporated into the monitors. The software in these systems is capable of diagnosing arrhythmias based on recognition of heart rate, variability, rhythm, intervals, segment lengths, QRS complex width, and morphology [124,125]. These systems have been validated in coronary care and general medical ICUs [123,126]. Computerized arrhythmia detection systems are well accepted by nursing personnel, who must work most closely with them [127].

ISCHEMIA MONITORING

Just as simple monitoring systems can miss episodes of ventricular tachycardia and ventricular fibrillation, they can fail to detect significant episodes of myocardial ischemia [128]. This is either because the episode is asymptomatic or because the patient's ability to communicate is impaired by intubation or altered mental status. ECG monitoring systems with automated ST segment analysis have been devised to attempt to deal with this problem.

In most ST segment monitoring systems, the computer initially creates a template of the patient's normal QRS complexes. It then recognizes the QRS complexes and the J points of subsequent beats and compares an isoelectric point just before the QRS with a portion of the ST segment 60 to 80 msec after the J point [129]. It compares this relationship to that of the same points in the QRS complex template. The system must decide whether the QRS complex in question was generated and conducted in standard fashion or whether the beats are aberrant, which negates the validity of comparison. Therefore, an arrhythmia detection system must be included in all ischemia monitoring systems designed for use in the ICU. Standard systems can monitor three leads simultaneously. These leads are usually chosen to represent the three major axes (anteroposterior, left-right, and craniocaudal). The machine can either display these axes individually or sum up the ST segment deviations and display them in a graph over time [129].

Automated ST segment analysis has gained widespread popularity among cardiologists. Since 1989, the American Heart Association has recommended that ischemia monitoring should be included in new monitoring systems developed for use in the coronary care unit [130]. In patients admitted for suspected acute coronary syndromes, ischemia is frequently both silent and strongly associated with adverse events after discharge [108,131]. While noting that no randomized clinical trials document improved patient outcomes when automated ST segment monitoring is used to detect ischemia, the American Heart Association recommends ST segment monitoring for patients with a number of primary cardiac issues (e.g., acute coronary syndromes), based on expert opinion. The guidelines make no statement regarding ST segment monitoring for ICU patients [108].

NEWER TECHNIQUES

Because conventional 3-lead monitoring detects only about one-third of transient ischemic events in patients with unstable coronary syndromes [132], some authors now advocate the use of continuous 12-lead ECG systems in the care of acute coronary syndromes [133,134]. Although 12-lead monitoring detects additional arrhythmias, studies have not compared outcomes between standard and 12-lead monitoring approaches in ICU patients. Other proposed enhancements to continuous ECG monitoring include signal-averaged ECG, QT dispersion, QT interval beat-to-beat variability, and heart rate variability [135]. Although associated with subsequent arrhythmic events, these have not yet reached common clinical use.

TECHNICAL CONSIDERATIONS

As with any other biomedical measurement, technical problems can arise when monitoring cardiac rhythms. Standards have been devised to guide manufacturers and purchasers of ECG monitoring systems [130,136].

The possibility of electrical shock exists whenever a patient is directly connected to an electrically operated piece of equipment by a low-resistance path. Electrical shocks would most commonly occur with improper grounding of equipment when a device such as a pacemaker is in place. Necessary precautions to avoid this potential catastrophe include (a) periodic checks to ensure that all equipment in contact with the patient is at the same ground potential as the power ground line, (b) insulating exposed lead connections, and (c) using appropriately grounded plugs [137,138].

The size of the ECG signal is important for accurate recognition of cardiac rate and rhythm. Several factors may affect signal size. The amplitude can be affected by mismatching between skin-electrode and preamplifier impedance. The combination of high skin-electrode impedance, usually the result of poor contact between the skin and electrode, with low-input impedance of the preamplifier can decrease the size of the ECG signal. Good skin preparation, site selection, and conducting gels can promote low skin-electrode impedance. A high preamplifier input impedance or the use of buffer amplifiers can also improve impedance matching and thereby improve the signal obtained. Another factor that affects complex size is critical damping, the system's ability to respond to changes in the input signal. An underdamped system responds to changes in input with displays that exaggerate the signal, called *overshoot*. An overdamped system responds slowly to a given change and may underestimate actual amplitude. The ECG signal can also be affected by the presence of inherent, unwanted voltages at the point of input. These include the common mode signal, a response to surrounding electromagnetic forces; the direct current skin potential produced by contact between the skin and the electrode; and a potential caused by internal body resistance. Finally, the ECG system must have a frequency response that is accurate for the signals being monitored. Modern, commercially available systems have incorporated features to deal with each of these problems.

PERSONNEL

The staff's ability to interpret the information received is crucial to effective ECG monitoring [130]. Primary interpretation may be made by nurses or technicians under the supervision of a physician. All personnel responsible for interpreting ECG monitoring should have formal training developed cooperatively by the hospital's medical and nursing staffs. At a minimum, this training should include basic ECG interpretation skills and arrhythmia recognition. Hospitals should also establish and adhere to formal protocols for responding to and verifying alarms. Finally, a physician should be available in the hospital to assist with interpretation and make decisions regarding therapy.

PRINCIPLES OF TELEMETRY

Intensive care patients frequently continue to require ECG monitoring after they are released from the ICU, and many postoperative critical care patients begin mobilization while in the ICU. At this point, increased mobility is important to allow physical and occupational therapy, as well as other rehabilitation services. Telemetry systems can facilitate this.

Telemetry means measurement at a distance [139]. Biomedical telemetry consists of measuring various vital signs, including heart rhythm, and transmitting them to a distant terminal [140]. Telemetry systems in the hospital consist of four major components [140]: (a) a signal transducer detects heart activity through skin electrodes and converts it into electrical signals, (b) a radio transmitter broadcasts the electrical signal, (c) a radio receiver detects the transmission and converts it back into an electrical signal, and (d) the signal converter and display unit present the signal in its most familiar format. Continuous telemetry requires an exclusive frequency so the signal can be transmitted without interruption from other signals [141], which means the hospital system must have multiple frequencies available to allow simultaneous monitoring of several patients. The telemetry signal may be received in one location or simultaneously in multiple locations, depending on staffing practices. The signal transducer and display unit should also be equipped with an automatic arrhythmia detection and alarm system to allow rapid detection and treatment of arrhythmias.

Notably, telemetry systems may be subject to interference by cellular phones [142] or other radio equipment.

SUMMARY

The American Heart Association recommends continuous ECG monitoring for the detection of arrhythmias as a class I intervention for all ICU patients [108]. Because ICU staff can miss a large percentage of arrhythmias when they use monitors without computerized arrhythmia detection systems, these computerized systems should be standard equipment in ICUs, especially those that care for patients with acute myocardial infarction. It appears that computerized monitoring devices can also detect a significant number of arrhythmias not noted manually in noncardiac patients, frequently leading to an alteration in patient care. Automated ST segment analysis facilitates the early detection of ischemic episodes. Telemetry provides close monitoring of recuperating patients while allowing them increased mobility.

RESPIRATORY MONITORING

Critical care personnel should monitor several primary respiratory parameters, including respiratory rate, tidal volume or minute ventilation, and oxygenation in critically ill patients. Routine monitoring of carbon dioxide levels would be desirable, but the technology for monitoring these parameters is not yet developed enough to consider mandatory continuous monitoring. In mechanically ventilated patients, many physiologic functions can be monitored routinely and continuously by the ventilator. This section does not discuss monitoring by the mechanical ventilator (see Chapter 33) but examines devices that might be routinely used to monitor the aforementioned parameters continuously and noninvasively.

RESPIRATORY RATE, TIDAL VOLUME, AND MINUTE VENTILATION

Clinical examination of the patient often fails to detect clinically important changes in respiratory rate and tidal volume [143]. Physicians, nurses, and hospital staff frequently report inaccurate respiratory rates, possibly because they underestimate the measurement's importance [144]. In another study, ICU staff had a greater than 20% error more than one-third of the time when the recorded respiratory rate was compared with objective tracings [145]. This is particularly surprising as the respiratory rate is an especially important predictor of outcome in many severity of illness scores [146–149]. Two studies in which physicians and staff were asked to assess tidal volume and minute ventilation indicate that tidal volume is (a) assessed poorly, (b) frequently overestimated, and (c) not reproducible on repeat assessment [150,151]. Objective monitoring must be used because clinical evaluation is inaccurate.

Impedance Monitors

ICUs commonly use impedance monitors to measure respiratory rates and approximate tidal volume. These devices typically use ECG leads and measure changes in impedance generated by the change in distance between leads as a result of the thoracoabdominal motions of breathing. Obtaining a quality signal requires placing the leads at points of maximal change in thoracoabdominal contour or using sophisticated computerized algorithms. Alarms can then be set for a high and low rate or for a percentage drop in the signal that is thought to correlate with a decrease in tidal volume.

In clinical use, impedance monitors suffer confounding problems. They have failed to detect obstructive apnea when it has occurred and falsely detected apnea when it has not [152,153]. Computerized impedance monitors have an approximately 30% false-positive alarm rate, while still failing to detect all apneas [154]. In situations with moving patients, they may be less accurate for the quantification of respiratory rate [155]. Impedance monitors are poor detectors of obstructive apnea because they may count persistent chest wall motion as breaths when the apneic patient struggles to overcome airway obstruction [152,153]. Impedance monitors offer the advantage of being very inexpensive when ECG is already in use but lack accuracy when precise measurements of apnea, respiratory rate, or tidal volume are required.

Respiratory Inductive Plethysmography

Respiratory inductive plethysmography (RIP) measures changes in the cross-sectional area of the chest and abdomen that occur with respiration, and processes these signals into respiratory rate and tidal volume. Typically, two elastic bands with embedded wire are placed above the xiphoid and around the abdomen. As the cross-sectional area of the bands changes with respiration, the self-inductance of the coils changes the frequency of attached oscillators. The signals from the oscillator pass through a demodulator, yielding a voltage signal. These signals are generally calibrated to a known gas volume, or may be internally calibrated so that further measurements reflect a percentage change from baseline rather than an absolute volume. RIP can accurately measure respiratory rate and the percentage change in tidal volume, as well as detect obstructive apnea [156–158]. RIP has been used to follow lung volumes in patients undergoing high-frequency oscillatory ventilation [159]. These measurements are more accurate than impedance measurements [153]. However, some studies have found problems with estimation of lung volumes by RIPs. Notably, RIP must be calibrated against a known gas volume in order to provide tidal volume estimates. This calibration is not always accurate and may result in errors of more than 10% in 5% to 10% of patients, even in highly controlled circumstances [156,160]. In mechanically ventilated patients, RIP had significant measurement drift (25 mL per minute) and imprecise volume estimates. Only about two-thirds of tidal volume estimates were accurate to within 10% of the reference value [161].

In addition to displaying respiratory rate and percentage change in tidal volume, RIP can provide asynchronous and paradoxic breathing measurements and alarms, which are common during early weaning and may be helpful in predicting respiratory failure [162,163]. The noninvasive nature of the tidal volume measurement may be helpful in patients in whom technical problems or leaks makes it difficult to directly measure expired volume (e.g., patients with bronchopleural fistulas). In addition, RIP can display changes in functional residual capacity, which permits health care providers to assess the effect of changing positive end-expiratory pressure (PEEP). Providers can determine the presence and estimation of the amount of auto (intrinsic) PEEP by observing the effect of applied (extrinsic) PEEP on functional residual capacity [164], with the caveats noted here regarding possible inaccuracy of volume measurements.

RIP systems are available with central station configurations, which have been used in noninvasively monitored respiratory care units; these units have allowed ICU-level patients to be safely moved to a less-expensive level of care [165,166]. Compared with inductance methods, RIP is more accurate and offers a variety of other useful measurements, but is less convenient and more expensive.

OTHER METHODS

Although health care providers can also use pneumotachometers, capnographs, and electromyography to accurately measure respiratory rate, these methods are not commonly used in the ICU. A pneumotachometer requires complete collection of exhaled gas and, therefore, either intubation or use of a tight-fitting face mask. This inconvenience and difficulties with calibration and maintenance limit the use of pneumotachometers in the ICU to measure either respiratory rate or tidal volume. A second alternative, capnography, works exceedingly well as a respiratory rate monitor. Because it does not require intubation or a face mask, it can be a useful tool in many circumstances. Capnography is discussed in more detail later. A third option, surface electromyography of respiratory muscles, can be used to calculate respiratory rate accurately [167] but cannot detect obstructive apnea or provide a measure of tidal volume. Electromyography works well in infants but presents difficulties in adults, especially in obese adults and those with edema.

MEASUREMENTS OF GAS EXCHANGE

Pulse Oximetry

Clinical estimation of hypoxemia is exceptionally unreliable [168,169]. Since the early 1980s, commercially available pulse oximeters have offered noninvasive determination of oxygen saturation and its response to therapy [170]. Pulse oximeters measure the saturation of hemoglobin in the tissue during the arterial and venous phases of pulsation and mathematically derive arterial saturation. Metaanalysis of 74 oximeter studies suggests that these estimates are usually accurate within 5% of simultaneous gold standard measurements [171]. However, up to 97% of physicians and nurses who use pulse oximeters do not understand their underlying fundamental principles [172]. This section reviews the essential technology involved in pulse oximetry, practical problems that limit its use, and indications for the use of oximeters in critically ill patients.

THEORY. Oximeters distinguish between oxyhemoglobin and reduced hemoglobin on the basis of their different absorption of light. Oxyhemoglobin absorbs much less red (± 660 nm) and slightly more infrared (± 910 to 940 nm) light than nonoxygenated hemoglobin. Oxygen saturation thereby determines the ratio of red to infrared absorption. When red and infrared light are directed from light-emitting diodes to a photodetector across a pulsatile tissue bed, the absorption of each wavelength by the tissue bed varies cyclically with pulse. During diastole, absorption is due to the nonvascular tissue components (e.g., bone, muscle, and interstitium) and venous blood. During systole, absorption is determined by all of these components and

arterialized blood. The pulse amplitude accounts for only 1% to 5% of the total signal [173]. Thus, the difference between absorption in systole and diastole is in theory due to the presence of arterialized blood. The change in ratio of absorption between systole and diastole can then be used to calculate an estimate of arterial oxygen saturation. Absorption is typically measured hundreds of times per second. Signals usually are averaged during several seconds and then displayed numerically. The algorithm used for each oximeter is determined by calibration on human volunteers. Most oximeters under ideal circumstances measure the saturation indicated by the pulse oximeter (SpO_2) to within 2% of arterial oxygen saturation [174].

Cooximeters perform measurements on whole blood obtained from an artery or a vein. They frequently measure absorbance at multiple wavelengths and compute the percentage of oxyhemoglobin, deoxyhemoglobin, methemoglobin, and carboxyhemoglobin (COHb) in total hemoglobin based on different absorption spectra. They are mostly free of the artifacts that limit the accuracy of tissue oximeters and are regarded as the gold standard by which other methods of assessing saturation are measured.

TECHNOLOGY. Many manufacturers now market pulse oximeters. Because of the variety of manufacturers, the numerous algorithms used, and the diverse patient populations studied, it is difficult to generalize the studies performed with one particular instrument, with its specific version of software, in one defined group of patients, to critically ill patients in general. The reader should always check with an oximeter's manufacturer before generalizing the following discussion to his or her oximeter and patient population.

PROBLEMS ENCOUNTERED IN USE. Because pulse oximeters are ubiquitous, all ICU providers must understand their limitations. A metaanalysis of problems encountered in pulse oximetry trials found that severe hypoxemia, dyshemoglobinemia, low perfusion states, skin pigmentation, and hyperbilirubinemia may affect the accuracy of pulse oximeter readings [171]. Any process that affects or interferes with the absorption of light between the light-emitting diodes and photodetector, alters the quality of pulsatile flow, or changes the hemoglobin has the potential to distort the oximeter's calculations. Pulse oximeters should be able to obtain valid readings in 98% of patients in an operating room or postanesthesia care unit [175]. Up to 9% of patients undergoing surgery may have a 10-minute or longer interruption in monitoring because of technical difficulty with oximetric measurement [176]. Table 27-1 lists the problems that must be considered in clinical use.

CALIBRATION. Because early attempts to calibrate pulse oximeters in accord with the principles of Beer's law of absorbance proved unsuccessful, manufacturers now use healthy volunteers to derive calibration algorithms. This creates three problems. First, manufacturers use different calibration algorithms, which results in a difference in SpO_2 of up to 2.7% between different manufacturers' oximeters used to measure the same patient [177]. Second, manufacturers define SpO_2 differently for calibration purposes. Calibration may or may not account for the interference of small amounts of dyshemoglobinemia (e.g., methemoglobin or COHb). For example,

TABLE 27-1. Conditions Adversely Affecting Accuracy of Oximetry

---

May result in poor signal detection
  Probe malposition
  Motion
  Hypothermia
  No pulse
  Vasoconstriction
  Hypotension
  Dark skin
Falsely lowers SpO$_2$
  Nail polish
  Ambient light
  Elevated serum lipids
  Methylene blue
  Indigo carmine
  Indocyanine green
Falsely raises SpO$_2$
  Elevated carboxyhemoglobin
  Elevated methemoglobin
  Ambient light
  Hypothermia

SpO$_2$, saturation indicated by the pulse oximeter.

---

if an oximeter is calibrated on the basis of a study of nonsmokers with a 2% COHb level, the measured SpO$_2$ percentage would differ depending on whether the value used to calibrate SpO$_2$ included or excluded the 2% COHb [177]. Third, it is difficult, for ethical reasons, for manufacturers to obtain an adequate number of validated readings in people with an SpO$_2$ of less than 70% to develop accurate calibration algorithms in this saturation range. Most oximeters give less precise readings and underestimate saturation in this saturation range [178]. Until better calibration algorithms are available, oximeters should be considered unreliable when SpO$_2$ is less than 70%, although this may have little clinical impact because emergent intervention is usually required for all SpO$_2$ readings less than 70%. Practitioners can check a unit's accuracy by systematically comparing the oximetry values of the oximeter with simultaneous cooximeter values measured from arterial blood.

MEASUREMENT SITES. Careful sensor positioning is crucial to obtaining accurate results from a pulse oximeter [179]. Practitioners can obtain accurate measurements from fingers, forehead, and earlobes [180,181]. The response time from a change in the partial pressure of arterial oxygen (Pao$_2$) to a change in displayed SpO$_2$ is delayed in finger and toe probes compared with ear, cheek, or glossal probes [180,182]. Forehead edema, wetness, and head motion may result in inaccurate forehead SpO$_2$ values [183]. Motion and perfusion artifacts are the greatest problems with finger or toe measurements. Glossal pulse oximetry has been useful in some patients in whom no other measuring site was available [184]. The earlobe is believed to be the site least affected by vasoconstriction artifact [185], but paradoxically the finger may give a better signal in times of hypoperfusion [171]. Although currently at an early stage of development, esophageal oximetry may address some of these limitations and is an area of active research [186].

FINGERNAILS. Long fingernails may prevent correct positioning of the finger pulp over the light-emitting diodes used in inflexible probes and therefore produce inaccurate SpO$_2$ readings without affecting the pulse rate [187]. Synthetic nails have produced erroneous results [174]. Adhesive tape, even when placed over both sides of a finger, did not affect measured SpO$_2$ [188]. Because pulse oximetry depends fundamentally on color, nail polish may falsely lower SpO$_2$. In a 1988 study, blue, green, and black polish showed greater decreases than red or purple [189]. However, a 2002 study with a newer-generation oximeter did not find this effect [190]. In addition, placing the probe sideways across the fingernail bed appeared to ameliorate any effect of fingernail polish in one study [191].

SKIN COLOR. The effect of skin color on SpO$_2$ was assessed in a study of 655 patients [192]. Although patients with the darkest skin had significantly less accurate SpO$_2$ readings, the mean inaccuracy in SpO$_2$ (compared with cooximetry) between subjects with light skin and those with the darkest skin was only 0.5%, a clinically insignificant difference. Pulse oximeters, however, encountered difficulties in obtaining readings in darker-skinned patients; 18% of patients with darker skin triggered warning lights or messages versus 1% of lighter-skinned patients. A study of 284 patients with a newer-generation oximeter also found that skin color did not affect measurement accuracy. Poor-quality readings were found more often in darker-skinned patients, although this was a rare event (less than 1% of all patients) [193]. At oxygen saturations between 60% and 70%, newer-generation oximeters overestimate oxygen saturations by 2% to 4% in darker-pigmented but not lighter-pigmented patients [194]. Thus, dark skin may prevent a measurement from being obtained, but when the oximeter reports an error-free value, the value is generally accurate enough for clinical use [195].

AMBIENT LIGHT. Ambient light that affects absorption in the 660- or 910-nm wavelengths, or both, may affect calculations of saturation and pulse. Xenon arc surgical lights [196], fluorescent lights [197], and fiberoptic light sources [198] have caused falsely elevated saturation but typically obvious dramatic elevations in pulse. An infrared heating lamp [199] has produced falsely low saturations and a falsely low pulse, and a standard 15-W fluorescent bulb resulted in falsely low saturation without a change in heart rate [200]. Interference from surrounding lights should be suspected by the presence of pulse values discordant from the palpable pulse or ECG, or changes in the pulse-saturation display when the probe is transiently shielded from ambient light with an opaque object. Most manufacturers have now modified their probes to minimize this problem. Studies report that ambient lighting has little or no effect on newer-generation oximeters [201], although this varies among manufacturers [202].

HYPERBILIRUBINEMIA. Bilirubin's absorbance peak is maximal in the 450-nm range but has tails extending in either direction [203]. Bilirubin, therefore, does not typically affect pulse oximeters that use the standard two-diode system [203,204]. However, it may greatly interfere with the measurement of saturation by cooximeters. Cooximeters typically use four to six wavelengths of light and measure absolute absorbance to quantify the percentage of all major hemoglobin variants. Serum bilirubin values as high as 44 mg per dL had no effect on the accuracy of pulse oximeters but led to falsely low levels of oxyhemoglobin measured by cooximetry [203].

DYSHEMOGLOBINEMIAS. Conventional(two-diode)pulse oximeters cannot detect the presence of methemoglobin, COHb, or fetal hemoglobin. Fetal hemoglobin may confound readings in neonates but is rarely a problem in adults. On the other hand, acquired methemoglobinemia, although still uncommon, is seen in routine practice, largely due to the use of methemoglobinemia-inducing drugs such as topical anesthetics [205–207]. Because methemoglobin absorbs more light at 660 nm than at 990 nm, it affects pulse oximetry readings when methemoglobin levels exceed 6% [208]. Moreover, higher levels of methemoglobin tend to bias the reading toward 85% to 90% [209]. COHb is typically read by a two-diode oximeter as 90% oxyhemoglobin and 10% reduced hemoglobin [210], resulting in false elevations of SpO_2. In the emergency department setting or shortly after ICU admission, a gap between pulse oximetry and Po_2 or cooximetrically measured oxygen saturation may suggest elevated COHb levels, particularly in patients with smoke inhalation or potential carbon monoxide poisoning [211,212]. Because COHb may routinely be 10% in smokers, pulse oximetry may fail to detect significant desaturation in this group of patients. Oxygen saturation in smokers, when measured by cooximetry, was on average 5% lower than pulse oximetric values [213]. Hemolytic anemia may also elevate COHb up to 2.6% [214]. Because other etiologies of COHb are rare in the hospital and the half-life of COHb is short, this problem is unusual in the critical care setting except in newly admitted patients, patients with active hemolysis, or those on COBh-inducing drugs such as sodium nitroprusside [215].

ANEMIA. Few clear data are available on the effect of anemia on pulse oximetry. In dogs, there was no significant degradation in accuracy until the hematocrit was less than 10% [216]. In one study of humans who had hemorrhagic anemia, there appeared to be little effect on pulse oximetry accuracy [217]. In patients with very low SpO_2 (less than 70%), anemia may cause pulse oximeters to underestimate the oxygen saturation; this effect is clinically minimal at higher saturations (less than 3% bias) [218].

LIPIDS. Patients with elevated chylomicrons and those receiving lipid infusions may have falsely low SpO_2 because of interference in absorption by the lipid [219]. This also affects cooximetry and may lead to spurious methemoglobin readings [220].

HYPOTHERMIA. Good-quality signals may be unobtainable in 10% of hypothermic patients (i.e., those with temperature less than 35°C) [221], and signal detection fails at temperatures less than 26.5°C [222]. The decrease in signal quality probably results from hypothermia-induced vasoconstriction. When good-quality signals could be obtained, SpO_2 differed from cooximetry-measured saturation by only 0.6% in one series [221] and tended to be falsely elevated by 0.9% to 3.0% SpO_2 in another [222].

INTRAVASCULAR DYES. Methylene blue, used to treat methemoglobinemia, has a maximal absorption at 670 nm

and therefore falsely lowers measured SpO_2 [223]. Indocyanine green and indigo carmine also lower SpO_2, but the changes are minor and brief [224]. Fluorescein has no effect on SpO_2 [224]. Because of the rapid vascular redistribution of injected dyes, the effect on oximetry readings typically lasts only 5 to 10 minutes [225]. Patent $\dot{V}$ dye, which is used to visualize lymphatics in sentinel node mapping, confounds pulse oximetry [226], an effect that may persist for more than 90 minutes [227].

MOTION ARTIFACT. Shivering and other motions that change the distance from diode to receiver may result in artifact. Oximeters account for motion by different algorithms. Some oximeters display a warning sign, others stop reporting data, and others display erroneous values. The display of a plethysmographic waveform rather than a signal strength bar helps to indicate that artifact has distorted the pulse signal and lowered the quality of the subsequent SpO_2 analysis [228]. Newer-generation oximeters appear to have significantly less susceptibility to motion artifact than earlier models [229].

HYPOPERFUSION. During a blood pressure cuff inflation model of hypoperfusion, most oximeters remained within 2% of control readings [230]. Increasing systemic vascular resistance and decreasing cardiac output can also make it more difficult to obtain a good-quality signal. In one series, the lowest cardiac index and highest systemic vascular resistance at which a signal could be detected were 2.4 L per minute per m^2 and 2,930 dynes second per cm^5 per m^2, respectively [222]. Warming the finger [231], sympathetic digital block [232], or applying a vasodilating cream [222] tended to extend the range of signal detection in individual patients. The ability of the oximeter to display a waveform and detect perfusion degradation of the signal was crucial in determining when the readings obtained were valid [230].

PULSATILE VENOUS FLOW. In physiologic states in which venous and capillary flows become pulsatile, the systolic pulse detected by the oximeter may no longer reflect just the presence of arterial blood. In patients with severe tricuspid regurgitation, the measured saturation may be falsely low, especially with ear probes [233,234].

INDICATIONS. The Society of Critical Care Medicine considers pulse oximetry (or transcutaneous oxygen measurement) essential monitoring for all ICU patients receiving supplemental oxygen [235]. Unsuspected hypoxemia is common in critically ill patients. Sixteen percent of patients not receiving supplemental oxygen in the recovery room have saturations of less than 90% [236]. In 35% of patients, saturations of less than 90% develop during transfer out of the operating room [237]. Because of the high frequency of hypoxemia in critically ill patients, the frequent need to adjust oxygen flow, and the unreliability of visual inspection to detect mild desaturation, oximeters should be used in most critically ill patients for routine, continuous monitoring. In one study that randomized more than 20,000 operative and perioperative patients to continuous or no oximetric monitoring, the authors concluded that oximetry permitted detection of more hypoxemic events, prompted increases in the fraction of oxygen in inspired air, and significantly decreased the incidence of myocardial ischemia, but did not significantly decrease mortality or complication rates [238].

Oximeters have been used in the ICU for reasons other than continuous monitoring. For example, oximeters may be helpful during difficult intubations. Once desaturation occurs, attempts to intubate should be postponed until manual ventilation restores saturation. Note, however, that oximetry is not helpful in promptly detecting inadvertent esophageal intubation because desaturation may lag significantly behind apnea in preoxygenated patients [239]. Oximeters can be useful in detecting systolic blood pressure (see the section Arterial Blood Pressure Monitoring). In trauma patients, an abrupt, sustained 10% drop in saturation in the presence of a stable chest radiograph and static compliance was highly predictive of pulmonary embolism [240], although massive pulmonary emboli may sometimes present without hypoxemia [241] and the presence of hypoxemia in other populations is not necessarily a useful diagnostic clue for pulmonary embolism [242,243]. Oximetry has had low sensitivity when used to evaluate potential compartment syndromes [244].

Capnography

Capnography involves the measurement and display of expired P_{CO_2} concentrations. This section reviews the technology, the sources of difference between end-tidal P_{CO_2} ($ETCO_2$) and $Paco_2$, and the indications for capnography in the ICU.

TECHNOLOGY. Expired P_{CO_2} concentration is usually determined by infrared absorbance or mass spectrometry. The infrared technique relies on the fact that carbon dioxide has a characteristic absorbance of infrared light, with maximal absorbance near a wavelength of 4.28 mm. A heated wire with optical filters is used to generate an infrared light of appropriate wavelength. When carbon dioxide passes between a focused beam of light and a semiconductor photodetector, an electronic signal can be generated that, when calibrated, accurately reflects the P_{CO_2} of the tested gas.

A mass spectrometer bombards gas with an electron stream. The ion fragments that are generated can be deflected by a magnetic field to detector plates located in precise positions to detect ions that are characteristic of the molecule being evaluated. The current generated at the detector can be calibrated to be proportional to the partial pressure of the molecule being evaluated.

The two techniques have different strengths. Mass spectrometers can detect the partial pressures of several gases simultaneously and can monitor several patients at once. Infrared techniques measure only P_{CO_2} and are usually used on only one patient at a time. The calibration and analysis time required for mass spectrometry is significantly longer than with infrared techniques. Infrared systems respond to changes in approximately 100 msec, whereas mass spectrometers take 45 seconds to 5 minutes to respond [245]. Although costs vary widely, mass spectrometers are generally far more expensive and are most frequently purchased to be the central component of a carbon dioxide monitoring system. In the operating room, mass spectrometry has the advantage of being able to measure the partial pressure of anesthetic gases, and the need for a technical specialist to oversee its operation can be more easily justified. For these reasons, mass spectrometry has achieved much more popularity in the operating room than in the ICU.

Gases can be sampled by mainstream or sidestream techniques. Mainstream sampling involves placing the capnometer directly in line in the patient's respiratory circuit. All air leaving the patient passes through the capnometer. The sidestream sampling techniques pump 100 to 300 mL of expired air per minute through thin tubing to an adjacent analyzing chamber.

The mainstream method can be used only on patients who are intubated or wearing a tight-fitting face or nose mask. Mainstream sampling offers the advantage of almost instantaneous analysis of sampled air, but it increases the patient's dead space and adds weight to the endotracheal tube. Sidestream sampling removes air from the expiratory circuit, altering measurement of tidal volume. Slower aspirating flow rates and longer tubing lengths significantly worsen the ability to detect a rapid rise in carbon dioxide and cause delay between physiologic changes in the patient and the display of changes on the monitor [246]. When the delay exceeds the respiratory cycle time, the generated data are inaccurate [246]. Located near the mouth or nose, sidestream sampling lines are also prone to clogging with secretions, saliva, or water condensation. Sidestream sampling can be used in nonintubated patients to detect cyclic changes in carbon dioxide concentrations. Because of these issues, accurate sidestream sampling requires short sampling tubes and attention to the possibility of clogged sample lines.

DIFFERENCES BETWEEN END-TIDAL AND ARTERIAL CARBON DIOXIDE. The P_{CO_2} in exhaled air measured at the mouth changes in a characteristic pattern in healthy people, which reflects the underlying physiologic changes in the lung (Fig. 27-1). During inspiration, the P_{CO_2} is negligible, but it rises abruptly with expiration. The rapid rise reflects mixing and the washout of dead-space air with air from perfused alveoli, which contain higher levels of CO_2. A plateau concentration is reached after dead-space air has been exhaled. The plateau level is determined by the mean alveolar P_{CO_2}, which is in equilibrium with pulmonary artery P_{CO_2}. The end-alveolar plateau level of P_{CO_2} measured during the last 20% of exhalation is the end-tidal P_{CO_2}. In healthy people at rest, the difference between end-tidal P_{CO_2} and $Paco_2$ is ±1.5 mm Hg. A difference exists because of the presence of dead space and a normal physiologic shunt. Changes in dead space or pulmonary perfusion alters ventilation-perfusion ratio and changes the relationship between end-tidal and arterial P_{CO_2} values. As dead space increases, the end-tidal P_{CO_2} represents more the (lower) P_{CO_2} of nonperfused alveoli, thereby diverging from the $Paco_2$ value. As perfusion decreases, fewer alveoli are perfused, creating a similar effect.

In most equipment, the end-tidal P_{CO_2} level is determined by a computerized algorithm. Because algorithms are imperfect, a waveform display is considered essential for accurate interpretation of derived values [246,247]. In slowly breathing patients, cardiac pulsations may cause the intermittent exhalation of small amounts of air at the end of the lungs' expiratory effort. This results in oscillations that may obscure the plateau phase. An irregular respiratory pattern or large increases in dead space can also distort the plateau phase. Visual inspection of traces can detect situations in which algorithms are prone to produce errors [245].

INDICATIONS. In the ICU, capnography is most useful for (a) detection of extubation, (b) determining the presence or absence of respiration, and (c) detecting return of spontaneous circulation after cardiac arrest. Such determinations do not require

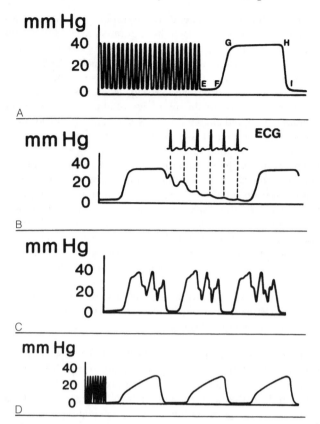

FIGURE 27-1. Normal and abnormal capnograms. In the normal capnogram **(A)**, on the right of the trace, the paper speed has been increased. The *EF* segment is inspiration. The *FG* segment reflects the start of expiration with exhalation of dead-space gas. The *GH* segment is the alveolar plateau. End-tidal values are taken at point *H. HI* is the beginning of inspiration. In the abnormal capnograms, the alveolar plateau is distorted and the end-tidal point cannot be clearly determined because of cardiac oscillations **(B)**, erratic breathing **(C)**, and obstructive airway disease **(D)**. ECG, electrocardiogram. [Modified from Stock MC: Noninvasive carbon dioxide monitoring. *Crit Care Clin* 4:511, 1988.]

that end-tidal Pco_2 be measured accurately, only that changes be detected reliably. Alarms for apnea and tachypnea can be set and relied on, although capnography cannot discriminate between obstructive and central apnea. Capnography is a useful adjunct for detecting unintentional extubation, malposition of the endotracheal tube, or absence of perfusion. Cyclic variation of end-tidal Pco_2 is absent in esophageal intubation or disconnection from the ventilator [248], although pharyngeal intubation with adequate ventilation may produce a normal capnogram. Capnography can demonstrate the return of circulation after cardiopulmonary arrest or bypass. In full cardiac arrest, $ETCO_2$ is low because of lack of perfusion; a rapid rise in $ETCO_2$ indicates return of circulation and successful delivery of CO_2 to the alveoli [249–251]. Capnography or capnometry is also frequently used to help detect esophageal intubation [252]; similarly, these methods can detect inadvertent bronchial placement of feeding tubes [253].

$ETCO_2$ measurements are unreliable indicators of $Paco_2$ in critically ill patients. Because these patients undergo rapid changes in dead-space fraction and pulmonary perfusion, the relationship of end-tidal Pco_2 to arterial $Paco_2$ may change rapidly and unpredictably. In one study of anesthetized, stable, generally healthy adults, $Paco_2$ could not be reliably determined from

end-tidal values [254]. In patients undergoing weaning from mechanical ventilation, end-tidal Pco_2 was also shown to have no predictable relationship to $Paco_2$ [255,256]. Although end-tidal and arterial values correlated well ($r = 0.78$) and rarely differed by more than 4 mm Hg, changes in end-tidal Pco_2 correlated poorly with changes in arterial Pco_2 ($r^2 = 0.58$). Because of changes in dead space and perfusion, arterial and end-tidal measurements at times moved unpredictably in opposite directions. Although theoretically attractive, the use of end-tidal carbon dioxide measurements to evaluate changes in ventilation-perfusion mismatch in response to ventilator changes has failed to yield consistent clinical benefits [257].

Capnography has been helpful in the operating room in detecting air and pulmonary embolism as well as malignant hyperthermia [245,251]. In these situations, the capnograph does not provide a diagnosis; it records a change that, if limits are exceeded, signals an alarm. The responsibility for accurately interpreting the subtleties of changes in the capnogram remains the task of an experienced physician.

SUMMARY. Capnography is of limited use in the critically ill patient. In any patient with changing cardiac output, fluctuating respiratory function, or chronic lung disease, it should not be used to replace $Paco_2$ monitoring. It has been used to assess correct endotracheal tube placement (or inadvertent extubation) and offers rapid information about the return of spontaneous circulation after cardiac arrest. Although it monitors respiratory rate accurately, it is far more expensive and inconvenient than other types of respiratory rate monitors. Capnography may be better suited to the operating room, where its value is increased because of its ability to help detect endotracheal tube malposition, air embolism, pulmonary embolism, and malignant hyperthermia, and where there is a highly skilled anesthesiologist immediately available to interpret subtle changes in the capnogram.

NONINVASIVE TISSUE PERFUSION MONITORING

Bedside providers usually monitor tissue perfusion based on clinical signs such as skin temperature and capillary refill time. However, several noninvasive technologies provide quantitative data about overall or regional tissue perfusion. Unlike most of the other monitoring technologies described in this chapter, clinical adoption of these techniques has been relatively limited and heterogenous [258]. This section reviews three such technologies that measure local Pco_2 or Po_2: Gastric tonometry, sublingual capnometry, and transcutaneous oxygen and carbon dioxide monitoring. Measurements from each of these techniques correlate meaningful clinical outcomes such as patient survival.

PHYSIOLOGY: WHY REGIONAL Po_2 AND Pco_2 REFLECTS TISSUE PERFUSION AND NOT JUST GLOBAL GAS EXCHANGE

At first glance, it would appear that measurement of Po_2 or Pco_2 in the skin, stomach, or tongue would reflect global gas exchange and might be used for noninvasive blood gas estimation. In some cases, this is true. In healthy adults, for example, transcutaneously measured Po_2 and Pco_2 ($P_{tc}O_2$ and

$P_{tc}CO_2$) accurately reflect PaO_2 and $PaCO_2$[259,260]. The measured transcutaneous values of oxygen and carbon dioxide are typically 10 mm Hg lower [261] and 5 to 23 mm Hg higher [262,263] than arterial values, respectively.

However, local PO_2 and PCO_2 therefore depend not only on global gas exchange, cardiac output, and oxygen content, but also on regional blood flow and oxygen delivery to the site of measurement. Under normal circumstances, oxygen delivery far exceeds consumption. In critical illness, however, regional hypoperfusion or inadequate regional delivery of oxygen may occur for any number of reasons, such as hypotension, regional vasoconstriction, low cardiac output states, anemia, and vascular occlusion. If there is no flow to the region, there can be no delivery of oxygen and no elimination of carbon dioxide by the vasculature, thus creating lower local PO_2 and higher local PCO_2 than in the arterial circulation. When tissue is hypoperfused, local metabolism then further alters local PO_2 and PCO_2. As cellular processes use available oxygen for the production of adenosine triphosphate, local PO_2 falls. When these cells use adenosine triphosphate faster than they replenish it, they liberate hydrogen ions (H+) and reduce local pH. (Alternatively, cells may produce lactic acid through the anaerobic metabolic pathway.) These additional hydrogen ions are then buffered by tissue bicarbonate, generating CO_2: $H^+ + HCO_3^- \rightarrow H_2O_3 \rightarrow H_2O + CO_2$. This increases local PCO_2 above corresponding global/arterial values [258,264–266]. For these reasons, local PO_2 and PCO_2 therefore vary not only with global gas exchange, but also with local tissue perfusion.

GASTRIC TONOMETRY

Gastric tonometry, probably the most commonly used of the three perfusion monitoring techniques discussed in this section, assesses regional splanchnic perfusion based on the stomach's mucosal PCO_2. The splanchnic circulation has several properties that make this region particularly useful to assess in critically ill patients. Early in the development of shock states, the splanchnic circulation vasoconstricts, shunting cardiac output toward other core organs. Although this helps to prevent circulatory collapse, it may also result in intestinal mucosal ischemia, increasing the risk of gastric stress ulceration, mesenteric ischemia, and translocation of gut bacteria into the systemic circulation [267–269]. The gut is particularly sensitive to hypoperfusion and so may provide earlier warning of occult hypoperfusion than other vascular beds, leading some to liken it to a coal miner's canary [270]. Gastric tonometry measures gastric luminal PCO_2 and estimates gastric intramucosal PCO_2 and pH (pHi).

Technical Considerations

DEVELOPMENT. Early measurements of visceral mucosal pH required operative implantation of monitors and focused on the gallbladder, urinary bladder, and small bowel [271,272]. Development of silastic tubing [273], which is exceptionally permeable to O_2 and CO_2, and confirmation that gases in tissue equilibrate rapidly with fluid in the lumen of a hollow viscus [274] allowed development of the modern gastrointestinal tonometer.

TECHNIQUE. Most current gastric tonometry catheters consist of a fluid-filled silicone balloon attached near the end of a nasogastric or sigmoid tube. Before insertion, the balloon is re-

peatedly infused with fluid until all air is eliminated. The upper gastrointestinal catheter is inserted with standard technique for nasogastric tube placement, and placement is confirmed radiographically. The stopcock is flushed with fluid to eliminate any trapped air, the balloon is filled to the manufacturer's specifications with fluid, and the tonometer lumen is closed to the outside environment. The fluid is allowed to equilibrate with the fluid in the lumen of the organ being monitored, a process believed to require approximately 90 minutes, although formulas are available to correct the values obtained with 30 to 90 minutes of equilibration [275]. After adequate time for equilibration, the dead space (usually 1.0 mL) is aspirated and discarded, and the fluid in the balloon is completely aspirated under anaerobic conditions. An arterial blood gas sample is taken simultaneously, and both samples are sent for analysis. The PCO_2 of the tonometer sample is measured directly. Providers can then calculate an arterial/mucosal PCO_2 gap or, using the HCO_3^- of arterial blood and the modified Henderson-Hasselbalch equation, pHi [276,277].

More recently, an air-based tonometer has gained clinical and research popularity. This device operates on the same principles as the saline-based tonometer, but automatically aspirates small amounts of air from a semipermeable balloon. This is substantially more convenient than the saline-based device, and allows semicontinuous measurement of gastric mucosal PCO_2. Results are generally similar to saline-based tonometry [265].

TECHNICAL LIMITATIONS. Several issues may confound the clinical use of gastric tonometry. Two of these apply only to saline-based tonometry. The fluid in the tonometer balloon requires 90 minutes for full equilibration with the fluid in the stomach. In a rapidly changing patient, this time window may not be appropriate. Additionally, manufacturers calibrate blood gas analyzers to measure PCO_2 in blood, not saline. PCO_2 measurements in tonometer saline, therefore, may vary based on the blood gas analyzer used [278]. Other limitations apply to the general principle of measuring gastric luminal PCO_2 to estimate mucosal perfusion. Tonometrically derived gastric pHi can be affected by the acid-secretory status of the stomach. In one study, mean gastric pHi was 7.30 in untreated healthy volunteers but 7.39 in a similar group treated with ranitidine [279]. This was because the PCO_2 in the gastric fluid of the treated patients was 42 ± 4 mm Hg, compared with 52 ± 14 mm Hg in the untreated group. The difference in carbon dioxide content of the fluid is thought to be due to production of carbon dioxide by the conversion of secreted H^+ and HCO_3^- into water and carbon dioxide. Enteral feeding may also affect pHi reading. Tube feedings may lead to increased production of carbon dioxide through the interaction of secreted hydrogen ions and HCO_3^-. Some suggest temporarily discontinuing tube feeds before taking pHi measurements [280], although the PCO_2 effect appears to diminish after 24 hours of continuous feeding [281]. Finally, pHi is a calculated variable that uses the systemic arterial bicarbonate value; this probably does not reflect regional perfusion [277]. The present consensus favors the use of arterial-gastric PCO_2 gap rather than pHi [265,282].

CLINICAL USEFULNESS AND LIMITATIONS. pHi correlates well with a number of clinically important end points. Changes in pHi during weaning from mechanical ventilation predict weaning failure [283]. Intraoperative and postoperative cardiac surgery patients have been particularly well studied, and in that group gastric pHi appears to predict complications well [284,285]. Most importantly, pHi predicts mortality in septic [286], acutely injured [287], and general ICU patients [288,289], among others [290–292].

For a diagnostic tool to be *therapeutically* useful, however, we must be able to act on its results in a way that improves patient outcome [293]. Therapeutic protocols based on gastric tonometry have produced conflicting results. A randomized, controlled trial of 260 ICU patients, reported in 1992, found that gastric pHi-based therapy had no effect on mortality of patients with a low admission pHi but was associated with reduced mortality in patients with a normal admission pHi [294]. However, interpretation of this finding is severely limited because the authors did not analyze the results in an intention-to-treat fashion, thus abandoning many of the benefits of randomization [295], and 21 patients were withdrawn from the study due to protocol noncompliance by treating physicians. A subsequent randomized, controlled trial of 210 general ICU patients, reported in 2000, found no difference between intervention and control arms [296]. In patients with a normal initial pHi, there was a nonsignificant trend toward increased 30-day mortality in the group treated based on pHi. One patient in the intervention group was excluded from analysis due to a conversion to comfort-measures-only status 5 hours after enrollment. A 2005 study randomized 151 trauma patients to pHi-driven therapy, splanchnic ischemia/reperfusion-based protocol, or usual care. The authors found no significant differences in mortality, organ dysfunction, ventilator days, or length of stay. Analysis was intention-to-treat [297]. Other, smaller randomized trials have generally found no effect [298,299].

ALTERNATIVE REGIONAL PCO2 MEASUREMENT: SUBLINGUAL CAPNOMETRY. Sublingual capnometry operates on the same fundamental principles as gastric tonometry. A sensor is placed under the tongue and CO_2 diffuses across a semipermeable membrane into a dye that fluoresces differently based on CO_2 concentration. A fiberoptic cable transmits light of the appropriate wavelength and detects the resulting fluorescence, which is proportional to CO_2 concentration in the sensor [258]. Results from this technique correlate with gastric tonometry [300] and patient outcome [301]. No randomized intervention trials based on sublingual capnometry have yet been published. Although sublingual capnometry was entering nonresearch clinical use, the manufacturer recalled the commercially available sublingual capnometry device in 2004 after an outbreak of *Burkholderia cepacia* related to contaminated sublingual probes [302].

SUMMARY. Although gastric tonometry predicts many important clinical outcomes, high-quality data do not support gastric tonometry-based resuscitation. The 2004 guidelines for hemodynamic management of septic shock from the Surviving Sepsis Campaign, representing 11 international professional societies, concludes that these results make gastric tonometry "of interest largely as a research tool rather than as a useful clinical monitor for routine use" [282]. Researchers are actively investigating the use of sublingual capnometry, a similar technology, as a potential resuscitation endpoint.

TRANSCUTANEOUS OXYGEN AND CARBON DIOXIDE MEASUREMENT IN ADULTS

Transcutaneous measurements of the partial pressures of oxygen ($P_{tc}O_2$) and carbon dioxide ($P_{tc}CO_2$) are frequently used for neonatal blood gas monitoring but have not gained widespread clinical acceptance in adult ICUs [258]. Similar to gastric tonometry, $P_{tc}O_2$ and $P_{tc}CO_2$ in adults reflect *local* tissue oxygen and carbon dioxide levels and therefore blur the boundary between assessment of global gas exchange and regional tissue perfusion monitoring.

This section examines the technology used to measure transcutaneous partial pressures, technical problems encountered with this monitoring, and clinical studies and correlations of such measurements. This section refers only to transcutaneous monitoring in adults.

Technique

Oxygen and carbon dioxide diffuse out of the capillaries, into the interstitium, and through the skin. The skin usually resists oxygen and carbon dioxide diffusion, but heating the skin promotes diffusion by changing the structure of the stratum corneum, shifting the oxygen dissociation curve, and promoting arterialization of dermal capillaries [258]. Transcutaneous systems take advantage of these properties to measure partial pressures of oxygen ($P_{tc}O_2$) and carbon dioxide ($P_{tc}CO_2$). Typically, a unit less than 1 inch in diameter is attached with an airtight seal to the skin with an adhesive. An electrode heats the skin to improve gas exchange; a temperature sensor measures skin temperature at the skin surface and adjusts the heater to provide a constant temperature, typically about 44°C. Oxygen and carbon dioxide diffuse out of the capillaries into the interstitium and through the skin to measuring electrodes. The diffusing distance from capillary to sensor may be as small as 0.3 mm. Then, precalibrated Clarke- and Severinghaus-type electrodes, similar to those used in blood gas machines, measure the partial pressure of oxygen and carbon dioxide. These signals are then electronically averaged and converted into a continuous digital display. Many units also display trend signals to indicate whether and in which direction changes occur.

Technical Limitations

Because units use electrodes for partial pressure measurement, problems with calibration and electrode drift during prolonged monitoring can clearly alter measurements. Drift may alter readings by up to 12% over a 2-hour period [259]. Because of the heating requirement, probe sites must be changed at least every 4 hours to prevent burns [303]. Units must be recalibrated whenever the probe temperature is changed, and every 4 to 6 hours to prevent artifact from electrode drift. Many units take 15 to 60 minutes to warm the skin and establish stable readings. Probes must be firmly attached to the skin, or resultant leaks from the surrounding atmosphere lower $P_{tc}CO_2$ and alter $P_{tc}O_2$ values. Adhesion is a problem in diaphoretic patients. Patient motion may produce tension on the cable that connects the sensor to the processing unit, causing leaks or disconnection. These factors can combine in many patients to make transcutaneous measurements very inconvenient, although newer sensors may be less time-consuming [304].

Thick or edematous skin provides a diffusion barrier that amplifies differences between arterial and transcutaneous Po_2

and Pco_2. The longer the distance the gases must diffuse to be measured, the more important are the effects of temperature, perfusion, and local metabolism. This appears to be the fundamental reason why transcutaneous measurements are usually more closely related to arterial values in neonates than in adults. Edema, burns, abrasions, or scleroderma would all be expected to alter transcutaneous values.

Clinical Usefulness and Limitations

Because $P_{tc}O_2$ and $P_{tc}CO_2$ reflect local Po_2 and Pco_2, they change in response both to regional perfusion/oxygen delivery and to global derangements. In stable, healthy adults without hemodynamic or respiratory instability, $P_{tc}O_2$ and $P_{tc}CO_2$ accurately reflect arterial Po_2 and Pco_2 [259,260]. The measured transcutaneous values of oxygen and carbon dioxide are typically 10 mm Hg lower [261] and 5 to 23 mm Hg higher [262,263] than arterial values, respectively. In stable patients, it may be reasonable to use transcutaneously measured values as surrogates for arterial Po_2 and Pco_2. However, systemic hypoperfusion due to low cardiac output, regional hypoperfusion due to sepsis or shock, and local hypoperfusion due to cutaneous vasoconstriction caused by medication or cold produces discrepancies. In these cases, transcutaneous measurements cease to reflect arterial values and are better for tracking oxygen delivery and tissue metabolism [305,306]. For these reasons, many authors have argued against relying on $P_{tc}O_2$ and $P_{tc}CO_2$ to estimate arterial Po_2 and Pco_2 in critically ill adults [306–309].

Several studies have demonstrated the value of transcutaneous oxygen measurements as indices of perfusion or oxygen delivery. When arterial Po_2 remains constant, a decrease in $P_{tc}O_2$ is probably due to changes in perfusion. Changes in local perfusion and metabolism may cause $P_{tc}O_2$ values to fall to zero and $P_{tc}CO_2$ values to climb to more than 30 mm Hg above arterial values [262]. During cardiac decompensation and arrest, $P_{tc}O_2$ correlates best with cardiac output [305]. In hemorrhagic shock, the ratio of $P_{tc}O_2$ to arterial Po_2 decreases, even though arterial Po_2 may remain normal [310,311]. Because the measurements are very sensitive to changes in flow, they can be useful in predicting or warning of imminent change before a blood pressure response is seen. In a small series of high-risk perioperative patients, declines in the transcutaneous to arterial Po_2 ratio predicted subsequent hemodynamic collapse [312]. Transcutaneous $P_{tc}O_2$ also correlates with mortality. In emergency department patients with severe sepsis or septic shock, $P_{tc}O_2$ was lower in nonsurvivors than survivors [313]. In trauma patients, $P_{tc}O_2$ values were significantly higher in survivors than nonsurvivors ($p < 0.001$) with an area under the receiver operating characteristics curve of 0.74 for predicting in-hospital mortality [314].

Ongoing Development

Recently, research has focused on a new device that is applied to the earlobe. This sensor received Food and Drug Administration marketing approval in 2005 and combines a pulse oximeter and $P_{tc}CO_2$ sensor. The $P_{tc}CO_2$ sensor, the Stow-Severinghaus-type CO_2 sensor, determines the pH of an electrolyte solution; pH changes are proportional to the logarithm of the Pco_2 solution [315]. The sensor is calibrated to a gas of known CO_2 concentration in the unit's storage chamber, and includes an element that heats the earlobe to 42°C [316]. In a small pilot study of volunteers and patients undergoing general anesthesia, its values correlated very well with blood gas Pco_2 and finger-clip SpO_2

[317]. Another study of 18 ICU patients with respiratory or heart failure found that the oximeter correlated very well with cooximetric values. $P_{tc}CO_2$ and arterial Pco_2 also correlated well ($r = 0.88$), with a bias of 3 ± 7 mm Hg [316]. No difference was seen between the nine patients on vasopressors and on those not on vasopressors. A more "real-world" study of 55 ICU patients investigated the performance of this sensor when applied by bedside providers, rather than a study team. $P_{tc}CO_2$ and arterial Pco_2 also correlated well ($r = 0.88$). However, 17% of the 417 paired measurements were outside the authors' clinically acceptable limits of agreement of 7.5 mm Hg [318]. Further evaluation is required both to confirm the device's performance in clinical practice and to verify its performance in patients with fluctuating hemodynamics.

Summary

Transcutaneous monitors have little role in the ICU as simple tools to replace other means of measuring arterial gas. Their application in practice is not complex but is far from simple. They predictably reflect arterial Po_2 and Pco_2 values only in hemodynamically stable patients, who are least likely to demand intensive care or to benefit from ICU monitoring. As monitors of trends in Pco_2 and Po_2, they can be regarded as effective only in the sense that they typically do not produce false-negative alarms; that is, if the arterial values change, the transcutaneous values reflect the change. So many other factors, such as changes in tissue edema and perfusion, may result in alterations in transcutaneous trends that the supervising staff can initially determine only that *something* has changed. An accurate interpretation of the clinical event usually requires reassessment of either cardiac status or arterial gases.

Therefore, transcutaneous monitors are inadequate cardiac monitors and inadequate pulmonary monitors but are good cardiopulmonary monitors. When perfusion is stable, values reflect gas exchange. When gas exchange is stable, values reflect perfusion. When both are unstable, the results cannot be interpreted without additional information.

REFERENCES

1. Barie PS, Hydo LJ, Eachempati SR: Causes and consequences of fever complicating critical surgical illness. *Surg Infect (Larchmt* 5:145, 2004.
2. Peres Bota D, Lopes Ferreira F, Melot C, et al: Body temperature alterations in the critically ill. *Intensive Care Med* 30:811, 2004.
3. Kholoussy AM, Sufian S, Pavlides C: Central peripheral temperature gradient: its value and limitations in the management of critically ill surgical patients. *Am J Surg* 140:609, 1980.
4. Perry PA: Banned in Boston. Medical mercury is on the way out. *Mater Manag Health Care* 10:15, 2001.
5. Harvey PD, Smith CM: The mercury's falling: the Massachusetts approach to reducing mercury in the environment. *Am J Law Med* 30(2-3):245, 2004.
6. Burgess GE, III, Cooper JR, Marino RJ: Continuous monitoring of skin temperature using a liquid-crystal thermometer during anesthesia. *South Med J* 71:516, 1978.
7. Roberts NH: The comparison of surface and core temperature devices. *J Am Assoc Nurse Anesth* 48:53, 1980.
8. Silverman RW, Lomax P: The measurement of temperature for thermoregulatory studies. *Pharmacol Ther* 27:233, 1985.
9. Vale RJ: Monitoring of temperature during anesthesia. *Int Anesthesiol Clin* 19:61, 1981.
10. Terndrup TE: An appraisal of temperature assessment by infrared emission detection tympanic thermometry. *Ann Emerg Med* 21:1483, 1992.
11. Terndrup TE, Rajk J: Impact of operator technique and device on infrared emission detection tympanic thermometry. *J Emerg Med* 10:683, 1992.
12. Myny D, De Waele J, Defloor T, et al: Temporal scanner thermometry: a new method of core temperature estimation in ICU patients. *Scott Med J* 50:15, 2005.
13. Suleman MI, Doufas AG, Akca O, et al: Insufficiency in a new temporal-artery thermometer for adult and pediatric patients. *Anesth Analg* 95:67, 2002.
14. Schuh S, Koma r L, Stephens D, et al: Comparison of the temporal artery and rectal thermometry in children in the emergency department. *Pediatr Emerg Care* 20:736, 2004.

15. Erickson R: Thermometer placement for oral temperature measurement in febrile adults. *Int J Nurs Stud* 13:199, 1976.

16. Heinz J: Validation of sublingual temperatures in patients with nasogastric tubes. *Heart Lung* 14:128, 1985.

17. Tandberg D, Sklar D: Effect of tachypnea on the estimation of body temperature by an oral thermometer. *N Engl J Med* 313:945, 1985.

18. Cork RC, Vaughan RW, Humphrey LS: Precision and accuracy of intraoperative temperature monitoring. *Anesth Analg* 62:211, 1983.

19. Bone ME, Feneck RO: Bladder temperature as an estimate of body temperature during cardiopulmonary bypass. *Anaesthesia* 43:181, 1988.

20. Ramsay JG, Ralley FE, Whalley DG: Site of temperature monitoring and prediction of afterdrop after open heart surgery. *Can Anaesth Soc J* 32:607, 1985.

21. Moorthy SS, Winn BA, Jallard MS: Monitoring urinary bladder temperature. *Heart Lung* 14:90, 1985.

22. Crocker BD, Okumura F, McCuaig DI: Temperature monitoring during general anaesthesia. *Br J Anaesth* 52:1223, 1980.

23. Severinghaus JW: Temperature gradients during hypothermia. *Ann N Y Acad Sci* 80:515, 1962.

24. Webb GE: Comparison of esophageal and tympanic temperature monitoring during cardiopulmonary bypass. *Anesth Analg* 52:729, 1973.

25. Fulbrook P: Core body temperature measurement: a comparison of axilla, tympanic membrane and pulmonary artery blood temperature. *Intensive Crit Care Nurs* 13:266, 1997.

26. Giuliano KK, Giuliano AJ, Scott SS, et al: Temperature measurement in critically ill adults: a comparison of tympanic and oral methods. *Am J Crit Care* 9:254, 2000.

27. Giuliano KK, Scott SS, Elliot S, et al: Temperature measurement in critically ill orally intubated adults: a comparison of pulmonary artery core, tympanic, and oral methods. *Crit Care Med* 27:2188, 1999.

28. Hoffman C, Boyd M, Briere B, et al: Evaluation of three brands of tympanic thermometer. *Can J Nurs Res* 31:117, 1999.

29. Farnell S, Maxwell L, Tan S, et al: Temperature measurement: comparison of non-invasive methods used in adult critical care. *J Clin Nurs* 14:632, 2005.

30. Amoateng-Adjepong Y, Del Mundo J, Manthous CA: Accuracy of infrared tympanic thermometer. *Chest* 115:1002, 1999.

31. Wallace CT, Marks WE, Adkins WY: Perforation of the tympanic membrane: a complication of tympanic thermometry during anesthesia. *Anesthesiology* 41:290, 1974.

32. Nierman DM: Core temperature measurement in the intensive care unit. *Crit Care Med* 19:818, 1991.

33. Lefrant JY, Muller L, de La Coussaye JE, et al: Temperature measurement in intensive care patients: comparison of urinary bladder, oesophageal, rectal, axillary, and inguinal methods versus pulmonary artery core method. *Intensive Care Med* 29:414, 2003.

34. Brooks SE, Veal RO, Kramer M: Reduction in the incidence of Clostridium difficile associated diarrhea in an acute care hospital and a skilled nursing facility following replacement of electronic thermometers with single-use disposables. *Infect Control Hosp Epidemiol* 13:98, 1992.

35. Livnorese LL, Dias S, Samel C: Hospital-acquired infection with vancomycin-resistant Enterococcus faecium transmitted by electronic thermometers. *Ann Intern Med* 117:112, 1992.

36. Haupt MT, Bekes CE, Brilli RJ, et al: Guidelines on critical care services and personnel: Recommendations based on a system of categorization of three levels of care. *Crit Care Med* 31:2677, 2003.

37. Roguin A: Scipione Riva-Rocci and the men behind the mercury sphygmomanometer. *Int J Clin Pract* 60:73, 2006.

38. Pierce EC: Percutaneous arterial catheterization in man with special reference to aortography. *Surg Gynecol Obstet* 93:56, 1951.

39. Donald DC Jr, Kesmodel KF Jr, Rollins SL Jr: An improved technique for percutaneous cerebral angiography. *Arch Neurol Psychiatry* 65:500, 1951.

40. Bruner JMR, Krenis LJ, Kunsman JM: Comparison of direct and indirect methods of measuring arterial blood pressure: Pt III. *Med Instrum* 15:182, 1981.

41. Reder RF, Dimich I, Cohen ML: Evaluating indirect blood pressure measurement techniques: a comparison of three systems in infants and children. *Pediatrics* 62:326, 1978.

42. Nystrom E, Reid KH, Bennett R: A comparison of two automated indirect arterial blood pressure meters: with recordings from a radial arterial catheter in anesthetized surgical patients. *Anesthesiology* 62:526, 1985.

43. DeGowin RL, Brown DD: Thorax: respiratory, cardiovascular, and lymphatic systems, in DeGowin RL, ed: *Diagnostic Examination*. 7th ed. New York, McGraw-Hill, 2000, p 247.

44. Hirschl MM, Binder M, Herkner H: Accuracy and reliability of noninvasive continuous finger blood pressure measurement in critically ill patients. *Crit Care Med* 24:1684, 1996.

45. Carrol GC: Blood pressure monitoring. *Crit Care Clin* 4:411, 1988.

46. Van Bergen FH, Weatherhead S, Treloar AE: Comparison of direct and indirect methods of measuring arterial blood pressure. *Circulation* 10:481, 1954.

47. Bailey RH, Knaus VL, Bauer JH: Aneroid sphygmomanometers: an assessment of accuracy at a university hospital and clinics. *Arch Intern Med* 151:1409, 1991.

48. O'Keefe KM, Bookman L: The portable Doppler: practical applications in EMS care. *JACEP* 5:987, 1976.

49. Weaver LK, Howe S: Noninvasive Doppler blood pressure in the monoplace hyperbaric chamber. *J Clin Monit* 7:304, 1991.

50. Talke PO: Measurement of systolic blood pressure using pulse oximetry during helicopter flight. *Crit Care Med* 19:934, 1991.

51. Talke P, Nichols RJ Jr, Traber DL: Does measurement of systolic blood pressure with a pulse oximeter correlate with conventional methods? *J Clin Monit* 6:5, 1990.

52. Zagzebski JA: Physics and instrumentation in Doppler and B-mode ultrasonography, in Zwiebel WJ, ed: *Introduction to Vascular Ultrasonography*. Orlando, FL, Grune & Stratton, 1986, p 21.

53. Kirby RR, Kemmerer WT, Morgan JL: Transcutaneous Doppler measurement of blood pressure. *Anesthesiology* 31:86, 1969.

54. Hochberg HM, Salomon H: Accuracy of automated ultrasound blood pressure monitor. *Curr Ther Res* 13:129, 1971.

55. Zezulka AV, Sloan PJ, Davies P, et al: Clinical evaluation of the Infrasonde D4000 blood pressure monitor. *Postgrad Med J* 61(714):321, 1985.

56. Cullen PM, Dye J, Hughes DG: Clinical assessment of the neonatal Dinamap 847 during anesthesia in neonates and infants. *J Clin Monit* 3:229, 1987.

57. Borow KM, Newberger JW: Non-invasive estimation of central aortic pressure using the oscillometric method for analyzing systemic artery pulsatile blood flow: comparative study of indirect systolic, diastolic, and mean brachial artery pressure with simultaneous direct ascending aortic pressure measurements. *Am Heart J* 103:879, 1982.

58. Van Egmond J, Hasenbros M, Crul JF: Invasive v. non-invasive measurement of arterial pressure. *Br J Anaesth* 57:434, 1985.

59. Bogert LW, van Lieshout JJ: Non-invasive pulsatile arterial pressure and stroke volume changes from the human finger. *Exp Physiol* 90:437, 2005.

60. O'Rourke MF, Adji A: An updated clinical primer on large artery mechanics: implications of pulse waveform analysis and arterial tonometry. *Curr Opin Cardiol* 20:275, 2005.

61. Steiner LA, Johnston AJ, Salvador R, et al: Validation of a tonometric noninvasive arterial blood pressure monitor in the intensive care setting. *Anaesthesia* 58:448, 2003.

62. Janelle GM, Gravenstein N: An accuracy evaluation of the T-Line Tensymeter (continuous noninvasive blood pressure management device) versus conventional invasive radial artery monitoring in surgical patients. *Anesth Analg* 102:484, 2006.

63. Wipperman CF, Schranz D, Huth RG: Evaluation of the pulse wave arrival time as a marker for pressure changes in critically ill infants and children. *J Clin Monit* 11:324, 1995.

64. Sharwood-Smith G, Bruce J, Drummond G: Assessment of pulse transit time to indicate cardiovascular changes during obstetric spinal anaesthesia. *Br J Anaesth* 96:100, 2006.

65. Chen W, Kobayashi T, Ichikawa S, et al: Continuous estimation of systolic blood pressure using the pulse arrival time and intermittent calibration. *Med Biol Eng Comput* 38:569, 2000.

66. Edwards RC, Goldberg AD, Bannister R: The infrasound blood pressure monitor: a clinical evaluation. *Lancet* 2:398, 1976.

67. Rutten AJ, Isley AH, Skowronski GA: A comparative study of the measurement of mean arterial blood pressure using automatic oscillometers, arterial cannulation and auscultation. *Anaesth Intensive Care* 14:58, 1986.

68. Yelderman M, Ream AK: Indirect measurement of mean blood pressure in the anesthetized patient. *Anesthesiology* 50:253, 1979.

69. Modesti PA, Gensini GF, Conti C: Clinical evaluation of an automatic blood-pressure monitoring device. *J Clin Hyper* 3:631, 1987.

70. Baker LK: Dinamap monitor versus direct blood pressure measurements. *Dimens Crit Care Nurs* 5:228, 1986.

71. Amoore JN, Geake WB, Scott DHT: Oscillometric non-invasive blood pressure measurements: the influence of the make of instrument on readings. *Med Biol Eng Comput* 35:131, 1997.

72. Derrico DJ: Comparison of blood pressure measurement methods in critically ill children. *Dimens Crit Care Nurs* 12:31, 1993.

73. Latman NS: Evaluation of finger blood pressure monitoring instruments. *Biomed Instrum Technol* 26:52, 1992.

74. Aitken HA, Todd JG, Kenny GNC: Comparison of the Finapres and direct arterial pressure monitoring during profound hypotensive anesthesia. *Br J Anaesth* 67:36, 1991.

75. Kermode JL, Davis NJ, Thompson WR: Comparison of the Finapres blood pressure monitor with intra-arterial manometry during induction of anaesthesia. *Anaesth Intensive Care* 17:470, 1989.

76. Farquhar IK: Continuous direct and indirect blood pressure measurement (Finapres) in the critically ill. *Anaesthesia* 46:1050, 1991.

77. Bos WJW, Imholz BPM, van Goudoever J: The reliability of non-invasive continuous finger blood pressure measurement in patients with both hypertension and vascular disease. *Am J Hypertens* 5:529, 1992.

78. Pace NL, East TD: Simultaneous comparison of intraarterial, oscillometric, and finapres monitoring during anesthesia. *Anesth Analg* 73:213, 1991.

79. Epstein RH, Kaplan S, Leighton BL, et al: Evaluation of a continuous noninvasive blood pressure monitor in obstetric patients undergoing spinal anesthesia. *J Clin Monit* 5:157, 1989.

80. Gibbs NM, Larach DR, Derr JA: The accuracy of Finapres noninvasive mean arterial pressure measurements in anesthetized patients. *Anesthesiology* 74:647, 1991.

81. Stokes DN, Clutton-Brock T, Patil C, et al: Comparison of invasive and non-invasive measurements of continuous arterial pressure using the Finapres. *Br J Anaesth* 67:26, 1991.

82. Paulus DA: Noninvasive blood pressure measurement. *Med Instrum* 15:91, 1981.

83. Sy WP: Ulnar nerve palsy possibly related to use of automatically cycled blood pressure cuff. *Anesth Analg* 60:687, 1981.

84. Betts EK: Hazard of automated noninvasive blood pressure monitoring. *Anesthesiology* 55:717, 1981.

85. Bainbridge LC, Simmons HM, Elliot D: The use of automatic blood pressure monitors in the burned patient. *Br J Plast Surg* 43:322, 1990.

86. Hutton P, Prys-Roberts C: An assessment of the Dinamap 845. *Anaesthesia* 39:261, 1984.

87. Davis FM, Stewart JM: Radial artery cannulation. *Br J Anaesth* 52:41, 1980.

88. Gardner RM, Schwarz R, Wong HC: Percutaneous indwelling radial-artery catheters for monitoring cardiovascular function. *N Engl J Med* 290:1227, 1974.

89. McNulty J, Katz E, Kim KY: Thrombocytopenia following heparin flush. *Prog Cardiovasc Nurs* 20:143, 2005.

90. Schwid HA: Frequency response evaluation of radial artery catheter-manometer systems: sinusoidal frequency analysis versus flush method. *J Clin Monit* 4:181, 1988.

91. Bruner JMR, Krenis LJ, Kunsman JM: Comparison of direct and indirect methods of measuring arterial blood pressure: Pt II. *Med Instrum* 15:97, 1981.

92. Rothe CF, Kim KC: Measuring systolic arterial blood pressure: possible errors from extension tubes or disposable transducer domes. *Crit Care Med* 8:683, 1980.
93. Hughes VG, Prys-Roberts C: Intra-arterial pressure measurements: a review and analysis of methods relevant to anaesthesia and intensive care. *Anaesthesia* 26:511, 1971.
94. Shinozaki T, Deane RS, Mazuzan JE: The dynamic responses of liquid filled catheter systems for direct measurements of blood pressure. *Anesthesiology* 53:498, 1980.
95. Russell JA, Joel M, Hudson RJ: Prospective evaluation of radial and femoral artery catheterization sites in critically ill adults. *Crit Care Med* 11:936, 1983.
96. Colvin MP, Curran JP, Jarvis D: Femoral artery pressure monitoring. *Anaesthesia* 32:451, 1977.
97. Scheer B, Perel A, Pfeiffer UJ: Clinical review: complications and risk factors of peripheral arterial catheters used for haemodynamic monitoring in anaesthesia and intensive care medicine. *Crit Care* 6:199, 2002.
98. Frezza EE, Mezghebe H: Indications and complications of arterial catheter use in surgical or medical intensive care units: analysis of 4932 patients. *Am Surg* 64:127, 1998.
99. Bryan-Brown CW, Kwun KB, Lumb PD: The axillary artery catheter. *Heart Lung* 12:492, 1983.
100. Kahler AC, Mirza F: Alternative arterial catheterization site using the ulnar artery in critically ill pediatric patients. *Pediatr Crit Care Med* 3:370, 2002.
101. Dorman T, Breslow MJ, Lipsett PA, et al: Radial artery pressure monitoring underestimates central arterial pressure during vasopressor therapy in critically ill surgical patients. *Crit Care Med* 26:1646, 1998.
102. Arnal D, Garutti I, Perez-Pena J, et al: Radial to femoral arterial blood pressure differences during liver transplantation. *Anaesthesia* 60:766, 2005.
103. Mignini MA, Piacentini E, Dubin A: Peripheral arterial blood pressure monitoring adequately tracks central arterial blood pressure in critically ill patients: an observational study. *Crit Care* 10:R43, 2006.
104. Yazigi A, Madi-Jebara S, Haddad F, et al: Accuracy of radial arterial pressure measurement during surgery under controlled hypotension. *Acta Anaesthesiol Scand* 46:173, 2002.
105. Michard F, Boussat S, Chemla D, et al: Relation between respiratory changes in arterial pulse pressure and fluid responsiveness in septic patients with acute circulatory failure. *Am J Respir Crit Care Med* 162:134, 2000.
106. Thys DM: The normal ECG, in Thys DM, Kaplan JA, eds: *The ECG in Anesthesia and Critical Care.* New York, Churchill Livingstone, 1987, p 1.
107. Winters SR: Diagnosis by wireless. *Sci Am* 124:465, 1921.
108. Drew BJ, Califf RM, Funk M, et al: Practice standards for electrocardiographic monitoring in hospital settings: an American Heart Association scientific statement from the Councils on Cardiovascular Nursing, Clinical Cardiology, and Cardiovascular Disease in the Young: endorsed by the International Society of Computerized Electrocardiology and the American Association of Critical-Care Nurses. *Circulation* 110:2721, 2004.
109. Reinelt P, Karth GD, Geppert A, et al: Incidence and type of cardiac arrhythmias in critically ill patients: a single center experience in a medical-cardiological ICU. *Intensive Care Med* 27:1466, 2001.
110. Delle Karth G, Reinelt P, Buberl A, et al: Circadian variation in ventricular tachycardia and atrial fibrillation in a medical-cardiological ICU. *Intensive Care Med* 29:963, 2003.
111. Batra GS, Molyneux J, Scott NA: Colorectal patients and cardiac arrhythmias detected on the surgical high dependency unit. *Ann R Coll Surg Engl* 83:174, 2001.
112. Brathwaite D, Weissman C: The new onset of atrial arrhythmias following major noncardiothoracic surgery is associated with increased mortality. *Chest* 114:462, 1998.
113. Ciriaco P, Mazzone P, Canneto B, et al: Supraventricular arrhythmia following lung resection for non-small cell lung cancer and its treatment with amiodarone. *Eur J Cardiothorac Surg* 18:12, 2000.
114. Lown B, Klein MD: Coronary and precoronary care. *Am J Med* 46:705, 1969.
115. Yu PN, Fox SM, Imboden CA: A specialized intensive care unit for acute myocardial infarction. *Mod Concepts Cardiovasc Dis* 34:23, 1965.
116. Kimball JT, Killip T: Aggressive treatment of arrhythmias in acute myocardial infarction: procedures and results. *Prog Cardiovasc Dis* 10:483, 1968.
117. Henkel DM, Witt BJ, Gersh BJ, et al: Ventricular arrhythmias after acute myocardial infarction: a 20-year community study. *Am Heart J* 151:806, 2006.
118. Cercek B, Lew AS, Laramee P: Time course and characteristics of ventricular arrhythmias after reperfusion in acute myocardial infarction. *Am J Cardiol* 60:214, 1987.
119. Buckingham TA, Devine JE, Redd RM: Reperfusion arrhythmias during coronary reperfusion therapy in man: clinical and angiographic correlations. *Chest* 90:346, 1986.
120. Linnik W, Tintinalli JE, Ramos R: Associated reactions during and immediately after rtPA infusion. *Ann Emerg Med* 18:234, 1989.
121. Romhilt DW, Bloomfield SS, Chou T: Unreliability of conventional electrocardiographic monitoring for arrhythmia detection in coronary care units. *Am J Cardiol* 31:457, 1973.
122. Holmberg S, Ryden L, Waldenstrom A: Efficiency of arrhythmia detection by nurses in a coronary care unit using a decentralized monitoring system. *Br Heart J* 39:1019, 1977.
123. Vetter NJ, Julian DG: Comparison of arrhythmia computer and conventional monitoring in coronary-care unit. *Lancet* 1:1151, 1975.
124. Pierpoint GL: Pitfalls of computer use in acute care medicine. *Heart Lung* 16:207, 1987.
125. Watkinson WP, Brice MA, Robinson KS: A computer-assisted electrocardiographic analysis system: methodology and potential application to cardiovascular toxicology. *J Toxicol Environ Health* 15:713, 1985.
126. Alcover IA, Henning RJ, Jackson DL: A computer-assisted monitoring system for arrhythmia detection in a medical intensive care unit. *Crit Care Med* 12:888, 1984.
127. Badura FK: Nurse acceptance of a computerized arrhythmia monitoring system. *Heart Lung* 9:1044, 1980.
128. Cecchi AC, Dovellini EV, Marchi F: Silent myocardial ischemia during ambulatory electrocardiographic monitoring in patients with effort angina. *J Am Coll Cardiol* 1:934, 1983.
129. Clements FM, Bruijn NP: Noninvasive cardiac monitoring. *Crit Care Clin* 4:435, 1988.
130. Mirvis DM, Berson AS, Goldberger AL: Instrumentation and practice standards for electrocardiographic monitoring in special care units. *Circulation* 79:464, 1989.
131. Amanullah AM, Lindvall K: Prevalence and significance of transient—predominantly asymptomatic—myocardial ischemia on Holter monitoring in unstable angina pectoris, and correlation with exercise test and thallium-201 myocardial perfusion imaging. *Am J Cardiol* 72:144, 1993.
132. Drew BJ, Pelter MM, Adams MG, et al: 12-lead ST-segment monitoring vs single-lead maximum ST-segment monitoring for detecting ongoing ischemia in patients with unstable coronary syndromes. *Am J Crit Care* 7:355, 1998.
133. Fesmire FM, Wharton DR, Calhoun FB: Instability of ST segments in the early stages of acute myocardial infarction in patients undergoing continuous 12-lead ECG monitoring. *Am J Emerg Med* 13:158, 1995.
134. Pepine CJ: Prognostic markers in thrombolytic therapy: looking beyond mortality. *Am J Cardiol* 78[12A]:24, 1996.
135. Balaji S, Ellenby M, McNames J, et al: Update on intensive care ECG and cardiac event monitoring. *Card Electrophysiol Rev* 6:190, 2002.
136. Association for the Advancement of Medical Instrumentation: *American National Standard for Cardiac Monitors, Heart Rate Meters, and Alarms (EC 13-1983).* Arlington, VA, ANSI/AAMI, 1984.
137. Starmer CF, Whalen RE, McIntosh HD: Hazards of electric shock in cardiology. *Am J Cardiol* 14:537, 1964.
138. Bruner JMR: Hazards of electrical apparatus. *Anesthesiology* 28:396, 1967.
139. Hanley J: Telemetry in health care. *Biomed Eng* 11:269, 1976.
140. Pittman JV, Blum MS, Leonard MS: *Telemetry Utilization for Emergency Medical Services Systems.* Atlanta, Georgia Institute of Technology, 1974.
141. Anderson GJ, Knoebel SB, Fisch C: Continuous prehospitalization monitoring of cardiac rhythm. *Am Heart J* 82:642, 1971.
142. Tri JL, Severson RP, Firl AR, et al: Cellular telephone interference with medical equipment. *Mayo Clin Proc* 80:1286, 2005.
143. Mithoefer JC, Bossman OG, Thibeault DW, et al: The clinical estimation of alveolar ventilation. *Am Rev Respir Dis* 98:868, 1968.
144. McFadden JP, Price RC, Eastwood HD: Raised respiratory rate in elderly patients: a valuable physical sign. *Br J Med* 284:626, 1982.
145. Krieger B, Feinerman D, Zaron A: Continuous noninvasive monitoring of respiratory rate in critically ill patients. *Chest* 90:632, 1986.
146. Knaus WA, Draper EA, Wagner DP, et al: APACHE II. a severity of disease classification system. *Crit Care Med* 13:818, 1985.
147. Knaus WA, Wagner DP, Draper EA, et al: The APACHE III prognostic system. Risk prediction of hospital mortality for critically ill hospitalized adults. *Chest* 100:1619, 1991.
148. Boyd CR, Tolson MA, Copes WS: Evaluating trauma care: the TRISS method. Trauma Score and the Injury Severity Score. *J Trauma* 27:370, 1987.
149. Groeger JS, Lemeshow S, Price K, et al: Multicenter outcome study of cancer patients admitted to the intensive care unit: a probability of mortality model. *J Clin Oncol* 16:761, 1998.
150. Mithoefer JC, Bossman OG, Thibeault DW: The clinical estimation of alveolar ventilation. *Am Rev Respir Dis* 98:868, 1968.
151. Semmes BJ, Tobin MJ, Snyder JV, et al: Subjective and objective measurement of tidal volume in critically ill patients. *Chest* 87:577, 1985.
152. Shelly MP, Park GR: Failure of a respiratory monitor to detect obstructive apnea. *Crit Care Med* 14:836, 1986.
153. Sackner MA, Bizousky F, Krieger BP: Performance of impedance pneumograph and respiratory inductive plethysmograph as monitors of respiratory frequency and apnea. *Am Rev Respir Dis* 135:A41, 1987.
154. Wiklund L, Hok B, Stahl K, et al: Postanesthesia monitoring revisited: frequency of true and false alarms from different monitoring devices. *J Clin Anesth.* 6:182, 1994.
155. Lovett PB, Buchwald JM, Sturmann K, et al: The vexatious vital: neither clinical measurements by nurses nor an electronic monitor provides accurate measurements of respiratory rate in triage. *Ann Emerg Med* 45:68, 2005.
156. Chadha TS, Watson H, Birch S, et al: Validation of respiratory inductive plethysmography using different calibration procedures. *Am Rev Respir Dis* 125:644, 1982.
157. Sackner MA, Watson H, Belsito AS: Calibration of respiratory inductive plethysmograph during natural breathing. *J Appl Physiol* 66:410, 1989.
158. Tobin MJ, Jenouri G, Lind B: Validation of respiratory inductive plethysmography in patients with pulmonary disease. *Chest* 83:615, 1983.
159. Wolf GK, Arnold JH: Noninvasive assessment of lung volume: respiratory inductance plethysmography and electrical impedance tomography. *Crit Care Med* 33[3 Suppl]:S163, 2005.
160. Stradling JR, Chadwick GA, Quirk C, et al: Respiratory inductance plethysmography: calibration techniques, their validation and the effects of posture. *Bull Eur Physiopathol Respir* 21:317, 1985.
161. Neumann P, Zinserling J, Haase C, et al: Evaluation of respiratory inductive plethysmography in controlled ventilation: measurement of tidal volume and PEEP-induced changes of end-expiratory lung volume. *Chest* 113:443, 1998.
162. Tobin MJ, Jenouri G, Birch S: Effect of positive end-expiratory pressure on breathing patterns of normal subjects and intubated patients with respiratory failure. *Crit Care Med* 11:859, 1983.
163. Tobin MJ, Guenther SM, Perez W: Konno-Mead analysis of ribcage-abdominal motion during successful and unsuccessful trials of weaning from mechanical ventilation. *Am Rev Respir Dis* 135:1320, 1987.
164. Hoffman RA, Ershowsky P, Krieger BP: Determination of auto-PEEP during spontaneous and controlled ventilation by monitoring changes in end-expiratory thoracic gas volume. *Chest* 96:613, 1989.

165. Krieger BP, Ershowsky P, Spivack D: Initial experience with a central respiratory monitoring unit as a cost-saving alternative to the intensive care unit for Medicare patients who require long-term ventilator support. *Chest* 93:395, 1988.

166. Krieger BP, Ershowsky P, Spivack D: One year's experience with a noninvasively monitored intermediate care unit for pulmonary patients. *JAMA* 264:1143, 1990.

167. O'Brien MJ, Van Eykern LA, Oetomo SB, et al: Transcutaneous respiratory electromyographic monitoring. *Crit Care Med* 15:294, 1987.

168. Mower WR, Sachs C, Nicklin EL: A comparison of pulse oximetry and respiratory rate in patient screening. *Respir Med* 90:593, 1996.

169. Brown LH, Manring EA, Korengay HB: Can prehospital personnel detect hypoxemia without the aid of pulse oximetry. *Am J Emerg Med* 14:43, 1996.

170. Aoyagi T: Pulse oximetry: its invention, theory, and future. *J Anesth* 17:259, 2003.

171. Jensen LA, Onyskiw JE, Prasad NG: Meta-analysis of arterial oxygen saturation monitoring by pulse oximetry in adults. *Heart Lung*. 27:387, 1998.

172. Stoneham MD, Saville GM, Wilson IH: Knowledge about pulse oximetry among medical and nursing staff. *Lancet* 344:1339, 1994.

173. Huch A, Huch R, Konig V: Limitations of pulse oximetry. *Lancet* 2:357, 1988.

174. New W: Pulse oximetry. *J Clin Monit* 1:126, 1985.

175. Moller JT, Pederen T, Rasmussen LS: Randomized evaluation of pulse oximetry in 20,802 patients: I. Design, demography, pulse oximeter failure rate, and overall complications rate. *Anesthesiology* 78:436, 1993.

176. Reich DL, Timcenko A, Bodian CA: Predictors of pulse oximetry data failure. *Anesthesiology* 84:859, 1996.

177. Choe H, Tashiro C, Fukumitsu K: Comparison of recorded values from six pulse oximeters. *Crit Care Med* 17:678, 1989.

178. Severinghaus JW, Naifeh KH, Koh SO: Errors in 14 pulse oximeters during profound hypoxia. *J Clin Monit* 5:72, 1989.

179. Barker SJ, Hyatt J, Shah NK: The effect of sensor malpositioning on pulse oximetry accuracy during hypoxemia. *Anesthesiology* 79:248, 1993.

180. Severinghaus JW, Naifeh KH: Accuracy of responses of six pulse oximeters to profound hypoxia. *Anesthesiology* 67:551, 1987.

181. Cheng EY, Stommel KA: Quantitative evaluation of a combined pulse oximetry and end-tidal CO2 monitor. *Biomed Instrum Technol* 23:216, 1989.

182. Reynolds LM, Nicolson SC, Steven JM: Influence of sensor site location on pulse oximetry kinetics in children. *Anesth Analg* 76:751, 1993.

183. Cheng EY, Hopwood MB, Kay J: Forehead pulse oximetry compared with finger pulse oximetry and arterial blood gas measurement. *J Clin Monit* 4:223, 1988.

184. Hickerson W, Morrell M, Cicala RS: Glossal pulse oximetry. *Anesth Analg* 69:72, 1989.

185. Evans ML, Geddes LA: An assessment of blood vessel vasoactivity using photoplethysmography. *Med Instrum* 22:29, 1988.

186. Kyriacou PA: Pulse oximetry in the oesophagus. *Physiol Meas* 27:R1, 2006.

187. Tweedie IE: Pulse oximeters and finger nails. *Anaesthesia* 44:268, 1989.

188. Read MS: Effect of transparent adhesive tape on pulse oximetry. *Anesth Analg* 68:701, 1989.

189. Cote CJ, Goldstein EA, Fuchsman WH: The effect of nail polish on pulse oximetry. *Anesth Analg* 67:683, 1988.

190. Brand TM, Brand ME, Jay GD: Enamel nail polish does not interfere with pulse oximetry among normoxic volunteers. *J Clin Monit Comput* 17:93, 2002.

191. Chan MM, Chan MM, Chan ED: What is the effect of fingernail polish on pulse oximetry? *Chest* 123:2163, 2003.

192. Ries AL, Prewitt LM, Johnson JJ: Skin color and ear oximetry. *Chest* 96:287, 1989.

193. Adler JN, Hughes LA, Vivilecchia R, et al: Effect of skin pigmentation on pulse oximetry accuracy in the emergency department. *Acad Emerg Med* 5:965, 1998.

194. Bickler PE, Feiner JR, Severinghaus JW: Effects of skin pigmentation on pulse oximeter accuracy at low saturation. *Anesthesiology* 102:715, 2005.

195. Bothma PA, Joynt GM, Lipman J: Accuracy of pulse oximetry in pigmented patients. *S Afr Med J* 86:594, 1996.

196. Costarino AT, Davis DA, Keon TP: Falsely normal saturation reading with the pulse oximeter. *Anesthesiology* 67:830, 1987.

197. Hanowell L, Eisele JH Jr, Downs D: Ambient light affects pulse oximeters. *Anesthesiology* 67:864, 1987.

198. Block FE, Jr: Interference in a pulse oximeter from a fiberoptic light source. *J Clin Monit* 3:210, 1987.

199. Brooks TD, Paulus DA, Winkle WE: Infrared heat lamps interfere with pulse oximeters. *Anesthesiology* 61:630, 1984.

200. Amar D, Neidzwski J, Wald A: Fluorescent light interferes with pulse oximetry. *J Clin Monit* 5:135, 1989.

201. Fluck RR Jr, Schroeder C, Frani G, et al: Does ambient light affect the accuracy of pulse oximetry? *Respir Care* 48:677, 2003.

202. Gehring H, Hornberger C, Matz H, et al: The effects of motion artifact and low perfusion on the performance of a new generation of pulse oximeters in volunteers undergoing hypoxemia. *Respir Care* 47:48, 2002.

203. Beall SN, Moorthy SS: Jaundice, oximetry, and spurious hemoglobin desaturation. *Anesth Analg* 68:806, 1989.

204. Veyckemans F, Baele P, Guillaume JE: Hyperbilirubinemia does not interfere with hemoglobin saturation measured by pulse oximetry. *Anesthesiology* 70:118, 1989.

205. Ash-Bernal R, Wise R, Wright SM: Acquired methemoglobinemia: a retrospective series of 138 cases at 2 teaching hospitals. *Medicine (Baltimore)* 83:265, 2004.

206. Moore TJ, Walsh CS, Cohen MR: Reported adverse event cases of methemoglobinemia associated with benzocaine products. *Arch Intern Med* 164:1192, 2004.

207. Novaro GM, Aronow HD, Militello MA, et al: Benzocaine-induced methemoglobinemia: experience from a high-volume transesophageal echocardiography laboratory. *J Am Soc Echocardiogr* 16:170, 2003.

208. Watcha MF, Connor MT, Hing AV: Pulse oximetry in methemoglobinemia. *Am J Dis Child* 143:845, 1989.

209. Reynolds KJ, Palayiwa E, Moyle JTB: The effect of dyshemoglobins on pulse oximetry: I. Theoretical approach. II. Experimental results using an in vitro system. *J Clin Monit* 9:81, 1993.

210. Barker SJ, Tremper KK: The effect of carbon monoxide inhalation on pulse oximetry and transcutaneous Po$_2$. *Anesthesiology* 66:677, 1987.

211. Buckley RG, Aks SE, Eshom JL: The pulse oximetry gap in carbon monoxide intoxication. *Ann Emerg Med* 24:252, 1994.

212. Hampson NB: Pulse oximetry in severe carbon monoxide poisoning. *Chest* 114:1036, 1998.

213. Glass KL, Dillard TA, Phillips YY: Pulse oximetry correction for smoking exposure. *Milit Med* 16:273, 1996.

214. Coburn RF, Williams WJ, Kahn SB: Endogenous carbon monoxide production in patients with hemolytic anemia. *J Clin Invest* 45:460, 1966.

215. Lopez-Herce J, Borrego R, Bustinza A, et al: Elevated carboxyhemoglobin associated with sodium nitroprusside treatment. *Intensive Care Med* 31:1235, 2005.

216. Lee SE, Tremper KK, Barker SJ: Effects of anemia on pulse oximetry and continuous mixed venous oxygen saturation monitoring in dogs. *Anesth Analg* 67:S130, 1988.

217. Jay GD, Hughes L, Renzi FP: Pulse oximetry is accurate in acute anemia from hemorrhage. *Ann Emerg Med* 24:32, 1994.

218. Severinghaus JW, Koh SO: Effect of anemia on pulse oximeter accuracy at low saturation. *J Clin Monit* 6:85, 1990.

219. Cane RD, Harrison RA, Shapiro BA: The spectrophotometric absorbance of intralipid. *Anesthesiology* 53:53, 1980.

220. Sehgal LR, Sehgal HL, Rosen AL, et al: Effect of Intralipid on measurements of total hemoglobin and oxyhemoglobin in whole blood. *Crit Care Med* 12:907, 1984.

221. Gabrielczyk MR, Buist RJ: Pulse oximetry and postoperative hypothermia: an evaluation of the Nellcor N-100 in a cardiac surgical intensive care unit. *Anaesthesia* 43:402, 1988.

222. Palve H, Vuori A: Pulse oximetry during low cardiac output and hypothermia states immediately after open heart surgery. *Crit Care Med* 17:66, 1989.

223. Rieder HU, Frei FJ, Zbinden AM: Pulse oximetry in methemoglobinemia: failure to detect low oxygen saturation. *Anaesthesia* 44:326, 1989.

224. Scheller MS, Unger RJ, Kelner MJ: Effects of intravenously administered dyes on pulse oximetry readings. *Anesthesiology* 65:550, 1986.

225. Unger R, Scheller MS: More on dyes and pulse oximeters. *Anesthesiology* 67:148, 1987.

226. Larsen VH, Freudendal-Pedersen A, Fogh-Andersen N: The influence of patent blue V on pulse oximetry and haemoximetry. *Acta Anaesthesiol Scand Suppl* 107:53, 1995.

227. Koivusalo AM, Von Smitten K, Lindgren L: Sentinel node mapping affects intraoperative pulse oximetric recordings during breast cancer surgery. *Acta Anaesthesiol Scand* 46:411, 2002.

228. Taylor MB: Erroneous actuation of the pulse oximeter. *Anaesthesia* 42:1116, 1987.

229. Barker SJ: "Motion-resistant" pulse oximetry: a comparison of new and old models. *Anesth Analg* 95:967, 2002.

230. Morris RW, Nairn M, Torda TA: A comparison of fifteen pulse oximeters: I: a clinical comparison. II. a test of performance under conditions of poor perfusion. *Anaesth Intensive Care* 17:62, 1989.

231. Paulus DA: Cool fingers and pulse oximetry. *Anesthesiology* 71:168, 1989.

232. Mineo R, Sharrock NE: Pulse oximeter waveforms from the finger and the toe during lumbar epidural anesthesia. *Reg Anesth* 18:106, 1993.

233. Broome IJ, Mills GH, Spiers P: An evaluation of the effect of vasodilatation on oxygen saturations measured by pulse oximetry and venous blood gas analysis. *Anaesthesia* 48:415, 1993.

234. Stewart KG, Rowbottom SJ: Inaccuracy of pulse oximetry in patients with severe tricuspid regurgitation. *Anaesthesia* 46:668, 1991.

235. American College of Critical Care Medicine of the Society of Critical Care Medicine. Critical care services and personnel: recommendations based on a system of categorization into two levels of care. *Crit Care Med* 27:422, 1999.

236. Smith DC, Canning JJ, Crul JF: Pulse oximetry in the recovery room. *Anaesthesia* 44:345, 1989.

237. Tyler IL, Tantisera B, Winter PM: Continuous monitoring of arterial oxygen saturation with pulse oximetry during transfer to the recovery room. *Anesth Analg* 64:1108, 1985.

238. Moller JT, Johannenssen NW, Espersen K: Randomized evaluation of pulse oximetry in 20,802 patients: II. Perioperative events and postoperative complications. *Anesthesiology* 78:423, 1993.

239. Guggenberger H, Lenz G, Federle R: Early detection of inadvertent esophageal intubation: pulse oximetry vs. capnography. *Acta Anaesthesiol Scand* 33:112, 1989.

240. Brathwaite CEM, OMalley KF, Ross SE: Continuous pulse oximetry and the diagnosis of pulmonary embolism in critically ill trauma patients. *J Trauma* 33:528, 1992.

241. Baird JS, Greene A, Schleien CL: Massive pulmonary embolus without hypoxemia. *Pediatr Crit Care Med* 6:602, 2005.

242. Jones JS, VanDeelen N, White L, et al: Alveolar-arterial oxygen gradients in elderly patients with suspected pulmonary embolism. *Ann Emerg Med* 22:1177, 1993.

243. Stein PD, Goldhaber SZ, Henry JW, et al: Arterial blood gas analysis in the assessment of suspected acute pulmonary embolism. *Chest* 109:78, 1996.

244. Mars M, Maesjo S, Thompson S: Can pulse oximetry detect raised intracompartmental pressure. *S Afr J Surg* 32:48, 1994.

245. Stock MC: Noninvasive carbon dioxide monitoring. *Crit Care Clin* 4:511, 1988.

246. Schena J, Thompson J, Crone R: Mechanical influences on the capnogram. *Crit Care Med* 12:672, 1984.

247. Paulus DA: Capnography. *Int Anesthesiol Clin* 27:167, 1989.

248. Murray IP, Modell JM: Early detection of endotracheal tube accidents by monitoring of carbon dioxide concentration in respiratory gas. *Anesthesiology* 59:344, 1983.

249. Steedman DJ, Robertson CE: Measurement of end-tidal carbon dioxide concentration during cardiopulmonary resuscitation. *Arch Emerg Med* 7:129, 1990.

250. Garnett AR, Ornato JP, Gonzalez ER, et al: End-tidal carbon dioxide monitoring during cardiopulmonary resuscitation. *JAMA* 257:512, 1987.

251. Falk JL, Rackow EC, Weil MH: End tidal carbon dioxide concentration during cardiopulmonary resuscitation. *N Engl J Med* 318:607, 1988.

252. Grmec S: Comparison of three different methods to confirm tracheal tube placement in emergency intubation. *Intensive Care Med* 28:701, 2002.

253. Araujo-Preza CE, Melhado ME, Gutierrez FJ, et al: Use of capnometry to verify feeding tube placement. *Crit Care Med* 30:2255, 2002.

254. Raemer DB, Francis D, Philip JH: Variation in PCO₂ between arterial blood and peak expired gas during anesthesia. *Anesth Analg* 62:1065, 1983.

255. Hoffman RA, Krieger BP, Kramer MR: End-tidal carbon dioxide in critically ill patients during changes in mechanical ventilation. *Am Rev Respir Dis* 140:1265, 1989.

256. Morley TF, Giaimo J, Maroszan E: Use of capnography for assessment of the adequacy of alveolar ventilation during weaning from mechanical ventilation. *Am Rev Respir Dis* 148:339, 1993.

257. Jardin F, Genevray B, Pazin M: Inability to titrate PEEP in patients with acute respiratory failure using end tidal carbon dioxide measurements. *Anesthesiology* 62:530, 1985.

258. Lima A, Bakker J: Noninvasive monitoring of peripheral perfusion. *Intensive Care Med* 31:1316, 2005.

259. Wimberley PD, Pedersen KG, Thode J: Transcutaneous and capillary PCO₂ and PO₂ measurements in healthy adults. *Clin Chem* 29:1471, 1983.

260. Rooth G, Hedstrand U, Tyden H: The validity of the transcutaneous oxygen tension method in adults. *Crit Care Med* 4:162, 1976.

261. Gothgen I, Jacobsen E: Transcutaneous oxygen tension measurement: I. Age variation and reproducibility. *Acta Anaesthesiol Scand* 67:66, 1978.

262. Eletr S, Jimison H, Ream AK: Cutaneous monitoring of systemic PCO₂ on patients in the respiratory intensive care unit being weaned from the ventilator. *Acta Anaesthesiol Scand* 68:123, 1978.

263. Tremper KK, Waxman K, Shoemaker WC: Use of transcutaneous oxygen sensors to titrate PEEP. *Ann Surg* 193:206, 1981.

264. Cerny V, Cvachovec K: Gastric tonometry and intramucosal pH–theoretical principles and clinical application. *Physiol Res* 49:289, 2000.

265. Marshall AP, West SH: Gastric tonometry and monitoring gastrointestinal perfusion: using research to support nursing practice. *Nurs Crit Care.* 9:123, 2004.

266. Brinkmann A, Calzia E, Trager K, et al: Monitoring the hepato-splanchnic region in the critically ill patient. Measurement techniques and clinical relevance. *Intensive Care Med* 24:542, 1998.

267. Fiddian-Green RG, McGough E, Pittenger G, et al: Predictive value of intramural pH and other risk factors for massive bleeding from stress ulceration. *Gastroenterology* 85:613, 1983.

268. Reilly PM, Wilkins KB, Fuh KC, et al: The mesenteric hemodynamic response to circulatory shock: an overview. *Shock* 15:329, 2001.

269. Rossi M, Sganga G, Mazzone M, et al: Cardiopulmonary bypass in man: role of the intestine in a self-limiting inflammatory response with demonstrable bacterial translocation. *Ann Thorac Surg* 77:612, 2004.

270. Dantzker DR: The gastrointestinal tract. The canary of the body? *JAMA* 270:1247, 1993.

271. Bergofsky EM: Determination of tissue O₂ tensions by hollow visceral tonometers: effects of breathing enriched O₂ mixtures. *J Clin Invest* 43:193, 1964.

272. Dawson AM, Trenchard D, Guz A: Small bowel tonometry: assessment of small gut mucosal oxygen tension in dog and man. *Nature* 206:943, 1965.

273. Kivisaari J, Niinikoski J: Use of Silastic tube and capillary sampling technic in the measurement of tissue PO₂ and PCO₂. *Am J Surg* 125:623, 1973.

274. Fiddian-Green RG, Pittenger G, Whitehouse WM: Back-diffusion of CO2 and its influence on the intramural pH in gastric mucosa. *J Surg Res* 33:39, 1982.

275. Fiddian-Green RG: Tonometry: theory and applications. *Intensive Care World* 9:1, 1992.

276. Fiddian-Green RG: Gastric intramucosal pH, tissue oxygenation and acid-base balance. *Br J Anaesth* 74:591, 1995.

277. Schlichtig R, Mehta N, Gayowski TJ: Tissue-arterial PCO₂ difference is a better marker of ischemia than intramural pH (pHi) or arterial pH-pHi difference. *J Crit Care* 11:51, 1996.

278. Riddington D, Venkatesh B, Clutton-Brock T, et al: Measuring carbon dioxide tension in saline and alternative solutions: quantification of bias and precision in two blood gas analyzers. *Crit Care Med* 22:96, 1994.

279. Heard SO, Helsmoortel CM, Kent JC: Gastric tonometry in healthy volunteers: effect of ranitidine on calculated intramural pH. *Crit Care Med* 19:271, 1991.

280. Marik PE, Lorenzana A: Effect of tube feedings on the measurement of gastric intramucosal pH. *Crit Care Med* 24:1498, 1996.

281. Marshall AP, West SH: Gastric tonometry and enteral nutrition: a possible conflict in critical care nursing practice. *Am J Crit Care* 12:349, 2003.

282. Beale RJ, Hollenberg SM, Vincent JL, et al: Vasopressor and inotropic support in septic shock: an evidence-based review. *Crit Care Med* 32[11 Suppl]:S455, 2004.

283. Mohsenifar Z, Hay A, Hay J, et al: Gastric intramural pH as a predictor of success or failure in weaning patients from mechanical ventilation. *Ann Intern Med* 119:794, 1993.

284. Fiddian-Green RG, Baker S: Predictive value of the stomach wall pH for complications after cardiac operations: comparison with other monitoring. *Crit Care Med* 15:153, 1987.

285. Landow L, Phillips DA, Heard SO: Gastric tonometry and venous oximetry in cardiac surgery patients. *Crit Care Med* 19:1226, 1991.

286. Friedman G, Berlot G, Kahn RJ, et al: Combined measurements of blood lactate concentrations and gastric intramucosal pH in patients with severe sepsis. *Crit Care Med* 23:1184, 1995.

287. Kirton OC, Windsor J, Wedderburn R, et al: Failure of splanchnic resuscitation in the acutely injured trauma patient correlates with multiple organ system failure and length of stay in the ICU. *Chest* 113:1064, 1998.

288. Maynard N, Bihari D, Beale R, et al: Assessment of splanchnic oxygenation by gastric tonometry in patients with acute circulatory failure. *JAMA* 270:1203, 1993.

289. Doglio GR, Pusajo JF, Egurrola MA, et al: Gastric mucosal pH as a prognostic index of mortality in critically ill patients. *Crit Care Med* 19:1037, 1991.

290. Lorente JA, Ezpeleta A, Esteban A, et al: Systemic hemodynamics, gastric intramucosal PCO2 changes, and outcome in critically ill burn patients. *Crit Care Med* 28:1728, 2000.

291. Maynard ND, Taylor PR, Mason RC, et al: Gastric intramucosal pH predicts outcome after surgery for ruptured abdominal aortic aneurysm. *Eur J Vasc Endovasc Surg* 11:201, 1996.

292. Theodoropoulos G, Lloyd LR, Cousins G, et al: Intraoperative and early postoperative gastric intramucosal pH predicts morbidity and mortality after major abdominal surgery. *Am Surg* 67:303, 2001.

293. Keenan SP, Guyatt GH, Sibbald WJ, et al: How to use articles about diagnostic technology: gastric tonometry. *Crit Care Med* 27:1726, 1999.

294. Gutierrez G, Palizas F, Doglio G, et al: Gastric intramucosal pH as a therapeutic index of tissue oxygenation in critically ill patients. *Lancet* 339:195, 1992.

295. Heritier SR, Gebski VJ, Keech AC: Inclusion of patients in clinical trial analysis: the intention-to-treat principle. *Med J Aust* 179:438, 2003.

296. Gomersall CD, Joynt GM, Freebairn RC, et al: Resuscitation of critically ill patients based on the results of gastric tonometry: a prospective, randomized, controlled trial. *Crit Care Med* 28:607, 2000.

297. Miami Trauma Clinical Trials Group: Splanchnic hypoperfusion-directed therapies in trauma: a prospective, randomized trial. *Am Surg* 71:252, 2005.

298. Ivatury RR, Simon RJ, Islam S, et al: A prospective randomized study of end points of resuscitation after major trauma: global oxygen transport indices versus organ-specific gastric mucosal pH. *J Am Coll Surg* 183:145, 1996.

299. Pargger H, Hampl KF, Christen P, et al: Gastric intramucosal pH-guided therapy in patients after elective repair of infrarenal abdominal aneurysms: is it beneficial? *Intensive Care Med* 24:769, 1998.

300. Marik PE: Sublingual capnography: a clinical validation study. *Chest* 120:923, 2001.

301. Marik PE, Bankov A: Sublingual capnometry versus traditional markers of tissue oxygenation in critically ill patients. *Crit Care Med* 31:818, 2003.

302. Nellcor, Inc (Pleasanton, CA): Nellcor announces nationwide voluntary recall of all CapnoProbe sublingual sensors (Press Release). Issued August 24, 2004. Available at http://www.fda.gov/cdrh/recalls/recall-082404-pressrelease.html. Accessed April 21, 2006.

303. Wimberley PD, Burnett RW, Covington AK, et al: Guidelines for transcutaneous p O2 and p CO2 measurement. *J Int Fed Clin Chem* 2:128, 1990.

304. American Association for Respiratory Care: Clinical practice guideline. Transcutaneous blood gas monitoring for neonatal and pediatric patients. *Respir Care* 39:1176, 1994.

305. Tremper KK, Waxman K, Bowman R, et al: Continuous transcutaneous oxygen monitoring during respiratory failure, cardiac decompensation, cardiac arrest, and CPR. Transcutaneous oxygen monitoring during arrest and CPR. *Crit Care Med* 8:377, 1980.

306. Tremper KK, Shoemaker WC: Transcutaneous oxygen monitoring of critically ill adults, with and without low flow shock. *Crit Care Med* 9:706, 1981.

307. Hasibeder W, Haisjackl M, Sparr H, et al: Factors influencing transcutaneous oxygen and carbon dioxide measurements in adult intensive care patients. *Intensive Care Med* 17:272, 1991.

308. Green GE, Hassell KT, Mahutte CK: Comparison of arterial blood gas with continuous intra-arterial and transcutaneous PO₂ sensors in adult critically ill patients. *Crit Care Med* 15:491, 1987.

309. Abraham E, Smith M, Silver L: Continuous monitoring of critically ill patients with transcutaneous oxygen and carbon dioxide and conjunctival oxygen sensors. *Ann Emerg Med* 13:1021, 1984.

310. Shoemaker WC, Fink S, Ray CW: Effect of hemorrhagic shock on conjunctival and transcutaneous oxygen tensions in relation to hemodynamic and oxygen transport changes. *Crit Care Med* 12:949, 1984.

311. Abraham E, Oye R, Smith M: Detection of blood volume deficits through conjunctival oxygen tension monitoring. *Crit Care Med* 12:931, 1984.

312. Nolan LS, Shoemaker WC: Transcutaneous O₂ and CO₂ monitoring of high risk surgical patients during the perioperative period. *Crit Care Med* 10:762, 1982.

313. Shoemaker WC, Wo CC, Yu S, et al: Invasive and noninvasive haemodynamic monitoring of acutely ill sepsis and septic shock patients in the emergency department. *Eur J Emerg Med* 7:169, 2000.

314. Shoemaker WC, Wo CC, Lu K, et al: Outcome prediction by a mathematical model based on noninvasive hemodynamic monitoring. *J Trauma* 60:82, 2006.

315. Sensors LM: 510(K) Summary for TOSCA 500 PCO2, SpO2, and pulse rate monitoring system. October 20, 2004. Available at http://www.fda.gov/cdrh/pdf4/K043357.pdf. Accessed April 22, 2006.

316. Senn O, Clarenbach CF, Kaplan V, et al: Monitoring carbon dioxide tension and arterial oxygen saturation by a single earlobe sensor in patients with critical illness or sleep apnea. *Chest* 128:1291, 2005.

317. Eberhard P, Gisiger PA, Gardaz JP, et al: Combining transcutaneous blood gas measurement and pulse oximetry. *Anesth Analg* 94[1 Suppl]:S76, 2002.

318. Bendjelid K, Schutz N, Stotz M, et al: Transcutaneous PCO₂ monitoring in critically ill adults: clinical evaluation of a new sensor. *Crit Care Med* 33:2203, 2005.

Nicholas A. Smyrnios
Frederick J. Curley

CHAPTER **28**

Indirect Calorimetry

Indirect calorimetry is a technique that uses measurements of inspired and expired gas flows, volumes, and concentrations to measure oxygen consumption and carbon dioxide production. Energy expenditure, respiratory quotient (RQ), and other values can be derived from the measured values. Indirect calorimetry provides a noninvasive, accurate method of measuring caloric requirements and oxygen consumption. This chapter focuses on the technique of performing indirect calorimetry in the intensive care unit (ICU) setting. Indirect calorimetry is the subject of a clinical practice guideline that was revised in 2004 by the American Association of Respiratory Care [1].

THEORETICAL BASIS OF INDIRECT CALORIMETRY

Indirect calorimetry systems rely on measurements of inhaled and exhaled airflow, volume, and concentrations of oxygen and carbon dioxide. Indirect calorimetry systems can be classified as *open-circuit systems*, which measure the difference between inspired and expired gas concentrations, or *closed-circuit systems*, which measure changes in the amount of gases in a fixed reservoir over time [2]. This chapter reviews only open-circuit systems because closed circuit systems are rarely used in critical care.

DEFINITIONS

Chemical energy used to fuel the human body is directly provided by adenosine triphosphate, which is formed by the oxidation of carbohydrate, protein, and lipid. The stores of adenosine triphosphate in the body are small, but they are in a constant, high-volume, well-balanced state of formation and utilization. Indirect calorimetry measures the oxygen used and carbon dioxide produced when carbohydrate, protein, and lipid are oxidized to produce adenosine triphosphate. Therefore, it is the *production* of chemical energy that is indirectly measured by the gas-exchange parameters. Despite this, it is the convention to describe this quantity as energy expended. Therefore, we use the term *energy expenditure* to describe the amount of energy quantified by indirect calorimetry.

In any discussion of energy expenditure, it is important to define what level of energy expenditure is being considered. Basal metabolic rate or basal energy expenditure (BEE) is the energy used by the body at complete rest and in the postabsorptive state (absence of active nutritional intake for at least 4 to 6 hours). This measurement can be obtained reliably only in deep sleep. If such a measurement is made, BEE does take into account the effects of illness and stress. However, BEE often is taken to be a value calculated from a standardized equation that does not account for stress, such as the Harris-Benedict equation. Resting energy expenditure (REE) is obtained from an awake person at rest and includes the energy used at rest in the awake state plus the energy used to metabolize foodstuffs, also called *diet-induced thermogenesis*. It is expected to be approximately 10% greater than BEE [3–5]. Total energy expenditure (TEE) is REE plus the energy used during activity. TEE and REE are closer in value for ICU patients than for patients in other settings because most ICU patients are bedridden. In most cases, we wish to know the 24-hour REE or TEE rather than the BEE.

CALCULATION OF ENERGY EXPENDITURE

Most indirect calorimetry systems use the modified de Weir equation to calculate energy expenditure. In its more complete form, this equation uses oxygen consumption ($\dot{V}_{O_2}$), carbon dioxide production ($\dot{V}_{CO_2}$), and nonprotein urinary nitrogen (UN):

$$\text{Energy expenditure} = 3.9(\dot{V}_{O_2}) - 1.1(\dot{V}_{CO_2}) - 2.17(\text{UN g/day})$$

The de Weir equation is not experimentally derived from measurements on humans but is mathematically derived. The derivation relies on the knowledge that (a) TEE is equal to the sum of the energy expended from the combustion of carbohydrate, fat, and protein; (b) the caloric equivalents of glucose (3.7 kcal per g), fat (9.5 kcal per g), and protein (4.1 kcal per g) are known; (c) the oxygen consumed and carbon dioxide produced in metabolizing each of these fuels is known; and (d) therefore, the equation for energy expenditure can be expressed in terms of oxygen consumption and carbon dioxide production by solving the system of equations that describes the stoichiometry of fuel combustion. The reader is referred to other sources for a complete derivation of the equation [6]. In practice, the amount of urea nitrogen in the urine is usually not measured because of the fact that its contribution to TEE is considered minimal.

CALCULATION OF OXYGEN CONSUMPTION

The essential measurements of indirect calorimetry are the inspired and expired oxygen fractions (F_{IO_2} and F_{EO_2}, respectively), carbon dioxide fractions (F_{ICO_2} and F_{ECO_2}, respectively), and minute ventilation. Oxygen consumption and carbon dioxide production can be calculated using similar equations, which compute the difference between inspired (I) and expired (E) volumes:

$$\text{Oxygen consumption} = \dot{V}O_2 = \dot{V}_I(F_{IO_2}) - \dot{V}_E(F_{EO_2})$$
$$\text{Carbon dioxide production} = \dot{V}CO_2 = \dot{V}_E(F_{ECO_2}) - \dot{V}_I(F_{ICO_2})$$

To avoid the need to measure the volumes of expiratory and inspiratory gases, techniques have been developed that preferentially measure only exhaled volumes and mathematically derive the inhaled volume. Any assumption that the volume exhaled is equal to the volume inhaled is erroneous whenever $\dot{V}CO_2$ and $\dot{V}O_2$ are not equal (i.e., RQ is not equal to 1) and becomes more erroneous as F_{IO_2} increases. A mathematic relationship of $\dot{V}_E$ to $\dot{V}_I$ called the *Haldane transformation* can be used to explain this phenomenon. It takes advantage of the fact that nitrogen is an essentially inert gas. Therefore,

$$\text{Volume inspired} (\dot{V}_I) \times F_{IN_2} = \text{volume expired} (\dot{V}_E) \times F_{EN_2}$$

Rearranged, this reads

$$\dot{V}_I = \dot{V}_E \times F_{EN_2}/F_{IN_2}$$

Because $F_{IO_2} + F_{IN_2} = 1$ and $F_{EO_2} + F_{ECO_2} + F_{EN_2} = 1$,

$$F_{IN_2} = 1 - F_{IO_2}$$

and

$$F_{EN_2} = 1 - F_{ECO_2} - F_{EO_2}$$

If we substitute back into the previous equation,

$$\dot{V}_I = \dot{V}_E \times (1 - F_{ECO_2} - F_{EO_2})/(1 - F_{IO_2})$$

As the inspired oxygen concentration increases, the denominator decreases and the difference between inspired and expired gas volume becomes greater. The Haldane equation can therefore be used to determine the value of $\dot{V}_I$ without measuring inspired volume.

The use of the Haldane equation during indirect calorimetry leads to some important and practical technical considerations. Most significantly, the accuracy of the Haldane equation in estimating inspired volume, and thereby oxygen consumption and energy expenditure, depends greatly on the accuracy of measurement of F_{IO_2} and $\dot{V}_E$. Any error in measuring exhaled volumes or gas concentrations directly produces an error of a greater magnitude in the calculation of oxygen consumption, carbon dioxide production, and energy expenditure. At a minute ventilation of 10 L per minute and an inspired-to-expired oxygen concentration difference of 0.03, the oxygen consumption would be 300 mL per minute. If the F_{IO_2} was measured to be 0.46 instead of 0.45 and the F_{EO_2} remained at 0.42, the oxygen consumption would be 400 mL per minute, a 33% change. If the measured minute ventilation was 10.1 L per minute and the actual value was 10 L per minute, there would be an error in the oxygen consumption of 30 mL per minute, or 10%. To prevent such errors, the analysis system must be free of leaks, and extremely accurate sensors must be used. Because most oxygen sensors are less accurate at higher F_{IO_2}, indirect calorimetry studies are usually limited to patients on 60% oxygen or less. Although some systems have provided accurate results in vitro with higher levels of oxygen, there have been no studies to date that prove the accuracy of any system above FiO_2 60% in critically ill patients [7,8]. The 2004 American Association of Respiratory Care guideline also confirms the limitation of F_{EO_2} to 0.6 [1].

EQUIPMENT AND TECHNIQUE

Open-circuit indirect calorimetry systems all involve certain basic components, typically an oxygen analyzer, a carbon dioxide analyzer, and a flowmeter (usually a pneumotach). Most systems also use masks, canopies, mixing chambers, tubing, desiccants, and pumps. Some newer systems developed for use on ambulatory patients are small enough to be held in one hand. These ambulatory devices are not validated for use on critically ill patients.

METHODS OF MEASUREMENT

Oxygen sensors in commercially available systems are either zirconium or differential paramagnetic sensors. The zirconium oxide sensor is coated with an oxygen-permeable substance. At temperatures of approximately 800°C, oxygen diffuses across this outer layer and an electrical signal that is proportional to the partial pressure of oxygen is created [2,9]. Differential paramagnetic analyzers measure the difference in concentration of the gas between the inspiratory and expiratory lines. These analyzers typically have an accuracy of ±0.02% and a response time of 130 msec or less. Essentially all available carbon dioxide analyzers are nondispersed infrared devices. A gas sample in the path of infrared energy creates an alteration in an electrical signal that is proportional to the concentration of carbon dioxide. These analyzers have an accuracy of ±0.02% with a response time of 110 msec. Some systems measure inspired and expired carbon dioxide, and some measure only expired, assuming the inspired value to be negligible. Volume is calculated by measuring flow and integrating the result over time to obtain volume. Flow is usually either measured with a pneumotach or a mass flow sensor or generated by the device and kept constant in response to changes in ventilation.

Gas concentrations are measured using one of three techniques: mixing chamber, breath-by-breath, and dilution. All devices must have well-validated calibration procedures for essential components. Newer machines have automated much of this process.

Mixing Chamber Method

The mixing chamber is the best-established method and has been considered the gold standard. A mixing chamber is an automated Douglas bag that mixes expired gases over a predetermined interval and provides the material to be sampled [9]. Expired gas is passed from a mouthpiece or the ventilator exhalation port into a collection chamber, which is in series with the flowmeter and gas analyzers. Inside the chamber, baffles interrupt airflow to create a more even mixing of gases. A sample of mixed gas is withdrawn from the chamber, the gas concentrations are analyzed, and the sample is returned to the chamber. Depending on the design, the gas is either vented or passed through the flowmeter. The concentrations of inspiratory gas are sampled from the inspiratory side of a mouthpiece or a ventilator circuit. Inspiratory volumes are calculated from expiratory volumes as explained previously. A computer compares mixed expired versus inspired concentrations and multiplies by volume to yield a measure of consumption or production. The results reflect the values of gases mixed over time and are reported as values per time interval of measurement (e.g., milliliters of oxygen consumed per minute).

Breath-by-Breath Method

The collection and analysis of gases in the breath-by-breath method are similar to those in the mixing chamber technique, but each breath is analyzed. A sample of gases is taken for analysis from each inspiration and expiration. These samples are coupled with flow measurements for each breath to calculate $\dot{V}O_2$, $\dot{V}CO_2$, and REE. The concentrations of expiratory gases are measured directly from samples drawn from the expiratory side of the mouthpiece or ventilator circuit. Inspired concentrations are measured from samples drawn from the inspiratory side of a mouthpiece or ventilator circuit. Oxygen consumption and carbon dioxide production values are usually expressed as milliliters per minute and energy expenditure as kilocalories per day for each breath and can be averaged or summed over varying periods, depending on the clinician's needs. The crucial component in these measurements is the alignment of various signals. If the time needed for the gases to reach the analyzer and the expiratory flow to reach the flowmeter is known, the $\dot{V}O_2$, $\dot{V}CO_2$, and $\dot{V}E$ signals can be precisely aligned and accurate measurements made. Instruments that use breath-by-breath analysis align the signals automatically by computer. Improper alignment can render the measurements useless. Oxygen and carbon dioxide sensors must have a very rapid response time. The placement of the gas analysis line just distal to the endotracheal tube can standardize transit time and eliminate artifact, which assists in this process.

Dilution Method

The dilution method is the only technique that can be used in intubated patients as well as nonintubated patients who cannot use a mouthpiece. A predetermined flow of gas containing known oxygen and carbon dioxide concentration passes through a face shield mask or a hoodlike canopy. The exhaled gases are diluted into the passing stream of known gas. The amount of gas the machine puts into the stream is adjusted to keep the flow constant as the patient alters his or her own ventilation. Samples of the diluted gases are removed for analysis and the values obtained are multiplied by the flow rate to yield a measure of volume. Oxygen consumption and carbon dioxide production are calculated by comparing concentrations in and out of the system.

FACTORS AFFECTING ACCURACY

Accurate measurements require close attention to technique. The following issues are frequently encountered in the ICU setting.

Leaks. In the mixing chamber and breath-by-breath methods, even a small error in measuring volume can produce a large error in calculated values. All connections to the metabolic cart and in the ventilator circuit must be checked for leaks. In intubated patients, it may be necessary to eliminate the small leak at the endotracheal tube cuff by overdistending the cuff for the brief duration of the study. It may be impossible to eliminate this leak in patients with high peak pressures. In general, leaks in the inspiratory circuit lower FIO_2 values, falsely lower oxygen consumption and energy expenditure measurements, and falsely elevate RQ. Leaks in the expira-

tory circuit falsely decrease volume measurements. Leaks in the breath-by-breath sampling line produce marked variability in the derived values.

Inspired and expired gas concentrations are typically sampled with long, narrow tubes leading from taps into the respiratory circuit. Tubing can easily clog with patient secretions and invalidate collected data. Most systems also somehow condition the gas from these sample tubings to standardize for temperature and water vapor. Failure to follow the manufacturer's advice on desiccant change or timing of tubing change alters the accuracy of the data.

Care must also be taken to interface the metabolic cart with the ventilator and associated equipment carefully. Disruption of the normal ventilator circuit with inappropriately placed sampling devices may lead to ventilator malfunction or trigger alarms. All connections to ventilators must be according to manufacturer's specifications.

Inappropriate location of sampling tubes may also lead to artifacts in flow or concentration measurements.

The use of positive end-expiratory pressure may variably alter the ventilator circuit compressible volume, leading to errors in volume and concentration measurements. Techniques to isolate sensors from the effects of positive end-expiratory pressure have been incorporated into the current generation of equipment.

Traditionally, children had not been monitored with indirect calorimetry because of leaks due to uncuffed endotracheal tubes, frequent use of high-frequency ventilation, the common use of high FIO_2, and low ventilator flows and gas exchange rates. Studies indicate that certain devices may be accurate even at very low rates of oxygen consumption [10]. Recent studies have emphasized the large variation between energy needs estimated by predictive equations and those determined by indirect calorimetry [11,12]. Therefore, indirect calorimetry is considered a more valuable tool in critically ill or injured children than ever before.

The presence of anesthetic gases or gases other than O_2, CO_2, or nitrogen can alter the calculations used to determine energy expenditure [1].

Very few measures can be used to determine whether the data obtained are reliable. The RQ can act as a quality control when the values obtained are outside the physiologic range (approximately 0.65 to 1.30 in the ICU) [2]. The variability of measurements of $\dot{V}O_2$ and $\dot{V}CO_2$ should not be greater than 5% during a 5-minute period [1]. Inspiratory values, which should be stable, should be frequently measured and displayed during the test to minimize the effect of any changes in those values.

USES OF INDIRECT CALORIMETRY IN THE ICU

The primary role of indirect calorimetry in the ICU is to assess energy expenditure and nutritional requirements. Indirect calorimetry can determine also the proportions of different substrates used for energy production. Indirect calorimetry can be used to measure oxygen consumption in shock states. The value of that is unproven. Indirect calorimetry is also useful for research into the pathophysiology of critical illness [13].

NUTRITIONAL ASSESSMENT

In most ICUs, the patient's caloric intake is determined by estimating a daily TEE. BEE is calculated from a standard equation and adjusted for level of illness, diet-induced thermogenesis, and amount of activity. Studies comparing this practice with indirect calorimetry have produced inconsistent results. Some studies conclude that estimates of energy expenditure routinely overestimate caloric need [14–17]; others conclude that estimates of energy expenditure are inaccurate but in no consistent direction [18–20], and still others conclude that clinical estimates are as accurate as measured values [21–24]. The results may differ because of the different techniques and patient populations in each study.

Indirect calorimetry studies have no standard length and frequency. Studies from 5 minutes to 24 hours in duration have been used [17,25,26]. It has been shown that a 30-minute study can predict 24-hour energy expenditure well in medical ICU patients [27]. However, even if the test accurately determines that day's energy expenditure, it is unclear whether it can predict caloric need for subsequent days. Weissman et al. [28] found day-to-day changes of 12% to 46%, depending on the patient's clinical condition.

If energy expenditure can be measured more accurately than it can be estimated, does it alter clinical outcome? Some investigators believe providing an average energy requirement suffices for most patients, and that indirect calorimetry can be reserved for the 10% to 20% with more complex nutritional problems [29]. Others believe that accurate determination of energy requirements is crucial [30]. No study has demonstrated a benefit in mortality or other clinically significant outcomes related to the use of indirect calorimetry. Until that information is available, the exact role of indirect calorimetry in the ICU will remain uncertain.

SUBSTRATE USE

An elevated RQ may indicate excessive levels of carbohydrate metabolism or net lipogenesis due to excess calorie intake [31–35]. Although the impact of altering substrate composition has not been shown in most diseases, in complicated cases of hepatic or renal failure an analysis of substrate use can be used quickly to assess the efficacy of a change in diet.

OXYGEN CONSUMPTION

The use of the pulmonary artery catheter declined in recent years due to the lack of evidence of any impact on outcome. Indirect calorimetry may have played a role in this change in practice because it was instrumental in demonstrating that the implied correlation of oxygen delivery (Do_2) and $\dot{V}o_2$ was due to mathematic coupling [36–40]. However, clinicians still often have interest in measurements of cardiac function. Continuous indirect calorimetry can provide an accurate and noninvasive measurement of oxygen consumption that, together with arterial and venous oxygen content measurements made with hemoglobin values and blood gases, can be used to calculate the cardiac output via the Fick equation [41]. It is unclear whether this determination of cardiac output has any more impact on outcomes than invasively measured values.

OUTCOME PREDICTION

One study has demonstrated that indirect calorimetry findings were associated with outcome in burn patients. Serial metabolic cart measurements that were performed on 250 severely burned patients revealed that declining energy expenditure predicted mortality in the very early (within 1 week after injury) and late (beyond 1 month after injury) postburn periods [42]. The clinical usefulness of this information has yet to be proven.

RESEARCH AND FUTURE APPLICATIONS

Although this discussion has focused primarily on the indirect calorimeter as a monitor of oxygen consumption and energy expenditure, other values measured by the calorimeter have potential value in the ICU. Many computerized indirect calorimetry systems permit inputs from other monitoring equipment into the system's computer. Values derived from the combination of device inputs have not been adequately studied to recommend routine clinical use. For example, the value of oxygen pulse, defined as oxygen consumption divided by heart rate, correlates well as an index of left ventricular stroke volume. The ventilatory equivalents of oxygen and carbon dioxide, calculated by dividing minute ventilation by oxygen consumption or carbon dioxide production, respectively, can serve as indices of ventilation-perfusion mismatch. As technology improves and high-quality equipment becomes more available, the use of indirect calorimeters as short-term monitors of complex physiologic changes resulting from disease and treatment may markedly increase.

REFERENCES

1. McArthur CD: Metabolic measurement using indirect calorimetry during mechanical ventilation—2004 revision and update. *Respir Care* 49:1073, 2004.
2. Branson RD: The measurement of energy expenditure: instrumentation, practical considerations, and clinical application. *Respir Care* 35:640, 1990.
3. Feurer ID, Crosby LO, Mullen JL: Measured and predicted resting energy expenditure in clinically stable patients. *Clin Nutr* 3:27, 1984.
4. Kinney J: Indirect calorimetry: the search for clinical relevance. *Nutr Clin Prac* 7:203, 1992.
5. Weissman C, Kemper M: Metabolic measurements in the critically ill. *Crit Care Clin* 11:169, 1995.
6. Ferrannini E: The theoretical bases of indirect calorimetry: a review. *Metabolism* 37:287, 1988.
7. Takala J, Keinanen O, Vaisanen P, et al: Measurement of gas exchange in intensive care: laboratory and clinical validation of a new device. *Crit Care Med* 17:1041, 1989.
8. Weissman C, Sardar A, Kemper M: An in vitro evaluation of an instrument designed to measure oxygen consumption and carbon dioxide production during mechanical ventilation. *Crit Care Med* 22:1995, 1994.
9. Teirlinck HC: Sensormedics 2900 metabolic measurement cart: technical and fundamental considerations in gas exchange measurements. *Cardiopulmonary Review* 1991, Yorba Linda, CA, Sensormedics Corporation.
10. Joosten KF, Jacobs FI, van Klaarwater E, et al: Accuracy of an indirect calorimeter for mechanically ventilated infants and children: the influence of low rates of gas exchange and varying F$_{IO_2}$. *Crit Care Med* 28:3014, 2000.
11. Taylor RM, Cheeseman P, Preedy V, et al: Can energy expenditure be predicted in critically ill children? *Pediatr Crit Care Med* 4:176, 2003.
12. Martinez JLV, Martinez-Romillo PD, Sebastian JD, et al: Predicted versus measured energy expenditure by continuous, online indirect calorimetry in ventilated, critically ill children during the early postinjury period. *Pediatr Crit Care Med* 5:19, 2004.
13. McManus C, Newhouse H, Seitz S, et al: Human gradient-layer calorimeter: development of an accurate and practical instrument for clinical studies. *JPEN J Parenter Enteral Nutr* 8:317, 1984.
14. Daly JM, Heymsfield SB, Head CA, et al: Human energy requirements: overestimation by widely used prediction equation. *Am J Clin Nutr* 42:1170, 1985.
15. Cortes V, Nelson LD: Errors in estimating energy expenditure in critically ill surgical patients. *Arch Surg* 124:287, 1989.
16. Mann S, Westenkow DR, Houtchens BA: Measured and predicted caloric expenditure in the acutely ill. *Crit Care Med* 13:173, 1985.

17. Makk LJK, McClave SA, Creech PW, et al: Clinical application of the metabolic cart to the delivery of total parenteral nutrition. *Crit Care Med* 18:1320, 1990.

18. Saffle JR, Medina E, Raymond J, et al: Use of indirect calorimetry in the nutritional management of burned patients. *J Trauma* 25:32, 1985.

19. Weissman C, Kemper M, Askanazi J, et al: Resting metabolic rate of the critically ill patient: measured versus predicted. *Anesthesiology* 64:673, 1986.

20. Smyrnios NA, Curley FJ, Jederlinic PJ, et al: Indirect calorimetry in the medical ICU comparison with traditional practice and effect on cost of care. *Am Rev Respir Dis* 141:A581, 1990.

21. Hunter DC, Jaksic T, Lewis D, et al: Resting energy expenditure in the critically ill: estimations versus measurement. *Br J Surg* 75:875, 1988.

22. Van Lanschot JB, Feenstra BWA, Vermeij CG, et al: Calculation versus measurement of total energy expenditure. *Crit Care Med* 14:981, 1986.

23. Saffle JR, Larson CM, Sullivan J: A randomized trial of indirect calorimetry-based feedings in thermal injury. *J Trauma* 30:776, 1990.

24. Liggett SB, Renfro AD: Energy expenditures of mechanically ventilated nonsurgical patients. *Chest* 98:682, 1990.

25. Vermeij CG, Feenstra BW, Van Lanschot JB, et al: Day-to-day variability of energy expenditure in critically ill surgical patients. *Crit Care Med* 17:623, 1989.

26. Rumpler WV, Seale JL, Conway JM, et al: Repeatability of 24-h energy expenditure measurements in humans by indirect calorimetry. *Am J Clin Nutr* 51:147, 1990.

27. Smyrnios NA, Curley FJ, Shaker KG: Accuracy of 30 minute indirect calorimetry studies in predicting 24-hour energy expenditure in mechanically ventilated, critically ill patients. *JPEN J Parenter Enteral Nutr* 21:168, 1997.

28. Weissman C, Kemper M, Hyman AI: Variation in the resting metabolic rate of mechanically ventilated critically ill patients. *Anesth Analg* 68:457, 1989.

29. Bursztein S, Elwyn DH: Measured and predicted energy expenditure in critically ill patients. *Crit Care Med* 21:312, 1993.

30. Mullen JL: Indirect calorimetry in critical care. *Proc Nutr Soc* 50:239, 1991.

31. Gieske T, Gurushanthaiah G, Glauser FL: Effects of carbohydrates on carbon dioxide excretion in patients with airway disease. *Chest* 71:55, 1977.

32. Covelli HD, Black JW, Olsen MS, et al: Respiratory failure precipitated by high carbohydrate loads. *Ann Intern Med* 95:579, 1981.

33. Herve P, Simmonneau G, Girard P, et al: Hypercapneic acidosis induced by nutrition in mechanically ventilated patients: glucose versus fat. *Crit Care Med* 13:537, 1985.

34. Sherman BW, Hamilton C, Panacek EA: Adequacy of early enteral nutrition support by the enteral route in patients with acute respiratory failure. *Chest* 98:104S, 1990.

35. Guenst JM, Nelson LD: Predictors of total parenteral nutrition induced lipogenesis. *Chest* 105:553, 1997.

36. Archie JP Jr: Mathematic coupling of data: a common source of error. *Ann Surg* 193:296, 1981.

37. Stratton HH, Feustel PJ, Newell JC. Regression of calculated variables in the presence of shared measurement error. *J Appl Physiol* 62:2083, 1987.

38. Ronco JJ, Fenwick JC, Wiggs BR, et al: Oxygen consumption is independent of increases in oxygen delivery by dobutamine in septic patients who have normal or increased plasma lactate. *Am Rev Respir Dis* 147:25, 1993.

39. Phang PT, Cunningham KF, Ronco JJ, et al: Mathematical coupling explains dependence of oxygen consumption on oxygen delivery in ARDS. *Am J Respir Crit Care Med* 150:308, 1994.

40. Yu M, Burchell S, Takiguchi SA, et al: The relationship of oxygen consumption measured by indirect calorimetry to oxygen delivery in critically ill patients. *J Trauma* 41:41, 1996.

41. Peyton PJ, Robinson GJB: Measured pulmonary oxygen consumption: difference between systemic oxygen uptake measured by the reverse Fick method and indirect calorimetry in cardiac surgery. *Anaesthesia* 60:146, 2005.

42. Hart DW, Wolf SE, Herndon DN, Chinkes DL, et al: Energy expenditure and caloric balance after burn: Increased feeding leads to fat rather than lean mass accretion. *Ann Surg* 235:152, 2002.

Andrew J. Goodwin
Ednan K. Bajwa
Atul Malhotra

CHAPTER **29**

Minimally Invasive Cardiology

The assessment of cardiac output has historically been vital to the management of critically ill or hemodynamically unstable patients. The underlying nature of shock in a hypotensive patient may not be obvious and is often multifactorial. In these circumstances, it is crucial to characterize what type of shock (i.e., distributive, cardiogenic, hypovolemic) is playing a role in a patient's presentation as well as how he or she will respond to interventions, such as volume loading. Determination of cardiac output is thought to be a critical component of this process and has been the center of research for decades.

The physical examination has proven to be a largely unreliable means of assessing hemodynamics in systolic heart failure [1] and in critically ill patients without recent myocardial infarction [2]. As such, more dependable measurements may be required to optimally treat such patients. Since its introduction [3], the pulmonary artery catheter (PAC) has been useful in obtaining measurements of cardiac output and has been used both diagnostically as well as to gauge response to treatment. For many years, the thermodilution PAC was considered to be the "gold standard" of intensive care unit (ICU) hemodynamic measurement. This philosophy has been called into question during the last several years in light of mounting evidence that clinicians may be using the PAC ineffectively [4] and that morbidity and mortality in a variety of clinical situations are not improved with its use [5,6], but instead may be worsened [7,8].

In light of these studies, many clinicians have begun to question the importance and the credibility of the PAC. Some postulate that the lack of improvement on morbidity and mortality stems from the deleterious complications that are inherently associated with an invasive procedure. Others have shown that even when the balance of oxygen supply and demand in critically ill patients is known and is optimized, even to supranormal levels, there is no improvement in outcomes [9]. This gives rise to the notion that once tissue hypoperfusion results in organ dysfunction, a cycle of inflammation ensues that leads to irreversible organ damage if not corrected early. This concept has been described as "cytopathic hypoxia," wherein hypoperfusion leads to the disruption of the intracellular utilization of oxygen to the point that delivery of normal or supranormal amounts of oxygen to a cell will not restore its function [10,11]. Some data have emerged that suggest that correction of hypoperfusion and inadequate oxygen delivery early in the course of sepsis yields beneficial mortality outcomes [12,13]. Interestingly, these studies did not use PACs, but instead used central venous oxygen saturation as a surrogate for cardiac output and volume responsiveness.

While we await more data to clarify the usefulness of directly monitoring cardiac output in critically ill patients and the timing at which it is best to use this monitoring, many are focusing on alternative and less-invasive methods of determining cardiac function. These methods can be divided into two broad categories: Measurements of cardiac output and measurements of indices of oxygen delivery and/or tissue perfusion as surrogates for cardiac output. The goal of this research has been to develop minimally invasive yet reliable and accurate techniques that can be easily applied to critically ill patients. In some cases, these studies have focused on adapting monitoring technology that is already routinely used in this patient population.

In this chapter, we focus on several emerging technologies being used to determine cardiac output and tissue perfusion in the critically ill patient. The bulk of the discussion will involve the methods of Doppler echocardiography, pulse contour analysis (PCA), partial carbon dioxide rebreathing, and gastric tonometry as these represent the modalities best studied to date. Consideration will also be given to new and developing methods such as thoracic bioimpedance, sublingual capnometry, and biomarkers. We will conclude with a summary of practice recommendations and future directions.

CARDIAC OUTPUT

Cardiac output is the amount of blood flow through the cardiovascular system during a period of time. Traditionally, it is reported in liters per minute and can be normalized for a person's body surface area to provide the cardiac index. In the healthy subject, cardiac output is directly related to that subject's metabolic rate and oxygen consumption ($\dot{V}o_2$). The therapy for a hypotensive patient with diminished cardiac output (cardiogenic shock) is fundamentally different from the therapy for a patient with diminished systemic vascular resistance (distributive shock). Therefore, an accurate knowledge of these variables is vital to the effective treatment of the hypotensive, critically ill patient. As the systemic vascular resistance can be challenging to measure directly, it is calculated from the ratio of pressure gradient (mean arterial pressure minus central venous pressure) and flow rate (cardiac output). This formula assumes an ohmic resistor (i.e., one with a linear pressure-flow relationship). Because a fall in systemic vascular resistance could represent a decrease in blood pressure or a rise in cardiac output, we favor the use of the primary measured variables in hemodynamic assessments. We would also caution against the use of the systemic vascular resistance in isolation, without consideration for the factors leading to its fluctuations (e.g., changes in cardiac output).

Traditionally, a number of techniques have been used for the assessment of cardiac function. Jugular venous pulsations, the presence of an S_3 gallop, and skin temperature have all been studied as means of using the physical examination to estimate cardiac output with mixed results [14–16]. The pulmonary artery occlusion pressure (PAOP) and central venous pressure (CVP) have also been used as surrogates for left and right ventricular function, respectively. The PAOP is commonly used to establish the diagnosis of left heart failure in the hypotensive patient and is often used to guide resuscitation. Magder and colleagues [17,18] demonstrated that the CVP could provide useful information about the volume status of critically ill patients. Because the majority of the blood volume is in the systemic veins, and the right ventricle is the major determinant of cardiac output, some would argue that the CVP should receive more attention as the focus of hemodynamic resuscitation protocols. Unfortunately, PAOP and CVP only represent the end-diastolic pressures of their respective chambers. These variables do not always accurately translate into systolic function and cardiac output. In addition, invasive assessment of PAOP [19,20] and clinical assessment of CVP [21] have been notoriously difficult to assess accurately and reliably.

During the last few decades, considerable research has been devoted to the accurate measurement of cardiac output by minimally invasive means. At present, there exist several modalities that are able to provide estimates of cardiac output on a continuous or near-continuous basis. Each is based on unique strategies and each has notable advantages and disadvantages. Although some have been established enough to warrant increasing use in clinical settings (esophageal Doppler [ED], PCA), the clinical usefulness of others is still being determined (partial carbon dioxide rebreathing, thoracic bioimpedance). Here, we describe each of these four modalities and summarize the evidence regarding their use.

ESOPHAGEAL DOPPLER

To date, the ED has been one of the most rigorously studied noninvasive cardiac output measurement modalities. It was first described by Side and Gosling [22] in 1971 and was later refined by Singer et al. [23]. This technique uses a Doppler probe placed in the esophagus to measure blood flow in the descending thoracic aorta. The ED uses the Doppler shift principle, which implies that when a transmitted sound wave is impeded by a structure, the reflected sound wave will vary in a frequency-dependent manner with the structure's characteristics. In the case of a fluid-filled tube, such as the aorta, the magnitude of Doppler shift will vary in direct proportion to the velocity of flow in the tube (Fig. 29-1). Thus, the reflected sound wave can be used to determine flow velocity in the descending aorta. Multiplying this flow velocity by the ejection time and the cross-sectional area of the aorta provides an estimate of the stroke volume (SV). As this measurement does not account for the component of total SV that travels to the coronary, carotid, and subclavian arteries, a correction factor must be applied to estimate the total SV. Cardiac output is then calculated by multiplying corrected SV by the heart rate. The original versions of the ED system only provided Doppler shift data; therefore, the cross-sectional area

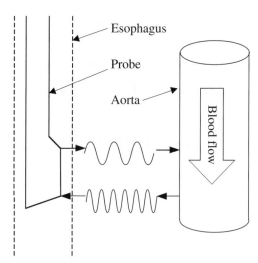

FIGURE 29-1. Esophageal Doppler probe using the Doppler Shift principle. Transmitted ultrasound waves are reflected back at varying frequencies, which depend on the velocity of flow of the red blood cells they encounter.

of the aorta was estimated from a nomogram based on a patient's height, weight, and age. Subsequently, a newer model with both a Doppler and ultrasound probe has been introduced that can simultaneously provide estimates of both aortic flow velocity and cross-sectional area [24]. The descending aortic cross-sectional area measured by this model correlated very well with that measured by transesophageal echocardiography. In addition, the aortic blood flow measured with this model was also well correlated with cardiac output as measured by thermodilution [24].

Beyond providing an estimate of cardiac output, ED systems can provide information about the preload and the contractility of the heart. Singer et al. [23] and Singer and Bennett [25] analyzed the flow-velocity waveform derived from an ED system and discovered that the corrected flow time correlated with preload (Fig. 29-2). These studies further demonstrated that as preload was increased or decreased, the corrected flow time increased or decreased, respectively [23,25]. Wallmeyer and colleagues [26] described a correlation between the peak velocity measured by a Doppler and contractility measured by electromagnetic catheter measured flow. Singer et al. [27] further substantiated this finding by demonstrating that dobutamine infusions increased peak flow velocities measured by an ED system in a dose-dependent fashion. These observations suggest that an experienced operator may be able to extrapolate useful hemodynamic parameters, beyond the cardiac output, through careful interpretation of the generated data.

Clinical Utility

The clinical usefulness of the ED system is still being determined. The majority of recent studies that have compared this system to the gold standard of thermodilution have been performed in either intraoperative or postoperative settings and have revealed mixed results. One single-center study of 35 patients that compared ED measurements of cardiac output with simultaneous measurements of cardiac output by thermodilution during off-pump coronary artery bypass grafting showed very poor

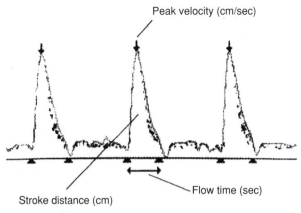

Peak velocity (cm/sec)

Flow time (sec)

Stroke distance (cm)

Minute distance (stroke distance × heart rate)

FIGURE 29-2. Esophageal Doppler flow-velocity waveform. [Adapted from Marik PE: Pulmonary artery catheterization and esophageal Doppler monitoring in the ICU. *Chest* 116:1085, 1999, with permission.]

TABLE 29-1. Advantages and Disadvantages of the Esophageal Doppler System for Cardiac Output Monitoring

Concept: Doppler probe in the esophagus measures stroke volume in the descending aorta to estimate cardiac output.

Advantages
  Continuous
  Short setup time
  Low incidence of iatrogenic complications
  Ability to leave in place for extended periods
  Minimal training period required
  Minimal infection risk
Disadvantages
  High up-front cost
  Can only be used in the intubated patient
  May require frequent repositioning if patient is moved
  High interobserver variability

correlation between the two techniques [28]. Other studies, including a metaanalysis of 11 trials, have shown that ED systems are better at following changes in cardiac output in response to fluid challenges than they are at measuring the absolute cardiac output [29–31]. The authors of the metaanalysis also made an important point when discussing the reliability of comparing ED systems with thermodilution. They argued that the poor reproducibility inherent to the use of the thermodilution technique will likely affect the limits of agreement between ED systems and thermodilution, irrespective of the performances of the ED systems [29]. Stated simply, because the measurements of cardiac output by thermodilution vary significantly even when drawn temporally close to each other, ED systems will not have close agreement to thermodilution systems even if their measurements are reliable. This concept was described by Bland and Altman [32] and has important implications when trying to interpret the degree of accuracy of absolute cardiac output measured by any system when compared to thermodilution.

Advantages and Disadvantages

While comparing ED systems to thermodilution, it is also important to consider the technical advantages and disadvantages (Table 29-1). One advantage of the ED system is that it is continuous. Unlike the traditional bolus thermodilution techniques, an ED system can continuously display cardiac output, which allows earlier recognition of hemodynamic deterioration or improvement in system responsiveness to a therapeutic intervention. Additionally, an ED probe can be placed in minutes and has not been associated with important iatrogenic complications [33,34]. Some in situ data suggest that, once inserted, an esophageal probe can be left in place safely for more than 2 weeks [35]. One study determined that the training required to become proficient in the use of ED consisted of no more than 12 patients [36]. Furthermore, as the esophagus is a nonsterile environment, it is logical to assume that the infectious risk of ED probe use is less than that of a PAC placed in normally sterile tissues.

There are also technical disadvantages to the ED system. One is the high up-front cost of the system itself as compared to the PAC apparatus. This cost may represent a very real limitation in the number of systems that a facility can purchase and maintain.

This financial obstacle must be balanced with the likelihood that multiple patients would have need of this system simultaneously, which would necessitate multiple systems. Another disadvantage of this system is that it can be used only in the intubated patient. Although a large percentage of critically ill and/or surgical patients who would benefit from this system fit this criterion, the nonintubated patient would have to be excluded as a candidate. Additional concerns would include the likely need for repositioning or recalibrating the ICU patient. Although a surgical patient is often paralyzed and remains immobile, ICU patients are often repositioned frequently in order to prevent skin breakdown or to facilitate improved oxygenation. Such movements will increase the chance of probe position changes that will require frequent calibration and repositioning. Finally, Roeck et al. [31] suggested that there is significant interobserver variability when measuring changes in SV in response to fluid challenges with ED. Without a reproducible interpretation of data, the clinical usefulness of the ED system will be limited. We also believe that extensive clinical experience with this technique is important and would caution against the implementation of ED technique without adequate training.

Future Research

As the ED is used more widely, it will be critical to establish whether its use will actually improve patient care. To date, the majority of research on this technique has focused on validating its data and determining if it is a technically feasible modality of measuring cardiac output. Very little data exist at present about whether the use of this technique affects patient outcomes. One notable study that compared intraoperative ED use with "conventional" monitoring during femoral neck fracture repair found a faster recovery time and significantly shorter hospital stay in the ED group [37]. Although this study is encouraging, its results have not been reliably repeated as of yet. As previous trials have shown us, even the gold standard has not had a positive effect on patient care [7,8]. Future research on ED should begin to focus more on outcome data.

PULSE CONTOUR ANALYSIS

PCA is another modality for measuring cardiac output noninvasively that has been extensively studied. This method relies on the theory, first described by Frank [38] in the early part of the 20th century, that SV and cardiac output can be derived from the characteristics of an aortic pressure waveform. Wesseling and colleagues [39] eventually published in 1983 an algorithm to mathematically link SV and the pressure waveform. This original version calculated SV continuously by dividing the area under the curve of the aortic pressure waveform by the aortic impedance. Because aortic impedance varies between patients, it had to be measured using another modality to initially calibrate the PCA system. The calibration method usually employed was arterial thermodilution. Aortic impedance, however, is not a static property. It is based on the complex interaction of the resistive and compliant elements of each vascular bed, which are often dynamic, especially in hemodynamically unstable patients. Since the first PCA algorithm was introduced, several unique algorithms have been created in an attempt to accurately model the properties of the human vascular system for use in PCA systems.

PCA involves the use of an arterially placed catheter with a pressure transducer, which can measure pressure tracings on a beat-to-beat basis. Such catheters are now routinely used in operating rooms and ICUs as they provide a continuous measurement of blood pressure that is believed to be superior to intermittent noninvasive measurements in hemodynamically unstable patients. These catheters are interfaced with a PCA system, which uses its unique algorithm as well as the initial aortic impedance calibration data from a thermodilution measurement of cardiac output to provide a continuously displayed measurement of cardiac output. Obviously, the reliability of a PCA system depends on the accuracy of the algorithm that it employs. Because each algorithm is unique in the weight that it ascribes to each element of vascular conductivity, it is impossible to ensure that a system will be able to reproduce the results of another system under similar conditions [40]. Keeping this in mind, one cannot conclude that all systems are equally reliable.

One particular PCA system has received considerable attention in the literature. Numerous studies have demonstrated good correlation between this system and pulmonary thermodilution in both critically ill and surgical patients [41–45]. Notably, this system did not require recalibration during these study periods, which were performed under static ventricular loading conditions. The system involves the placement of a femoral arterial catheter that is passed into the abdominal aorta. In addition to a pressure transducer, the catheter also contains a thermistor for arterial thermodilution. The system is calibrated by injecting cold saline via a central venous catheter at the right atrium in a manner similar to pulmonary arterial thermodilution. Instead of using a thermistor in the pulmonary artery, however, the thermistor on the arterial catheter allows calculation of cardiac output. This initial value of cardiac output is then used to calibrate the PCA system that is attached to the arterial catheter. Because the arterial catheter is used for calibration, a PAC is not necessary. When compared to pulmonary artery thermodilution, the arterial thermodilution method was found to be accurate, implying that it is an acceptable method for calibration of a PCA system [41–43].

Clinical Utility

As mentioned previously, the initial trials studying this system used data from static ventricular loading conditions. Both the critically ill and the surgical patient, however, often experience rapid changes in ventricular preload. The validity of this sys-

tem with changes in preload was addressed in a subsequent study, which used an updated version of the previous algorithm. Felbinger and colleagues [46] showed that changes in cardiac output in response to preload could be accurately measured in a cardiac surgical ICU population when compared to pulmonary thermodilution.

Although being able to monitor cardiac output during volume loading is important, being able to determine when a patient would benefit from increased preload has major clinical benefit. Pulse pressures commonly vary throughout the respiratory cycle. Pulse pressure variation (PPV) is defined as the result of the minimum pulse pressure subtracted from the maximum pulse pressure divided by the mean of these two pressures.

$$PPV = \frac{Pulse\ Pressure_{max} - Pulse\ Pressure_{min}}{Pulse\ Pressure_{mean}}$$

It has been observed that the magnitude of the pulse pressure variation in a patient can predict preload responsiveness [47–49]. Analogous to pulse pressure variation, an additional piece of data that PCA systems can provide is the stroke volume variation (SVV). The SVV represents the change in percentage of SV over a preceding time period as a result of changes in SV due to ventilation. Thus far, the ability to use SVV to determine preload responsiveness has yielded mixed results. Reuter et al. [50] found that SVV reliably decreased as cardiac index increased in response to preloading with colloids in ventilated postoperative cardiac surgical patients. This finding supports the argument that the magnitude of SVV may be used to predict preload responsiveness. It is important to note that the tidal volumes used in this study were supraphysiologic (15 mL/kg), which results in a larger SVV and a resultant increase in the accuracy of this approach. Subsequently, another study used a smaller tidal volume (10 mL/kg) in a similar patient population and could not demonstrate a reliable relationship between SVV and an increase in cardiac index in response to preloading [51]. This finding suggests that when using lower tidal volume ventilation strategies, which are optimal for acute respiratory distress syndrome (ARDS), PCA-derived SVV should not be used to estimate preload responsiveness.

Advantages and Disadvantages

Overall, the PCA system offers several advantages over the traditional gold standard of pulmonary artery thermodilution (Table 29-2). It requires the use of an arterial catheter as well as a central venous catheter, which are both commonly already in place in critically ill and surgical patients for monitoring and therapeutic purposes. Because these systems can be reliably calibrated by the arterial thermodilution method, the potential risk of a PAC can be avoided. The PCA system also provides a continuous measurement of cardiac output as opposed to the intermittent nature of traditional thermodilution systems.

As with any system, there are disadvantages to the PCA system as well. The ability to use this system to determine preload responsiveness is questionable in patients who are being managed with common ventilatory strategies. In addition, some data suggest that in patients who have marked changes in blood pressure, the algorithm is not able to model adequately the changes in vascular resistance and compliance and, therefore, the accuracy of the measured cardiac output declines [52]. Furthermore, a similar breakdown in the accuracy of measured cardiac output has

TABLE 29-2. Advantages and Disadvantages of the Pulse Contour Analysis Method for Cardiac Output Monitoring

Concept: Arterial catheter used to determine stroke volume from aortic pressure waveforms.

Advantages
  Continuous
  Uses catheters that are already commonly used in patients in the intensive care unit
  Does not require calibration with pulmonary artery catheter

Disadvantages
  Likely unable to determine preload responsiveness during low tidal volume ventilation
  Questionable accuracy during large changes in blood pressure
  Questionable accuracy during vasoconstrictor use

been suggested during the administration of vasoconstrictors [53], which are common in the critically ill patient.

Future Research

The clinical utility of the PCA system is still being determined. Future studies that may help in defining the system's clinical role could focus on several points. First, a better understanding of how changes in blood pressure and vasoconstrictor use affect the accuracy of a particular system's algorithm will help to determine a schedule for when a system needs to be recalibrated in order to maintain its accuracy. Additionally, an analysis of how SVV predicts preload responsiveness at tidal volumes that are commonly used in the ARDS patient population will provide more applicable information than what is currently available. Finally, a paucity of data regarding how PCA systems affect patient outcomes exists at present. Comparisons between the outcomes seen with this system and pulmonary artery thermodilution may provide convincing evidence about the real usefulness of PCA.

PARTIAL CARBON DIOXIDE REBREATHING METHOD

The Fick equation for calculating cardiac output has been known for more than 100 years. Its underlying principle states that for a gas (X) whose uptake in the lung is transferred completely to the blood, the ratio of that gas's consumption (VX) to the difference between the arterial (C_aX) and venous (C_vX) contents of the gas will equal the cardiac output. In its original form, Fick used the example of oxygen (O_2) and described the following equation:

$$\text{Cardiac Output} = \frac{\dot{V}O_2}{C_aO_2 - C_vO_2}$$

For this equation to be accurate, several conditions must exist. The first is that blood flow through the pulmonary capillaries must be constant. In order for this to occur, the right and left ventricular outputs must be equal and there must be no respiratory variation of pulmonary capillary flow. Another condition critical to this method's accuracy is an absence of shunts. As this method depends on using gas exchange to calculate cardiac output, any blood that does not participate in gas exchange will result in underestimation of cardiac output. Furthermore, oxygen uptake by the lung itself must be minimal to maintain the integrity of this equation.

Although possible, the accurate measurement of $\dot{V}O_2$ is clinically challenging, especially in patients who require high

F_{IO_2} [54]. This prompted some investigators to focus on using carbon dioxide production ($\dot{V}CO_2$) in place of $\dot{V}O_2$ [55–57]. As $\dot{V}O_2$ is equal to $\dot{V}CO_2$ divided by the respiratory quotient, they determined that cardiac output could be calculated by $\dot{V}CO_2$ divided by the arteriovenous difference between O_2 concentrations as well as the respiratory quotient (R). In order to measure O_2 concentrations continuously, arterial and venous oximeters were used to measure oxygen saturation (SO_2) and concentration was determined based on measured hemoglobin (Hgb) levels. This technique, therefore, relied upon the assumption that both R and Hgb levels remained constant during the measurement period.

$$\dot{V}O_2 = \frac{\dot{V}CO_2}{R}$$

$$C_aO_2 = 13.4 \times Hgb \times S_aO_2$$

$$co = \frac{\dot{V}CO_2}{13.4 \times Hgb \times R \times [S_aO_2 - S_vO_2]}$$

Using this method, one study found good correlation with cardiac output determined by thermodilution [57]. The drawback to this approach, however, is the need for an invasive central venous catheter to accurately measure venous oxygen saturations as well as to initially calibrate the system and determine R. Subsequently, the partial carbon dioxide rebreathing method was introduced in an attempt to avoid the need for such catheters.

The partial CO_2 rebreathing method is based upon the Fick equation for CO_2 [58]:

$$co = \frac{\dot{V}CO_2}{C_vCO_2 - C_aCO_2}$$

When using this method, a disposable rebreathing loop is placed between the endotracheal tube and the ventilator, resulting in the rebreathing of carbon dioxide. A carbon dioxide sensor, an airflow sensor, and an arterial noninvasive pulse oximeter are then used to gather data before and after a period of CO_2 rebreathing. The CO_2 sensor and airflow monitor allow for the calculation of $\dot{V}CO_2$ both before and during the rebreathing period. Because cardiac output does not change from baseline during rebreathing conditions [59], one can generate the following equation [58]:

$$co = \frac{\dot{V}CO_{2_{baseline}}}{C_vCO_{2_{baseline}} - C_aCO_{2_{baseline}}} = \frac{\dot{V}CO_{2_{rebreathing}}}{C_vCO_{2_{rebreathing}} - C_aCO_{2_{rebreathing}}}$$

Gedeon et al. [60] determined that subtracting the rebreathing ratio from the baseline ratio yields the following equation [58]:

$$co = \frac{\dot{V}CO_{2_{baseline}} - \dot{V}CO_{2_{rebreathing}}}{[C_vCO_{2_{baseline}} - C_aCO_{2_{baseline}}] - [C_vCO_{2_{rebreathing}} - C_aCO_{2_{rebreathing}}]}$$

As CO_2 diffuses rapidly into the blood, one can further assume that the mixed venous CO_2 concentration (C_vCO_2) remains unchanged between baseline and rebreathing conditions; that is, $C_vCO_{2_{baseline}} = C_vCO_{2_{rebreathing}}$. This allows for further simplification of the equation to the following [58]:

$$co = \frac{\Delta\dot{V}CO_2}{\Delta C_aCO_2}$$

C_aCO_2 can be estimated from end-tidal carbon dioxide ($etCO_2$) and the carbon dioxide dissociation curve. Therefore, ΔC_aCO_2 can be substituted for by $\Delta etCO_2$ multiplied by the slope (S) of the dissociation curve [58]:

$$co = \frac{\Delta \dot{V}co_2}{\Delta etco_2 \times S}$$

An estimate of cardiac output can now be calculated using data that can be measured before and after a period of rebreathing, in addition to S, which can be determined from a carbon dioxide dissociation curve. It is important to note that the estimate of cardiac output calculated using this final equation only accounts for the blood that is able to participate in gas exchange. Any blood involved in a right-to-left intrapulmonary shunt is not considered by this equation; therefore, a correction factor must be incorporated to account for this shunted blood. This is determined by a partial rebreathing system by using the data collected from the noninvasive arterial oximeter, the Fio_2, and the Pao_2 as determined by arterial blood gases. These data allow one to determine an estimate of shunted blood using the Nunn's isoshunt tables of Benatar et al. [61].

Clinical Utility

Thus far, the results of comparisons between partial co_2 rebreathing techniques and alternative methods of measuring cardiac output have been mixed at best. Some studies have demonstrated decent agreement with the gold standard of thermodilution [62–64], but others have shown poor agreement [44,65,66]. One of these studies did demonstrate good reproducibility of the results obtained from the partial rebreathing method despite the fact that they did not correlate with results obtained by thermodilution [66]. One could infer from this that the method may have been appropriately precise but that something in its algorithm (i.e., estimation of shunt or estimation of C_aco_2 from etco_2) prevented it from obtaining accurate results. This may be encouraging evidence that the partial rebreathing method can be an acceptable technique in certain clinical situations as the accuracy of currently marketed systems is improved.

Determining which clinical situations are appropriate for the partial rebreathing method is critical when considering its use. Because the method's accuracy depends on an estimate of C_aco_2 from etco_2 as well as an estimate of shunt, clinical situations that affect these estimates may not be appropriate for using this method. For instance, postoperative cardiac surgical patients tend to have increased pulmonary dead space and shunt [67] and may not be an appropriate population for partial co_2 rebreathing monitor use [66]. In addition, some data suggest that the correlation between this method and thermodilution declines as the amount of venous admixture from shunting increases in animal models [68]. In order for C_aco_2 to be accurately estimated by etco_2, gas exchange needs to be somewhat homogenous throughout the lung. One of the hallmarks of acute lung injury (ALI) and ARDS is a heterogeneous pattern of damage and fibrosis. This heterogeneity results in a large variation of gas exchange throughout the lung. Consequently, the etco_2 may be a poor estimate of C_aco_2 leading to an important source of error. Indeed, one study, which compared the partial co_2 rebreathing method to thermodilution in patients with varying degrees of ALI, found poor agreement between the two methods [69]. The disagreement intensified with worsening severity of ALI. Finally, significant variations in tidal volume during a period of measurement will often dramatically affect the accuracy of $\dot{V}co_2$ on a breath-to-breath basis. Consequently, the accuracy of measured cardiac output is limited in situations

TABLE 29-3. Advantages and Disadvantages of the Partial Carbon Dioxide Rebreathing Method for Cardiac Output Monitoring

Concept: Using exhaled carbon dioxide to determine cardiac output using a modified fick equation
Advantages
Truly noninvasive
Nearly continuous
Disadvantages
High up-front cost
Can only be used in the intubated patient
Questionable accuracy in patients with lung injury
Unclear risk in patients with hypercapnia or increased intracranial pressure

of varying tidal volume, such as pressure-support ventilation [70].

Advantages and Disadvantages

The most notable advantage of the partial co_2 rebreathing method is its true noninvasive nature. With the exception of the arterial blood gases used to estimate shunt, this method does not require any additional invasive procedures. Additionally, cardiac output can be measured on a near-continuous basis. The disadvantages of the system are substantial, however (Table 29-3). It is challenging to use in patients who are not intubated, or in intubated patients with spontaneous ventilation. Its accuracy is questionable in patients with intrapulmonary shunt and lung injury, which are both common findings in the critically ill patient. Because the technique raises arterial Pco_2, its safety in patients with hypercapnia or increased intracranial pressure is unknown. Each system also represents an important up-front cost but can only be used by one patient at any given time. The limited clinical utility of these systems may not justify this expenditure.

Future Research

At present, the clinical applicability of partial co_2 rebreathing systems is not completely known. Future research should focus on further examining the accuracy of these systems in patients with lung injury as the current data are limited. Improvements of existing algorithms for shunt and C_aco_2 estimation could also aid in increasing this method's generalizability. Finally, determining if this method's noninvasive nature truly makes a difference in clinical outcomes should be an important focus of upcoming investigation. In critically ill patients, there may be no major advantage to using monitoring techniques that avoid central lines and arterial lines because these are nearly ubiquitous in the ICU.

THORACIC BIOIMPEDANCE

The thoracic bioimpedance technique was first developed by Kubicek et al. [71] as a means of noninvasively measuring the cardiac output of astronauts. It involves the delivery of a low-amplitude, high-frequency electrical current across the thorax. A series of sensing electrodes, which measure the resistance of the thorax, are placed along the path of this current (Fig. 29-3). Because of the conductive properties of fluid, the bioimpedance of a thorax is inversely proportional to the amount of fluid in the

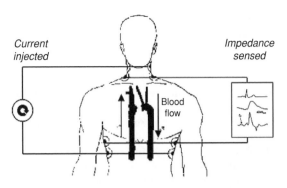

Current injected

Impedance sensed

Blood flow

FIGURE 29-3. Lead placement in thoracic bioimpedance. [Adapted from Summers RL, Shoemaker WC, Peacock WF, et al: Bench to bedside: electrophysiologic and clinical principles of noninvasive hemodynamic monitoring using impedance cardiography. *Acad Emerg Med* 10:669, 2003, with permission.]

thorax at the time of measurement. Thus, as intrathoracic fluid volume increases during each cardiac cycle, the bioimpedance measured by the sensing electrodes decreases. This principle provides the basis for measuring the SV and, hence, cardiac output using this technique. In order to estimate cardiac output accurately, however, aortic blood flow must be distinguished from other sources of intrathoracic fluid movement. Simultaneously recording the electrocardiogram and using a computer algorithm to filter electrical noise caused by other fluid movement can accomplish this.

Since its inception, a variety of modifications have been made to the original technique in order to improve its accuracy. The original version used a cylindrical model of the thorax, and later models changed to a conical model for improved accuracy [72]. Furthermore, early versions used coefficients based on "ideal body" proportions derived from mean measurements of the population. Systems using these estimates of body shape were found to be imprecise and tended to overestimate cardiac output [73]. More recent models now use measurements of chest circumference, weight, height, and sex to more accurately model the thorax in an attempt to improve the accuracy of cardiac output measurement [74]. Additionally, a more accurate estimate of the impedance of blood based on hematocrit may also improve accuracy [74]. Finally, the use of nonlinear algorithms to analyze the impedance waveform is thought to improve accuracy in critically ill patients with left and right heart asynchrony [74].

Clinical Utility

Overall, the validation studies comparing thoracic bioimpedance with thermodilution have yielded variable results to date. One large metaanalysis revealed a broad range of correlation between the two techniques with correlation coefficients (r) ranging from 0.44 to 0.74 [75]. The diversity of patient population studied likely accounts for some of this variation. One population in which many clinicians question the accuracy of thoracic bioimpedance is patients with ALI. One of the hallmarks of ALI is pulmonary edema, and many patients with this syndrome also have pneumonia or pleural effusions. The presence of each of these conditions increases intrathoracic fluid levels, which may generate enough "noise" to affect the accuracy of bioimpedance measurements. One small, prospective study compared thoracic

bioimpedance to thermodilution in patients with ALI during ventilation both with and without positive end-expiratory pressure. It showed poor correlation between the techniques, which was not improved with the use of positive end-expiratory pressure [76]. In addition, a large multicenter trial comparing the two techniques found that correlation improved when patients with high thoracic fluid volume were excluded [77]. Another population in which concern regarding the accuracy of thoracic bioimpedance has been expressed is among obese patients. Sageman and Amundson [78] found no correlation ($r^2 = .00$) between invasive cardiac index measurements and those measured by thoracic bioimpedance in a subset of obese patients following coronary bypass. In contrast, a retrospective review of a prospective database revealed that patients with a body mass index greater than 30 kg per m^2 actually had equivalent correlation and less bias between thoracic bioimpedance and thermodilution when compared to patients with a body mass index less than 30 kg per m^2 [79]. Given the increasing prevalence of obesity, further clarification of the accuracy of thoracic bioimpedance in obese patients will be clinically relevant.

Future Research

As with many noninvasive methods of monitoring cardiac output, the utility of thoracic bioimpedance to change patient outcome has not been well studied. As the accuracy of the many commercially available systems continues to improve, further studies should focus on their effect on clinical outcome. Additionally, focusing on improving accuracy in patients with increased intrathoracic fluid volume could result in clinical benefit.

OXYGEN DELIVERY AND TISSUE PERFUSION

Although directly measuring cardiac output can provide information vital to the management of critically ill patients, one can also argue that accurate knowledge of oxygen delivery and/or adequacy of tissue perfusion can be similarly useful. Proponents of this concept are less interested in the absolute cardiac output as long as adequate oxygen is delivered to tissues. One of the traditional techniques used to assess oxygen delivery is the mixed venous oxygen saturation ($S_{mv}O_2$). The $S_{mv}O_2$ is measured by sampling blood from the pulmonary artery, which is representative of the venous return from both the superior and inferior vena cava after sufficient mixing. It depends on both systemic oxygen delivery ($\dot{D}O_2$) as well as systemic oxygen consumption ($\dot{V}O_2$). Because $\dot{V}O_2$ does not dramatically change in the absence of major metabolic derangements, decreases in $S_{mv}O_2$ can be considered to be due to decreases in $\dot{D}O_2$ (and, thereby, cardiac output) in most patients. As a result, investigators have focused on the clinical utility of measuring $S_{mv}O_2$ as a surrogate means of monitoring cardiac output [80,81]. Pearson et al. [82] found that $S_{mv}O_2$ monitoring did not improve length of ICU stay or length of vasopressor requirement when compared to traditional PAC use and CVP monitoring. In addition, $S_{mv}O_2$ monitoring cost more.

Another potential drawback of $S_{mv}O_2$ monitoring is the need for pulmonary artery catheterization and the inherent risks associated with it. Because many critically ill patients receive central venous catheters, some research has focused on using central venous oxygen saturations ($S_{cv}O_2$) rather than $S_{mv}O_2$.

One early study found that $S_{cv}O_2$ tended to be approximately 5% to 10% lower than $S_{mv}O_2$ in humans [83]. While studying dogs, Reinhart and colleagues [84] found good correlation ($r = 0.96$) between the two. Thus far, clinical data using this variable are limited; however, the previously mentioned landmark trial by Rivers et al. [12] used $S_{cv}O_2$ among other variables with success and was recently validated [13].

In addition to estimating oxygen delivery, recent research has focused on estimating tissue perfusion as a guide for resuscitative therapy. With this approach, the adequacy of blood and oxygen delivery is assessed by measuring markers of hypoperfusion of accessible organs. We will focus on three modalities that have demonstrated considerable promise in this field to date: gastric tonometry, sublingual capnometry, and cardiac biomarkers.

GASTRIC TONOMETRY

Mounting evidence that early correction of hypoperfusion in shock improves mortality [12,13,85] has lead investigators to focus on the development of methods for its early detection. It is known that tissue levels of CO_2 rise early in the setting of hypoperfusion [86–88]. The level of CO_2 in a tissue is determined by the balance between the concentration of arterial CO_2 (C_aCO_2), blood flow to the tissue, and CO_2 production by the tissue. In a state of hypoperfusion, CO_2 increase is thought to be multifactorial. Carbon dioxide production increases in hypoperfused tissue in order to buffer the increase in hydrogen ions generated by the hydrolysis of adenosine triphosphate during glycolysis [89]. Additionally, the low flow state seen in hypoperfusion results in an impaired clearance of CO_2, causing a further increase in tissue CO_2 concentrations [90]. The complex mucosal circulation of the gut results in the recirculation of CO_2 as well as arteriovenous O_2 shunting, which is exacerbated by the low-flow state of hypoperfusion. As a result, the gut mucosa is one of the earliest regions in the body affected by hypoperfusion. This characteristic combined with the relatively easy accessibility of the gut makes gastric tonometry an appealing choice for the early detection of shock [91].

Tonometry is based on the principle that gases will equilibrate between semipermeable compartments over time. Gastric tonometry involves placing a nasogastric tube tipped with a fluid or air-filled balloon into the lumen of the stomach and allowing its contents to equilibrate with the fluid in the stomach. This gastric fluid, in turn, is in equilibrium with the mucosal lining the stomach. Therefore, by sampling the contents of the balloon after sufficient time for equilibration, one can estimate the partial pressure of CO_2 in the gastric mucosa ($P_{gm}CO_2$). The original setups used saline in the balloon, which required approximately 90 minutes for equilibration. Once equilibrated, the saline was aspirated and its P_{CO_2} was determined. Newer automated models use air in place of saline, which results in shorter equilibration times (less than 20 minutes) and improved precision [92–94]. Many of the early studies performed with gastric tonometry used the $P_{gm}CO_2$ to determine the intramucosal pH (pH_i) by estimating the tissue bicarbonate levels from serum bicarbonate and solving the Henderson-Hasselbach equation. Recent focus has shifted away from this approach due to the introduction of error by estimating intramucosal bicarbonate from serum bicarbonate. Instead, the P_{CO_2} gap ($P_{gm}CO_2 - P_aCO_2$) has been proposed

as an alternative measure of tissue perfusion that is not influenced by the systemic acid-base status [95].

Clinical Utility

Given its relatively noninvasive nature, gastric tonometry would be an ideal candidate for a safe modality for the guidance of resuscitation in shock. Indeed, many studies have attempted to explore this technique's ability to guide therapy in situations of hypoperfusion. Silva et al. [96] measured changes in P_{CO_2} gap in addition to changes in systemic hemodynamic variables in response to fluid challenges in septic patients. They found that while cardiac index increased in response to fluid loading, indices of global oxygen delivery such as $S_{mv}O_2$ did not. The P_{CO_2} gap, however, was noted to significantly fall in response to fluid challenges. This implies that gastric tonometry may provide a more reliable and less invasive means of monitoring response to resuscitation than monitoring traditional global variables of oxygenation. In perhaps the best-known trial using this modality, Guitierrez and colleagues [97] randomized 260 critically ill patients in the ICU to a standard therapy arm and a protocol arm in which patients received additional therapy aimed at improving oxygen delivery whenever pH_i fell below 7.35. These authors found a significant increase in 28-day survival in a subset of the protocol group whose pH_i was greater than 7.35 on admission. Although this study suggested that gastric tonometry could be used to improve survival in a select group of patients, perhaps its most relevant point is that early correction of hypoperfusion is crucial to improving survival. Barquist et al. [98] compared the effects of a pH_i-guided splanchnic therapy with that of a non-pH_i–guided therapy in trauma patients. They found that patients in the splanchnic therapy group had fewer organ failures, which was associated with shorter length of both ICU and hospital stays.

Not all studies, however, have demonstrated the usefulness of gastric tonometry as a resuscitative guide. In one notable article comparing pH_i-guided therapy to therapy that was guided by global oxygen delivery indices in trauma patients, Ivatury and colleagues [99] did not find any significant difference in overall mortality. In their analysis, however, they pointed out that the time to optimization of pH_i was significantly longer in nonsurvivors. This implies that the resuscitative therapy used or the clinical condition of the nonsurvivors likely resulted in a delay of pH_i optimization and that this delay was most responsible for their outcome. Gomersall et al. [100] also compared pH_i-guided therapy to conventional treatment in 210 ICU patients. They too found no significant change in mortality, although some believe that this study was underpowered to detect a statistical difference [101].

Although the ideal use of gastric tonometry is guidance of resuscitation in shock, many studies using this modality have demonstrated its prognostic utility. Levy and colleagues [85] analyzed how pH_i and P_{CO_2} gap on admission to the ICU and at 24 hours correlated with outcome in 95 critically ill patients. They found that the nonsurvivor group had significantly lower pH_i values on admission and at 24 hours as compared to the survivor group. In addition, the P_{CO_2} gap at 24 hours independently predicted 28-day survival. These findings supported those of Maynard et al. [102], who compared pH_i to other global measures of perfusion in 83 patients with acute circulatory failure. In their study, pH_i was found to be a better predictor of outcome than lactate and other global measures of perfusion.

TABLE 29-4. Advantages and Disadvantages
of Gastric Tonometry

Concept: Using a semipermeable balloon in the lumen of the
  stomach to estimate gastric mucosal perfusion.

Advantages
  Low risk of infection
  May provide signs of early shock before traditional methods
  Provides evidence of response to therapy before traditional markers

Disadvantages
  Not continuous, takes up to 20 minutes per measurement
  Does not reveal the cause of hypoperfusion (i.e., cardiogenic vs.
    distributive)

Interestingly, mortality may not be the only outcome that can
be predicted through the use of gastric tonometry. The relationship between pH_i and outcome of ventilator weaning has also
been studied [103–106]. In these studies, a low baseline pH_i and
a significant drop in pH_i during weaning were associated with
failure to wean and failed extubations. It is not entirely clear if
the witnessed drop in pH_i is due to splanchnic ischemia from
diverted blood flow to facilitate increased work of breathing or
if it is related to increased P_aCO_2.

Thus far, studies have suggested that gastric tonometry may be
a promising modality for the treatment and prognosis of shock
with numerous advantages over traditional methods (Table
29-4). It is relatively noninvasive and can provide early information regarding the development of hypoperfusion that may
be more reliable than global indices of oxygen delivery. Insufficient sample sizes and the inability of some treatment protocols
to raise pH_i may explain some of the negative results derived
from the studies performed to date. Critics of this modality
question the validity of using gastric intramucosal pH as a surrogate for the entire splanchnic circulation [107]. Others wonder if the information obtained from gastric tonometry could
be determined less invasively by the base deficit/excess [108].
This particular question was partially addressed by Totapally and
colleagues [109], who showed that base excess responded very
slowly to changes in intravascular changes in hemorrhagic shock
in rats. Alternatively, esophageal PCO_2 gap was seen to reflect
changes in intravascular volume more closely.

Future Research

The future study of gastric tonometry should focus in several
directions. First, it should be used to help determine effective
protocols for increasing gut mucosal perfusion. Poorly outlined
and/or ineffective protocols were potential flaws in the studies
of both Guitierrez et al. [97] and Ivatury et al. [99]. A clearly
delineated and effective protocol for optimizing pH_i or PCO_2
gap would allow for a more meaningful comparison between
conventional and gastric tonometry-guided treatment. Furthermore, once a reliable protocol has been determined, gastric
tonometry may be used to further validate the increasing evidence that early restoration of perfusion and oxygen delivery
in shock is crucial to outcomes. Finally, the ability of gastric
tonometry to prognosticate not only mortality but also ability to
wean from mechanical ventilation should be further explored
as this may help to guide determining goals of care and family
decision-making.

SUBLINGUAL CAPNOMETRY

In attempts to further explore the clinical utility of guiding resuscitative therapy by tissue CO_2 levels, investigators have begun
to focus on using alternative sites for measurement. One site
that appears to be particularly promising due to its easy accessibility and, thus far, its accuracy, is the sublingual mucosa. After
Sato et al. [110] demonstrated that esophageal pH_i correlated
well with gastric pH_i in a rodent model, Jin and colleagues [111]
revealed that the more proximal sublingual mucosa developed
hypercapnia to a similar degree as gastric mucosa in a model of
hemorrhagic shock. These authors went on to show not only a
close correlation between increases in sublingual PCO_2 ($P_{sl}CO_2$)
and decreases in arterial pressure and cardiac index, [112] but
also demonstrated that reversal of shock led to a correction of
$P_{sl}CO_2$ comparable to that of $P_{gm}CO_2$ and more rapidly than the
traditional marker of hypoperfusion, lactate [113].

The most widely used sublingual capnometry system is composed of a CO_2-sensing optode. This device is a CO_2-permeable
capsule filled with a buffered solution of fluorescent dye. The
capsule is attached to an optic fiber and is placed under the
tongue. As CO_2 diffuses into the capsule, the pH of the buffered
solution is altered by production of carbonic acid (H_2CO_3). This
change in pH results in an alteration of the fluorescent emissions from the solution, which is ultimately sensed as a change
in projected light by the attached optic fiber. Hence, by calibrating wavelengths of light with known partial pressures of CO_2, one
can measure PCO_2 with this system. In order to ensure the highest
possible accuracy of the device, it must be placed securely under the tongue with the mouth closed. An open mouth allows
the entrance of light and ambient air to the optode, which can
significantly alter accuracy. The reliable range of a well-seated
and calibrated probe is 30 to 150 mm Hg [114].

Clinical Utility

Using this probe, researchers have begun to further investigate
the comparability of sublingual capnometry and gastric tonometry as well as the clinical utility of capnometry. In one validation study, Marik [115] demonstrated close correlation between
$P_{gm}CO_2$ and $P_{sl}CO_2$ ($r = 0.78$; $p < 0.001$) in a heterogeneous population of 76 ICU patients. Furthermore, Marik and Bankov
[116] went on to show that in another ICU population of 54
patients, $P_{sl}CO_2$ and $P_{sl}CO_2$-P_aCO_2 gap were better predictors of
outcome than lactate or $S_{mv}O_2$. These authors specifically found
that a $P_{sl}CO_2$-P_aCO_2 gap greater than 25 mm Hg was the best
discriminator of outcome. In addition, they found that $P_{sl}CO_2$
and $P_{sl}CO_2$-P_aCO_2 gap were more responsive to treatment measures than were lactate and $S_{mv}O_2$. Weil and colleagues [117] also
demonstrated the prognostic abilities of sublingual capnometry
when they found that a $P_{sl}CO_2$ less than 70 mm Hg had a positive
predictive value of 93% for survival.

Conclusion

In summary, the existing research regarding the clinical utility
of sublingual capnometry appears promising. This technique
may provide similar accuracy to gastric tonometry while being
less invasive and providing results on a more instantaneous basis. In addition, it does not require discontinuation of enteral
feeding during measurement periods, as some have advocated
for gastric tonometry. As sublingual capnometry use becomes
more widespread, it may replace the use of lactate and $S_{mv}O_2$

as markers of hypoperfusion and as resuscitative guides. Further research into this technique's effect on patient outcome is warranted and will likely occur in the near future.

CARDIAC BIOMARKERS

Cardiac biomarkers are molecules, usually proteins, that are specifically released from the heart into the blood and can be used to judge both cardiac function and dysfunction. Myocardial dysfunction is commonly seen early in the course of sepsis [118] and may be related to elevated levels of proinflammatory cytokines such as interleukin-1 and tumor necrosis factor-α, which have been shown to be cardiodepressant [119]. However, due to a concomitant increase in left ventricular ejection fraction caused by afterload reduction from systemic vasodilation, diagnosis of myocardial dysfunction early in sepsis can be difficult by traditional echocardiography. The study of cardiac biomarkers in the ICU setting is becoming an increasingly popular method of determining early cardiac dysfunction. As they can be obtained from a peripheral venous blood sample, they represent completely noninvasive and potentially valuable data that may assist in prognostication as well as in guiding management. To date, research has focused primarily on two proteins: troponin and B-type natriuretic peptide (BNP).

Troponin

Troponin T (TnT) and troponin I (TnI) are cardiac-specific contractile proteins that have been studied extensively in the context of myocardial ischemia. Both have been shown to be superior to the traditional creatinine kinase-MB in diagnosing myocardial injury in certain clinical contexts [120–122]. As such, they have become part of the mainstay for diagnosing acute myocardial infarction today. Less is known about their role in the ICU in patients who are not undergoing myocardial infarction due to coronary plaque rupture. Several authors have observed an elevated level of troponin in ICU patients who are not undergoing an acute coronary syndrome [123,124]. One recent prospective case control study showed that 17 of 20 patients (85%) with systemic inflammatory response syndrome, sepsis, or septic shock had elevations in TnI. Furthermore, of the six patients who died in the study, five had elevated TnI levels. Ten of the 17 patients with elevated TnI levels had no evidence of important coronary artery disease by coronary angiography, stress echocardiography, or autopsy [125]. Interestingly, in this study there were patients with a normal left ventricular ejection fraction by echocardiography who had increased TnI levels. This suggests that TnI may be able to detect myocardial dysfunction even when echocardiography cannot. Troponin has also been studied as a prognostic marker in sepsis. Spies and colleagues [126] measured serum TnT levels in 26 septic patients in a surgical ICU. They found that elevated TnT levels within the first 24 hours of sepsis were associated with a significantly higher mortality rate when compared to normal TnT levels. Thus, troponin may be useful for detection of occult myocardial dysfunction as well as for prognostication in ICU patients in the absence of an acute coronary syndrome. These promising early findings should lead to further research into the utility troponin in the ICU.

B-Type Natriuretic Peptide

The natriuretic peptides are a family of hormones that exert a wide range of biologic functions including diuresis and vasodi-lation. Two members of this family, atrial natriuretic peptide (ANP) and B-type (or brain) natriuretic peptide (BNP), are secreted by the atria and the ventricles, respectively. Their secretion is stimulated by myocardial stretch induced by increased filling volumes. Each hormone is derived from a prohormone that is cleaved into the biologically active C-terminal component and the biologically quiescent but longer lasting N-terminal component. In recent years, research has suggested that BNP can be a valuable surrogate for left ventricular end-diastolic pressure and left ventricular ejection fraction and can correlate with New York Heart Association heart failure class in patients with congestive heart failure [127–131]. Until recently, however, little was known about the role of BNP as a marker of myocardial dysfunction in the critically ill population. Prompted by data that suggest that BNP can correlate with PAOP in patients with severe congestive heart failure [132,133], Tung et al. [134] investigated the utility of using BNP as a surrogate for PAC placement in a heterogeneous population in shock. Although BNP levels did not correlate with cardiac index or PAOP in this study, they did find that a BNP level of less than 350 pg per mL had a 95% negative predictive value for the diagnosis of cardiogenic shock. This suggests that although BNP should not be used in place of PAOP, a low BNP level may obviate the need for PAC placement. This study also demonstrated that BNP levels have prognostic significance among the critically ill. The median BNP level at the time of PAC placement was significantly higher in the nonsurvivor population as compared with survivors. In addition, a multivariate analysis showed that a BNP concentration in the highest log-quartile was the strongest predictor of mortality with an odds ratio of 4.5. This was an even stronger predictor of mortality than the Acute Physiology and Chronic Health Evaluation (APACHE) II scores [134].

The prognostic utility of BNP was further validated by Brueckmann et al. [135] when these authors found that elevated N-terminal proBNP (NT-proBNP) levels on day 2 were significantly correlated with an increased mortality rate in patients with severe sepsis. However, these authors did not find prognostic significance with N-terminal proANP (NT-proANP). Interestingly, the levels of NT-proBNP, NT-proANP, and TnI were all found to be significantly lower in patients being treated with drotrecogin alfa (activated) than in those not receiving it [135]. This suggests that drotrecogin alfa (activated) may provide some cardioprotective effect in severe sepsis, perhaps through its proposed antiinflammatory properties. Due to sample size, however, these authors were not able to determine if these findings were correlated with mortality benefit.

Conclusion

In summary, the study of cardiac biomarkers in the ICU is still in the early stages. To date, the majority of data suggest that troponin and BNP may have some prognostic significance in critically ill patients without congestive heart failure. Neither has been shown to be able to guide management thus far, although some data suggest that low BNP levels may exclude cardiogenic shock, thereby preventing the need for a diagnostic PA line. Larger trials may further prove this concept in the future allowing for less invasive management of a select population of patients. Furthermore, a better understanding of the effect of drotrecogin alfa (activated) on cardiac biomarkers may provide some insight into the nature of the myocardial dysfunction seen in sepsis.

PRACTICE RECOMMENDATIONS

Independent of which cardiac monitoring technique is employed, a strategy that should be used in all patients with shock is early intervention. Mounting evidence suggests that "cytopathic hypoxia" may be playing a role in the pathogenesis of shock [10,11] and efforts to correct hemodynamic derangements and augment oxygen delivery early in shock have shown promising results thus far [12]. The optimal method for cardiac monitoring, however, is yet to be determined. At present, pulmonary artery thermodilution remains the gold standard; however, increasing interest has been given to less-invasive monitoring modalities. To date, the most substantial research has focused on ED, PCA, and gastric tonometry systems. Although there remains some question whether the absolute cardiac output determined by ED is accurate, most studies have proven its reliability in monitoring trends in cardiac output in response to therapeutic interventions. This ability to monitor trends may be sufficient for the management of patients in shock. Pulse contour analysis systems have also proven to be useful in monitoring trends in response to interventions. In addition, PCA systems do not require additional invasive procedures other than an arterial catheter, which is commonly used in patients with shock.

Despite these positive attributes, both ED and PCA systems do not provide a direct measure of tissue perfusion, which is, arguably, the most important variable to follow. Alternatively, gastric tonometry, and by extension sublingual capnometry, do not focus on the absolute cardiac output but instead measure indices of tissue perfusion. This quality, combined with their relatively noninvasive natures, makes these techniques perhaps the most appealing as replacements of thermodilution. The partial carbon dioxide rebreathing method and thoracic bioimpedance have not yet sufficiently demonstrated their applicability to the critically ill patient. Confounding clinical features such as ALI and pleural effusions are commonly found in this population and would likely impair the validity of existing systems. Finally, although BNP has not shown the ability to replace the PAC to date, there is some evidence that suggests that patients with a low BNP may not need one for diagnostic purposes.

It should be noted that, at present, use of any of these modalities must be performed with care. The majority of data available regarding these techniques have focused on comparing their accuracy with that of thermodilution. Very few studies have addressed patient outcomes. Ultimately, before definite recommendations can be made, further research focusing on clinical outcomes will be necessary.

FUTURE DIRECTIONS

As medical technology continues to advance at an explosive rate, it is easy to imagine that the practice of critical care medicine will completely change in the not-too-distant future. The next generation of intensivists and likely younger members of this generation may find themselves looking back with awe at the "archaic" methods of current practice. At present, there are many technologies that are still in their early stages of ICU practice but may one day provide useful clinical knowledge. A few of these deserve mention.

Magnetic resonance imaging (MRI) has become a common fixture in many large hospitals and is routinely used in a variety of clinical settings due to its improved accuracy over computed tomography in defining soft tissue structure. The role of MRI continues to expand as clinicians and researchers develop new ways to use its capabilities. One area in which MRI has shown particular promise is that of cardiac MRI. Although this technique is still being primarily used experimentally, early results have demonstrated its ability to assess both cardiac function as well as viability [136–138]. As more data become available, one can envision the possibility of more routine use of MRI to assess cardiac function. Additionally, advances in nuclear magnetic resonance spectroscopy have made it possible to estimate arterial oxygen supply ($\dot{D}o_2$) as well as skeletal muscle reoxygenation, mitochondrial ATP production, and oxygen consumption ($\dot{V}o_2$) [139]. Although cost and the technical difficulties of using MRI in critically ill patients may be prohibitive, there clearly exists potential in this arena.

Although traditional two-dimensional transthoracic echocardiography is certainly not a new technology, recently there has been new interest in this technique among intensivists. Echocardiography has historically fallen under the domain of cardiologists, who are formally trained to perform and interpret these useful studies. This technique can provide a wealth of information about systolic function, valvular dysfunction, and pericardial disease in critically ill patients [140]. More and more, noncardiology intensivists are now learning how to perform at least basic examinations to help quickly guide initial management decisions. For example, some bedside ultrasound devices used for central line placement, also have probes, which allow at least cursory examination of cardiac function (e.g., to exclude pericardial tamponade). However, the authors are aware of instances of erroneous information being gathered from such devices when used in untrained hands. Therefore, a more formal education in echocardiography would likely be beneficial for intensivists who do not have access to immediate echocardiography by a cardiologist.

Finally, emerging technology in combination with the completion of the human genome project will likely soon revolutionize critical care through the fields of proteomics and genomics. These techniques use mass spectroscopy and microarrays to isolate and compare which proteins and genes are preferentially expressed during different disease states. Through analysis of these proteins and genes, it may be possible to better understand the mechanisms behind diseases such as sepsis and ARDS and why some patients develop them and others do not. Additionally, because each person's pattern of gene expression is unique, it may one day be possible to tailor each patient's therapy according to what the genes suggest is the optimal treatment. Proteomics and genomics could, in theory, be used in the field of hemodynamic monitoring if it could be determined that specific proteins or genes are expressed in different types of shock. Ideally, a simple blood test could reveal a gene or protein expression pattern consistent with cardiogenic shock that would take the place of invasive measuring of cardiac output. Determining these expression patterns as well as refining the technique such that the information could be obtained in a timely manner will be important and challenging obstacles to overcome.

REFERENCES

1. Thomas JT, Kelly RF, Thomas SJ, et al: Utility of history, physical examination, electrocardiogram, and chest radiograph for differentiating normal from decreased systolic function in patients with heart failure. *Am J Med* 112:437, 2002.
2. Connors AF Jr, McCaffree DR, Gray BA: Evaluation of right-heart catheterization in the critically ill patient without acute myocardial infarction. *N Engl J Med* 308:263, 1983.

3. Swan HJ, Ganz W, Forrester J, et al: Catheterization of the heart in man with use of a flow-directed balloon-tipped catheter. *N Engl J Med* 283:447, 1970.
4. Iberti TJ, Fischer EP, Leibowitz AB, et al: A multicenter study of physicians' knowledge of the pulmonary artery catheter. Pulmonary Artery Catheter Study Group. *JAMA* 264:2928, 1990.
5. Richard C, Warszawski J, Anguel N, et al: Early use of the pulmonary artery catheter and outcomes in patients with shock and acute respiratory distress syndrome: a randomized controlled trial. *JAMA* 290:2713, 2003.
6. Gore JM, Goldberg RJ, Spodick DH, et al: A community-wide assessment of the use of pulmonary artery catheters in patients with acute myocardial infarction. *Chest* 92:721, 1987.
7. Connors AF Jr, Speroff T, Dawson NV, et al: The effectiveness of right heart catheterization in the initial care of critically ill patients. SUPPORT investigators. *JAMA* 276:889, 1996.
8. Binanay C, Califf RM, Hasselblad V, et al: Evaluation study of congestive heart failure and pulmonary artery catheterization effectiveness: the ESCAPE trial. *JAMA* 294:1625, 2005.
9. Gattinoni L, Brazzi L, Pelosi P, et al: A trial of goal-oriented hemodynamic therapy in critically ill patients. SvO2 collaborative group. *N Engl J Med* 333:1025, 1995.
10. Schwartz DR, Malhotra A, Fink M: Cytopathic hypoxia in sepsis: an overview. *Sepsis* 2:279, 1998.
11. Fink M: Cytopathic hypoxia in sepsis [review]. *Acta Anaesth Scand Suppl* 110:87, 1997.
12. Rivers E, Nguyen B, Havstad S, et al: Early goal-directed therapy in the treatment of severe sepsis and septic shock . *N Engl J Med* 345:1368, 2001.
13. Trzeciak S, Dellinger RPFCCP, Abate NL, et al: Translating research to clinical practice: a 1-year experience with implementing early goal-directed therapy for septic shock in the emergency department. *Chest* 129:225, 2006.
14. Rame JE, Dries DL, Drazner MH: The prognostic value of the physical examination in patients with chronic heart failure [review]. *Congest Heart Fail* 9:170, 2003.
15. Kaplan LJ, McPartland K, Santora TA, et al: Start with a subjective assessment of skin temperature to identify hypoperfusion in intensive care unit patients. *J Trauma* 50:620, 2001.
16. Joly HR, Weil MH: Temperature of the great toe as an indication of the severity of shock. *Circulation* 39:131, 1969.
17. Magder S, Georgiadis G, Tuck C: Respiratory variations in right atrial pressure predict response to fluid challenge. *J Crit Care* 7:76, 1992.
18. Magder S, Lagonidis D, Erice F: The use of respiratory variations in right atrial pressure to predict the cardiac output response to PEEP. *J Crit Care* 16:108, 2001.
19. Morris AH, Chapman RH, Gardner RM: Frequency of technical problems encountered in the measurement of pulmonary artery wedge pressure. *Crit Care Med* 12:164, 1984.
20. Marik P, Heard SO, Varon J: Interpretation of the pulmonary artery occlusion (wedge) pressure: physician's knowledge versus the experts' knowledge [comment]. *Crit Care Med* 26:1761, 1998.
21. Eisenberg PR, Jaffe AS, Schuster DP: Clinical evaluation compared to pulmonary artery catheterization in the hemodynamic assessment of critically ill patients. *Crit Care Med* 12:549, 1984.
22. Side CD, Gosling RG: Non-surgical assessment of cardiac function. *Nature* 232:335, 1971.
23. Singer M, Clarke J, Bennett ED: Continuous hemodynamic monitoring by esophageal doppler. *Crit Care Med* 17:447, 1989.
24. Cariou A, Monchi M, Joly LM, et al: Noninvasive cardiac output monitoring by aortic blood flow determination: evaluation of the sometec dynemo-3000 system. *Crit Care Med* 26:2066, 1998.
25. Singer M, Bennett ED: Noninvasive optimization of left ventricular filling using esophageal doppler. *Crit Care Med* 19:1132, 1991.
26. Wallmeyer K, Wann LS, Sagar KB, et al: The influence of preload and heart rate on Doppler echocardiographic indexes of left ventricular performance: comparison with invasive indexes in an experimental preparation. *Circulation* 74:181, 1986.
27. Singer M, Allen MJ, Webb AR, et al: Effects of alterations in left ventricular filling, contractility, and systemic vascular resistance on the ascending aortic blood velocity waveform of normal subjects. *Crit Care Med* 19:1138, 1991.
28. Sharma J, Bhise M, Singh A, et al: Hemodynamic measurements after cardiac surgery: transesophageal Doppler versus pulmonary artery catheter. *J Cardiothorac Vasc Anesth* 19:746, 2005.
29. Dark PM, Singer M: The validity of trans-esophageal doppler ultrasonography as a measure of cardiac output in critically ill adults [review]. *Intensive Care Med* 30:2060, 2004.
30. Kim K, Kwok I, Chang H, et al: Comparison of cardiac outputs of major burn patients undergoing extensive early escharectomy: esophageal Doppler monitor versus thermodilution pulmonary artery catheter. *J Trauma* 57:1013, 2004.
31. Roeck M, Jakob SM, Boehlen T, et al: Change in SV in response to fluid challenge: assessment using esophageal Doppler. *Intensive Care Med* 29:1729, 2003.
32. Bland JM, Altman DG: Statistical methods for assessing agreement between two methods of clinical measurement. *Lancet* 1:307, 1986.
33. Singer M: Esophageal Doppler monitoring of aortic blood flow: beat-by-beat cardiac output monitoring [review]. *Int Anesthesiol Clin* 31:99, 1993.
34. Valtier B, Cholley BP, Belot JP, et al: Noninvasive monitoring of cardiac output in critically ill patients using transesophageal Doppler. *Am J Respir Crit Care Med* 158:77, 1998.
35. Gan TJ, Arrowsmith JE: The oesophageal Doppler monitor [comment]. *BMJ* 315:893, 1997.
36. Lefrant JY, Bruelle P, Aya AG, et al: Training is required to improve the reliability of esophageal Doppler to measure cardiac output in critically ill patients. *Intensive Care Med* 24:347, 1998.
37. Sinclair S, James S, Singer M: Intraoperative intravascular volume optimisation and length of hospital stay after repair of proximal femoral fracture: randomised controlled trial. *BMJ* 315:909, 1997.
38. Frank O: Wellen- und windkesselthrorie [estimation of the stroke volume of the human heart using the "windkessel" theory]. *Zeitschr Biol* 90:405, 1930.
39. Wesseling KH, de Wit B, Weber JAP, et al: A simple device for the continuous measurement of cardiac output. *Adv Cardiovasc Phys* 5:16, 1983.
40. Pinsky MR: Probing the limits of arterial pulse contour analysis to predict preload responsiveness [comment]. *Anesth Analg* 96:1245, 2003.
41. Della Rocca G, Costa MG, Pompei L, et al: Continuous and intermittent cardiac output measurement: pulmonary artery catheter versus aortic transpulmonary technique. *Br J Anaesth* 88:350, 2002.
42. Della Rocca G, Costa MG, Coccia C, et al: Cardiac output monitoring: aortic transpulmonary thermodilution and pulse contour analysis agree with standard thermodilution methods in patients undergoing lung transplantation. *Can J Anaesth* 50:707, 2003.
43. Godje O, Hoke K, Goetz AE, et al: Reliability of a new algorithm for continuous cardiac output determination by pulse-contour analysis during hemodynamic instability. *Crit Care Med* 30:52, 2002.
44. Mielck F, Buhre W, Hanekop G, et al: Comparison of continuous cardiac output measurements in patients after cardiac surgery. *J Cardiothorac Vasc Anesth* 17:211, 2003.
45. Rauch H, Muller M, Fleischer F, et al: Pulse contour analysis versus thermodilution in cardiac surgery patients. *Acta Anaesthesiol Scand* 46:424, 2002.
46. Felbinger TW, Reuter DA, Eltzschig HK, et al: Cardiac index measurements during rapid preload changes: a comparison of pulmonary artery thermodilution with arterial pulse contour analysis. *J Clin Anesth* 17:241, 2005.
47. Gunn SR, Pinsky MR: Implications of arterial pressure variation in patients in the intensive care unit [review]. *Curr Opin Crit Care* 7:212, 2001.
48. Michard F, Teboul JL: Using heart-lung interactions to assess fluid responsiveness during mechanical ventilation [review]. *Crit Care* 4:282, 2000.
49. Michard F, Teboul JL: Predicting fluid responsiveness in ICU patients: a critical analysis of the evidence [review]. *Chest* 121:2000, 2002.
50. Reuter DA, Felbinger TW, Schmidt C, et al: Stroke volume variations for assessment of cardiac responsiveness to volume loading in mechanically ventilated patients after cardiac surgery. *Intensive Care Med* 28:392, 2002.
51. Wiesenack C, Prasser C, Rodig G, et al: Stroke volume variation as an indicator of fluid responsiveness using pulse contour analysis in mechanically ventilated patients. *Anesth Analg* 96:1254, 2003.
52. Goedje O, Hoeke K, Lichtwarck-Aschoff M, et al: Continuous cardiac output by femoral arterial thermodilution calibrated pulse contour analysis: comparison with pulmonary arterial thermodilution. *Crit Care Med* 27:2407, 1999.
53. Rodig G, Prasser C, Keyl C, et al: Continuous cardiac output measurement: pulse contour analysis vs thermodilution technique in cardiac surgical patients. *Br J Anaesth* 82:525, 1999.
54. Ultman JS, Bursztein S: Analysis of error in the determination of respiratory gas exchange at varying FIO_2. *J Appl Physiol* 50:210, 1981.
55. Mahutte CK, Jaffe MB, Sassoon CS, et al: Cardiac output from carbon dioxide production and arterial and venous oximetry. *Crit Care Med* 19:1270, 1991.
56. Mahutte CK, Jaffe MB, Chen PA, et al: Oxygen fick and modified carbon dioxide fick cardiac outputs. *Crit Care Med* 22:86, 1994.
57. Lynch J, Kaemmerer H: Comparison of a modified fick method with thermodilution for determining cardiac output in critically ill patients on mechanical ventilation. *Intensive Care Med* 16:248, 1990.
58. Berton C, Cholley B: Equipment review: new techniques for cardiac output measurement–oesophageal Doppler, fick principle using carbon dioxide, and pulse contour analysis [review]. *Crit Care* 6:216, 2002.
59. Murias GE, Villagra A, Vatua S, et al: Evaluation of a noninvasive method for cardiac output measurement in critical care patients. *Intensive Care Med* 28:1470, 2002.
60. Gedeon A, Forslund L, Hedenstierna G, et al: A new method for noninvasive bedside determination of pulmonary blood flow. *Med Biol Eng Comput* 18:411, 1980.
61. Benatar SR, Hewlett AM, Nunn JF: The use of iso-shunt lines for control of oxygen therapy. *Br J Anaesth* 45:711, 1973.
62. Neviere R, Mathieu D, Riou Y, et al: Carbon dioxide rebreathing method of cardiac output measurement during acute respiratory failure in patients with chronic obstructive pulmonary disease. *Crit Care Med* 22:81, 1994.
63. Odenstedt H, Stenqvist O, Lundin S. Clinical evaluation of a partial CO_2 rebreathing technique for cardiac output monitoring in critically ill patients. *Acta Anaesthesiol Scand* 46:152, 2002.
64. Binder JC, Parkin WG: Non-invasive cardiac output determination: comparison of a new partial-rebreathing technique with thermodilution. *Anaesth Intensive Care* 29:19, 2001.
65. Botero M, Kirby D, Lobato EB, et al: Measurement of cardiac output before and after cardiopulmonary bypass: comparison among aortic transit-time ultrasound, thermodilution, and noninvasive partial CO_2 rebreathing. *J Cardiothorac Vasc Anesth* 18:563, 2004.
66. Nilsson LB, Eldrup N, Berthelsen PG: Lack of agreement between thermodilution and carbon dioxide-rebreathing cardiac output. *Acta Anaesthesiol Scand* 45:680, 2001.
67. Hachenberg T, Tenling A, Nystrom SO, et al: Ventilation-perfusion inequality in patients undergoing cardiac surgery. *Anesthesiology* 80:509, 1994.
68. de Abreu MG, Quintel M, Ragaller M, et al: Partial carbon dioxide rebreathing: a reliable technique for noninvasive measurement of nonshunted pulmonary capillary blood flow. *Crit Care Med* 25:675, 1997.
69. Valiatti JL, Amaral JL: Comparison between cardiac output values measured by thermodilution and partial carbon dioxide rebreathing in patients with acute lung injury. *Sao Paulo Med J* 122:233, 2004.
70. Tachibana K, Imanaka H, Takeuchi M, et al: Noninvasive cardiac output measurement using partial carbon dioxide rebreathing is less accurate at settings of reduced minute ventilation and when spontaneous breathing is present. *Anesthesiology* 98:830, 2003.
71. Kubicek WG, Karnegis JN, Patterson RP, et al: Development and evaluation of an impedance cardiac output system. *Aerosp Med* 37:1208, 1966.

72. Sramek BB: Cardiac output by electrical impedance. *Med Electron* 13:93, 1982.
73. Penney BC: Theory and cardiac applications of electrical impedance measurements. [review]. *Crit Rev Biomed Eng* 13:227, 1986.
74. Barin E, Haryadi DG, Schookin SI, et al: Evaluation of a thoracic bioimpedance cardiac output monitor during cardiac catheterization. *Crit Care Med* 28:698, 2000.
75. Raaijmakers E, Faes TJ, Scholten RJ, et al: A meta-analysis of three decades of validating thoracic impedance cardiography. *Crit Care Med* 27:1203, 1999.
76. Genoni M, Pelosi P, Romand JA, et al: Determination of cardiac output during mechanical ventilation by electrical bioimpedance or thermodilution in patients with acute lung injury: effects of positive end-expiratory pressure. *Crit Care Med* 26:1441, 1998.
77. Shoemaker WC, Belzberg H, Wo CC, et al: Multicenter study of noninvasive monitoring systems as alternatives to invasive monitoring of acutely ill emergency patients. *Chest* 114:1643, 1998.
78. Sageman WS, Amundson DE: Thoracic electrical bioimpedance measurement of cardiac output in postaortocoronary bypass patients. *Crit Care Med* 21:1139, 1993.
79. Brown CV, Martin MJ, Shoemaker WC, et al: The effect of obesity on bioimpedance cardiac index. *Am J Surg* 189:547, 2005.
80. Cason CL, DeSalvo SK, Ray WT: Changes in oxygen saturation during weaning from short-term ventilator support after coronary artery bypass graft surgery. *Heart Lung* 23:368, 1994.
81. Magilligan DJ Jr, Teasdall R, et al: Mixed venous oxygen saturation as a predictor of cardiac output in the postoperative cardiac surgical patient. *Ann Thorac Surg* 44:260, 1987.
82. Pearson KS, Gomez MN, Moyers JR, et al: A cost/benefit analysis of randomized invasive monitoring for patients undergoing cardiac surgery. *Anesth Analg* 69:336, 1989.
83. Lee J, Wright F, Barber R, et al: Central venous oxygen saturation in shock: a study in man. *Anesthesiology* 36:472, 1972.
84. Reinhart K, Rudolph T, Bredle DL, et al: Comparison of central-venous to mixed-venous oxygen saturation during changes in oxygen supply/demand. *Chest* 95:1216, 1989.
85. Levy B, Gawalkiewicz P, Vallet B, et al: Gastric capnometry with air-automated tonometry predicts outcome in critically ill patients. *Crit Care Med* 31:474, 2003.
86. Fink MP: Tissue capnometry as a monitoring strategy for critically ill patients: just about ready for prime time. *Chest* 114:667, 1998.
87. Sato Y, Weil MH, Tang W: Tissue hypercarbic acidosis as a marker of acute circulatory failure (shock) [review]. *Chest* 114:263, 1998.
88. Marik P: Gastric tonometry: the canary sings once again. *Crit Care Med* 26:809, 1998.
89. Krebs HA, Woods HF, Alberti KGMM: Hyperlactataemia and lactic acidosis. *Essays Biochem* 1:81, 1970.
90. Neviere R, Chagnon JL, Teboul JL, et al: Small intestine intramucosal PCO(2) and microvascular blood flow during hypoxic and ischemic hypoxia. *Crit Care Med* 30:379, 2002.
91. Fiddian-Green RG, Baker S: Predictive value of the stomach wall pH for complications after cardiac operations: comparison with other monitoring. *Crit Care Med* 15:153, 1987.
92. Graf J, Konigs B, Mottaghy K, et al: In vitro validation of gastric air tonometry using perfluorocarbon FC 43 and 0.9% sodium chloride. *Br J Anaesth* 84:497, 2000.
93. Barry B, Mallick A, Hartley G, et al: Comparison of air tonometry with gastric tonometry using saline and other equilibrating fluids: an in vivo and in vitro study. *Intensive Care Med* 24:777, 1998.
94. Tzelepis G, Kadas V, Michalopoulos A, et al: Comparison of gastric air tonometry with standard saline tonometry. *Intensive Care Med* 22:1239, 1996.
95. Schlichtig R, Mehta N, Gayowski TJ: Tissue-arterial PCO$_2$ difference is a better marker of ischemia than intramural pH (pHi) or arterial pH-pHi difference. *J Crit Care* 11:51, 1996.
96. Silva E, De Backer D, Creteur J, et al: Effects of fluid challenge on gastric mucosal PCO$_2$ in septic patients. *Intensive Care Med* 30:423, 2004.
97. Gutierrez G, Palizas F, Doglio G, et al: Gastric intramucosal pH as a therapeutic index of tissue oxygenation in critically ill patients. *Lancet.* 339:195, 1992.
98. Barquist E, Kirton O, Windsor J, et al: The impact of antioxidant and splanchnic-directed therapy on persistent uncorrected gastric mucosal pH in the critically injured trauma patient. *J Trauma* 44:355, 1998.
99. Ivatury RR, Simon RJ, Islam S, et al: A prospective randomized study of end points of resuscitation after major trauma: global oxygen transport indices versus organ-specific gastric mucosal pH. *J Am Coll Surg* 183:145, 1996.
100. Gomersall CD, Joynt GM, Freebairn RC, et al: Resuscitation of critically ill patients based on the results of gastric tonometry: a prospective, randomized, controlled trial. *Crit Care Med* 28:607, 2000.
101. Heard SO: Gastric tonometry: the hemodynamic monitor of choice (pro). *Chest* 123[5 Suppl]:469S, 2003.
102. Maynard N, Bihari D, Beale R, et al: Assessment of splanchnic oxygenation by gastric tonometry in patients with acute circulatory failure. *JAMA* 270:1203, 1993.
103. Mohsenifar Z, Hay A, Hay J, et al: Gastric intramural pH as a predictor of success or failure in weaning patients from mechanical ventilation. *Ann Intern Med* 119:794, 1993.
104. Bouachour G, Guiraud MP, Gouello JP, et al: Gastric intramucosal pH: an indicator of weaning outcome from mechanical ventilation in COPD patients. *Eur Respir J* 9:1868, 1996.
105. Bocquillon N, Mathieu D, Neviere R, et al: Gastric mucosal pH and blood flow during weaning from mechanical ventilation in patients with chronic obstructive pulmonary disease. *Am J Respir Crit Care Med* 160[5 Pt 1]:1555, 1999.
106. Hurtado FJ, Beron M, Olivera W, et al: Gastric intramucosal pH and intraluminal Pco$_2$ during weaning from mechanical ventilation. *Crit Care Med* 29:70, 2001.
107. Uusaro A, Lahtinen P, Parviainen I, et al: Gastric mucosal end-tidal Pco$_2$ difference as a continuous indicator of splanchnic perfusion. *Br J Anaesth* 85:563, 2000.
108. Boyd O, Mackay CJ, Lamb G, et al: Comparison of clinical information gained from routine blood-gas analysis and from gastric tonometry for intramural pH. *Lancet* 341:142, 1993.
109. Totapally BR, Fakioglu H, Torbati D, et al: Esophageal capnometry during hemorrhagic shock and after resuscitation in rats. *Crit Care* 7:79, 2003.
110. Sato Y, Weil MH, Tang W, et al: Esophageal Pco$_2$ as a monitor of perfusion failure during hemorrhagic shock. *J Appl Physiol* 82:558, 1997.
111. Jin X, Weil MH, Sun S, et al: Decreases in organ blood flows associated with increases in sublingual Pco$_2$ during hemorrhagic shock. *J Appl Physiol* 85:2360, 1998.
112. Nakagawa Y, Weil MH, Tang W, et al: Sublingual capnometry for diagnosis and quantitation of circulatory shock. *Am J Respir Crit Care Med* 157[6 Pt 1]:1838, 1998.
113. Povoas HP, Weil MH, Tang W, et al: Comparisons between sublingual and gastric tonometry during hemorrhagic shock. *Chest* 118:1127, 2000.
114. Maciel AT, Creteur J, Vincent JL: Tissue capnometry: does the answer lie under the tongue?. *Intensive Care Med* 30:2157, 2004.
115. Marik PE: Sublingual capnography: a clinical validation study. *Chest* 120:923, 2001.
116. Marik PE, Bankov A: Sublingual capnometry versus traditional markers of tissue oxygenation in critically ill patients. *Crit Care Med* 31:818, 2003.
117. Weil MH, Nakagawa Y, Tang W, et al: Sublingual capnometry: a new noninvasive measurement for diagnosis and quantitation of severity of circulatory shock. *Crit Care Med* 27:1225, 1999.
118. Price S, Anning PB, Mitchell JA, et al: Myocardial dysfunction in sepsis: Mechanisms and therapeutic implications [review]. *Eur Heart J* 20:715, 1999.
119. Scire CA, Caporali R, Perotti C, et al: Plasma procalcitonin in rheumatic diseases [review]. *Reumatismo* 55:113, 2003.
120. Gerhardt W, Katus H, Ravkilde J, et al: S-troponin T in suspected ischemic myocardial injury compared with mass and catalytic concentrations of S-creatine kinase isoenzyme MB. *Clin Chem* 37:1405, 1991.
121. Katus HA, Remppis A, Neumann FJ, et al: Diagnostic efficiency of troponin T measurements in acute myocardial infarction. *Circulation* 83:902, 1991.
122. Parrillo JE. Myocardial depression during septic shock in humans. *Crit Care Med* 18:1183, 1990.
123. Fernandes CJ Jr, Iervolino M, Neves RA, et al: Interstitial myocarditis in sepsis. *Am J Cardiol* 74:958, 1994.
124. Piper RD: Myocardial dysfunction in sepsis [review]. *Clin Exp Pharmacol Physiol* 25:951, 1998.
125. Ammann P, Fehr T, Minder EI, et al: Elevation of troponin I in sepsis and septic shock. *Intensive Care Med* 27:965, 2001.
126. Spies C, Haude V, Fitzner R, et al: Serum cardiac troponin T as a prognostic marker in early sepsis. *Chest* 113:1055, 1998.
127. Omland T, Aakvaag A, Bonarjee VV, et al: Plasma brain natriuretic peptide as an indicator of left ventricular systolic function and long-term survival after acute myocardial infarction. Comparison with plasma atrial natriuretic peptide and N-terminal proatrial natriuretic peptide. *Circulation* 93:1963, 1996.
128. Krishnaswamy P, Lubien E, Clopton P, et al: Utility of B-natriuretic peptide levels in identifying patients with left ventricular systolic or diastolic dysfunction. *Am J Med* 111:274, 2001.
129. Maisel AS, Koon J, Krishnaswamy P, et al: Utility of B-natriuretic peptide as a rapid, point-of-care test for screening patients undergoing echocardiography to determine left ventricular dysfunction. *Am Heart J* 141:367, 2001.
130. Maisel AS, Krishnaswamy P, Nowak RM, et al: Rapid measurement of B-type natriuretic peptide in the emergency diagnosis of heart failure. *N Engl J Med* 347:161, 2002.
131. Vasan RS, Benjamin EJ, Larson MG, et al: Plasma natriuretic peptides for community screening for left ventricular hypertrophy and systolic dysfunction: te Framingham Heart Study. *JAMA* 288:1252, 2002.
132. Kazanegra R, Cheng V, Garcia A, et al: A rapid test for B-type natriuretic peptide correlates with falling wedge pressures in patients treated for decompensated heart failure: a pilot study. *J Card Fail* 7:21, 2001.
133. Park MH, Scott RL, Uber PA, et al: Usefulness of B-type natriuretic peptide levels in predicting hemodynamic perturbations after heart transplantation despite preserved left ventricular systolic function. *Am J Cardiol* 90:1326, 2002.
134. Tung RH, Garcia C, Morss AM, et al: Utility of B-type natriuretic peptide for the evaluation of intensive care unit shock. *Crit Care Med* 32:1643, 2004.
135. Brueckmann M, Huhle G, Lang S, et al: Prognostic value of plasma N-terminal pro-brain natriuretic peptide in patients with severe sepsis. *Circulation* 112:527, 2005.
136. Lee VS, Resnick D, Tiu SS, et al: MR imaging evaluation of myocardial viability in the setting of equivocal SPECT results with (99m)TC sestamibi. *Radiology* 230:191, 2004.
137. Chiu CW, So NM, Lam WW, et al: Combined first-pass perfusion and viability study at MR imaging in patients with non-ST segment-elevation acute coronary syndromes: feasibility study. *Radiology* 226:717, 2003.
138. Kitagawa K, Sakuma H, Hirano T, et al: Acute myocardial infarction: myocardial viability assessment in patients early thereafter comparison of contrast-enhanced MR imaging with resting (201)tl SPECT. Single photon emission computed tomography. *Radiology* 226:138, 2003.
139. Carlier PG, Brillault-Salvat C, Giacomini E, et al: How to investigate oxygen supply, uptake, and utilization simultaneously by interleaved NMR imaging and spectroscopy of the skeletal muscle. *Magn Reson Med* 54:1010, 2005.
140. Price S, Nicol E, Gibson DG, et al: Echocardiography in the critically ill: current and potential roles. *Intensive Care Med* 32:48, 2006.

Eric A. Bedell
Donald S. Prough

CHAPTER **30**

Neurologic and Intracranial Pressure Monitoring

Options for evaluating and monitoring neurologic function have increased steadily in the past 10 years and provide the clinician a wide array of tools for the evaluation of the critically ill patient with neurologic diseases such as traumatic brain injury (TBI), subarachnoid hemorrhage (SAH), stroke, and encephalopathy. These include intracranial pressure (ICP) monitoring, electrophysiologic monitoring, and brain oxygenation monitoring.

The basic requirements and limitations of physiologic monitoring—both neurologic and nonneurologic—are unchanged and require the end-user to balance the risks of a monitoring technique against any benefits (whether proven or inferred) that are conferred by the information gathered. Important characteristics of monitoring devices include the ability to detect important abnormalities (sensitivity), to differentiate between dissimilar disease states (specificity), and to prompt changes in care that alter long-term prognosis (Table 30-1). Limitations of techniques include risks to patients (during placement, use, and removal), variability errors in generation of data (e.g., calibration and drift), and inherent trade-offs between specificity and sensitivity. Monitors with high specificity—values fall outside of threshold levels only when a disease state is unequivocally present—are unlikely to detect less profound levels of disease, while monitors with high sensitivity (will detect any value outside of the normal range) are likely to demonstrate small deviations from normal that may be trivial in individual patients. Therefore, clinicians who rely on monitoring devices must understand those devices, with their potential value and limitations, and correctly apply and interpret the monitored data within the context of individual patients. In addition, clinicians must understand integration of multiple techniques to improve sensitivity and specificity of monitoring brain function—this is the concept of "multimodal monitoring." The theoretical importance of brain monitoring is based on the high vulnerability of the brain to hypoxic and ischemic injuries. The brain uses more oxygen and glucose per weight of tissue than any large organ, yet has no appreciable reserves of oxygen or glucose. The brain is thus completely dependent on uninterrupted cerebral blood flow (CBF) to supply metabolic substrates that are required for continued function and survival and to remove toxic by-products. Even transient interruptions in CBF, whether local or global, can injure or kill neural cells. These perturbations may not result in immediate cell death, but can initiate metabolic or cellular processes (e.g., gene transcription) that may lead to cell

death days, months, or years after the insult. Therefore, clinical monitoring of neuronal well-being should emphasize early detection and reversal of potentially harmful conditions. Although there is limited conclusive data to demonstrate that morbidity and mortality are reduced by the information gathered from current neurologic monitoring techniques, most clinicians caring for patients with critical neurologic illness have confidence that their use improves management. In this chapter, we will review currently available techniques with emphasis on current scientific literature and indications for utilization.

GOALS OF BRAIN MONITORING

Monitoring devices cannot independently improve outcome. Instead, they contribute physiologic data that can be integrated into a care plan that, while frequently adding risks (associated with placement, use, and removal), may lead to an overall decrease in morbidity and mortality. The risks inherent in the monitoring technique cannot be overemphasized and must be individualized to the patients' conditions and acuity. Neurologic monitoring falls into two general categories: qualitative measurements (e.g., Glasgow Coma Scale [GCS] scoring, cranial nerve testing, electroencephalographic [EEG], and evoked-potential [EP] monitoring) and quantitative/semiquantitative monitors (e.g., ICP, transcranial Doppler ultrasonography, jugular bulb venous oxygen saturation [$SjvO_2$], brain tissue oxygen tension [$PbtO_2$], and brain microdialysis). Qualitative monitoring provides information as to the integrated functioning of the brain/nervous system, whereas quantitative monitoring provides specific measurements that may be useful in directing specific therapeutic interventions and gauging therapeutic effectiveness.

Nonneurologic examples of qualitative and quantitative monitors include, respectively, peripheral nerve stimulation for assessing neuromuscular blockade and continuous electrocardiography (ECG). Peripheral nerve stimulation assesses the qualitative function of the neuromuscular junction by depolarizing a peripheral nerve and evaluating the muscle response. It provides information about overall function, but does not uniquely identify or quantify the nature of abnormalities. Continuous ECG provides specific and quantitative information about heart rate and rhythm and facilitates evaluation of interventions, such as beta-blocker administration for the treatment of sinus tachycardia, but does not provide information about the adequacy of

TABLE 30-1. Glossary of Neurologic Monitor Characteristics

Term	Definition
Bias	Average difference (positive or negative) between monitored values and "gold standard" values
Precision	Standard deviation of the differences (bias) between measurements
Sensitivity	Probability that the monitor will demonstrate cerebral ischemia when cerebral ischemia is present
Positive predictive value	Probability that cerebral ischemia is present when the monitor suggests cerebral ischemia
Specificity	Probability that the monitor will not demonstrate cerebral ischemia when cerebral ischemia is not present
Negative predictive value	Probability that cerebral ischemia is not present when the monitor reflects no cerebral ischemia
Threshold value	The value used to separate acceptable (i.e., no ischemia present) from unacceptable (i.e., ischemia present)
Speed	The time elapsed from the onset of actual ischemia or the risk of ischemia until the monitor provides evidence

cardiac function with respect to systemic needs. For each example, the limitations of the devices are well known and information should only be interpreted within that context. Failure to appreciate these limitations can interfere with patient management. Indeed, few clinicians would assess cardiac well-being based only on the ECG. In the same way, care must be taken when applying information gathered from neurologic monitoring.

CEREBRAL ISCHEMIA

Virtually all neurologic monitors detect actual or possible cerebral hypoxia/ischemia, defined as cerebral delivery of oxygen (CDO_2) insufficient to meet metabolic needs. Cerebral ischemia is traditionally characterized as global or focal, and complete or incomplete (Table 30-2). Systemic monitors readily detect most global cerebral insults, such as hypotension, hypoxemia, or cardiac arrest. Therefore, brain-specific monitors can provide additional information primarily in situations, such as stroke, SAH with vasospasm, and TBI, in which systemic oxygenation and perfusion appear to be adequate but focal cerebral oxygenation may be impaired.

The severity of ischemic brain damage has traditionally been thought to be proportional to the magnitude and duration of reduced CDO_2. For monitoring to influence long-term patient morbidity and mortality, prompt recognition of reversible cerebral hypoxia/ischemia is essential. In monkeys, potentially re-

TABLE 30-2. Characteristics of Types of Cerebral Ischemic Insults

Characteristics	Examples
Global, incomplete	Hypotension, hypoxemia, cardiopulmonary resuscitation
Global, complete	Cardiac arrest
Focal, incomplete	Stroke, subarachnoid hemorrhage with vasospasm

versible paralysis develops if regional CBF declines below about 23 mL per 100 g per minute; whereas infarction of brain tissue generally requires that CBF remain below 18 mL per 100 g per minute [1]. More recently, similar results were demonstrated in humans with TBI [2]. The tolerable duration of more profound ischemia is inversely proportional to the severity of CBF reduction (Fig. 30-1). More recent studies have demonstrated the importance of protein synthesis, enzymatic function, and gene expression resulting from hypoxia/ischemia, and the development of cellular dysfunction or death from different types and levels of cellular stress. Alterations in gene expression occur following periods of neurologic stress and may influence long-term neurologic function [3], for instance, the production of inflammatory mediators in response to stress [4] may contribute to neuronal injury and death. Other proteins synthesized in response to altered oxygen delivery, such as hypoxia inducible factors (HIF), have been identified as adaptive mechanisms that respond to variations in oxygen partial pressure [5] and may be protective. This interaction between protein synthesis/gene expression, inducible protective mechanisms, and long-term outcome after hypoxia/ischemia is an area of potential monitoring and therapeutic intervention. When a cerebral monitor detects ischemia, the results must be carefully interpreted. Often, all that is known is that cerebral oxygenation in the region of brain that is assessed by that monitor has fallen below a critical threshold. Such information does not specifically imply that ischemia will necessarily progress to infarction, nor does it clearly define what biochemical or genetic transcriptional changes may subsequently occur. Also, because more severe ischemia produces neurologic injury more quickly

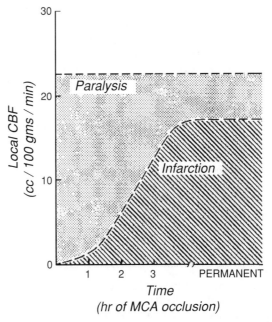

FIGURE 30-1. Schematic representation of ischemic thresholds in awake monkeys. The threshold for reversible paralysis occurs at local cerebral blood flow (Local CBF) of approximately 23 mL per 100 m per minute. Irreversible injury (infarction) is a function of the magnitude of blood flow reduction and the duration of that reduction. Relatively severe ischemia is potentially reversible if the duration is sufficiently short. [From Jones TH, Morawetz RB, Crowell RM, et al: Thresholds of focal cerebral ischemia in awake monkeys. *J Neurosurg* 54:773–782, 1981, with permission.]

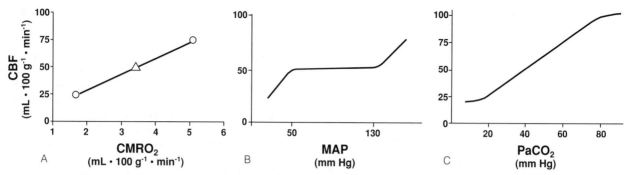

FIGURE 30-2. **A:** The normal relationship between the cerebral metabolic rate of oxygen consumption ($CMRO_2$) and cerebral blood flow (CBF) is characterized by closely couple changes in both variables. Normally, CBF is 50 mL per 100 g per minute in adults (*open triangle*). As $CMRO_2$ increases of decreases, CBF changes in a parallel fashion (*solid line*). **B:** Effect of mean arterial pressure (MAP) on CBF. Note that changes in MAP produce little change in CBF over a broad range of pressures. If intracranial pressure (ICP) exceeds normal limits, substitute cerebral perfusion pressure on the horizontal axis. **C:** Effect of $PaCO_2$ on CBF. Changes in $PaCO_2$ exert powerful effects on cerebral vascular resistance across the entire clinically applicable range of values.

than less severe ischemia, time and dose effects must be considered. Therefore, it is impossible to use a threshold monitor (i.e., one that becomes abnormal with mild cerebral ischemia) to predict with certainty whether changes in neurologic function will be followed by irreversible cerebral injury. More important, if regional ischemia involves structures that are not components of the monitored variable, then infarction could develop without warning.

In healthy persons, CBF is tightly regulated through multiple pathways such that CDO_2 is adjusted to meet the metabolic requirements of the brain. In the normal, "coupled" relationship, CBF is dependent on the cerebral metabolic rate for oxygen ($CMRO_2$), which varies directly with body temperature and with the level of brain activation (Fig. 30-2A). As $CMRO_2$ increases or decreases, CBF increases or decreases to match oxygen requirements with oxygen delivery. Pressure autoregulation maintains CBF at a constant rate (assuming unchanged metabolic needs) over a wide range of systemic blood pressures (Fig. 30-2B). If pressure autoregulation is intact, changes of cerebral perfusion pressure (CPP) do not alter CBF over a range of pressures of 50 to 130 mm Hg [6]. CPP can be described by the equation CPP = MAP – ICP, where MAP equals mean arterial pressure. After neurologic insults (e.g., TBI), autoregulation of the cerebral vasculature may be impaired such that CBF may not increase sufficiently in response to decreasing CPP [7–9]. This failure to maintain adequate CDO_2 can lead to ischemia and add to preexisting brain injury, a process termed secondary injury, at blood pressures that would not normally be associated with cerebral ischemia/injury. Normally, arterial partial pressure of carbon dioxide, ($PaCO_2$) significantly regulates cerebral vascular resistance over a range of $PaCO_2$ of 20 to 80 mm Hg (Fig. 30-2C). CBF is acutely halved if $PaCO_2$ is halved, and doubled if $PaCO_2$ is doubled. This reduction in CBF (via arteriolar vasoconstriction) results in a decrease in cerebral blood volume and a decrease in ICP. Conceptually, decreasing $PaCO_2$ to decrease ICP may appear to be desirable. Hyperventilation as a clinical tool was described by Lundberg et al. [10] in 1959 as a treatment for increased ICP, and was a mainstay of treatment for over 40 years. However, in healthy brain, there are limits to maximal cerebral vasoconstriction with falling $PaCO_2$ (as well as vasodilation with

increasing $PaCO_2$), such that, as CBF decreases to the point of producing inadequate CDO_2, local vasodilatory mechanisms tend restore CBF and CDO_2. As a consequence, in healthy brain, hyperventilation does not produce severe cerebral ischemia; however, after TBI, hypocapnia can generate cerebral ischemia as reflected in decreased $PbtO_2$ and $SjvO_2$ [11–14]. Thus, one indication for cerebral oxygenation monitoring includes the decision to use therapeutic hyperventilation in treatment of TBI, in which case monitoring data can be used to determine the endpoint of hyperventilation [15,16]. If hyperventilation is required to acutely reduce ICP, administration of an increased inspired oxygen concentration can markedly increase $SjvO_2$ (Fig. 30-3) [16]. In response to decreasing arterial oxygen content (CaO_2), whether the reduction is secondary to a decrease of hemoglobin (Hgb) concentration or of arterial oxygen saturation (SaO_2), CBF normally increases, although injured brain tissue has impaired ability to increase CBF [17,18].

TECHNIQUES OF NEUROLOGIC MONITORING

NEUROLOGIC EXAMINATION

Frequent and accurately recorded neurologic examinations remain an important aspect of medical care, but are of limited utility in patients with moderate to severe neurologic compromise. Neurologic examination quantifies three key characteristics: level of consciousness, focal brain dysfunction, and trends in neurologic function. Recognition of changing consciousness may warn of a variety of treatable conditions, such as progression of intracranial hypertension, and systemic complications of intracranial pathology, such as hyponatremia.

The GCS score, originally developed as a tool for the assessment of impaired consciousness [19], has also been used as a prognostic tool for patients with TBI [20]. The GCS score at the time of initial hospitalization is used to characterize the severity of TBI, with severe TBI defined as a GCS score less than or equal to 8, moderate TBI as a GCS score of 9 to 12, and mild TBI as that associated with a GCS score greater than 12 [21]. Lower GCS scores are generally associated with poorer long-term outcomes

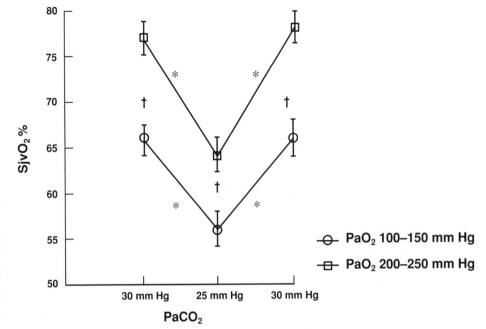

FIGURE 30-3. The effect of hyperoxia on percentage of oxygen saturation of jugular venous blood ($SjvO_2$) at two levels of $PaCO_2$. *P <0.001 for $SjvO_2$ at $PaCO_2$ 25–30 mm Hg at each PaO_2. †P <0.001 for $SjvO_2$ between PaO_2 at each $PaCO_2$ level. [From Thiagarajan A, Goverdhan PD, Chari P, et al: The effect of hyperventilation and hyperoxia on cerebral venous oxygen saturation in patients with traumatic brain injury. *Anesth Analg* 87:850–853, 1998, with permission.]

[11], although correlation to individual patients with TBI is difficult because of the significant variations in mortality rates and functional outcome [22], and some have recommended that its use as a prognostic tool is no longer warranted in TBI [23]. The GCS score is popular as a quick, reproducible estimate of level of consciousness (Table 30-3), has become a common tool for the serial monitoring of consciousness, and has been incorporated into various outcome models, such as the Trauma score, APACHE II, and the Trauma-Injury Severity score. The GCS score, which includes eye opening, motor responses in the best functioning limb, and verbal responses, should be supplemented by recording pupillary size and reactivity and the presence of other abnormal neurologic findings. Even so, the use of serial GCS determinations remains a common tool in the management of patients with neurologic dysfunction.

SYSTEMIC MONITORING

Although not specific to neurologic monitoring, systemic parameters, including blood pressure, arterial oxygen saturation (SaO_2), $PaCO_2$, serum glucose concentration, and temperature, have clinical relevance in the management of patients with neurologic dysfunction or injury. The relationships between these systemic variables and long-term outcome after neurologic insults are closely linked and are subject to continuing research.

Perhaps the most important systemic monitor is blood pressure, as CBF is dependent on the relationship between CPP and cerebral vascular resistance (CVR), and can be modeled generally by the equation: CBF = CPP/CVR. As previously discussed, CBF is maintained relatively constant over a wide range of blood pressures (pressure autoregulation) through arteriolar changes in resistance (assuming no change in brain metabolism) in healthy individuals. After brain injury, autoregulation may become impaired, especially in traumatically brain-injured patients. Chesnut et al. [24,25] reported that even brief periods of hypotension (systolic blood pressure less than 90 mm Hg) worsened outcome after TBI, and recommended that systolic blood pressure be maintained greater than 90 mm Hg (with possible benefit from higher pressures). These recommendations have also been promoted by the Brain Trauma Foundation for patients with severe TBI [26]. To achieve this goal, the use of vasoactive substances, such as norepinephrine, may be required [27]. Nevertheless, optimal blood pressure management for patients with TBI has yet to be defined. Some clinical data suggest that the influence of hypotension on outcome after TBI is equivalent to the influence of hypotension on outcome after nonneurologic trauma [28]. Proposed treatment protocols include CPP greater than 70 mm Hg [29,30], greater than

TABLE 30-3. Glasgow Coma Scale

Component	Response	Score
Eye opening	Spontaneously	4
	To verbal command	3
	To pain	2
	None	1
		Subtotal: 1–4
Motor response (best extremity)	Obeys verbal command	6
	Localizes pain	5
	Flexion-withdrawal	4
	Flexor (decorticate posturing)	3
	Extensor (decerebrate posturing)	2
	No response (flaccid)	1
		Subtotal: 1–6
Best verbal response	Oriented and converses	5
	Disoriented and converses	4
	Inappropriate words	3
	Incomprehensive sounds	2
	No verbal response	1
		Subtotal: 1–5
		Total: 3–15

60 mm Hg [31,32], or greater than 50 mm Hg [33]. The augmentation of CPP above 70 mm Hg with fluids and vasosuppressors has, however, been associated with increased risk of acute respiratory distress syndrome and is not universally recommended [32].

Another essential step in insuring adequate CDO_2 is the maintenance of adequate CaO_2, which in turn is dependent on Hgb and SaO_2; therefore, anemia and hypoxemia can reduce CDO_2, which would normally result in compensatory increases in CBF. However, these compensatory mechanisms are limited. As SaO_2 (or PaO_2) decreases below the compensatory threshold, $SjvO_2$ and jugular venous oxygen content ($CjvO_2$), which reflect the ability of CDO_2 to supply $CMRO_2$, also decrease (Fig. 30-4A) [34]. The correlation is most evident below a PaO_2 of approximately 60 mm Hg, the PaO_2 at which SaO_2 is 90% and below which SaO_2 rapidly decreases. In contrast, as Hgb is reduced by normovolemic hemodilution, $SjvO_2$ remains relatively constant unless severe anemia is produced (Fig 30-4B) [34].

The management of arterial CO_2 in patients with neurologic injury has changed dramatically in the past 10 years. Although hyperventilation as a management strategy for increased ICP was routine in the 1990s, it is now reserved for acute or life-threatening increases in the intensive care unit (ICU) and is no longer recommended for routine use. Having been associated with cerebral ischemia in children [12] and adults [13,14] with severe TBI, hyperventilation is least likely to be harmful when combined with monitoring, such as $SjvO_2$ or $PbtO_2$, that can identify cerebral ischemia.

Hyperglycemia increased injury in experimental TBI [35,36] and was associated with worse outcome in clinical TBI [37,38], although it is difficult to distinguish between elevated glucose causing worsened outcome versus increased severity of TBI inducing more elevated glucose levels [39]. In critically ill patients requiring mechanical ventilation, elevated glucose levels were associated with worsened outcomes [40], and current recommendations are to tightly control serum glucose in all critically ill patients [41], although more evidence is necessary to support this recommendation and to clarify the importance of glucose control in various subgroups.

The monitoring and management of body temperature remains an important aspect of care for critically ill patients. Hypothermia and hyperthermia should be considered separately in this context. The use of hypothermia as a treatment for brain injury, while demonstrating benefit in animals [42–44] and in some phase II human studies [45], has not shown consistent benefit in larger studies [46] and is not recommended for general use in TBI [47,48]. In contrast, induced hypothermia

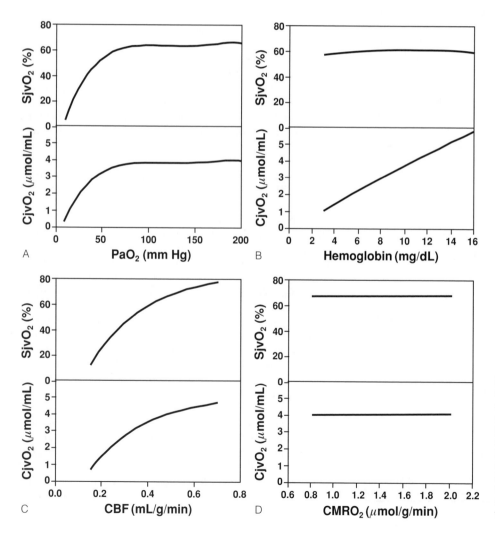

FIGURE 30-4. Changes in jugular venous saturation ($SjvO_2$) and jugular venous oxygen content ($CjvO_2$) in a normal subject in response to **(A)** hypoxia; **(B)** normovolemic anemia; **(C)** reduced cerebral blood flow (CBF); and **(D)** increased cerebral metabolic rate of oxygen ($CMRO_2$). [From Feldman Z, Robertson CS: Monitoring of cerebral hemodynamics with jugular bulb catheters. *Crit Care Clin* 13:51–77, 1997, with permission.]

after resuscitation from cardiac arrest (secondary to ventricular tachycardia or fibrillation) has improved outcome in some trials [49,50] and may be indicated for clinical use. Research into this complex area is ongoing, and clinical practice is likely to undergo further refinement.

Hyperthermia is common in critically ill patients, occurring in up to 90% of patients with neurologic disease, related both to diagnosis and length of stay [51–53]. Hyperthermia is generally associated with poorer outcome when associated with neurologic injury in adults and children [54,55], but a causal link with adverse outcome (as with serum glucose levels) is lacking. It is unclear whether increased temperatures result in worsened long-term neurologic outcome, or whether a greater severity of brain injury is associated with more frequent or severe increases in systemic temperature.

The method of temperature monitoring is important. Thermal gradients exist throughout the body, and the site of measurement influences the diagnosis of hypothermia, normothermia, or hyperthermia. Measurements of systemic temperature may underestimate brain temperature. In studies of temperature monitoring by site, variations of up to 3°C have been identified between the brain and other routinely used monitoring sites [56–58], emphasizing the importance of monitoring site selection in patients with neurologic injury and the need to appreciate the difference between brain temperature and the active site of measurement used clinically for a given patient. Electroencephalographic (EEG) monitoring has long been used in neurology for diagnosis, but has less frequently been used as a neurologic monitoring technique in critically ill patients. Rather, EEG is indicated in response to suspicion of a new or progressive abnormality such as cerebral ischemia or new onset of seizures. The cortical EEG, which is altered by mild cerebral ischemia and abolished by profound cerebral ischemia, can be used to indicate potentially damaging cerebral hypoperfusion. Likewise, the EEG can document seizures, either convulsive or nonconvulsive, and provide information as to the efficacy of antiseizure therapy. Other functions include defining the depth or type of coma, documenting focal or lateralizing intracranial abnormalities, and the diagnosis of brain death.

If the EEG is to be used for monitoring, care must be taken and weaknesses of the technique appreciated [59]. In the ICU, electrical noise from other equipment may interfere with technically adequate tracings. Continuous EEG recording is cumbersome owing to the sheer volume of data (300 pages per hour of hard copy on as many as 16 channels), although techniques for networking direct computer recording of EEG data are now available given adequate computer power and storage. Scalp fixation has also been a significant limiting factor, although newer fixation techniques are easier to apply and more stable. Techniques of mathematical data analysis, such as rapid Fourier analysis, can be used to determine the relative amplitude in each frequency band (delta—less than 4 Hz, theta—4 to 8 Hz, alpha—8 to 13 Hz, beta—greater than 13 Hz), which can then be displayed graphically in formats such as the compressed spectral array or density spectral array [60,61]. Analytic software has been developed that processes the raw EEG signal to provide single number interpretation of the "depth of sedation." These devices have been recommended for use during general anesthesia as a means to reduce the risk of awareness [62], although the scientific justification for this claim is not conclusive. The American

Society of Anesthesiologists has developed a practice advisory on this issue [63]. Use of this type of monitoring has also been implemented by some for use in the ICU for monitoring sedation levels in the critically ill, the utility of which has yet to be proven [64,65]. All devices use proprietary analysis of an EEG signal (either spontaneous or evoked, with or without electromyogram monitoring), which is converted to a single number that is intended to correspond to an awareness level based on an arbitrary scale. The future role and evidence of improved patient outcomes with this monitoring modality are unknown. Technical information on EEG processing can be found in a recent review [66].

EVOKED POTENTIALS

Sensory evoked potentials (EPs), which include somatosensory evoked potentials (SSEPs), brainstem auditory EPs, and visual EPs, can be used as qualitative threshold monitors to detect severe neural ischemia. Whereas the EEG records the continuous, spontaneous activity of the brain, EPs evaluate the responses of the brain to specific stimuli. To record SSEPs, stimuli are applied to a peripheral nerve, usually the median nerve at the wrist or posterior tibial nerve at the ankle, by a low-amplitude current of approximately 20 msec in duration. The resultant sensory (afferent) nerve stimulation and resultant cortical response to the stimulus are recorded at the scalp. Repeated identical stimuli are applied and signal averaging is used to remove the highly variable background EEG and other environmental electrical noise and thereby visualize reproducible evoked responses (Fig. 30-5) [67].

EPs are described in terms of the amplitude of cortical response peaks and the conduction delay (latency) between the stimulus and the appearance of response waveform. Because peripheral nerve stimulation can be uncomfortable, SSEPs are usually obtained from sedated or anesthetized patients. SSEPs are unaffected by neuromuscular blocking agents but may be significantly influenced by sedative, analgesic, and anesthetic agents, often in a dose-dependent manner [68–70]. In general, however, the doses of drugs required to influence EPs are sufficient to produce general anesthesia and are not usually clinically important in the ICU. If a patient is undergoing EP monitoring and requires large doses of analgesic or sedative agents, potential impairment of monitoring should be considered. Motor EPs represent a method of selectively evaluating descending motor tracts. Stimulation of proximal motor tracts (cortical or spinal) and evaluation of subsequent responses yield information that can be used for intraoperative and early postoperative neurosurgical management. Induction of motor EP and its interpretation is exquisitely sensitive to sedative, analgesic, and anesthetic drugs [71], making clinical use difficult when drugs are given concurrently. Despite these limitations, motor EP evaluation has been successfully used for the management of neuro-ICU patients and may become more common as techniques and equipment improve [72,73].

The sensitivity of EP monitoring is similar to that of EEG monitoring. EPs, especially brainstem auditory EPs, are relatively robust, although they can be modified by trauma, hypoxia, or ischemia. Because obliteration of EPs occurs only under conditions of profound cerebral ischemia or mechanical trauma, EP monitoring is one of the most specific ways in which to assess neurologic integrity in specific monitored pathways. However, as

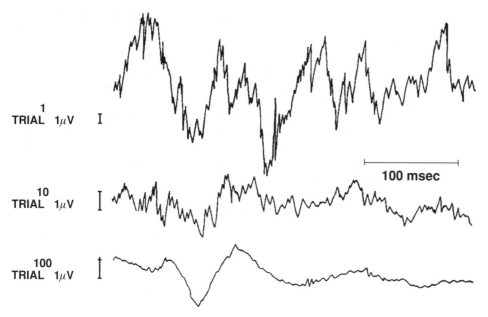

TRIAL 1   1μV

TRIAL 10   1μV

100 msec

TRIAL 100   1μV

FIGURE 30-5. Averaging reduces background noise. After 100 trials, this visual evoked potential (EP) is relatively noise-free. The same EP is hard to distinguish after only 10 trials and would be impossible to find in the original unaveraged data. [From Nuwer MR: *Evoked Potential Monitoring in the Operating Room.* New York, Raven Press, 1986, p 29, with permission.]

with the discussion of cerebral ischemia, there is a dose-time interaction that ultimately determines the magnitude of cerebral injury. As a result, neurologic deficits occur that have not been predicted by changes in EPs [74], and severe changes in EPs may not be followed by neurologic deficits [75]. Even so, loss of cortical SSEPs remains a strong indicator of poor outcome [76,77].

INTRACRANIAL PRESSURE MONITORING

The symptoms and signs of intracranial hypertension are neither sensitive nor specific. Usually, the physical findings associated with increasing ICP (e.g., Cushing's response–hypertension and Cushing's triad–hypertension, reflex bradycardia, and alterations in respiratory function) become apparent only when intracranial hypertension has become sufficiently severe to injure the brain. Likewise, papilledema is a late development and is often difficult to identify clinically. Because ICP cannot otherwise be adequately assessed, direct measurement and monitoring of ICP has become a common intervention, especially in the management of TBI [78], and less commonly after critical illnesses such as SAH or stroke. Even so, there is no conclusive evidence that the use of this technique improves outcomes. Continuing debate centers on how to use ICP data to change patient care and reduce morbidity and mortality. ICP monitoring is generally recommended for the management of patients who are comatose after TBI [79] and for patients at risk of increased ICP with GCS less than 8 [80]. Because pressure gradients may exist among various sites within the calvarium, it may be advantageous to monitor in or adjacent to the most severely damaged hemisphere [81], although some even recommend bilateral ICP monitoring to circumvent this problem [82].

ICP functions as the outflow pressure apposing MAP (CPP = MAP − ICP) when ICP exceeds jugular venous pressure. Because the skull is not distensible, the brain, cerebrospinal fluid (CSF), and cerebral blood volume have little room to expand without increasing ICP. It is important to appreciate that some increase in intracranial volume is possible without much change

in ICP, but when the compensatory mechanisms are exhausted, even small changes in volume can lead to significant increases in pressure. Although CBF cannot be directly inferred from knowledge of MAP and ICP, severe increases in ICP reduce CPP and CBF. ICP monitoring provides temporally relevant, quantitative information. The problems associated with ICP monitoring fall generally into three categories: direct morbidity due to monitor placement (e.g., intracranial hemorrhage, cortical damage, and infection), inaccurate measurement, and misinterpretation or inappropriate use of the data. Clinically, one of three sites is used to measure ICP: a lateral ventricle, the subdural space, or the brain parenchyma. Ventricular catheterization, when performed using strict asepsis, is the method of choice for ICP monitoring and CSF drainage [83] in patients with acute intracranial hypertension and excess CSF (i.e., acute hydrocephalus). In practice, intraventricular catheters may be difficult to place if cerebral edema or brain swelling has compressed the ventricular system. Intraventricular pressure monitoring can also be performed with fiber-optic catheters (instead of a hollow catheter) that use a variable reflectance pressure sensing system (transducer tip) to measure pressure (Camino Laboratories, San Diego, CA). These fiber-optic catheters are less susceptible to short-term malfunction than conventional, fluid-filled catheters [84,85] but may slowly and unpredictably drift over days to weeks [86].

Pressure monitoring from the subdural space may use a fluid-coupled bolt (simple transcranial conduit), fluid-coupled subdural catheters (or reservoirs), or fiber-optic transducer-tipped catheters (see above). Because subdural bolts are open tubes facing end-on against the brain surface, brain tissue may herniate into the system, obstructing the system, distorting measurements, and potentially damaging the cerebral cortex. Reservoir systems require surgical placement into the subdural space. Fiber-optic systems do not have these specific problems, but fixation and equipment reliability are practical issues [84].

Intraparenchymal placement of a fiber-optic catheter is also possible and is associated with complications similar to ventricular fiber-optic catheters. Complications are generally noted to be highest with ventriculostomies (when compared with fiber-optic catheter usage) and complication of ICP monitoring are associated with a worse GCS score [87].

Management decisions based on ICP data are the focus of ongoing debate and study. Clinical studies after TBI have demonstrated that increased ICP is associated with worsened outcome [88]. Therefore, control of ICP has been considered by some clinicians to be the primary focus of treatment [33], while other clinicians have considered restoration of CPP (by increasing MAP) to be the primary goal of medical management [29,89]. To date, the ideal approach has not been established by outcome trials; therefore, practice patterns remain variable [90,91]. Clinical experience with ICP monitoring of head-injured patients has resulted in publication of clinical guidelines using an evidence-based approach (Fig. 30-6) [92].

CEREBRAL BLOOD FLOW MONITORING

The first quantitative clinical method of measurement of CBF, the Kety-Schmidt [93] technique, calculated global CBF from the difference between the arterial and jugular bulb concentration curves of an inhaled, inert gas as it equilibrated with blood and brain tissue. Later techniques used extracranial gamma detectors to measure regional cortical CBF from washout curves after intracarotid injection of a radioisotope such as 133-xenon (Xe 133) [94]. Carotid puncture was avoided by techniques that measured cortical CBF after inhaled [95] or intravenous administration of Xe 133, using gamma counting of exhaled gas to correct clearance curves for recirculation of Xe 133. Because Xe is radiodense, saturation of brain tissue increases radiographic density in proportion to CBF. Imaging of the brain after equilibration with stable (nonradioactive) Xe provides a regional estimate of CBF that includes deep brain structures [96]. Clinical studies of CBF after TBI performed using stable xenon computed tomography (CT) have prompted a radical revision of conventional understanding by demonstrating that one-third of patients had evidence of cerebral ischemia within 8 hours of trauma [8]. Although slow in becoming a routine clinical tool, Xe CT is becoming a more common technique for monitoring CBF in patients. The use of helical and spiral CT scanners (with very short acquisition times) reduces the radiation exposure to the patient and decreases the time needed for a scan, improving clinical utility [97]. Another CT-based technique, perfusion CT, uses iodinated contrast infusion with repeated images to calculate local CBF. This technique is limited to smaller regions and may not provide uniform results between brain regions [98]. Other techniques, such as single photon emission CT (SPECT) and magnetic resonance perfusion imaging also can provide information about CBF, but are not as clinically useful at this time [97]. Transcranial Doppler ultrasonography can be used to estimate changes in CBF. In most patients, cerebral arterial flow velocity can be measured easily in intracranial vessels, especially the middle cerebral artery, using transcranial Doppler ultrasonography. Doppler flow velocity uses the frequency shift, proportional to velocity, which is observed when sound waves are reflected from moving red blood cells. Blood moving toward the transducer shifts the transmitted frequency to higher frequencies; blood moving away, to lower frequencies. Velocity is a function both of blood flow rate and vessel diameter. If diameter remains constant, changes in velocity are proportional to changes in CBF; however, intersubject differences in flow velocity correlate poorly with intersubject differences in CBF [99]. Entirely noninvasive, transcranial Doppler measurements can be repeated at frequent intervals or even applied continuously. The detection and monitoring of post-SAH vasospasm remains the most common use of transcranial Doppler (Fig. 30-7) [100,101]. However, further clinical research is necessary to define those situations in which the excellent capacity for rapid trend monitoring can be exploited.

JUGULAR BULB VENOUS OXYGEN SATURATION

Several measurements of cerebral oxygenation are clinically useful, including measurement of $SjvO_2$. To insert a retrograde jugular venous bulb catheter, the internal jugular vein can be located by ultrasound guidance or by external anatomic landmarks and use of a "seeker" needle, namely, the same technique used for antegrade placement of jugular venous catheters. Once the vessel is identified, the catheter is directed cephalad, toward the mastoid process, instead of centrally. A lateral cranial radiograph can confirm the position just superior to the base of the skull. The decision to place a jugular bulb catheter in the left or right jugular bulb is important. Simultaneous measurements of $SjvO_2$ in the right and left jugular bulb demonstrates differences in saturation [102,103], suggesting that one jugular bulb frequently is dominant, carrying the greater portion of cerebral venous blood [104]. Differences in the cross-sectional areas of the vessels that form the torcula and the manner in which blood is distributed to the right and left lateral sinus contribute to differences between the two jugular bulbs [104]. Ideally, a jugular bulb catheter should be placed on the dominant side, which can be identified as the jugular vein that, if compressed, produces the greater increase in ICP or as the vein on the side of the larger jugular foramen as detected by CT [105,106].

In general $SjvO_2$ reflects the adequacy of CDO_2 to support $CMRO_2$, but mixed cerebral venous blood, like mixed systemic blood, represents a global average of cerebral venous blood from regions that are variably perfused and may not reflect marked regional hypoperfusion/ischemia of small regions. In contrast to ICP and CPP, which provide only indirect information concerning the adequacy of CDO_2 to support $CMRO_2$, $SjvO_2$ directly reflects the balance between these variables on a global or hemispheric level. CBF, $CMRO_2$, CaO_2, and $CjvO_2$ are modeled by the equation: $CMRO_2 = CBF (CaO_2 - CjvO_2)$. In healthy brain, if $CMRO_2$ remains constant as CBF decreases, $SjvO_2$ and $CjvO_2$ decrease (Fig. 30-4C) [34]. If flow-metabolism coupling is intact, decreases in $CMRO_2$ result in parallel decreases in CBF while $SjvO_2$ and $CjvO_2$ remain constant (Fig. 30-4D) [34]. Abnormally low $SjvO_2$ (i.e., less than 50%, compared to a normal value of 65%) suggests the possibility of cerebral ischemia; but normal or elevated $SjvO_2$ does not prove the adequacy of cerebral perfusion because of possible saturation averaging between normal and abnormal areas of perfusion. This is especially true for focal areas of hypoperfusion. Therefore, the negative predictive value of a normal $SjvO_2$ is poor. After placement of a jugular catheter, monitoring of $SjvO_2$ can be achieved through repeated blood sampling. However, repeated blood sampling yields only "snapshots" of cerebral oxygenation [107] and thus provides discontinuous data that may miss rapid changes in saturation. To achieve continuous monitoring of $SjvO_2$, indwelling fiber-optic

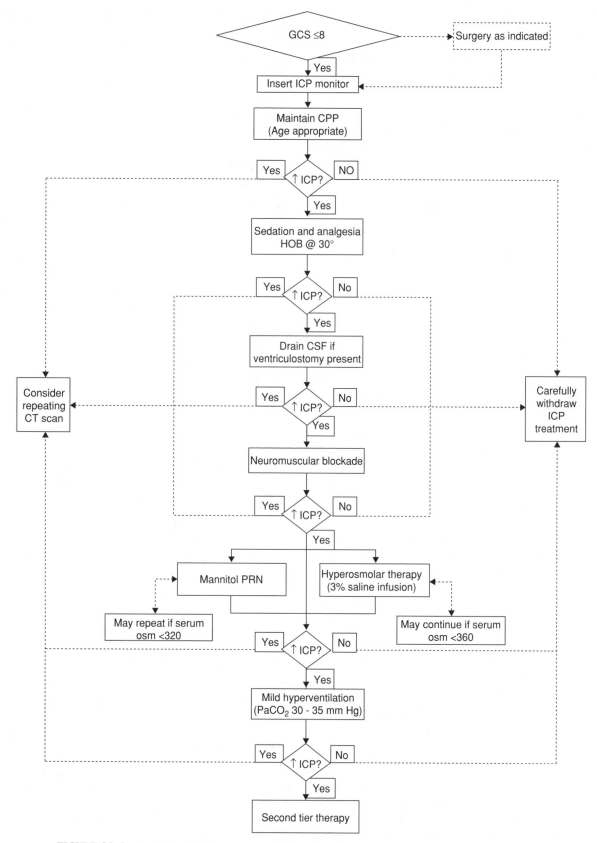

FIGURE 30-6.   Critical pathway for treatment of intracranial hypertension in the pediatric patient with severe head injury. [From Adelson PD, Bratton SL, Carney NA, et al: Chapter 17. Critical pathway for the treatment of established intracranial hypertension in pediatric traumatic brain injury. *Ped Crit Care Med* 4(3) [Suppl]:S65–67, July 2003, with permission.]

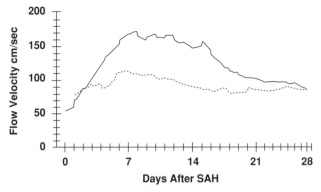

FIGURE 30-7.   Mean flow velocity (FV, in cm/sec) curves of 18 patients with laterally localized aneurysms (arising from the internal carotid and middle cerebral arteries). The side of the ruptured aneurysm (*continuous line*) shows a higher FV than the unaffected side (*dotted line*). SAH = subarachnoid hemorrhage. [From Seiler RW, Grolimund P, Aaslid R, et al: Cerebral vasospasm evaluated by transcranial ultrasound correlated with clinical grade and CT-visualized subarachnoid hemorrhage. *J Neurosurg* 64:594–600, 1986, with permission.]

oximetric catheters have been used. Because oxyhemoglobin and deoxyhemoglobin absorb light differently, $SjvO_2$ can be determined from differential absorbance. Oximetric jugular bulb catheters have proven somewhat challenging to maintain, requiring frequent recalibration, repositioning, and confirmation of measured saturation by analyzing blood samples in a co-oximeter [108]. The highest frequency of confirmed desaturation episodes occurs in patients with intracerebral hematomas, closely followed by those with SAH. In patients with TBI, the number of jugular desaturations is strongly associated with poor neurologic outcome; even a single desaturation episode is associated with a doubling of the mortality rate (Fig. 30-8) [109]. Clinical application of jugular venous bulb cannulation has been limited, perhaps in part because the technique is invasive, although

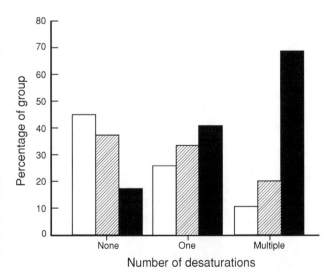

FIGURE 30-8.   Occurrence of jugular venous desaturation was strongly associated with a high mortality rate and a poor outcome; 3-month Glasgow Outcome Scale: white bars represent percentage of patients who had good recovery/moderate disability; striped bars represent percentage of patients who had severe disability/persistent vegetative state; black bars represent percentage of patients who died. [From Gopinath SP, Robertson CS, Contant CF, et al: Jugular venous desaturation and outcome after head injury. *J Neurol Neurosurg Psychiatry* 57:717–723, 1994, with permission.]

the risks of cannulation injury, including hematoma and injury to the adjacent carotid, are low [110]. Several modifications of jugular venous oxygen monitoring have been proposed. Cerebral extraction of oxygen, which is the difference between SaO_2 and $SjvO_2$ divided by SaO_2, is less confounded by anemia than the cerebral A-VDO_2 [111]. Another concept, termed cerebral hemodynamic reserve, is defined as the ratio of percentage of change in global cerebral extraction of oxygen (reflecting the balance between $CMRO_2$ and CBF) to percentage of change in CPP [112]. This equation attempts to integrate cerebral hemodynamics and metabolism with intracranial compliance. Cruz et al. [111] found that cerebral hemodynamic reserve decreased as intracranial compliance decreased, even as a consequence of minor elevations in ICP. Theoretically, this variable may allow more precise management of cerebral hemodynamics in patients with decreased intracranial compliance.

BRAIN TISSUE OXYGEN TENSION

Another promising technique for monitoring the adequacy of CDO_2 is direct assessment of $PbtO_2$. Monitoring of $PbtO_2$ overcomes one important limitation of $SjvO_2$ monitoring, which is that the global saturation measurements provide no information about regional or focal tissue oxygenation. Only relatively profound focal global ischemia causes $SjvO_2$ to decrease to less than the accepted critical threshold of 50%. Even severe regional ischemia may not result in desaturation if venous effluent from other regions is normally saturated, in part because the absolute flow of poorly saturated blood returning from ischemic regions is by definition less per volume of tissue than flow from well-perfused regions, resulting in a smaller percentage of poorly oxygenated to well-oxygenated blood. Intracranial, intraparenchymal probes have been developed that monitor only $PbtO_2$ or that also monitor brain tissue PCO_2 and pH [112]. Modified from probes designed for continuous monitoring of arterial blood gases, intraparenchymal probes can be inserted through multiple-lumen ICP monitoring bolts. Although these probes provide no information about remote regions, they nevertheless provide continuous information about the region that is contiguous to the probe. They also carry the theoretical risk of hematoma formation, infection, and direct parenchymal injury. Evaluation of $PbtO_2$ after TBI has shown that low partial pressures ($PbtO_2$ less than 10 mm Hg for greater than 30 minutes) powerfully predict poor outcomes [113]. Both $PbtO_2$ and $SjvO_2$ may reflect changes in cerebral oxygenation secondary to alterations in CBF (Fig. 30-9) [114]. However, comparisons of simultaneous $PbtO_2$ and $SjvO_2$ monitoring suggest that each monitor detects cerebral ischemia that the other fails to detect. In 58 patients with severe TBI, the two monitors detected 52 episodes in which $SjvO_2$ decreased to less than 50% or $PbtO_2$ decreased to less than 8 mm Hg; of those 52 episodes, both monitored variables fell below the ischemic threshold in 17, only $SjvO_2$ reflected ischemia in 19, and only $PbtO_2$ reflected ischemia in 16 (Fig. 30-10) [115]. Ongoing research will determine the role of $PbtO_2$ monitoring and the relationship between $PbtO_2$ monitoring and $SjvO_2$ monitoring in critical neurologic illness.

NEUROCHEMICAL MONITORING

Neuronal injury is associated with the release or production of chemical markers such as free radicals, inflammatory mediators, metabolic products, and excitatory amino acids [4].

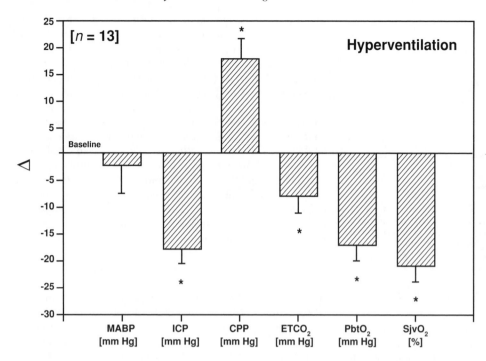

FIGURE 30-9. The effect of hyperventilation-induced hypocapnia on changes in mean arterial blood pressure (MABP), intracranial pressure (ICP), cerebral perfusion pressure (CPP), end-tidal CO_2 (ETCO$_2$), PtiO$_2$, and jugular bulb oximetry (SjvO$_2$). *$p < 0.05$; before hyperventilation versus 10 minutes later. [From Unterberg AW, Kiening KL, Härtl R, et al: Multimodal monitoring in patients with head injury: evaluation of the effects of treatment on cerebral oxygenation. *J Trauma* 42:S32–S37, 1997, with permission.]

Neurochemical monitoring via microdialysis allows assessment of the chemical milieu of cerebral extracellular fluid, provides valuable information about neurochemical processes in various neuropathologic states [116,117], and is used clinically in the management of severe TBI [118,119] and SAH [120–122]. Substances monitored via microdialysis include energy-related metabolites such as glucose, lactate, pyruvate, adenosine, and xanthine; neurotransmitters such as glutamate, aspartate, gamma-amino butyric acid; markers of tissue damage such as glycerol and potassium [116,123], and alterations in membrane phospholipids by oxygen radicals [124]. The magnitude of release of these substances correlates with the extent of ischemic

damage [125]. The time-dependent changes of these substances and the clinical implications are being evaluated, and their incorporation into standard practice is being studied.

NEAR-INFRARED SPECTROSCOPY

Theoretically, the best monitor of brain oxygenation would be a noninvasive device that characterizes brain oxygenation in real time: near-infrared spectroscopy (NIRS) might eventually offer the opportunity to assess the adequacy of brain oxygenation continuously and noninvasively, although to date the use of the technique in adults has been limited.

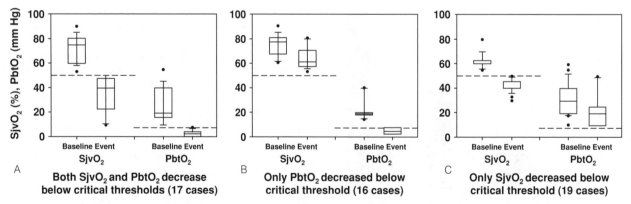

FIGURE 30-10. Changes in jugular venous oxygen saturation (SjvO$_2$) and brain tissue PO$_2$ (PbtO$_2$) during 52 episodes of cerebral hypoxia/ischemia. The horizontal line across the box plot represents the median, and the lower and upper ends of the box plot are the 25th percentile and 75th percentile, respectively. The error bars mark the 10th and 90th percentiles. The closed circles indicate any outlying points. **Left:** summary of the 17 cases in which both SjvO$_2$ and PbtO$_2$ decreased to less than their respective thresholds, as defined in the text. **Middle:** Summary of the 16 cases in which PbtO$_2$ decreased to less than the defined threshold; but SjvO$_2$; although decreased, did not decrease to less than 50%. **Right:** Summary of the 19 cases in which SjvO$_2$ decreased to less than the threshold, but PbtO$_2$ remained at greater than 10 torr. [From Gopinath SP, Valadka AB, Uzura M, et al: Comparison of jugular venous oxygen saturation and brain tissue PO$_2$ as monitors of cerebral ischemia after head injury. *Crit Care Med* 27:2337–2345, 1999, with permission.]

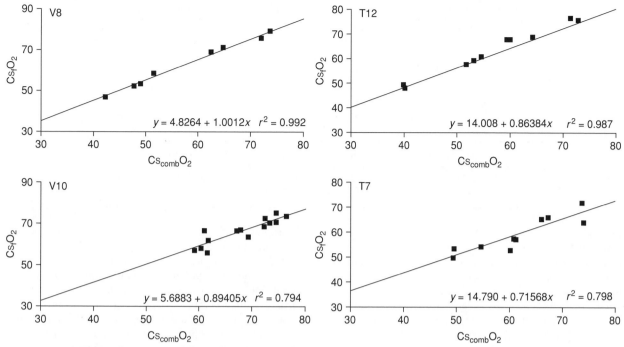

FIGURE 30-11.   Cerebral oximeter signal (Cs_fO_2) and estimated global brain oxygen saturation ($Cs_{comb}O_2$) are closely correlated for the training group ($r^2 = 0.798 - 0.987$) for individual subjects. The number in the upper left corner represents the individual subjects' identities. T, training set; V, validation set. The best and worst examples are represented. [From Pollard V, Prough DS, DeMelo AE, et al: Validation in volunteers of a near infrared spectroscope for monitoring brain oxygenation in vivo. *Anesth Analg* 82:269–277, 1996, with permission.]

Near-infrared light penetrates the skull and, during transmission through or reflection from brain tissue, undergoes changes in intensity that are proportional to the relative concentrations of oxygenated and deoxygenated hemoglobin in the arteries, capillaries, and veins within the field [126,127]. The absorption (A) of light by a chromophore (i.e., hemoglobin) is defined by Beer's Law: $A = abc$, where a is the absorption constant, b is the path length of the light, and c is the concentration of the chromophore, namely, oxygenated and deoxygenated hemoglobin. Because it is impossible to measure the path length of NIRS light in tissue, approximations as to relative lengths and arterial versus venous contribution must be made.

Extensive preclinical and clinical data demonstrate that NIRS detects qualitative changes in brain oxygenation (Fig. 30-11) [128–130]. However, despite promise, many problems remain with the technology [131,132], and brain saturation measured using NIRS correlated poorly with continuous $SjvO_2$ in patients with severe closed-head injury [133]. Therefore, validation studies suggest that NIRS may be more useful for qualitatively monitoring trends of brain tissue oxygenation than for actual

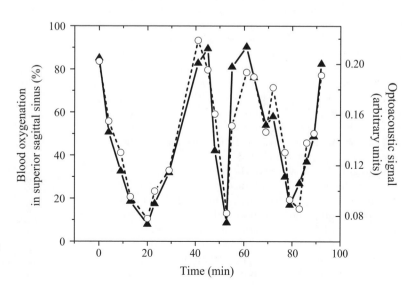

FIGURE 30-12.   Optoacoustic signal intensity (*dashed line*) and superior sagittal sinus hemoglobin saturation in (*solid line*) as a function of time.

TABLE 30-4. Outcome at Discharge in Relation to Intracranial Diagnosis (% of patients)

Outcome	DI I	DI II	DI III	DI IV	Evacuated Mass	Nonevacuated Mass
GR	27.0	8.5	3.3	3.1	5.1	2.8
MD	34.6	26.0	13.1	3.1	17.7	8.3
SD	19.2	40.7	26.8	18.8	26.0	19.4
PVS	9.6	11.2	22.9	18.8	12.3	16.7
Death	9.6	13.5	34.0	56.2	38.8	52.8
Total	100	100	100	100	100	100

GR, good recovery; MD, moderate disability; SD, severe disability; PVS, persistent vegetative state; DI, diffuse injury; DI categories I–IV represent increasingly severe classes of diffuse brain injury.
From Marshall LF, Marshall SB, Klauber MR, et al: A new classification of head injury based on computerized tomography. *J Neurosurg* 75:S14–S20, 1991, with permission.

quantification [130,134,135]. Some of the liabilities of near-infrared spectroscopy may be overcome by optoacoustic monitoring of cerebral venous saturation. Optoacoustic monitoring of cerebral venous saturation depends on the generation by near-infrared light of ultrasonic signals in blood. The acoustic signals are then transmitted linearly through tissue and bone and provide a focused, depth-resolved signal that reflects venous oxygenation (Fig. 30-12) [136].

NEUROIMAGING

Magnetic resonance imaging (MRI), positron emission spectroscopy (PET) scans, cerebral angiography, and radionuclide scans do not function as monitors per se. Rather, they are indicated in response to suspicion of a new or progressive anatomic lesion, such as a subdural or intracerebral hematoma or cerebral arterial vasospasm, that requires altered treatment. Most neuroimaging modalities provide static, discontinuous data and require moving a critically ill patient from the ICU to a remote location. Even so, these techniques play an important role in the overall management of patients with brain injury [137]. With the introduction of portable CT scanners and the development of ultrafast helical and spiral CT scanners, availability and acquisition time for evaluations have significantly decreased and can now be used for serial monitoring of ongoing neurologic processes and for evaluation of changes in CBF (see above).

CT scans obtained at the time of admission to the hospital can provide valuable prognostic information. Marshall et al. [138] predicted outcome of head-injured patients in relation to four grades of increasingly severe diffuse brain injury and the presence of evacuated or nonevacuated intracranial mass lesions (Table 30-4). Normal CT scans at admission in patients with GCS scores less than 8 are associated with a 10% to 15% incidence of ICP elevation [139–141]; however, the risk of ICP elevation increases in patients older than age 40 years, those with unilateral or bilateral motor posturing, or those with systolic blood pressure less than 90 mm Hg [139].

Although MRI often provides better resolution than CT scans, the powerful magnetic fields make the use of ferrous metals impractical (and dangerous), a ubiquitous component of life-support equipment. To address this issue, MRI-compatible ventilators, monitors, and infusion pumps have been developed, although the logistics of transport and the time required for scans continues to make this technique difficult for repeated monitoring. Recent advances in MRI technology, such as

diffusion-weighted imaging, magnetic resonance spectroscopy (carbon, phosphorus, and nitrogen-labeled), and phase contrast angiography provide information about brain function, oxidative metabolic pathways, cerebral blood volume, and functional CBF [137,142–144]. These techniques, while undergoing further evaluation and validation, may one day prove useful in evaluating brain injury and its management. Recent clinical evidence of brain mitochondrial dysfunction after TBI, despite apparently adequate CDO_2, suggests that functional cellular evaluation and associated therapy may someday be as important as maintaining CDO_2 [145].

MULTIMODAL MONITORING STRATEGIES

Advanced clinical practice takes into account the limitations of each monitoring modality and compensates by combining different techniques into a generalized strategy. This concept of multimodal monitoring is not new (consider the operating room and the role of the anesthesiologist) but is becoming more common in the management of brain injury [31,146,147], and the use of these regimented techniques may lead to improvements in patient outcome [148].

REFERENCES

1. Jones TH, Morawetz RB, Crowell RM, et al: Thresholds of focal cerebral ischemia in awake monkeys. *J Neurosurg* 54:773–782, 1981.
2. Cunningham AS, Salvador R, Coles JP, et al: Physiological thresholds for irreversible tissue damage in contusional regions following traumatic brain injury. *Brain* 128:1931–1942, 2005.
3. Carmichael ST: Gene expression changes after focal stroke, traumatic brain and spinal cord injuries. *Curr Opin Neurol* 16:699–704, 2003.
4. Enriquez P, Bullock R: Molecular and cellular mechanisms in the pathophysiology of severe head injury. *Curr Pharm Des* 10:2131–2143, 2004.
5. Acker T, Acker H: Cellular oxygen sensing need in CNS function: physiological and pathological implications. *J Exp Biol* 207:3171–3188, 2004.
6. Strandgaard S, Paulson OB: Cerebral autoregulation. *Stroke* 15:413–416, 1984.
7. Bouma GJ, Muizelaar JP, Choi SC, et al: Cerebral circulation and metabolism after severe traumatic brain injury: the elusive role of ischemia. *J Neurosurg* 75:685–693, 1991.
8. Bouma GJ, Muizelaar JP, Stringer WA, et al: Ultra-early evaluation of regional cerebral blood flow in severely head-injured patients using xenon-enhanced computerized tomography. *J Neurosurg* 77:360–368, 1992.
9. Hlatky R, Furuya Y, Valadka AB, et al: Dynamic autoregulatory response after severe head injury. *J Neurosurg* 97:1054–1061, 2002.
10. Lundberg N, Kjällquist Å, Bien C: Reduction of increased intracranial pressure by hyperventilation. *Acta Psychiatr Neurol (Scand)* 34[Suppl]:5–57, 1959.
11. Muizelaar JP, Marmarou A, Ward JD, et al: Adverse effects of prolonged hyperventilation in patients with severe head injury: a randomized clinical trial. *J Neurosurg* 75:731–739, 1991.
12. Skippen P, Seear M, Poskitt K, et al: Effect of hyperventilation on regional cerebral blood flow in head-injured children. *Crit Care Med* 25:1402–1409, 1997.

13. Marion DW, Puccio A, Wisniewski SR, et al: Effect of hyperventilation on extracellular concentrations of glutamate, lactate, pyruvate, and local cerebral blood flow in patients with severe traumatic brain injury. *Crit Care Med* 30:2619–2625, 2002.

14. Coles JP, Minhas PS, Fryer TD, et al: Effect of hyperventilation on cerebral blood flow in traumatic head injury: clinical relevance and monitoring correlates. *Crit Care Med* 30:1950–1959, 2002.

15. Matta BF, Lam AM, Mayberg TS: The influence of arterial oxygenation on cerebral venous oxygen saturation during hyperventilation. *Can J Anaesth* 41:1041–1046, 1994.

16. Thiagarajan A, Goverdhan PD, Chari P, et al: The effect of hyperventilation and hyperoxia on cerebral venous oxygen saturation in patients with traumatic brain injury. *Anesth Analg* 87:850–853, 1998.

17. Tommasino C, Moore S, Todd MM: Cerebral effects of isovolemic hemodilution with crystalloid or colloid solutions. *Crit Care Med* 16:862–868, 1988.

18. DeWitt DS, Prough DS, Taylor CL, et al: Reduced cerebral blood flow, oxygen delivery, and electroencephalographic activity after traumatic brain injury and mild hemorrhage in cats. *J Neurosurg* 76:812–821, 1992.

19. Teasdale G, Jennett B: Assessment of coma and impaired consciousness: a practical scale. *Lancet* 2:81–84, 1974.

20. Langfitt TW: Measuring the outcome from head injuries. *J Neurosurg* 48:673–678, 1978.

21. Miller JD: Head injury. *J Neurol Neurosurg Psychiatry* 56:440–447, 1993.

22. Udekwu P, Kromhout-Schiro S, Vaslef S, et al: Glasgow Coma Scale score, mortality, and functional outcome in head-injured patients. *J Trauma* 56:1084–1089, 2004.

23. Balestreri M, Czosnyka M, Chatfield DA, et al: Predictive value of Glasgow Coma Scale after brain trauma: change in trend over the past ten years. *J Neurol Neurosurg Psychiatry* 75:161–162, 2004.

24. Chesnut RM, Marshall SB, Piek J, et al: Early and late systemic hypotension as a frequent and fundamental source of cerebral ischemia following severe brain injury in the traumatic coma data bank. *Acta Neurochir* 59:121–125, 1993.

25. Chesnut RM, Ghajar J, Mass AIR, et al. Management and prognosis of severe traumatic brain injury. Part II. Early indications of prognosis in severe traumatic brain injury. *J Neurotrauma* 17:555–627, 2000.

26. Bullock RM, Chesnut RM, Clifton GL, et al: Resuscitation of blood pressure and oxygenation. *J Neurotrauma* 17:471–478, 2000.

27. Johnston AJ, Steiner LA, Chatfield DA, et al: Effect of cerebral perfusion pressure augmentation with dopamine and norepinephrine on global and focal brain oxygenation after traumatic brain injury. *Intensive Care Med* 30:791–797, 2004.

28. Shafi S, Gentilello L: Hypotension does not increase mortality in brain-injured patients more than it does in non-brain-injured patients. *J Trauma* 59:830–834, 2005.

29. Rosner MJ, Rosner SD, Johnson AH: Cerebral perfusion pressure: management protocol and clinical results. *J Neurosurg* 83:949–962, 1995.

30. Bullock RM, Chesnut RM, Clifton GL, et al: Guidelines for cerebral perfusion pressure. *J Neurotrauma* 17:507–511, 2000.

31. Vincent JL, Berre J: Primer on medical management of severe brain injury. *Crit Care Med* 33:1392–1399, 2005.

32. Brain Trauma Foundation, American Association of Neurological Surgeons Congress of Neurological Surgeons Joint Section on Neurotrauma and Critical Care. Guidelines for the management of severe traumatic brain injury: cerebral perfusion pressure. 3-14-2003. Brain Trauma Foundation, Inc. Available from the Agency for Healthcare Research and Quality (AHRQ), http://www.guideline.gov/summary/summary.aspx?doc_id=3794 Retrieved December 5, 2006.

33. Grande PO, Asgeirsson B, Nordstrom CH. Physiologic principles for volume regulation of a tissue enclosed in a rigid shell with application to the injured brain. *J Trauma* 42:S23–S31, 1997.

34. Feldman Z, Robertson CS: Monitoring of cerebral hemodynamics with jugular bulb catheters. *Crit Care Clin* 13:51–77, 1997.

35. Cherian L, Goodman JC, Robertson CS: Hyperglycemia increases brain injury caused by secondary ischemia after cortical impact injury in rats. *Crit Care Med* 25:1378–1383, 1997.

36. Kinoshita K, Kraydieh S, Alonso O, et al: Effect of posttraumatic hyperglycemia on contusion volume and neutrophil accumulation after moderate fluid-percussion brain injury in rats. *J Neurotrauma* 19:681–692, 2002.

37. Jeremitsky E, Omert LA, Dunham CM, et al: The impact of hyperglycemia on patients with severe brain injury. *J Trauma* 58:47–50, 2005.

38. Cochran A, Scaife ER, Hansen KW, et al: Hyperglycemia and outcomes from pediatric traumatic brain injury. *J Trauma* 55:1035–1038, 2003.

39. Rovlias A, Kotsou S: The influence of hyperglycemia on neurological outcome in patients with severe head injury. *Neurosurgery* 46:335–343, 2000.

40. Van den Berghe G, Wouters P, Weekers F, et al: Intensive insulin therapy in critically ill patients. *N Engl J Med* 345:1359–1367, 2001.

41. Van Den BG, Wouters PJ, Bouillon R, et al: Outcome benefit of intensive insulin therapy in the critically ill: insulin dose versus glycemic control. *Crit Care Med* 31:359–366, 2003.

42. Dietrich WD, Busto R, Alonso O, et al: Intraischemic but not postischemic brain hypothermia protects chronically following global forebrain ischemia in rats. *J Cereb Blood Flow Metab* 13:541–549, 1993.

43. Clifton GL, Jiang JY, Lyeth BG, et al: Marked protection by moderate hypothermia after experimental traumatic brain injury. *J Cereb Blood Flow Metab* 11:114–121, 1991.

44. Globus MYT, Alonso O, Dietrich WD, et al: Glutamate release and free radical production following brain injury: Effects of posttraumatic hypothermia. *J Neurochem* 65:1704–1711, 1995.

45. Marion DW, Penrod LE, Kelsey SF, et al: Treatment of traumatic brain injury with moderate hypothermia. *N Engl J Med* 336:540–546, 1997.

46. Clifton G: Hypothermia and severe brain injury. *J Neurosurg* 93:718–719, 2000.

47. McIntyre LA, Fergusson DA, Hebert PC, et al: Prolonged therapeutic hypothermia after traumatic brain injury in adults: a systematic review. *JAMA* 289:2992–2999, 2003.

48. Henderson WR, Dhingra VK, Chittock DR, et al: Hypothermia in the management of traumatic brain injury. A systematic review and metaanalysis. *Intensive Care Med* 29:1637–1644, 2003.

49. Hypothermia after cardiac arrest study group: mild therapeutic hypothermia to improve the neurologic outcome after cardiac arrest. *N Engl J Med* 346:549–556, 2002.

50. Bernard SA, Gray TW, Buist MD, et al. Treatment of comatose survivors of out-of-hospital cardiac arrest with induced hypothermia. *N Engl J Med* 346:557–563, 2002.

51. Kilpatrick MM, Lowry DW, Firlik AD, et al: Hyperthermia in the neurosurgical intensive care unit. *Neurosurgery* 47:850–856, 2000.

52. Schwarz S, Hafner K, Aschoff A, et al: Incidence and prognostic significance of fever following intracerebral hemorrhage. *Neurology* 54:354–361, 2000.

53. Albrecht RF, Wass CT, Lanier WL: Occurrence of potentially detrimental temperature alterations in hospitalized patients at risk for brain injury. *Mayo Clin Proc* 73:629–635, 1998.

54. Azzimondi G, Bassein L, Nonino F, et al: Fever in acute stroke worsens prognosis. A prospective study. *Stroke* 26:2040–2043, 1995.

55. Natale JE, Joseph JG, Helfaer MA, et al: Early hyperthermia after traumatic brain injury in children: risk factors, influence on length of stay, and effect on short-term neurologic status. *Crit Care Med* 28:2608–2615, 2000.

56. Rumana CS, Gopinath SP, Uzura M, et al: Brain temperature exceeds systemic temperature in head-inured patients. *Crit Care Med* 26:562–567, 1998.

57. Mellergard P: Monitoring of rectal, epidural, and intraventricular temperature in neurosurgical patients. *Acta Neurochir Suppl* 60:485–487, 1994.

58. Crowder CM, Tempelhoff R, Theard MA, et al: Jugular bulb temperature: comparison with brain surface and core temperatures in neurosurgical patients during mild hypothermia. *J Neurosurg* 85:98–103, 1996.

59. Nuwer M: Assessment of digital EEG, quantitative EEG, and EEG brain mapping: report of the American Academy of Neurology and the American Clinical Neurophysiology Society. *Neurology* 49:277–292, 1997.

60. Levy WJ, Shapiro HM, Maruchak G, et al: Automated EEG processing for intraoperative monitoring: a comparison of techniques. *Anesthesiology* 53:223–236, 1980.

61. Sloan TB: Electrophysiologic monitoring in head injury. *New Horizons* 3:431–438, 1995.

62. Preventing and managing the impact of anesthesia awareness. JCAHO Sentinel Event Alert 2004. Available from the Joint Commission on Accreditation of Healthcare Organizations, http://www.jointcommission.org/SentinelEvents/SentinelEventAlert/seq_32.htm Retrieved December 5, 2006.

63. American Society of Anesthesiologists practice advisory for intraoperative awareness and brain function monitoring. House of Delegates. 10-25-2005. Available from the American Society of Anesthesiologists, http://www.asahg.org/publicationsAndServices/AwareAdvisoryFinalOct5.pdf Retrieved December 5, 2006.

64. Nasraway SA Jr, Wu EC, Kelleher RM, et al: How reliable is the bispectral index in critically ill patients? A prospective, comparative, single-blinded observer study. *Crit Care Med* 30:1483–1487, 2002.

65. Bruhn J, Bouillon TW, Shafer SL: Electromyographic activity falsely elevates the bispectral index. *Anesthesiology* 92:1485–1487, 2000.

66. Rampil IJ: A primer for EEG signal processing in anesthesia. *Anesthesiology* 89:980–1002, 1998.

67. Nuwer MR. *Evoked Potential Monitoring in the Operating Room.* New York, Raven, 1986.

68. Scheepstra GL, De Lange JJ, Booij LHD, et al: Median nerve evoked potentials during propofol anaesthesia. *Br J Anaesth* 62:92–94, 1989.

69. Pathak KS, Amaddio MD, Scoles PV, et al: Effects of halothane, enflurane, and isoflurane in nitrous oxide on multilevel somatosensory evoked potentials. *Anesthesiology* 70:207–212, 1989.

70. Sloan TB, Fugina ML, Toleikis JR: Effects of midazolam on median nerve somatosensory evoked potentials. *Br J Anaesth* 64:590–593, 1990.

71. Lotto ML, Banoub M, Schubert A: Effects of anesthetic agents and physiologic changes on intraoperative motor evoked potentials. *J Neurosurg Anesthesiol* 16:32–42, 2004.

72. Schwarz S, Hacke W, Schwab S: Magnetic evoked potentials in neurocritical care patients with acute brainstem lesions. *J Neurol Sci* 172:30–37, 2000.

73. Rohde V, Irle S, Hassler WE: Prediction of the post-comatose motor function by motor evoked potentials obtained in the acute phase of traumatic and nontraumatic coma. *Acta Neurochir* 141:841–848, 1999.

74. Lesser RP, Raudzens P, Luders H: Postoperative neurological deficits may occur despite unchanged intraoperative somatosensory evoked potentials. *Ann Neurol* 19:22–25, 1986.

75. Guerit JM: Medical technology assessment EEG and evoked potentials in the intensive care unit. *Neurophysiol Clin* 29:301–317, 1999.

76. Berkhoff M, Donati F, Bassetti C: Postanoxic alpha (theta) coma: a reappraisal of its prognostic significance. *Clin Neurophysiol* 111:297–304, 2000.

77. Madl C, Kramer L, Domanovits H, et al: Improved outcome prediction in unconscious cardiac arrest survivors with sensory evoked potentials compared with clinical assessment. *Crit Care Med* 28:721–726, 2000.

78. Marion DW, Spiegel TP: Changes in the management of severe traumatic brain injury: 1991–1997. *Crit Care Med* 28:16–18, 2000.

79. Bullock RM, Chesnut RM, Clifton GL, et al: Management and prognosis of severe traumatic brain injury. Part I. Guidelines for the management of severe traumatic brain injury. *J Neurotrauma* 17:449–553, 2000.

80. Bullock RM, Chesnut RM, Clifton GL, et al: Indications for intracranial pressure monitoring. *J Neurotrauma* 17:479–491, 2000.

81. Sahuquillo J, Poca MA, Arribas M, et al: Interhemispheric supratentorial intracranial pressure gradients in head-injured patients: are they clinically important? *J Neurosurg* 90:16–26, 1999.

82. Chambers IR, Kane PJ, Signorini DF, et al: Bilateral ICP monitoring: its importance in detecting the severity of secondary insults. *Acta Neurochir Suppl* 71:42–43, 1998.

83. Bullock RM, Chesnut RM, Clifton GL, et al: Recommendations for intracranial pressure monitoring technology. *J Neurotrauma* 17:497–506, 2000.

84. Munch E, Weigel R, Schmiedek P, et al: The Camino intracranial pressure device in clinical practice: reliability, handling characteristics and complications. *Acta Neurochir (Wien)* 140:1113–1119, 1998.

85. Crutchfield JS, Narayan RK, Robertson CS, et al: Evaluation of a fiberoptic intracranial pressure monitor. *J Neurosurg* 72:482–487, 1990.

86. Martinez-Manas RM, Santamarta D, de Campos JM, et al: Camino intracranial pressure monitor: prospective study of accuracy and complications. *J Neurol Neurosurg Psychiatry* 69:82–86, 2000.

87. Guyot LL, Dowling C, Diaz FG, et al: Cerebral monitoring devices: analysis of complications. *Acta Neurochir Suppl* 71:47–49, 1998.

88. Juul N, Morris GF, Marshall SB, et al: Intracranial hypertension and cerebral perfusion pressure: influence on neurological deterioration and outcome in severe head injury. *J Neurosurg* 92:1–6, 2000.

89. Ferring M, Berre J, Vincent JL: Induced hypertension after head injury. *Intensive Care Med* 25:1006–1009, 1999.

90. Robertson CS, Valadka AB, Hannay HJ, et al: Prevention of secondary ischemic insults after severe head injury. *Crit Care Med* 27:2086–2095, 1999.

91. Robertson CS: Management of cerebral perfusion pressure after traumatic brain injury. *Anesthesiology* 95:1513–1517, 2001.

92. Adelson PD, Bratton SL, Carney NA, et al: Guidelines for the acute medical management of severe traumatic brain injury in infants, children, and adolescents. Chapter 17. Critical pathway for the treatment of established intracranial hypertension in pediatric traumatic brain injury. *Pediatr Crit Care Med* 4:S65–S67, 2003.

93. Kety SS, Schmidt CF: The nitrous oxide method for the quantitative determination of cerebral blood flow in man: theory, procedure and normal values. *J Clin Invest* 27:476–483, 1948.

94. Olesen J, Paulson OB, Lassen NA: Regional cerebral blood flow in man determined by the initial slope of the clearance of intra-arterially injected 133Xe. Theory of the method, normal values, error of measurement, correction for remaining radioactivity, relation to other flow parameters and response to PaCO2 changes. *Stroke* 2:519–540, 1971.

95. Obrist WD, Thompson HK Jr, Wang HS, et al: Regional cerebral blood flow estimated by 133 Xenon inhalation. *Stroke* 6:245–256, 1975.

96. Tachibana H, Meyer JS, Okayasu H, et al: Changing topographic patterns of human cerebral blood flow with age measured by Xenon CT. *Am J Roentgenol* 142:1027–1034, 1984.

97. Latchaw RE: Cerebral perfusion imaging in acute stroke. *J Vasc Interv Radiol* 15:S29–S46, 2004.

98. Sase S, Honda M, Machida K, et al: Comparison of cerebral blood flow between perfusion computed tomography and xenon-enhanced computed tomography for normal subjects: territorial analysis. *J Comput Assist Tomogr* 29:270–277, 2005.

99. Bishop CCR, Powell S, Rutt D, et al: Transcranial Doppler measurement of middle cerebral artery blood flow velocity: a validation study. *Stroke* 17:913–915, 1986.

100. Lindegaard KF: The role of transcranial Doppler in the management of patients with subarachnoid haemorrhage—a review. *Acta Neurochir Suppl* 72:59–71, 1999.

101. Qureshi AI, Sung GY, Razumovsky AY, et al: Early identification of patients at risk for symptomatic vasospasm after aneurysmal subarachnoid hemorrhage. *Crit Care Med* 28:984–990, 2000.

102. Stocchetti N, Paparella A, Bridelli F, et al: Cerebral venous oxygen saturation studied with bilateral samples in the internal jugular veins. *Neurosurgery* 34:38–44, 1994.

103. Lam JMK, Chan MSY, Poon WS: Cerebral venous oxygen saturation monitoring: is dominant jugular bulb cannulation good enough? *Br J Neurosurg* 10:357–364, 1996.

104. Gibbs EL, Gibbs FA: The cross section areas of the vessels that form the torcula and the manner in which flow is distributed to the right and to the left lateral sinus. *Anat Rec* 59:419–426, 1934.

105. Andrews PJD, Dearden NM, Miller JD: Jugular bulb cannulation: description of a cannulation technique and validation of a new continuous monitor. *Br J Anaesth* 67:553–558, 1991.

106. Metz C, Holzschuh M, Bein T, et al: Monitoring of cerebral oxygen metabolism in the jugular bulb: reliability of unilateral measurements in severe head injury. *J Cereb Blood Flow Metab* 18:332–343, 1998.

107. Gupta AK, Hutchinson PJ, Al-Rawi P, et al: Measuring brain tissue oxygenation compared with jugular venous oxygen saturation for monitoring cerebral oxygenation after traumatic brain injury. *Anesth Analg* 88:549–553, 1999.

108. Sheinberg M, Kanter MJ, Robertson CS, et al: Continuous monitoring of jugular venous oxygen saturation in head-injured patients. *J Neurosurg* 76:212–217, 1992.

109. Gopinath SP, Robertson CS, Contant CF, et al: Jugular venous desaturation and outcome after head injury. *J Neurol Neurosurg Psychiatry* 57:717–723, 1994.

110. Coplin WM, O'Keefe GE, Grady MS, et al: Thrombotic, infectious, and procedural complications of the jugular bulb catheter in the intensive care unit. *Neurosurgery* 41:101–109, 1997.

111. Cruz J, Jaggi JL, Hoffstad OJ: Cerebral blood flow and oxygen consumption in acute brain injury with acute anemia: an alternative for the cerebral metabolic rate of oxygen consumption? *Crit Care Med* 21:1218–1224, 1993.

112. Zauner A, Doppenberg EMR, Woodward JJ, et al: Continuous monitoring of cerebral substrate delivery and clearance: initial experience in 24 patients with severe acute brain injuries. *Neurosurgery* 41:1082–1093, 1997.

113. van den Brink WA, van Santbrink H, Steyerberg EW, et al: Brain oxygen tension in severe head injury. *Neurosurgery* 46:868–878, 2000.

114. Unterberg AW, Kiening KL, Härtl R, et al: Multimodal monitoring in patients with head injury: evaluation of the effects of treatment on cerebral oxygenation. *J Trauma* 42:S32–S37, 1997.

115. Gopinath SP, Valadka AB, Uzura M, et al: Comparison of jugular venous oxygen saturation and brain tissue PO2 as monitors of cerebral ischemia after head injury. *Crit Care Med* 27:2337–2345, 1999.

116. Hillered L, Persson L, Ponten U: Neurometabolic monitoring of the ischaemic human brain using microdialysis. *Acta Neurochir* 102:91–97, 1990.

117. Landolt H, Langemann H, Alessandri B: A concept for the introduction of cerebral microdialysis in neurointensive care. *Acta Neurochir Suppl* 67:31–36, 1996.

118. Mazzeo AT, Bullock R: Effect of bacterial meningitis complicating severe head trauma upon brain microdialysis and cerebral perfusion. *Neurocrit Care* 2:282–287, 2005.

119. Bullock R, Zauner A, Woodward JJ, et al: Factors affecting excitatory amino acid release following severe human head injury. *J Neurosurg* 89:507–518, 1998.

120. Nilsson OG, Brandt L, Ungerstedt U, et al: Bedside detection of brain ischemia using intracerebral microdialysis: subarachnoid hemorrhage and delayed ischemic deterioration. *Neurosurgery* 45:1176–1185, 1999.

121. Sarrafzadeh AS, Sakowitz OW, Kiening KL, et al: Bedside microdialysis: a tool to monitor cerebral metabolism in subarachnoid hemorrhage patients? *Crit Care Med* 30:1062–1070, 2002.

122. Bellander BM, Cantais E, Enblad P, et al: Consensus meeting on microdialysis in neurointensive care. *Intensive Care Med* 30:2166–2169, 2004.

123. Johnston AJ, Gupta AK: Advanced monitoring in the neurology intensive care unit: microdialysis. *Cur Opin Crit Care* 8:121–127, 2002.

124. Peerdeman SM, Girbes AR, Vandertop WP: Cerebral microdialysis as a new tool for neurometabolic monitoring. *Intensive Care Med* 26:662–669, 2000.

125. Hillered L, Persson L, Carlson H, et al: Excitatory amino acids: basic pharmacology to clinical evaluation. *Clin Neuropharmacol* 15:695–696, 1992.

126. Pollard V, Prough DS. Cebral Oxygenation: Near-infrared spectroscopy, in Tobin MJ (ed): *Principles and Practice of Intensive Care Monitoring.* New York, McGraw-Hill, 1998, pp 1019–1033.

127. Ferrari M, Mottola L, Quaresima V: Principles, techniques, and limitations of near infrared spectroscopy. *Can J Appl Physiol* 29:463–487, 2004.

128. Delpy DT, Cope M, Cady EB, et al: Cerebral monitoring in newborn infants by magnetic resonance and near infrared spectroscopy. *Scand J Clin Lab Invest Suppl* 188:9–17, 1987.

129. Delpy DT, Cope M, van der Zee P, et al: Estimation of optical path length through tissue from direct time of flight measurement. *Phys Med Biol* 33:1433–1442, 1988.

130. Pollard V, Prough DS, DeMelo AE, et al: Validation in volunteers of a near-infrared spectroscope for monitoring brain oxygenation in vivo. *Anesth Analg* 82:269–277, 1996.

131. Nicklin SE, Hassan IA-A, Wickramasinghe YA, et al: The light still shines, but not that brightly? the current status of perinatal near infrared spectroscopy. *Arch Dis Child* 88:F263–F268, 2003.

132. Villringer A, Planck J, Hock C, et al: Near infrared spectroscopy (NIRS): a new tool to study hemodynamic changes during activation of brain function in human adults. *Neurosci Lett* 154:101–104, 1993.

133. Unterberg A, Rosenthal A, Schneider GH, et al. Validation of monitoring of cerebral oxygenation by near-infrared spectroscopy in comatose patients, in Tasubokawa T, Marmarou A, Robertson C, et al (eds): *Neurochemical Monitoring in the Intensive Care Unit.* New York, Springer-Verlag, 1995, pp 204–210.

134. Pollard V, DeMelo AE, Deyo DJ, et al: The influence of position change on near-infrared spectroscopic assessment of cerebral hemoglobin desaturation. *Anesthesiology* 81:A530, 1994.

135. Henson LC, Calalang C, Temp JA, et al: Accuracy of a cerebral oximeter in healthy volunteers under conditions of isocapnic hypoxia. *Anesthesiology* 88:58–65, 1998.

136. Petrov YY, Prough DS, Deyo DJ, et al: Optoacoustic, noninvasive, real-time, continuous monitoring of cerebral blood oxygenation: an in vivo study in sheep. *Anesthesiology* 102:69–75, 2005.

137. Newberg AB, Alavi A: Neuroimaging in patients with head injury. *Semin Nucl Med* 33:136–147, 2003.

138. Marshall LF, Marshall SB, Klauber MR, et al: A new classification of head injury based on computerized tomography. *J Neurosurg* 75:S14–S20, 1991.

139. Narayan RK, Kishore PRS, Becker DP, et al: Intracranial pressure: to monitor or not to monitor? A review of our experience with severe head injury. *J Neurosurg* 56:650–659, 1982.

140. Lobato RD, Sarabia R, Cordobes F, et al: Posttraumatic cerebral hemispheric swelling. Analysis of 55 cases studied with computerized tomography. *J Neurosurg* 68:417–423, 1988.

141. Eisenberg HM, Gary HE Jr, Aldrich EF, et al: Initial CT findings in 753 patients with severe head injury. A report from the NIH Traumatic Coma Data Bank. *J Neurosurg* 73:688–698, 1990.

142. Kemp GJ: Non-invasive methods for studying brain energy metabolism: what they show and what it means. *Dev Neurosci* 22:418–428, 2000.

143. Watson NA, Beards SC, Altaf N, et al: The effect of hyperoxia on cerebral blood flow: a study in healthy volunteers using magnetic resonance phase-contrast angiography. *Eur J Anaesthesiol* 17:152–159, 2000.

144. Zaharchuk G, Mandeville JB, Bogdanov AA Jr., et al: Cerebrovascular dynamics of autoregulation and hypoperfusion. An MRI study of CBF and changes in total and microvascular cerebral blood volume during hemorrhagic hypotension. *Stroke* 30:2197–2205, 1999.

145. Verweij BH, Muizelaar P, Vinas FC, et al: Impaired cerebral mitochondrial function after traumatic brain injury in humans. *J Neurosurg* 93:815–820, 2000.

146. Chan KH, Dearden NM, Miller JD, et al: Multimodality monitoring as a guide to treatment of intracranial hypertension after severe brain injury. *Neurosurgery* 32:547–553, 1993.

147. De Georgia MA, Deogaonkar A: Multimodal monitoring in the neurological intensive care unit. *Neurologist* 11:45–54, 2005.

148. Elf K, Nilsson P, Enblad P: Outcome after traumatic brain injury improved by an organized secondary insult program and standardized neurointensive care. *Crit Care Med* 30:2129–2134, 2003.

Achikam Oren-Grinberg
Adam B. Lerner
Daniel Talmor

CHAPTER **31**

Echocardiography in the Intensive Care Unit

Echocardiography was introduced to the operating suite in the 1970s, with epicardial echocardiography as its initial application. Transesophageal echocardiography (TEE) during surgery was first described in 1980 but did not become commonplace until the mid-1980s. Since then, TEE has evolved to become a widely used and versatile modality for diagnosis and monitoring of critically ill patients. As such, its use has expanded into the perioperative period and the intensive care unit (ICU). Echocardiography provides both anatomic and functional information about the heart; systolic and diastolic function, cavity size, and valvular function [1].

Ease of utilization, availability of diagnostic information within 10 to 15 minutes from the start of examination, high quality imaging in most patients, and low complication rates have all led to the pervasive use of echocardiography in the perioperative environment and increasing use in the ICU [2–8]. However, patient safety and optimal outcome depend heavily on a thorough understanding of both the strengths and limitations of the available technologies and their applications.

INDICATIONS AND GUIDELINES

The role of TEE has evolved and expanded, leading to the need for standardization of indications and practice. A task force created in 1993 conducted a literature review of 558 studies in search of evidence for the effectiveness of TEE in the perioperative setting. Three years later, the American Society of Anesthesiologists (ASA) and the Society of Cardiovascular Anesthesiologists (SCA) published guidelines regarding the indications for TEE [9]. Three categories of evidence-based clinical indications were identified. For indications grouped into category I, TEE was judged to be *frequently* useful in improving clinical outcomes. To date there is only a single category I indication for TEE in the ICU. That indication is for "unstable patients with unexplained hemodynamic disturbance, suspected valve disease, or thromboembolic problems (if other tests or monitoring techniques have not confirmed the diagnosis or patients are too unstable to undergo other tests)"[9]. This indication, however, encompasses a significant proportion of ICU patients.

As TEE utilization in the perioperative setting became more widespread, the need for consistency in imaging acquisition became increasingly evident. In 1999, the joint task force of the American Society of Echocardiography (ASE) and SCA pub-

lished guidelines defining a comprehensive cardiac exam using TEE [10]. Specifically, these guidelines defined a set of cross-sectional views and nomenclature that constitute a comprehensive intraoperative TEE examination. It is important to note that occasional deviation from the guidelines is needed in order to acquire optimum imaging. The expectation was that "the guidelines may enhance quality improvement by providing means to assess the technical quality and completeness of individual studies" and that "more consistent acquisition and description of intraoperative echocardiographic data will facilitate communication between centers and provide a basis for multicenter investigations" [10].

BASIC TERMINOLOGY OF ECHOCARDIOGRAPHY TECHNIQUES

A sonographer must use different echocardiographic imaging techniques and hemodynamic modalities in order to achieve a diagnosis or management plan. The following is a list of the basic techniques used during an echocardiographic study.

TWO-DIMENSIONAL ECHOCARDIOGRAPHY

Two-dimensional (2D) echocardiography is the backbone of the echocardiographic exam [11]. Using 2D, a complete visualization of the beating heart is achieved by displaying anatomic structures in real time tomographic images. By aiming the ultrasound probe at the heart, exactly oriented anatomic "slices" are obtained. Information acquired includes cardiac chamber sizes, global and regional systolic function, and valvular anatomy.

M-MODE ECHOCARDIOGRAPHY

M-mode or motion-mode images are a continuous one-dimensional graphic display that can be derived by selecting any of the individual sector lines from which a 2D image is constructed [11]. It is useful for quantification of myocardial wall and chambers sizes, which in turn can be used to estimate left ventricle (LV) mass and chamber volumes, respectively. In addition, since it has high temporal resolution, M-mode is helpful in assessing the motion of rapidly moving cardiac structures such as cardiac valves.

DOPPLER ECHOCARDIOGRAPHY

Doppler echocardiography is used to supplement 2D and M-mode echocardiography. It can provide functional information regarding intracardiac hemodynamics; systolic and diastolic flows, blood velocities and volumes, severity of valvular lesions, location and severity of intracardiac shunts, and assessment of diastolic function. The four types of Doppler modalities used include continuous-wave, pulsed-wave, color flow mapping, and tissue Doppler [11]. Continuous-wave Doppler is used for measuring high pressure gradient/high velocity flows such as seen in aortic stenosis. When using continuous-wave Doppler, the ultrasound probe continuously transmits and receives sound waves. This increases the maximum limit of blood velocity that can be evaluated before exceeding the Nyquist limit. The Nyquist limit represents the maximum flow velocity that can be evaluated by Doppler and is dependent on both equipment and imaging variables. Continuous-wave Doppler can evaluate higher flows but does so at the expense of spatial specificity. Pulsed-wave Doppler is used for measuring lower pressure gradient/lower velocity flows such as in mitral stenosis. In this mode, the ultrasound probe sends out a pulse of sound and then waits to receive reflected waves. This lowers the Nyquist limit and the maximum velocities that can be interrogated but allows for precise spatial resolution. Color flow mapping is useful for screening valves for stenosis or regurgitation, quantifying the degree of valvular regurgitation, imaging systolic and diastolic flow, and detection of intracardiac shunts. Doppler tissue imaging has been introduced as a new method of quantifying segmental and global left ventricular function. It records systolic and diastolic velocities within the myocardium and at the corners of the mitral annulus and is useful for studying diastolic function and contractile asynchrony of the left ventricle.

CONTRAST ECHOCARDIOGRAPHY

Contrast echocardiography is used to enhance the diagnostic quality of the echocardiogram [12]. It may be used to improve assessment of global function and regional wall motion abnormalities by 2D echocardiography. Although approved only for LV opacification, recent clinical studies suggest a potential use in assessing myocardial perfusion [13,14].

ECHOCARDIOGRAPHY COMPARED WITH TRADITIONAL MONITORING IN THE INTENSIVE CARE UNIT

For almost four decades, the pulmonary artery catheter (PAC) has been used as a mainstay of patient monitoring in the ICU setting. It provides direct information on pressure variables such as pulmonary artery pressure, pulmonary artery wedge pressure (PAWP), and central venous pressure. It can also provide flow related data such as cardiac output (CO) and mixed venous oxygen saturation. From these data, other hemodynamic variables, such as systemic vascular resistance, pulmonary vascular resistance, and stroke volume can be calculated. Despite its extensive use (more than 1.5 million PACs inserted annually in North America), the clinical value of data obtained from pulmonary artery catheters remains unproven [15]. One of the major drawbacks of the pressure measurements obtained from

PACs is the inability to definitively relate these measurements to intravascular and cardiac chamber volumes. This is due mainly to inter- and intrapatient variability of myocardial compliance. Early studies of the use of PAC in surgical patients yielded inconsistent results. While some studies demonstrated decreased mortality [16–18], others showed no effect [19,20]. In contrast, other studies demonstrated increased morbidity and mortality [21,22]. Two systematic reviews that included a mixed population of surgical and medical patients and patients with myocardial infarction demonstrated no overall benefit and increased morbidity and mortality from the use of PAC [23,24]. Finally, a recent randomized, prospective study of nearly 2,000 patients found no benefit to therapy directed by PAC in high-risk surgical patients requiring intensive care [15].

Hemodynamic optimization is a complex task requiring, among other things, monitoring of arterial and venous pressures, urine output, acid-base balance, and oxygen content/delivery. These parameters, however, reflect the overall circulatory state and not the basic physiologic determinants of CO, which include preload, afterload, and contractility. In many conditions, such as with pericardial and pleural effusions, pulmonary embolism, and valvular pathologies, current invasive monitors provide only minimal and indirect information to facilitate satisfactory management. In addition, the current monitoring modalities provide little to no information for assessment of ventricular compliance and relaxation. At present, echocardiography is the only method that can provide real-time bedside imaging of the heart [25,26]. It allows for the assessment of LV systolic and diastolic function, measurement of CO, and reliable assessment of other hemodynamic variables such as pulmonary artery pressure and PAWP [27]. Data obtained from TEE examination frequently differ from PAC assessments of LV preload and systolic function and, when used, can lead to a change in therapy in 40% to 60% of patients [7,28].

TRANSESOPHAGEAL VERSUS TRANSTHORACIC ECHOCARDIOGRAPHY

Although transthoracic echocardiography (TTE) is a less invasive way to image cardiac structures, suboptimal acoustic windows lead to low-quality images in many critically ill patients. These suboptimal acoustic windows are due to obesity, pulmonary disease, the presence of chest tubes, drains and wound dressings, and limitations on patient positioning. Using TTE in the ICU can be challenging; one report found the echocardiographic examination to be inadequate in approximately 50% of patients on mechanical ventilation and 60% of all ICU patients [8]. The relatively low percentage of adequate imaging improves when TTE is used as a *monitoring tool*, which does not require the same quality of images, and not as a diagnostic tool. In a report of more than 200 ICU patients, TTE used as a monitoring tool provided 2D images of acceptable quality in 97% of patients [25].

In contrast to transthoracic echocardiography, TEE is more invasive but consistently provides images of better quality. In up to 40% of patients, TEE may provide additional unexpected diagnoses that are missed by TTE [4,29]. Recent advances in ultrasound imaging, which include harmonic imaging, digital acquisition, and contrast endocardial enhancement, have improved the diagnostic yield of TEE [30,31]. TEE may also be used as a continuous monitor of heart function and, when indicated, the probe can be left in the esophagus or stomach for several hours.

CONTRAINDICATIONS TO PERFORMING TRANSESOPHAGEAL ECHOCARDIOGRAPHY

Although TEE is safe [32,33], there are several contraindications to probe insertion. These include significant esophageal or gastric pathology, mass or tumors, strictures, diverticulum, Mallory-Weiss tears, recent esophageal or gastric surgery, upper GI bleeding, and dysphagia or odynophagia not previously evaluated. Esophageal varices are not an absolute contraindication, and a risk/benefit analysis of each case must be done before performing TEE in any individual patient [34]. Practitioners must be aware of the potential for severe bleeding, in particular when a coagulation abnormality exists. Cervical spinal injury is another relative contraindication requiring careful risk/benefit analysis.

COMPLICATIONS AND SAFETY OF TRANSESOPHAGEAL ECHOCARDIOGRAPHY

TEE is considered a moderately invasive procedure and complications are rare. In one study of ICU patients, complication rates reached 1.6% and included hypotension following sedation for probe insertion, oropharyngeal bleeding in a coagulopathic patient, and aspiration during tracheal intubation performed prior to TEE [33]. Another study in 2,508 ICU patients reported a complication rate of 2.6%. In this study, as would be expected, there was no examination related mortality. Complications included transient hypotension or hypertension, circulatory deterioration, hypoxemia, arrhythmias, vomiting, coughing, superficial mucous membrane lesions, displacement of a tracheostomy tube, and accidental removal of a duodenal feeding tube [32]. A large European multicenter study of 10,419 exams reported a complication rate of 2.5% with one (0.01%) case of fatal hematemesis due to a malignant tumor [2]. In addition, in 0.88% of the reported cases, the TEE exam had to be prematurely terminated due either to patient intolerance or because of cardiac, pulmonary, or bleeding events [2].

COMMON INDICATIONS FOR TRANSESOPHAGEAL ECHOCARDIOGRAPHY IN THE INTENSIVE CARE UNIT

As mentioned, the only current category I indication for the performance of TEE in the ICU setting is in "unstable patients with unexplained hemodynamic disturbances, suspected valve disease, or thromboembolic problems (if other tests or monitoring techniques have not confirmed the diagnosis or patients are too unstable to undergo other tests)" [9]. In practice, however, clinicians use echocardiography in the ICU for many other indications. These are summarized in Table 31-1.

TABLE 31-1. Common Indications for Performing Transthoracic Echocardiography in the Intensive Care Unit

Assessment of left ventricle systolic function	Evaluation of valvular pathology
Hemodynamic management	Determination of source of emboli
Evaluation of pericardial tamponade	Evaluation of endocarditis
Evaluation of pulmonary embolism	Evaluation of chest trauma
Evaluation of aortic dissection	Evaluation of hypoxemia

ECHOCARDIOGRAPHY AS A HEMODYNAMIC MONITOR IN THE INTENSIVE CARE UNIT

Managing the hemodynamically unstable patient in the ICU remains an often challenging and time-consuming exercise. Echocardiography can be used effectively as a monitoring tool for management of these complex ICU patients. The FATE protocol is a relatively easy to use and efficient protocol for monitoring patients in the ICU [25]. The FATE examination is a rapid echocardiographic assessment performed to screen for significant pathology and obtain information about the volume and contractility of the heart. The steps of the protocol include [25]:

1. Excluding obvious pathology
2. Assessing wall thickness and chamber dimensions
3. Assessing contractility
4. Visualizing the pleura on both sides
5. Relating the information to the clinical context

The exam can be performed by physicians with only limited training in echocardiography. It requires imaging the heart and pleura in the most favorable sequence from one or more tomographic planes [25]. Different Doppler modalities can be used as needed to calculate CO, assess valvular pathologies, and to measure a variety of hemodynamic variables. Although it is possible to terminate the protocol once the clinical question has been answered, it is recommended that all imaging positions be obtained because of the possibility of further disorders that would otherwise be missed (Fig. 31-1).

Although the FATE protocol was described for TTE, its principles are readily applied to TEE as well. This systematic approach allows for a rapid assessment of myocardial load conditions, dimensions, and contractility and promotes the ability to properly diagnose and intervene expeditiously. The protocol has been shown to be a practical and useful hemodynamic monitoring tool in ICU patients. A study of the FATE protocol demonstrated that it added new information in 37.3% of patients and contributed decisive information in 24.5% of the patients. Only in 2.6% of the exams performed was the information too limited to aid in patient management [25]. These findings and other reports support the benefit of TEE exam when performed by a noncardiologist in the ICU [28,35–37].

ECHOCARDIOGRAPHIC EVALUATION OF HEMODYNAMIC INSTABILITY

Hemodynamic instability is an extremely common event in every ICU. Determining the cause of such can sometimes be more challenging than one would expect. Echocardiography can be used successfully in the diagnosis, monitoring, and management

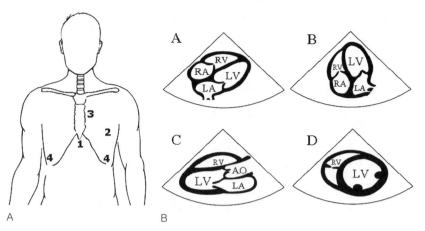

FIGURE 31-1. The FATE protocol. **A**: Transducer position; (1) subcostal view; (2) apical view; (3) parasternal view; (4) pleural view. **B**: Schematic drawing of the four most important image planes as they appear on the monitor during TTE. (A) Subcostal four-champer view (position 1). (B) Apical four chamber view (position 2). (C) Parasternal long-axis view (position 3). (D) Parasternal short-axis view (position 3). AO, aorta; LA, left ventricle; RA, right atrium; RV, right ventricle. [From Dr. Eric Sloth, Department of Anaesthesiology, Skejby Sygehus, Aarhus University Hospital, Denmark, with permission.]

of the unstable patient in the ICU. Using echocardiography to determine the etiology of hemodynamic instability requires assessment of cardiac function, volume status, valvular function, and extra-cardiac processes.

Assessment of Cardiac Function

Systolic dysfunction of either ventricular chamber must be considered in every unstable patient. The etiology of dysfunction may oftentimes be discerned from the echocardiographic evaluation allowing for appropriate therapy to be initiated.

Assessment of Left Ventricular Systolic Function

Utilization of several echocardiographic assessment modalities is necessary for evaluation of left ventricular systolic function. These modalities include quantitative as well as qualitative assessments.

QUANTITATIVE ASSESSMENT OF LEFT VENTRICULAR SYSTOLIC FUNCTION

Volumetric Method Utilizing Geometric Models. Quantitative assessment of left ventricular systolic function relies on volume assessment using 2D tomographic images. To determine the volume at end diastole (LVEDV) and end systole (LVESV), the endocardial borders in one or more tomographic planes are traced at end diastole and end systole. Several geometric assumptions and formulas have been developed (e.g., truncated ellipse, "bullet" formula, cylinder, and cone) to determine the LVEDV and LVESV based on these 2D images. Once LVEDV and LVESV have been determined, the stoke volume, and thus cardiac output can be calculated:

$$SV = LVEDV - LVESV$$
$$CO = SV \times HR$$

In addition, ejection fraction can be calculated from these volumes using the formula:

$$EF = SV/LVEDV \times 100\%$$

The advantage of the geometric assumption techniques is that they require only limited visualization for calculation of ventricular volumes. However, these formulas work only in a symmetrically contracting ventricle; the presence of regional wall motion abnormalities decreases their accuracy. In addition, foreshortening of the LV cavity is a common source of underestimation

of LV end diastolic and end systolic volumes and can similarly impact the accuracy of systolic function assessment with these formulas [1,38]. Finally, since the models depend on accurate endocardial border definition, their use requires adequate visualization. Incomplete endocardial definition is described in 10% to 20% of routine echocardiographic studies [39] and may reach 25% in ICU patients [40]. This challenge is even greater in patients requiring mechanical ventilation in which imaging can be particularly challenging. These challenges have limited the utilization of the geometric models and formulas for assessment of LV systolic function.

Discs Method (Simpson's Rule). Another method for volumetric assessment of LV systolic function is the discs method, which may be more accurate than the other volumetric methods described above, particularly in the presence of distorted LV geometry [41]. In this method the ventricle is divided into a series of discs of equal height and each disc volume is calculated as follows: Disc volume = disc height × disc area. The ventricular volume can be calculated from the sum of the volumes. This technique requires true apical images, which in clinical practice may be difficult to achieve. Foreshortening of the ventricular apex will result in inaccurate assessment of the left ventricular ejection fraction and cardiac output (Fig. 31-2).

QUALITATIVE ASSESSMENT OF LEFT VENTRICULAR SYSTOLIC FUNCTION

2D Evaluation of Ventricular Systolic Function. Using 2D imaging, two of the most important questions regarding hemodynamic stability can be rapidly answered: Are the ventricles contracting well and are they adequately filled? Using 2D, an experienced observer can qualitatively evaluate systolic function. This should be assessed from multiple tomographic planes, and attention must be made to obtaining adequate endocardial definition. Normal ventricular contraction consists of simultaneous myocardial thickening and endocardial excursion toward the center of the ventricle. It is important to look for this myocardial thickening; infarcted myocardium may be pulled inward by surrounding, normal myocardium. There is some regional heterogeneity of normal wall motion with the proximal lateral and inferolateral (or posterior) walls contracting somewhat later than the septum and inferior wall [42]. For qualitative assessment of overall systolic function, the echocardiographer integrates the degree of wall thickening and endocardial motion in all tomographic views and reaches a conclusion about overall LV systolic

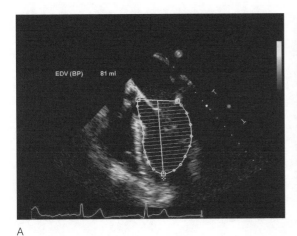

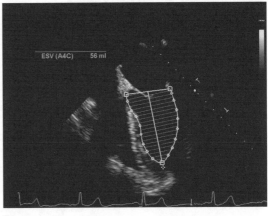

A   B

FIGURE 31-2.   Calculation of cardiac output using the disc method (Simpson's rule). TEE midesophageal four-chamber view in diastole **(A)** and systole **(B)** is shown. Using Simpson's rule, LVEDV (81 mL) and LVESV (56 mL) were calculated by the echocardiographic computer. From these volumes the cardiac output was calculated to be 1.7 L/min (81 mL – 56 mL) × 69 beats per minute.

function and ejection fraction (EF). Although different institutions use different standards, severe LV systolic dysfunction is usually defined as an EF less than 30%, moderate dysfunction 30% to 45%, mild depression 45% to 55%, and normal greater than 55%. This method of EF estimation is of great clinical utility and can be performed with good correlation to quantitative measurements. There are, however, a few potential pitfalls to 2D assessment of EF that must be considered:

Accurate assessment requires satisfactory endocardial border definition. Qualitative EF estimation becomes inaccurate when the endocardium is inadequately defined.

Accurate estimation of EF depends on the experience of the echocardiographer.

In asynchronous contraction (paced-rhythm, conduction defects, etc.), assessment of EF is more difficult.

Despite its limitations, 2D qualitative assessment is the most widely used technique for assessment of LV systolic function due to its ease of application in the clinical setting. In the operating room, after completing the TEE exam, most physicians monitor LV systolic function continuously with 2D imaging using the transgastric (TG) midpapillary short-axis view. This allows for quick assessment of regional wall motion abnormalities in all coronary arterial circulatory beds as well as rudimentary evaluation of volume status [43]. However, it is important to remember that this view alone is never satisfactory for assessing overall systolic function.

Regional Left Ventricular Function

Most commonly, abnormal regional wall motion is the result of coronary artery disease and resultant ischemia/infarction. Abnormal wall motion is a continuum of conditions consisting of hypokinesis, akinesis, and dyskinesis. With dyskinesis, the affected wall segment moves away from the center of the ventricle during systole. In order to standardize echocardiographic evaluations of wall motion, a 17-segment model of the LV has been defined [42]. These 17 segments are evaluated separately for the presence and degree of regional wall motion abnormality. When the etiology of the wall motion abnormality is coronary artery disease, the location of the coronary lesion can usually be

predicted from the location of the regional wall motion abnormality.

Contrast Echocardiography

Recent innovations have been made to overcome some of the technical obstacles related to endocardial border detection and image quality. Intravenous echocardiographic contrast agents that opacify the left side of the heart can markedly improve visualization of the LV cavity and enhance endocardial definition. These agents can aid assessment of regional and global LV function [44–47]. They also have the potential to "salvage" nondiagnostic TTEs in ICU patients. One study demonstrated a "salvage" rate of 51% [48], and another 77% of nondiagnostic TTEs [49]. Optison™, a sonicated Perfluoron propane-filled albumin microsphere contrast, and other similar agents have been used safely to improve endocardial border visualization [45,50]. In addition to improving visualization and assessment of LV function, assessment of myocardial perfusion defects with intravenous contrast has been reported with a variety of imaging techniques and modalities [51–53].

Doppler Assessment of Left Ventricular Systolic Function. Doppler spectral profiles can be used to quantitatively evaluate left ventricular function. This evaluation of left ventricular systolic function is based on calculation of stroke volume (SV) and cardiac output (CO). SV is the volume of blood ejected during each cardiac cycle and is a key indicator of cardiac performance. SV can be calculated by using pulse wave Doppler (PWD) to measure the instantaneous blood velocity recorded during systole from an area in the heart where a cross-sectional area (CSA) can be easily determined. The left ventricular outflow track (LVOT) is most commonly used because its cross section is essentially a circle. By measuring the diameter of the LVOT and assuming a circular geometry, the CSA is calculated as $\pi(D/2)^2$. Any cardiac chamber or structure that has a measurable CSA may be used; mitral valve annulus, right ventricular outflow tract and tricuspid annulus are examples. By tracing the outline of the PWD profile, the echocardiographic computer can calculate the integral of velocity by time or the velocity time integral (VTI). The VTI is the distance (commonly

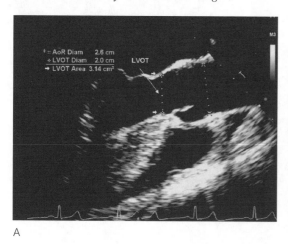
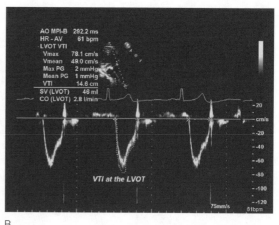

FIGURE 31-3. Calculation of CO using spectral Doppler approach. **A:** Midesophageal long axis view of LVOT. LVOT measurement is 2.0 cm. The CSA is calculated as $\pi(D/2)^2$, 3.14 cm^2 in this example. **B:** Transgastric long axis view using pulsed wave Doppler beam directed parallel to flow through the LVOT. By tracing the outer envelope of the spectral signal, VTI is calculated as 14.6 cm in this example. SV is the product of CSA and VTI: $3.14 \times 14.6 = 46$ mL. CO = SV × HR: $46 \times 61 = 2.8$ L/min.

referred as the *stroke distance*) that the average red cell has traveled during the systolic ejection phase. SV (cm^3) is then calculated by multiplying the VTI (stroke distance in cm) by the CSA in cm^2 of the conduit (i.e., LVOT, aorta, mitral valve annulus, pulmonary artery) through which the blood has traveled [54–60]; SV = CSA × VTI. CO is then easily derived by multiplying the calculated SV by the heart rate: CO (cm^3/min) = SV × HR (Fig. 31-3).

This approach to SV and CO calculations has shown very good correlation with thermodilution-derived cardiac output measurements [61]. There are several potential sources of error:

1. CSA determination often leads to the greatest source of error. When using any diameter for CSA determination, any error in measurement will be squared (CSA = $\pi(D/2)^2$). This translates to a 20% error in calculation of cardiac output for each 2-mm error when measuring a 2.0-cm diameter LV outflow tract [42]. Studies have shown that while the Doppler velocity curves can be recorded consistently with little interobserver measurement variability (2% to 5%), the variability in 2D LVOT diameter measurements for CSA is significantly greater (8% to 12%) [62].

2. The Doppler signal is assumed to have been recorded at a parallel or near parallel intercept angle, called θ, to blood flow. The Doppler equation has a cos θ term in its denominator. With an intercept angle of 0°, the cos θ term equals 1. Deviations up to 20 degrees in intercept angle are acceptable since only a 6% error in measurement is introduced.

3. Velocity and diameter measurements should be made at the same anatomic site. When the two are measured at different places the accuracy of SV and CO calculations are decreased.

4. While the pattern of flow is assumed to be laminar, in reality the flow profile is parabolic. This does have some impact on velocity based calculations [42]. However, in routine clinical practice this factor is of little significance and can be essentially ignored.

Determination of Left Ventricular dP/dt. The changing rate of left ventricular pressure (dP/dt) is an important parameter in the assessment of myocardial systolic function. Traditionally, dP/dt was derived from the left ventricular pressure curve acquired at cardiac catheterization using a micromanometer catheter recording. It has been shown that echocardiography can be used accurately and reliably to assess dP/dt by performing Doppler assessment of mitral regurgitant jet [63,64]. Using continuous wave Doppler, a spectral display of the mitral regurgitation jet is obtained. From the spectral display, information about the rate of pressure development within the left ventricle can be derived using measurements undertaken in the early phase of systole (the upstroke of the velocity curve is used for calculations). Determination of dP/dt using the mitral regurgitation spectral jet is done by calculation of the time required for the MR jet velocity to go from 1 msec to 3 msec. The time between these two points represents the time that it takes for a 32 mm Hg pressure change to occur in the left ventricular cavity. This is based on the modified Bernoulli equation ($P = 4v^2$), which relates pressure to velocity. Thus, in going from 1 msec to 3 msec:

$$P = 4v^2_B - 4v^2_A(4(3^2) - 4(1^2) = 32),$$

where V_B is velocity of 3 msec and V_A is velocity of 1 msec. dP/dt is then calculated using the formula:

$$dP/dt = 32 \text{ mm Hg} \div \text{time (seconds)}.$$

A depressed ventricle will take a longer time to develop this pressure gradient, and thus a lower dP/dt.

Assessment of Patient Volume Status

LEFT VENTRICULAR PRELOAD. Preload is defined as the myocardial fiber length at end diastole [61]. LVEDV is one of several clinical variables used to assess preload. Accurate preload estimation is one of the main challenges faced when caring for critically ill patients, even to the most experienced physician. Traditionally, preload has been assessed using physical examination, clinical assessment of end-organ perfusion, and direct measurement of intravascular pressures. Echocardiography can be used efficiently to supplement clinical assessment.

2D Echo Method. LV diameter measured with 2D echo can be used to extrapolate LV volume at end diastole, and thus estimate preload. These measurements can be compared with published estimates of normal ventricular dimensions to define degrees of ventricular enlargement. A single measurement, however, is of limited value in defining the preload state of any given patient. A patient with a history of cardiomyopathy, as an example, will have an increased LV end-diastolic diameter compared to a normal patient. To define such a patient as having adequate or excess preload is not justifiable. Serial measurements of LV diameter are more useful clinically in assessing changes over time and in response to therapies such as intravenous fluid challenge or diuresis. A number of studies that have compared echocardiographic estimates of preload with pulmonary artery occlusion pressure (PAOP) have shown the potential superiority of the echocardiographic method [65–67]. This method seems to perform well in detecting decreased end-diastolic volumes and hypovolemia. However, when used to diagnose high preload or fluid overload, they may not be as reliable [61]. In the operating room, both end-diastolic areas and volumes correlated well with thermodilution cardiac index in patients undergoing coronary artery bypass grafting [68] and liver transplantation [69], while PAWP showed no correlation.

Pulsed Wave Doppler Method. Preload estimation can be assessed by Doppler echocardiography. The velocity profile of blood flow through the mitral valve during diastole is normally biphasic. In a young individual with normal LV compliance and relaxation, the early, passive filling phase, represented by the E wave, exceeds the component of filling due to atrial contraction, represented by the A wave. The magnitude of theses flows and their ratio vary with age in normal individuals [42] (Fig. 31-4).

Using the peak *E/A velocity* ratio, LV end diastolic pressure (LVEDP) can be roughly estimated. With this technique, a ratio greater than 2 is associated with LVEDP greater than 20 mm Hg [70]. It is possible to more accurately estimate PAWP by using the equation [71] $PAWP = 18.4 + [17.1 \cdot \ln(E \text{ peak}/A \text{ peak})]$.

A recent study demonstrated that measurement of transmitral and pulmonary venous flows by Doppler can be used to estimate LV filling pressure in critically ill patients under mechanical ventilation [27]. In this study, an *E/A* ratio greater than 2 had a positive predictive value of 100% for a PAWP value greater than 18 mm Hg. However, a large *E/A* ratio may also be seen in young healthy subjects. In this population, LV elastic myocardial relaxation is rapid, which allows for almost complete LV filling during early diastole. This can lead to high *E/A* ratio without elevation of left arterial (LA) pressure [72]. Therefore, any interpretation of transmitral flow must take into account the patient's age. In addition, heart rate also modifies the transmitral flow pattern. Since tachycardia shortens diastolic filling time, atrial contraction may occur before early filling is completed. This will potentially result in a higher peak A-wave velocity than when the heart rate is slower. Furthermore, the transmitral E and A waves can overlap, making interpretation of the transmitral indices impossible [73]. Thus, in tachycardic patients a low *E/A* ratio does not necessarily relate to a low PAOP.

Evaluation of Right Ventricular Function and Preload

Right ventricular (RV) systolic dysfunction is another potential cause of hypotension. In practice, estimates of RV function are made from qualitative assessments of 2D imaging. Using either TEE (midesophageal four-chamber view) or TTE (apical and subcostal views), the right ventricular free wall can be visualized and its thickening and displacement noted. In situations where RV dysfunction is the sole cause of hypotension, whether directly from states causing myocardial dysfunction or as a result of a secondary issue such as a pulmonary embolus, the left ventricle is typically underfilled. Preload of the right ventricle is also estimated from either qualitative or quantitative assessment of ventricular size while again understanding that single measurements of such dimensions are of limited usefulness.

Assessment of Valvular Etiologies of Hemodynamic Instability

Abnormalities of valvular function can, on occasion, be the primary cause of hypotension. More frequently, however, chronic valvular dysfunction leads to abnormalities of ventricular function or difficulties with maintaining ventricular preload. Both of these issues can be assessed echocardiographically as outlined previously. In order to use echocardiography to its full potential, the practitioner must first understand the basics of valvular assessment. Although valvular stenoses can certainly have an impact on hemodynamics in the ICU patient, they are rarely the direct cause of hypotension. For this reason, this section will concentrate on evaluation of regurgitant valvular lesions.

ECHOCARDIOGRAPHIC EVALUATION OF MITRAL REGURGITATION. Echocardiographic evaluation of mitral regurgitation (MR) includes assessment of valve anatomy, severity of regurgitation, left atrial enlargement due to volume

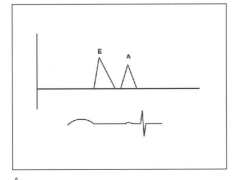
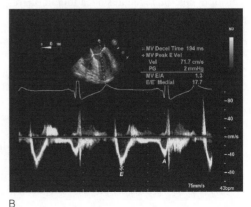

FIGURE 31-4. A: Schematic representation of transmitral inflow profile showing E and A waves during diastole. **B:** TEE midesophageal four-chamber view of transmitral inflow showing E and A waves.

A

B

TABLE 31-2.   Etiologies of Acquired Mitral Regurgitation

1. Leaflets abnormalities
   a. Myxomatous degeneration
   b. Rheumatic disease (may accompany mitral stenosis)
   c. Endocarditis (bacterial, viral, other)
   d. Cardiomyopathy (abnormal leaflet motion and anatomy)
      i. Hypertrophic
      ii. Dilated: ischemic, idiopathic, alcohol- or drug-related
   e. Marfan syndrome
   f. Infiltrative disease: amyloid, sarcoid, mucopolysaccharidosis, ankylosing spondylitis
   g. Collagen-vascular diseases: systemic lupus erythematosus, rheumatoid arthritis
2. Mitral annular dilation
   a. Left atrial dilation
   b. Left ventricular dilation
3. Chordal dysfunction
   a. Chordal tear
   b. Elongation
4. Papillary muscle
   a. Complete or partial tear
   b. Ischemia

overload, ventricular function, and the severity of pulmonary arterial hypertension. The mitral apparatus includes the anterior and posterior leaflets, the annulus, chordae tendineae, and the papillary muscles with their supporting LV walls. Dysfunction of any one of these components can result in mitral regurgitation and may be due to congenital or acquired abnormalities. Mitral valve leaflet pathology can be caused by rheumatic disease, endocarditis, myxomatous disease, infiltrative diseases such as amyloid, sarcoid, mucopolysaccharidosis, and collagen-vascular disorders such as systemic lupus erythematosus and rheumatoid arthritis [62]. Mitral annular dilation, which can occur secondary to left atrial as well as LV dilation, may result in mitral regurgitation due to incomplete leaflet coaptation. Mitral regurgitation can also occur as a result of chordal tear or elongation, which leads to inadequate tensile support of the closed leaflet(s) in systole with prolapse of the leaflet(s) into the left atrium [62]. Although complete papillary muscle rupture can occur in the setting of acute myocardial infarction and frequently leads to cardiogenic shock from acute, severe MR, partial rupture is more common and better tolerated. More commonly, temporary papillary muscle dysfunction can be caused by ischemia and may lead to significant MR (Table 31-2).

The Carpentier classification is commonly used to define the pathophysiologic mechanism leading to the regurgitation: normal, restrictive, or excessive leaflet motion [74].

• Class I. Normal leaflet motion: the most common causes of MR wherein leaflet motion is normal are mitral annular dilation and papillary muscle dysfunction due to myocardial ischemia. In most cases, the MR jet is centrally directed into the left atrium.
• Class II. Excessive leaflet motion: the severity of excessive leaflet motion ranges from leaflet *billowing*, wherein a portion of a leaflet projects above the annulus in systole while the coaptation point remains below the mitral annulus; to *prolapse*, wherein the excursion of a leaflet tip is above the level of the mitral annulus during systole; to *flail*, wherein a

leaflet flows freely into the left atrium, frequently as a consequence of ruptured chordae tendineae. Typically, the MR jet is eccentrically directed away from the affected leaflet.
• Class III. Restrictive leaflet motion: most commonly as a result of left ventricular dilation that displaces the papillary muscle away from the mitral valve annulus and in this way prevents leaflet coaptation. Restricted motion can also occur as a consequence of fibrosis or calcification. Restrictive processes may also lead to mitral stenosis. The direction of the MR jet may be central or eccentrically directed toward the side of the more affected leaflet. Mitral valvular systolic anterior movement, which will be discussed later, is also considered as an example of restricted leaflet motion.

SYSTOLIC ANTERIOR MOTION (SAM). SAM of the mitral valve represents an important diagnosis that must be considered in the unstable patient. MV SAM is caused when a venturi effect of blood flow at high velocity through a narrowed space between the anterior mitral valve leaflet and LV septum causes the MV leaflet(s) to be displaced toward the LVOT, causing obstruction to systolic flow. Patients at risk for developing SAM include those with hypertrophied LV septums, whether asymmetric or symmetric, patients with small LV diameters, patients with redundant mitral apparatus tissue, and patients with hypercontractile left ventricles. 2D imaging of the mitral leaflet and LVOT will show movement of the leaflet into the path of blood flow. Color Doppler imaging will reveal "color aliasing" of blood flow, the Doppler equivalence of turbulence, in the LVOT. In addition, SAM frequently prevents normal coaptation of the mitral leaflets, resulting in significant, usually anteriorly directed, eccentric MR. M-mode imaging of the aortic valve in the long axis will reveal midsystolic closure of the valve leaflets. Finally, continuous wave Doppler interrogation of the outflow tract from deep gastric windows will reveal a high velocity flow profile, often "dagger" shaped, which can be used to quantify a pressure gradient across the obstruction. The response of this process to therapeutic interventions can be followed using these echocardiographic assessments.

MITRAL REGURGITATION ASSESSMENT. There are two types of MR assessment:

1. *2D Examination*: Basic 2D assessment may provide clues for the presence of MR. Structural leaflet abnormality or coaptation defects may be obvious in some cases. Indirect signs of MR should also be sought. These include LV and left atrial enlargement and signs of pulmonary arterial hypertension and elevated PA pressures estimated from Doppler interrogation of TR jets, as an example.
2. *Doppler Flow Examination*: Doppler flow examination is the most common method used to screen and evaluate MR. MR is graded as trivial, mild, moderate, or severe, which corresponds to the angiography scores of 1+, 2+, 3+, and 4+ respectively. A visual assessment of the area of the MR color map provides a rough estimate of the severity of regurgitation. However, this simple visual assessment has limitations. As an example, eccentric MR jets that run along a left atrial wall may appear less severe (the Coanda effect). In addition, color gain settings—a technical issue—can have significant impact on the size of the MR

color map. Low color gains will increase the size; whereas high gains will reduce it. This is sometimes referred to as the "dial-a-jet" phenomenon. Typically, color flow velocity limits should be set in the 50 to 60 cm per second range when evaluating MR. As mentioned in the prior section, MR jet direction has important clinical implications. Centrally directed jets usually result from annular dilation or ischemic and dysfunctional papillary muscle. Eccentric jets are caused almost exclusively by structural abnormalities of the mitral apparatus. As a consequence, eccentric jets are unlikely to improve after improving myocardial ischemia.

Quantification of Mitral Regurgitation

VENA CONTRACTA WIDTH. The vena contracta is the narrow contracted portion of the MR jet seen just below the mitral leaflets. The width of this jet has been shown to correlate well with the severity of MR [75]. Widths of less than 3 mm correspond to mild MR, 3 to 5 mm with moderate MR, and over 5 mm with severe MR [76]. The limitations of this technique include situations where there may be several different MR jets or where the eccentricity of the jet makes vena contracta measurement difficult or impossible.

PULMONARY VEIN FLOW REVERSAL. Blunting or reversal of the systolic component of pulmonary venous inflow is one of the most reliable signs of hemodynamically significant MR. Frank reversal is associated with severe MR, whereas blunting is usually associated with moderate or moderate to severe MR. A limitation of this sign occurs in patients with atrial fibrillation. With the loss of left atrial relaxation in atrial fibrillation, there is a blunting of systolic pulmonary venous inflow independent to the effects of MR.

PROXIMAL ISOVELOCITY SURFACE AREA (PISA). The PISA method is based on the principle that a regurgitant jet accelerates in layers of concentric shells with equal velocity upstream from the valve (proximal to the regurgitant orifice). Immediately adjacent to the orifice, these shells have a small area with high-velocity flow, and at increasing distance from the orifice they have larger area and lower velocities [62]. By interrogating this area with color Doppler, the regurgitant volume can be calculated. First, PISA is calculated as $2\pi r^2$, where r is the distance from the aliasing velocity to the regurgitant orifice. Then the velocity of the PISA can be determined as the aliasing velocity from the color flow image where a distinct color interface is seen. At this interface the velocity equals the Nyquist limit, and this number can be obtained by reading the maximum velocity from the color scale on the echo screen. The regurgitant volume of blood is the product of the shell area (PISA) and the aliasing velocity. Since this regurgitant volume is passing through a defect in the mitral valve, the regurgitant orifice area (ROA) can be calculated as follows: ROA = regurgitant volume $\div$ VTI $_{MRjet}$.

Assessing Aortic Regurgitation

Causes of aortic regurgitation (AR) can be divided into abnormalities of the aortic valve leaflets and abnormalities of the aorta. Primary diseases of the valve leaflets include degenerative calcification, rheumatic fever, infective endocarditis, and congenital bicuspid aortic valve (which is usually associated with aortic stenosis) [77]. Dilation of the ascending aorta and aortic root may be due to chronic hypertension, aortic dissection, degenerative diseases of the aorta, cystic medial necrosis, Marfan syndrome, and several rare conditions including ankylosing spondylitis and syphilitic disease.

In response to chronic volume overload from AR, the LV undergoes progressive enlargement and increase in sphericity. With chronic and gradual increase of AR, the LV remains compliant in diastole. In contrast, acute AR is associated with significant increase in end-diastolic pressure because the LV compliance has not been able to adapt to the increase in volume. The causes of acute AR include aortic dissection and endocarditis. Echocardiography has a major role in the diagnosis of these pathologies

EVALUATION OF AORTIC REGURGITATION SEVERITY

Jet Width/LVOT Diameter Ratio. By viewing the LVOT in the long axis, the regurgitant jet width can be qualitatively compared to the diameter of the LVOT. A ratio of 1% to 24% is considered trivial AR (0–1+), 25% to 46% mild AR (1+–2+), 47% to 64% moderate (2+–3+), and greater than 65% severe (3+–4+) AR [78]. An alternative method uses color M-mode. The Doppler beam is placed perpendicular to the outflow tract and by activation of both M-mode and color Doppler; the regurgitant jet can be seen within the LVOT boundaries during diastole. Dividing the regurgitant jet width by the LVOT width can then be used as outlined to grade the AR.

Jet Area/LVOT Area Ratio. Using a short axis view of the aortic valve, the area of the regurgitant jet can be compared with the area of the LVOT. A ratio of greater than 4% is considered trivial AR (0–1+), 4% to 24% mild (1+–2+), 25% to 59% moderate (2+–3+), and greater than 60% severe (3+–4+) AR [79].

Vena Contracta. As with the assessment of MR, the vena contracta width of an AI jet can be measured in the long-axis view of the jet. A vena contracta width of more than 6 mm has been associated with severe AR [80].

Slope of Aortic Regurgitant Jet Velocity Profile. Since the velocity of the regurgitant jet is directly correlated to the pressure gradient between the aorta and the LV in diastole, the larger the defect in the aortic valve the faster the pressure difference between the aorta and LV will disappear. Thus the more severe the AR the faster the velocity profile will approach zero. Using this principle, the slope of the rate of decay of the velocity jet can be used as a measure of regurgitation severity. A measurement of the pressure half-time of this decay (i.e., the time interval (in milliseconds) between the time when the transvalvular AR pressure gradient is maximal and the time when it is half the maximum) can be calculated. A pressure half-time of less than 200 msec corresponds to severe, 200 to 500 msec moderate, and greater than 500 msec mild AR [81,82]. A potential pitfall of this grading technique is that it may be influenced by other pathologies that influence the gradient between the aorta and LV. These include issues that cause diastolic dysfunction of the LV.

Assessing Tricuspid Regurgitation

Tricuspid regurgitation (TR) may be the result of leaflet abnormalities due to myxomatous disease or destruction from endocarditis. More frequently, increases in TR may be secondary to processes that impact right ventricular and tricuspid annular dimensions. Such examples include both acute and chronic volume overload and acute and chronic increases to RV afterload. Examples of the latter include pulmonary embolus and primary or secondary pulmonary artery hypertension. TR is typically quantified by assessing color map area. Evaluation for RV enlargement and systolic function are important. Continuous-wave Doppler interrogation of the TR jet allows for quantification of systolic pulmonary arterial pressures and allows for partial assessment of RV afterload. This is performed by adding an actual or estimate of CVP to the maximum pressure of the TR jet.

EXTRACARDIAC CAUSES OF HEMODYNAMIC INSTABILITY

PERICARDIAL TAMPONADE

Cardiac tamponade is a clinical and hemodynamic diagnosis; echocardiography may, however, be of assistance in equivocal cases. Chronic or slowly accumulating effusions can become very large (greater than 1,000 mL) without significant increase in pericardial pressures. In the acute setting, however, even a small volume of fluid (50 to 100 mL) may lead to significant increase in pericardial pressure and tamponade physiology. The echocardiographic diagnosis of tamponade first requires demonstration of an effusion. From there, the examination should focus on identifying cardiac chamber collapse. As the pericardial pressure increases, the cardiac chambers will show collapse in sequence from lowest pressure to highest; the atria will collapse first, followed by the RV, and then LV. Furthermore, the collapse of each chamber will be most pronounced during the portion of the cardiac cycle during which the pressure is the lowest in that chamber; ventricular systole for the atria and ventricular diastole for the ventricles. This collapse can be evaluated with M-mode interrogation of the chamber walls. Pulsed-wave Doppler echocardiographic interrogation of ventricular inflow, across both the mitral and tricuspid valves, can also be used to assess for the effects of respiratory variation on ventricular filling—the echocardiographic equivalent of pulsus paradoxus. In the setting of tamponade, the peak LV inflow velocities will decrease by more than 25% with spontaneous inspiration, while peak RV velocities will decrease by more than 25% during expiration [62] (Fig. 31-5).

PULMONARY EMBOLUS

Diagnosis of pulmonary embolism (PE) in ICU patients can be extremely challenging. TTE has been described as a routine screening test in patients with suspected PE. When TTE is nondiagnostic and the clinician has a high level of suspicion, or there is evidence of RV overload or hemodynamic instability, TEE examination is indicated [83]. In these circumstances, TEE has a sensitivity of 80% and a specificity of 100%. Two-dimensional echo visualization of the main and proximal right and left pulmonary arteries may allow visualization of an embolus lodged in those locations. The left pulmonary artery may be difficult to visualize as the left bronchus is frequently interposed between the TEE probe and the artery. When the PE is not extensive and easily diagnosed by echocardiography, several indirect echocardiographic signs may suggest the presence of one. These include

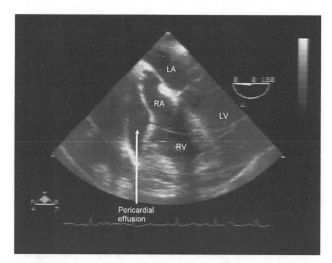

FIGURE 31-5. TEE midesophageal four-chamber view showing a large pericardial effusion and right atrial collapse in a patient with clinical tamponade. LA, left atrium; RA, right atrium; LV, left ventricle; RA, right ventricle.

evidence of acute right ventricular pressure overload with elevated PA pressures, right ventricular dilation, right ventricular systolic dysfunction, and increased tricuspid regurgitation. In situations where the echocardiogram cannot definitively make the diagnosis of PE, the exam findings can aid the clinician in guiding therapy.

AORTIC DISSECTION

Aortic dissection is a life-threatening condition where an intimal tear in the aortic wall allows passage of blood into a "false" lumen between the intima and the media. The mortality rate for acute aortic dissection is as high as a 1% per hour among untreated patients in the first 48 hours [84]. A rapid and correct diagnosis is paramount for improving survival rate. TEE has become a standard modality for the evaluation of suspected aortic dissection due to its availability, low cost, and noninvasiveness [85]. In addition, TEE can be used to diagnose other dissection-related cardiac and noncardiac complications such as aortic insufficiency, coronary occlusion, pericardial effusion with or without tamponade, and hemothorax.

Diagnosis of an ascending aortic dissection can prove to be very challenging due to imaging related issues. The ascending aorta and aortic arch are areas where imaging artifacts due to reverberation and refraction are common. These artifacts can mimic the appearance of dissection flaps. Furthermore, at the level of the distal ascending aorta and proximal arch, the left mainstem bronchus crosses between the esophagus and aorta, causing image degradation. As an end result, imaging from different tomographic planes and angles is mandatory to ensure accurate reporting. To distinguish artifact from dissection flap, the echocardiographer should establish whether or not the linear echodensity conforms to the limits of the aorta or if it seems to disregard such anatomic boundaries as would an artifact. Color Doppler imaging can be used to establish whether or not blood flow respects or ignores the echodensity.

Usually, an intimal flap creates a true and false lumen. Identification of these lumina is frequently an important goal of TEE evaluation but can create a diagnostic challenge for the

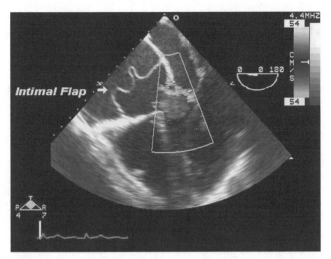

FIGURE 31-6. TEE midesophageal four-chamber view showing acute aortic dissection with an intimal flap in the proximal ascending aorta (*arrow*). Color Doppler imaging demonstrates aortic regurgitation.

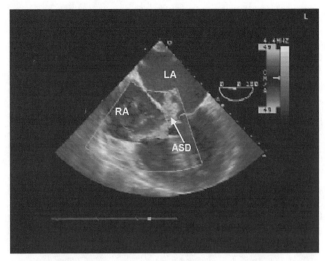

FIGURE 31-7. TEE midesophageal four-chamber view showing a left to right shunt through an atrial septal defect (*arrow*). LA, left atrium; RA, right atrium; ASD, atrial septal defect.

sonographer. There are several indirect findings that can help differentiate the lamina. First, the true lumen usually expands during systole and is slightly compressed during diastole [86]. Second, spontaneous echo contrast or thrombus may be seen in the false lumen as a result of stagnant flow; however, this may occasionally be misleading as in some instances it may be the true lumen where flow is stagnant. In addition, the true lumen is usually smaller than the false lumen, especially in chronic dissection [87,88]. Several communications between the true and false lamina can often be identified by color Doppler. Although some of these communications represent entry sites allowing blood to flow from the true to the false lumen, others are exit sites with bidirectional flow. Identification of the starting point of a dissection can have ramifications for deciding therapy (Fig. 31-6).

ECHOCARDIOGRAPHIC EVALUATION OF HYPOXEMIA

Assessment of unexplained hypoxemia and the inability to wean from ventilatory support are other potential uses of echocardiography in the ICU. Etiologies of hypoxemia that can be diagnosed by echocardiography include intracardiac right to left shunting, pulmonary embolus, and LV pathologies such as LV systolic and/or diastolic dysfunction and mitral valvular abnormalities that can lead to pulmonary edema. The echocardiographic evaluation of pulmonary embolus and of LV and mitral valvular pathologies has been previously discussed.

Intracardiac shunt is defined as an abnormal communication between two cardiac chambers and is characterized by blood flow across the defect [62]. The direction and volume of flow is determined by the pressure gradient across the defect and the size of the defect. A chronic left-to-right shunt may lead to right-sided volume overload and, over time, right-sided pressure overload from irreversible pulmonary arterial hypertension. This right-sided pressure increase may then lead to right-to-left shunting through the same defect. In clinical practice right-to-left shunt is more commonly seen in settings where right-sided pressure acutely increases over left-sided pressures

and typically involves defects in the interatrial septum. The diagnosis of an intracardiac shunt can be made with color flow Doppler. Typically the flow across an atrial septal defect (ASD) is of low velocity because of the small pressure difference between the chambers. A significant right-to-left shunt will occur when right atrial pressure exceeds left atrial as with severe pulmonary arterial hypertension. Other echocardiographic signs consistent with an ASD are biatrial and RV enlargement. The ratio of pulmonary to systemic blood flow, Q_p/Q_s, can be determined by Doppler flow measurements. To calculate Q_p/Q_s, it is necessary to measure stroke volume from the left and right sides of the heart. Transpulmonary flow, Q_p, can be calculated by measurement of the pulmonary artery CSA and VTI at the same site. Systemic flow, Q_s, is calculated from the measurement of LVOT CSA and VTI as outlined earlier (Fig. 31-7).

$$Q_p/Q_s = \frac{CSA_{PA} \times VTI_{PA}}{CSA_{LVOT} \times VTI_{LVOT}}$$

ECHOCARDIOGRAPHIC ASSESSMENT FOR SOURCES OF EMBOLI

Several disease processes, including intracardiac mass and shunt, are potential sources of systemic emboli leading to acute vascular occlusive events. Echocardiography can be very useful in the diagnosis or exclusion of the heart as a source of systemic emboli.

The three basic types of cardiac masses include vegetation, thrombus, and tumor, all of which are known causes of emboli. Infective endocarditis is a common indication for a TEE in the ICU, since critically ill patients are at a high risk for bacteremia. Endocarditis is a diagnosis based on a combination of findings from physical examination, laboratory findings (most importantly bacteremia), and echocardiographic examination. The purpose of the echocardiographic exam is to identify valvular lesions that may be consistent with endocarditis, to evaluate any functional abnormality associated with the affected valve, to assess the impact of the valvular disease on chamber function and dimensions, and to discover other complications of endocarditis such as paravalvular abscess and pericardial effusion.

All valves have to be carefully inspected as more than one valve can be involved. Echocardiographic evaluation of valvular endo-carditis involves multiple acoustic windows and 2D views, since the vegetation may be seen only in a certain tomographic planes. Most commonly, the vegetation is attached to the upstream, lower pressure side of the valve leaflet. It appears as an abnormal, echogenic, irregular mass attached to a leaflet [62]. Although vegetations can be attached to any part of the leaflet, attachment to the coaptation point is most common.

A thrombus mass is suspected when intracardiac thrombi form in areas of blood stasis or low flow. Examples of this within the ventricles include ventricular aneurysm, pseudoaneurysm, and areas adjacent to severely hypokinetic or akinetic wall segments. Left atrial thrombi are usually associated with atrial enlargement, mitral stenosis, and atrial fibrillation. Most left atrial thrombi are found in the left atrial appendage, which is best visualized by TEE. Thrombi are usually more echogenic than the underlying myocardium and have a shape distinct from the endocardial border. Imaging from several tomographic planes is frequently necessary to rule out artifact that may mimic thrombus. Again, color Doppler can be used to establish whether or not blood flow respects the apparent boundaries of the suspected thrombus to attempt to distinguish it from an echo artifact.

Nonprimary cardiac tumors are 20 times more common than primary cardiac tumors, and can involve the heart either by metastatic or lymphatic spread or invasion from neighboring malignancies. They can invade all structures of the heart: the pericardium, epicardium, myocardium, and endocardium. About 75% of metastatic cardiac tumors involve the pericardium and epicardium, and most commonly present as pericardial effusion. A definite diagnosis usually cannot be made from the echocardiographic images alone. A probable diagnosis can sometimes be made by incorporating the clinical information along with the echocardiographic images. Renal cell carcinoma has a propensity to develop "fingerlike" projections that may extend up the inferior vena cava into the right atrium. Occasionally, uterine tumors may present in a similar manner.

As described above, right-to-left shunting can play a role in hypoxemia. In addition, any right-to-left communications can allow for paradoxical emboli to travel from the systemic venous to arterial circulation. This can lead to stroke or vascular occlusive disease of one or several organs.

IMPACT OF INTENSIVE CARE UNIT ECHOCARDIOGRAPHY ON PATIENT MANAGEMENT

Indications for performing a TEE study vary significantly depending on patient type: For patients in the medical and neurosurgical ICUs, most TEE studies are performed to rule out or confirm bacterial endocarditis (medical ICU) and/or a cardiac source of emboli (neurosurgical ICU). In contrast, in medical-surgical and coronary ICU patients the most common indications are for diagnosing aortic dissection, valvular dysfunction, or hemodynamic instability [32].

A recent review of 21 studies evaluating the impact of TEE on patient management demonstrated that out of 2,508 critically ill patients, TEE findings had therapeutic implications, either surgical interventions or changes in medical therapy, in 68.5%

of patients [32]. Of these 5.6% of patients underwent a surgical intervention without additional investigations following their TEE. In 62.9% of patients, the TEE study had a therapeutic, non-surgical impact. Included within this group was the institution or dose adjustment of inotropic or vasopressor drugs, antibiotics, anticoagulation, thrombolysis, fluid administration, and the initiation of advanced hemodynamic monitoring. This represents the largest reported series evaluating the use of TEE in a noncardiac surgical ICU setting.

The current body of literature that focuses on the use of echocardiography in the ICU lacks prospective, randomized controlled studies demonstrating efficacy in decreasing morbidity and mortality and cost-effectiveness. However, this literature does point to the potential benefits that may be gained by the availability of echocardiography in ICUs. It also demonstrates the potential benefit of more widespread and advanced training in echocardiography for intensive care physicians.

FUTURE POTENTIAL USE OF ECHOCARDIOGRAPHY IN TRAUMA PATIENTS IN THE INTENSIVE CARE UNIT

Recently, hand-carried ultrasound (HCU) devices have been introduced into clinical use [89–91]. These devices are attractive because of their size, portability, and cost. They may be easily stored in the ICU, which makes them immediately available for bedside use. Portable echocardiograms performed at the bedside can help the physician diagnose and manage critically ill patients. Although overall image and color flow qualities of hand-carried echocardiographic devices are not equivalent to the standard full-featured machines, they have been found to compare well with standard platforms for the identification of cardiac pathology [92]. Reports in the literature regarding the use of these devices are mixed. Early reports showed favorable results in the outpatient setting [90], when used on hospital rounds [91], and in a small cohort of ICU patients [89]. Some of these reports have shown a good correlation between these devices and standard echocardiographic equipment for the evaluation of wall motion abnormalities and valvular regurgitation [93,94]. In addition, data from a few studies have shown a high level of agreement between hand-carried device examination and standard echocardiographic examination [89,91,95–97]. In one study, examination with a HCU device was able to evaluate and answer 85% of clinical questions presented by the referring physician. of those questions, 86% were later confirmed as correctly answered [98]. Although one study has demonstrated the relative equivalence of the HCU device with regards to 2D imaging, even in mechanically ventilated patients [99], other studies have shown it to be inferior to standard echocardiography when comparing spectral Doppler capabilities [100]. Other reports have shown that HCU imaging may lead to inadequate evaluation of pulmonary hypertension, valvular disease, and LV outflow tract obstruction in severely ill patients [98,99]. In ICU cohorts, several reports have demonstrated similar shortcomings [98,100].

In addition to cardiac evaluation, the HCU can be used in the ICU to aid in placing central venous catheters and arterial lines as well as for ultrasound guidance of pleurocentesis and paracentesis. The day when the HCU becomes an extension of the traditional physical exam may not be far off. It is also not unreasonable to imagine the HCU used by the hospital code team for better diagnosis and patient management during resuscitative efforts.

CONCLUSION

Echocardiography is an important tool for diagnosis and monitoring of the critically ill. With time, utilization of echocardiography is likely to become even more widespread. It is quickly establishing itself as a highly efficient and reliable clinical tool. The echo exam can be performed in numerous clinical settings and in a diverse patient population, including the most complex. Technical advancements in this field will potentially improve the imaging quality and clinical capabilities and allow for implementation of this tool in new situations and settings. With this in mind, proper education and implementation of utilization guidelines become increasingly important. To achieve optimal clinical results, clinicians must be well aware of the limitations as well as the benefits of each modality and when and how they should be used. An important step toward achieving this will be inclusion of echocardiographic training within critical care fellowships.

Acknowledgments

All TEE figures are courtesy of Feroze Mahmood, MD, Department of Anesthesia Critical Care and Pain Medicine, Beth Israel Deaconess Medical Center, Boston.

REFERENCES

1. Cahalan MK, Litt L, Botvinick EH: Advances in noninvasive cardiovascular imaging: implications for the anesthesiologist. *Anesthesiology* 66:356–372, 1987.
2. Daniel WE, Erbel R, Kasper W, et al: Safety of transesophageal echocardiography. A multicenter survey of 10,419 examinations. *Circulation* 83:817–821, 1991.
3. Sohn DW, Shin GJ, Oh JK, et al: Role of transesophageal echocardiography in hemodynamically unstable patients. *Mayo Clin Proc* 70:925–931, 1995.
4. Hwang JJ, Shyu KG, Chen JJ, et al: Usefulness of transesophageal echocardiography in the treatment of critically ill patients. *Chest* 104:861–866, 1993.
5. Khoury AF, Afridi I, Quinones MA, et al: Transesophageal echocardiography in critically ill patients: feasibility, safety and impact on management. *Am Heart J* 127:1363–1371, 1994.
6. Heidenreich PA, Stainback RF, Redberg RF, et al: Transesophageal echocardiography predicts mortality in critically ill patients with unexplained hypotension. *J Am Coll Cardiol* 26:152–158, 1995.
7. Poelaert JI, Trouerback J, De Buyzere M, et al: Evaluation of transesophageal echocardiography as a diagnostic and therapeutic aid in a critical care setting. *Chest* 107:774–779, 1995.
8. Vignon P, Mentec H, Terre S, et al: Diagnostic accuracy and therapeutic impact of transthoracic and transesophageal echocardiography in mechanically ventilated patients in the ICU. *Chest* 106:1829–1834, 1994.
9. Thys DM, Abel M, Bollen BA, et al: Practice guidelines for perioperative transesophageal echocardiography: a report by the American Society of Anesthesiologists and the Society of Cardiovascular Anesthesiologists task force on transesophageal echocardiography. *Anesthesiology* 84:986–1006, 1996.
10. Shanewise JS, Cheung AT, Aronson S: ASE/SCA guidelines for performing a comprehensive intraoperative multiplane transesophageal echocardiography examination: recommendations of the American Society of Echocardiography Council for intraoperative echocardiography and the Society of Cardiovascular Anesthesiologists task force for certification in perioperative transesophageal echocardiography. *J Am Soc Echocardiogr* 12:884–900, 1999.
11. Gottdiener JS, Bednarz J, Devereux R, et al: American Society of Echocardiography recommendations for use of echocardiography in clinical trials. *J Am Soc Echocardiogr* 17:1086–1119, 2004.
12. Mulvagh SL, De Maria AN, Feinstein SB, et al: Contrast echocardiography: current and future applications. *J Am Soc Echocardiogr* 13:331–342, 2000.
13. Mor-Avi V, Caiani EG, Collins KA, et al: Combined assessment of myocardial perfusion and regional left ventricular function by analysis of contrast-enhanced power modulation images. *Circulation* 104:352–357, 2001.
14. Porter TR, Xie F, Silver M, et al: Real-time perfusion imaging with low mechanical index pulse inversion Doppler imaging. *J Am Coll Cardiol* 10:748–753, 2001.
15. Sandham JD, Hull RD, Brant RF, et al: A randomized, controlled trial of the use of pulmonary-artery catheters in high-risk surgical patients. *N Engl J Med* 348:5–14, 2003.
16. Rao TLK, Jacobs KH, El-Etr AA: Reinfarction following anesthesia in patients with myocardial infarction. *Anesthesiology* 59:499–505, 1983.
17. Boyd O, Grounds RM, Bennett ED: A randomized clinical trial of the effect of deliberate perioperative increase of oxygen delivery on mortality in high-risk surgical patients. *JAMA* 370:2699–2707, 1993.
18. Del Guercio LRM, Cohen JD: Monitoring operative risk in the elderly. *JAMA* 243:1350–1355, 1980.
19. Wu AW, Rubin HR, Rosen MJ: Are elderly people less responsive to intensive care? *J Am Geriatr Soc* 38:621–627, 1990.
20. Tuman KJ, McCarthy RJ, Spiess BD, et al: Effect of pulmonary artery catheterization on outcome in patients undergoing coronary artery surgery. *Anesthesiology* 70:199–206, 1989.
21. Hayes MA, Timmins AC, Yau EHS, et al: Elevation of systemic oxygen delivery in the treatment of critically ill patients. *N Engl J Med* 330:1717–1722, 1994.
22. Polanczyk CA, Rohde LE, Goldman I, et al: Right heart catheterization and cardiac complications in patients undergoing non-cardiac surgery: an observational study. *JAMA* 286:309–314, 2001.
23. Heyland DK, Cook DJ, King D, et al: Maximizing oxygen delivery in critically ill patients: a methodologic appraisal of the evidence. *Crit Care Med* 24:517–524, 1996.
24. Ivanov RI, Allen J, Sandham JD, et al: Pulmonary artery catheterization: a narrative and systemic critique of randomized controlled trials and recommendations for the future. *New Horizons* 5:268–276, 1997.
25. Jensen MB, Sloth E, Larsen KM, et al: Transthoracic echocardiography for cardiopulmonary monitoring in intensive care. *Eur J Anaesthesiol* 21:700–707, 2004.
26. Jensen MB, Sloth E: Echocardiography for cardiopulmonary optimization in the intensive care unit: should we expand its use? *Acta Anaesthesiol Scand* 48:1069–1070, 2004.
27. Boussuges A, Blanc P, Molenat F, et al: Evaluation of left ventricular filling pressure by transthoracic Doppler echocardiography in the intensive care unit. *Crit Care Med* 30:362–367, 2002.
28. Benjamin E, Griffin K, Leibowitz AB, et al: Goal-directed transesophageal echocardiography performed by intensivists to assess left ventricular function: comparison with pulmonary artery catheterization. *J Cardiothorac Vasc Anesth* 12:10–5, 1998.
29. Pearson AC, Castello R, Labovitz AJ: Safety and utility of transesophageal echocardiography in the critically ill. *Am Heart J* 119:1083–1089, 1990.
30. Beaulieu Y, Marik PE: Bedside ultrasonography in the ICU part 1. *Chest* 128:881–895, 2005.
31. Joseph MX, Disney PJS, Da Costa R, et al: Transthoracic echocardiography to identify or exclude cardiac cause of shock. *Chest* 126:1592–1597, 2004.
32. Huttemann E, Schelenz C, Kara F, et al: The use and safety of transesophageal echocardiography in the general ICU—a minireview. *Acta Anaesthesiol Scand* 48:827–836, 2004.
33. Colreavy FB, Donovan K, Lee KY, et al: Transesophageal echocardiography in critically ill patients. *Crit Care Med* 30:989–996, 2002.
34. Lobato EB, Urdaneta F: Transesophageal echocardiography in the intensive care unit, in Perrino RSA Jr (ed): *A Practical Approach to Transesophageal Echocardiography*. Philadelphia, Lippincott Williams & Wilkins, 2003, pp 272–285.
35. Moore CL, Rose GA, Tayal VS, et al: Determination of left ventricular function by emergency physician echocardiography of hypotensive patients. *Acad Emerg Med* 9:186–193, 2002.
36. Willenheimer RB, Lsraelsson BA, Cline CM, et al: Simplified echocardiography in the diagnosis of heart failure. *Scand Cardiovasc J* 31:9–16, 1997.
37. Kimura BJ, Pezeshki B, Frack S, et al: Feasibility of "limited" echo imaging: characterization of incidental findings. *J Am Soc Echocardiogr* 11:746–750, 1998.
38. Chuang ML, Hibberd MG, Salton CJ, et al: Importance of imaging method over imaging modality in noninvasive determination of left ventricular volumes and ejection fraction: assessment by two- and three-dimentional echocardiography and magnetic resonance imaging. *J Am Coll Cardiol* 35:477–484, 2000.
39. Crouse IJ, Cheirif J, Hanly DE, et al: Opacification and border delineation improvement in patients with suboptimal endocardial border definition in routine echocardiography: results of the phase III Albunex multicenter trial. *J Am Coll Cardiol* 22:1494–1500, 1993.
40. Reilly JP, Tunick PA, Timmermans RJ, et al: Contrast echocardiography clarifies uninterpretable wall motion in intensive care unit patients. *J Am Coll Cardiol* 35:485–490, 2000.
41. Gottdiener JS, Bednarz J, Devereux R, et al: American Society of Echocardiography recommendations for use of echocardiography in clinical trials. *J Am Soc Echocardiog* 17:1086–1119, 2004.
42. Feigenbaum H, Armstrong WF, Ryan T. *Evaluation of Systolic and Diastolic Function of the Left Ventricle Feigenbaum's Echocardiography*. Philadelphia, Lippincott Williams & Wilkins, 2005, pp 138–180.
43. Walton SJ, Reeves ST, Dorman BH Jr: Ventricular systolic performance and pathology, in Perrino AJ, Reeves ST (eds): *Transesophageal Echocardiography*. Philadelphia, Lippincott Williams & Wilkins, 2003, pp 37–55.
44. Cohen JL, Cheirif J, Segar DS, et al: Improved left ventricular endocardial border delineation and opacification with OPTISON (FS069), a new echocardiographic contrast agent. Results of phase III multicenter trial. *J Am Coll Cardiol* 32:746–752, 1998.
45. Kitzman DW, Goldman ME, Gillam LD, et al: Efficacy and safety of the novel ultrasound contrast agent perflutren (Definity) in patients with suboptimal baseline left ventricular echocardiographic images. *Am J Cardiol* 86:669–674, 2000.
46. Malhotra V, Nwogu J, Bondmass MD, et al: Is the technically limited echocardiographic study an endangered species? Endocardial border definition with native tissue harmonic imaging and Optison contrast: a review of 200 cases. *J Am Soc Echocardiog* 13:771–773, 2000.
47. Spencer KT, Bednarz J, Mor-Avi V, et al: The role of echocardiographic harmonic imaging and contrast enhancement for improvement of endocardial border delineation. *J Am Soc Echocardiog* 13:131–138, 2000.
48. Nash PJ, Kassimatis KC, Borowski AG, et al: Salvage of nondiagnostic transthoracic echocardiograms on patients in intensive care units with intravenous ultrasound contrast. *Am J Cardiol* 94:409–411, 2004.

49. Costa JM, Tsutsui JM, Nozawa E, et al: Contrast echocardiography can save nondiagnostic exams in mechanically ventilated patients. *Echocardiography* 22:389–394, 2005.

50. Daniel GK, Chawla MK, Sawada SG, et al: Echocardiographic imaging of technically difficult patients in the intensive care unit: use of Optison in combination with fundamental and harmonic imaging. *J Am Soc Echocardiog* 14:917–920, 2001.

51. Heinle SK, Noblin J, Goree-Best P, et al: Assessment of myocardial perfusion by harmonic power Doppler imaging at rest and during adenosine stress. *Circulation* 102:55–60, 2000.

52. Porter TR, Li S, Kricsfeld D, et al: Detection of myocardial perfusion in multiple echocardiographic windows with one intravenous injection of microbubbles using transient response second harmonic imaging. *J Am Coll Cardiol* 29:791–799, 1997.

53. Porter TR, Li S, Jiang L, et al: Real-time visualization of myocardial perfusion and wall thickening in human beings with intravenous ultrasonographic contrast and accelerated intermittent harmonic imaging. *J Am Soc Echocardiog* 12:266–271, 1999.

54. Darmon PL, Hillel Z, Mograder, et al: Cardiac output by transesophageal echocardiography using continuous-wave Doppler across the aortic valve. *Anesthesiology* 80:796–805, 1994.

55. Gorcsan III J, Dianna P, Ball BS, et al: Intraoperative determination of cardiac output by transesophageal continuous wave Doppler. *Am Heart J* 123:171–176, 1992.

56. Maslow AD, Haering J, Comunale M, et al: Measurement of cardiac output by pulsed wave Doppler of the right ventricular outflow tract. *Anesth Analg* 83:466–471, 1996.

57. Muhiuden IA, Kuecherer HF, Lee E, et al: Intraoperative estimation of cardiac output by transesophageal pulsed Doppler echocardiography. *Anesthesiology* 74:9–14, 1991.

58. Perrino AC, Harris SN, Luther MA: Intraoperative determination of cardiac output using multiplane transesophageal echocardiography: a comparison to thermodilution. *Anesthesiology* 89:350–357, 1998.

59. Savino JS, Troianos CA, Aukbur S, et al: Measurements of pulmonary blood flow with transesophageal two-dimentional and Doppler echocardiography. *Anesthesiology* 75:445–451, 1991.

60. Steward WJ, Jiang L, Mich R, et al: Variable effects of changes in flow rate through the aortic, pulmonary, and mitral valves on valve area and flow velocity: impact on quantitative Doppler flow calculations. *J Am Coll Cardiol* 6:653–662, 1985.

61. Brown JM: Use of echocardiography for hemodynamic monitoring. *Crit Care Med* 30:1361–1364, 2002.

62. Otto CM: *Textbook of Clinical Echocardiography*. 2nd ed. Philadelphia, WB Saunders Company, 2000.

63. Bargiggia GS, Bertucci C, Recusani F, et al: A new method for estimating left ventricular dP/dt by continuous wave Doppler-echocardiography. Validation studies at cardiac catheterization. *Circulation* 80:1287–1292, 1989.

64. Pai RG, Bansal RC, Shah PM: Doppler-derived rate of left ventricular pressure rise. Its correlation with the postoperative left ventricular function in mitral regurgitation. *Circulation* 82:514–520, 1990.

65. Dalibon N, Schlumberger S, Saada M, et al: Haemodynamic assessment of hypovolaemia under general anaesthesia in pigs submitted to graded haemorrhage and retransfusion. *Br J Anaesth* 82:97–103, 1999.

66. Clements FM, Harpole DH, Quill T, et al: Estimation of left ventricular volume and ejection fraction by two-dimensional transesophageal echocardiography: comparison of short axis imaging and simultaneous radionuclide angiography. *Br J Anaesth* 64:331–336, 1990.

67. Jardin F, Valtier B, Beauchet A, et al: Invasive monitoring combined with two-dimensional echocardiographic study in septic shock. *Int Care Med* 20:550–554, 1994.

68. Thys DM, Hillel Z, Goldman ME, et al: A comparison of hemodynamic indices derived by invasive monitoring and two-dimensional echocardiography. *Anesthesiology* 67:630–634, 1987.

69. Tuchy GL, Gabriel A, Muller C, et al: Titrating the preload by using the rapid infusion system: Use of echocardiography during orthotopic liver transplantation. *Transplant Proc* 25:1858–1860, 1993.

70. Channer KS, Culling W, Wilde P, et al: Estimation of left ventricular end-diastolic pressure by pulsed Doppler ultrasound. *Lancet* 1:1005–1007, 1986.

71. Vanoverschelde JL, Robert AR, Gerbaus A, et al: Noninvasive estimation of pulmonary arterial wedge pressure with Doppler transmitral flow velocity pattern in patients with known heart disease. *Am J Cardiol* 75:383–389, 1995.

72. Appleton CP, Hatle LK: The natural history of left ventricular filling abnormalities: assessment by two-dimensional and Doppler echocardiography. *Echocardiography* 9:437–457, 1992.

73. Sohn DW, Choi YJ, Oh BH, et al: Estimation of left ventricular end-diastolic pressure with the difference in pulmonary venous and mitral A durations is limited when mitral E and A waves are overlapped. *J Am Soc Echocardiogr* 1999:106–112, 1999.

74. Carpentier A: Cardiac valve surgery—the "French correction." *J Thorac Cardiovasc Surg* 86:323–337, 1983.

75. Lambert AS: Mitral Regurgitation. Perrino AC, Jr (ed): *A Practical Approach to Transesophageal Echocardiography*. Philadelphia, Lippincott Williams & Wilkins, 2003.

76. Hall SA, Brickner E, Willet DWL, et al: Assessment of mitral regurgitation severity by Doppler color flow mapping of the vena contracta. *Circulation* 95:636–642, 1997.

77. Nyuan D, Johns RA: Anesthesia for cardiac surgery procedures, in Miller (ed) *Miller's Anesthesia*. Philadelphia, Elsevier Churchill Livingstone, 2005.

78. Perry J, Helmcke F, Nanda N, et al: Evaluation of aortic insufficiency by Doppler color flow mapping. *J Am Coll Cardiol* 9:952–959, 1987.

79. Cohen IS: *A Practical Approach to Transesophageal Echocardiography*, Perrino AC, Jr (ed.). Philadelphia, Lippincott Williams & Wilkins, 2003.

80. Willett DL, Hall SA, Jessen ME, et al: Assessment of aortic regurgitation by transesophageal color Doppler imaging of the vena contracta: validation against an intraoperative aortic flow probe. *J Am Coll Cardiol* 37:1450–1455, 2001.

81. Labovitz AJ, Ferrara RP, Kern MJ, et al: Quantitative evaluation of aortic insufficiency by continuous wave Doppler echocardiography. *J Am Coll Cardiol* 8:1341–1347, 1986.

82. Cohen IS: Aortic regurgitation, in Perrino AC Jr (ed): *A Practical Approach to Transesophageal Echocardiography*. Philadelphia: Lippincott Williams & Wilkins, 2003, pp 177–187.

83. Bobato EB, Urdanet F: Transesophageal echocardiography in the intensive care unit, in Perrino A Jr, (ed): *A Practical Approach to Transesophageal Echocardiography*. Philadelphia, Lippincott Williams & Wilkins, 2003, pp 272–285.

84. Hirst AE Jr, Johns VJ Jr, Kime SW Jr: Dissecting aneurysm of the aorta: a review of 585 cases. *Medicine* 37:217–279, 1985.

85. Payne KJ, Yarbrough WM, Ikonomidis JS, et al: Transesophageal echocardiography of the thoracic aorta, in Perrino AC Jr (ed): *A Practical Approach to Transesophageal Echocardiography*. Philadelphia, Lippincott Williams & Wilkins, 2003, pp 251–271.

86. Iliceto S, Nanda NC, Rizzon P, et al. Color Doppler evaluation of aortic dissection. *Circulation* 75:748–755, 1987.

87. Erbel R, Mohr-Kahaly S, Oelert H, et al. Diagnostic strategies in suspected aortic dissection: comparison of computed tomography, aortography, and transesophageal echocardiography. *Am J Card Imaging* 4:157–172, 1990.

88. Mohr-Kahaly S, Erbel R, Rennollet H, et al: Ambulatory follow-up of aortic dissection by transesophageal two-dimensional and color-coded Doppler echocardiography. *Circulation* 80:24–33, 1989.

89. Firstenberg MS, Cardon L, Jones P, et al: Initial clinical experience with an ultra-portable echocardiograph for the rapid diagnosis and evaluation of critically ill patients [abstract]. *J Am Soc Echocardiog* 13:489, 2000.

90. Bruce CJ, Zummach PL, Prince DP, et al: Personal ultrasound imager: utility in the cardiology outpatient setting [abstract]. *Circulation* 102:II364, 2000.

91. Pandian NG, Ramasamy S, Martin P, et al: Ultrasound stethoscopy as an extension of clinical examination during hospital patient rounds: preliminary experience with a hand-held miniaturized echocardiography instrument [abstract]. *J Am Soc Echocardiog* 13:486, 2000.

92. DeCara JM, Lang RM, Spencer KT: The hand-carried echocardiographic device as an aid to the physical examination. *Echocardiography* 20:477–485, 2003.

93. Masuyama T, Yamamoto K, Nishikawa N, et al: Accuracy of ultraportable hand-carried echocardiography system in assessing ventricular function and valvular regurgitation [abstract]. *Circulation* 102:II364, 2000.

94. Rugolotto M, Hu BS, Liang DH, et al: Validation of new small portable ultrasound device (SPUD): a comparison study with standard echocardiography [abstract]. *Circulation* 102:II364, 2000.

95. Rugolotto M, Hu BS, Liang DH, et al: Rapid assessment of cardiac anatomy and function with a new hand-carried ultrasound device (OptiGo): a comparison with standard echocardiography. *Eur J Echocardiogr* 2:262–269, 2001.

96. Pritchett AM, Bruce CJ, Bailey KR, et al: Personal ultrasound imager: Extension of the cardiovascular physical examination [abstract]. *J Am Soc Echocardiog* 13:485, 2000.

97. Alexander JH, Peterson ED, Chen Ay, et al: Feasibility of point-of-care echo by non-cardiologist physicians to assess left ventricular function, pericardial effusion, mitral regurgitation, and aortic valvular thickening [abstract]. *Circulation* II-334, 2001.

98. Goodkin GM, Spevack DM, Tunick PA, et al. How useful is hand-carried bedside echocardiography in critically ill patients? *J Am Coll Cardiol* 37:2019–2022, 2001.

99. Vignon P, Chastagner C, Francois B, et al: Diagnostic ability of hand-held echocardiography in ventilated critically-ill patients. *Crit Care Med* 7:R84–91, 2003.

100. Vignon P, Frank MBJ, Lesage J, et al: Hand-held echocardiography with doppler capability for the assessment of critically-ill patients: is it reliable? *Intensive Care Med* 30:718–723, 2004.

Ruben J. Azocar
Suresh Agarwal
Ishaq Lat

CHAPTER **32**

Monitoring Gastrointestinal Tract Function

Gastrointestinal system function is of paramount importance for the maintenance of the body's homeostasis, which is not only limited to the important functions of digestion and absorption but also closely related to immune function. Monitoring the gastrointestinal tract function remains largely based on clinical exam and a few diagnostic tests. The majority of the tests that are available have been primarily used for research purposes and are not available at the bedside of the critically ill patient (Table 32-1).

This chapter examines the diagnostic modalities available, on an organ system basis, for assessing abnormalities in the critically ill patient.

ESOPHAGUS

TESTS OF ESOPHAGEAL MOTILITY AND LOWER ESOPHAGEAL SPHINCTER FUNCTION

The evaluation of esophageal function may be performed with barium swallow and real-time fluoroscopy, yielding both functional and anatomic data about the esophagus and the swallowing mechanism. Similarly, an isotope swallow, utilizing a technetium-99 colloid and a gamma camera, may provide data regarding esophageal physiology. The ease of performing fluoroscopy usually outweighs benefits that may be had from nuclear radiography.

Esophageal manometry has been used extensively to study gastroesophageal reflux disease (GERD) in critically ill patients. One study, of 15 critically ill patients, demonstrated that low esophageal sphincter (LES) pressure (mean 2.2 ± 0.4 mm Hg) and poor motor response to reflux correlated with the presence of GERD. Furthermore, low LES pressures were associated with frequent reflux episodes (60% of untreated patients) and decreased esophageal motility [1].

Twenty-four–hour pH monitoring further elucidates the function of the LES and the amount of gastric reflux a patient is experiencing. Over a 24-hour period, the pH should not drop below 4 frequently or for a prolonged duration (6% of total time in the supine patient, 10% of total time in the upright patient). An indirect method by which to assess for gastric reflux is by treating with proton pump inhibitor and assessing for abatement of symptoms.

STOMACH

TESTS OF GASTRIC AND DUODENAL MOTILITY

Clinical measurement of gastric motility can be done by means of physical exam and quantification of gastric residual volumes via orogastric or nasogastric intubation. Despite being easy to perform, these tests are poor predictors of the patient's ability to tolerate enteral nutrition. In addition, a recent article suggests that the use of residual volumes as a marker of risk for aspiration in critically ill patients has poor validity [2]. Gastroduodenal manometry has been used as a more accurate method of assessing gastric emptying but has been largely used for research purposes.

Breath tests are a novel and useful bedside technique to assess gastric emptying of both solids and liquids by using 13C or 14C labeled octanoic acid. The absorption of the labeled octanoic acid in the small intestine and subsequent metabolism in the liver produce $13CO_2$, which can be measured in the exhaled air. The delivery of the 13-octanoic acid into the duodenum is the rate-limiting step for these processes. As such, measurement of $13CO_2$ levels correlates with the rate of gastric emptying. Ritz et al. [3] founded that gastric emptying of a caloric-dense liquid meal is slow in 40 to 45 of unselected mechanically ventilated patients by using the 13-octanoic acid breath test. They concluded that this test is a useful bedside adjunct to measure gastric emptying in ventilated, critically ill patients. Other investigative modalities, such as reflectometry of gastric contents, have also described valuable complementary information to the adequacy of gastric emptying [4].

The acetaminophen absorption test may also be used to assess gastric emptying, by administering 1,000 mg of acetaminophen and measuring serum concentrations of acetaminophen over a 1-hour period to construct an area under the curve (AUC) absorption model. This AUC is then compared to a known AUC model constructed from healthy volunteers. The utility of this test may be quite variable in the critically ill patient given differences in volume of distribution, hepatic metabolism, and renal clearance [5].

Finally, gamma scintigraphy presents a quantitative method to measuring gastric motility by administering radiolabeled solid food (usually greater than 200 kcal) and measuring transit after 2 to 4 hours. The administration of liquids may not be

TABLE 32-1. Tests for Monitoring Gastrointestinal Function

Organ	Function	Test
Esophagus	Motility/LES function	Barium swallow
		Isotope swallow
		Esophageal manometry
		Esophageal pH
Stomach	Motility	Gastric residuals
		Gastroduodenal manometry
		Breath tests
		Acetaminophen absorption test
	Mucosal permeability and ischemia	Gastric tonometry
		Laser Doppler flowmetry
		Near infrared spectrometry
		Positron emission tomography
		Microdyalisis
Small intestine	Absorption	Stool analysis: fecal pH, fecal osmotic gap, steatorrhea
		Carbohydrates absorption tests (D-xylose, L-rhamnose)
		Acetaminophen absorption test
		Breath tests
Pancreas:	Exocrine functions	Fecal fat concentration
		Amylase/lipase
		Secretin tests
Liver	Liver function test	**Static tests**
		Transaminases
		Bilirubin
		Albumin
		Lactate
		Coagulation tests
		Dynamic test
		MEGX
		ICG
		Breath tests
	Hepatic blood flow tests	ICG
		MEGX
	Cholestasis	Transaminases
		Bilirubin
		Alkaline phosphatase
		Gamma glutamyl transpeptidase
		Ultrasound
		HIDA

relevant as liquids may empty from the stomach even as solid food remains behind. The feasibility of scintigraphy testing for the critically ill patient makes the test less relevant as it is often impractical to transport these individuals to the nuclear radiology suite.

TESTS OF MUCOSAL PERMEABILITY AND ISCHEMIA

Gastric Tonometry

Although the diagnosis of bowel ischemia may be done by a variety of different methods, gastric tonometry is the simplest, most practical, and least invasive [6]. It attempts to determine the perfusion status of the gastric mucosa by measuring the local PCO_2 [7]. Carbon dioxide diffuses from the mucosa into the lumen of the stomach and subsequently into the silicone balloon of the tonometer. The CO_2 in the balloon is used as a reflection of the mucosal CO_2 and can be measured by either saline tonometry or air tonometry. In the saline tonometry technique, a saline solution is injected into the balloon and af-

ter an equilibration period, the CO_2 is measured using a blood gas analyzer. For the air tonometry technique, air is pumped through the balloon and an infrared detector measures the PCO_2 continuously. As perfusion to the stomach decreases, the PCO_2 in the tonometer will increase. Once cellular anaerobic respiration starts, the hydrogen ions titrate with bicarbonate, with the end result of more CO_2 production by mass action. Initially, most investigators calculated the intramucosal pH (pHi) using the Henderson-Hasselbach equation and assumed that arterial bicarbonate was equal to the mucosal bicarbonate. Experimental evidence has shown that a lower pHi was associated with lower mucosal flow by laser Doppler, demonstrating that mucosal bicarbonate is not equal to arterial bicarbonate [8]. Furthermore, it has been shown that respiratory acid/base disturbances affect pHi calculation [9]. Therefore, the use of the PCO_2 gap (the difference between gastric mucosa and arterial CO_2) is considered a better way to assess gastric perfusion [10].

The use of the technique has not gained widespread popularity despite many clinical studies that have validated gastric tonometry as a valuable and easily accessible prognostic tool [11,12]. This may be explained by the possibility of error in the determination of the PCO_2 and interoperator variability [13,14]. Other pitfalls include multiple local effects, including increased gastric secretions and refluxed duodenal contents; both of which can increase CO_2 measurement and lead to false PCO_2 measurement, and that this technique may only represent one region of perfusion [7].

Laser Doppler Flowmetry

Laser Doppler flowmetry, which estimates gastric blood perfusion by integrating red blood cell content and velocity, is highly correlated with absolute blood flow. The flowmeter consists of a laser source, a fiberoptic probe, and a photodetector with a signal-processing unit. The laser conducts through the tissue by a flexible fiberoptic guide. The probe contains an optic fiber for transmission of laser light to the tissue and two fibers for collecting the reflected scattered light. The signal-processing unit consists of a photodetector and an analog circuit to analyze the frequency spectrum of the scattered light. By determining the instantaneous mean Doppler frequency and the fraction of backscattered light that is Doppler shifted, the signal-processing unit provides a continuous output proportional to the number of red blood cells moving in the measuring volume and the mean velocity of these cells. Measurements are considered satisfactory if: (a) the measurement is stable for 15 seconds; (b) the measurement is free of motion artifacts; (c) pulse waves can be clearly identified; and (d) the reading is reproducible [8].

Other Techniques

Near infrared spectrometry (NIRS) has been used to measure local tissue blood flow and oxygenation at the cellular level [15]. Local oxygen delivery and oxygen saturation can be determined by comparing the differences in absorption spectrum of oxyhemoglobin with its deoxygenated counterpart, deoxyhemoglobin [16]. Puyana et al. [17] reported using NIRS to measure tissue pH in a model of experimental shock and showed that NIRS gut pH correlated with the pH obtained by microelectrodes.

Positron emission tomography (PET) may also be used to evaluate regional blood flow. Fluoromisonidazole accumulation has been used to demonstrate abdominal splanchnic perfusion and regional oxygenation of the liver in pigs; however, the lack of portability of this technique makes it difficult to use for monitoring in the intensive care unit (ICU) [15].

Microdialysis measurement of mucosal lactate is a novel way to assess gut mucosal ischemia. Tenhunen et al. [18] inserted microdialysis catheters into the lumen of the jejunum, the jejunal wall, and the mesenteric artery and vein of pigs. Subsequently, the animals were subjected to nonischemic hyperlactatemia or an episode of mesenteric ischemia and reperfusion. The lactate levels from the jejunal wall and the jejunal lumen were compared. The gut wall lactate was increased in both the nonischemic and the ischemic lactatemia, whereas the lactate measured from the jejunal lumen only was altered significantly during true ischemia.

Microdialysates of other substances have also been measured, including glucose and glycerol, showing that, while lactate levels increase with ischemia, intestinal wall glucose levels drop with the same stressor. Glycerol was increased, but the changes were seen later than the changes in lactate [19]. Similarly, increases in the lactate/pyruvate ratio in both intraperitoneal or intraluminal placed microdialysis catheters have correlated with hypoperfusion [20]. As glucose from the splanchnic circulation is inhibited, pyruvate accumulates in the tissue and, in the setting of inadequate oxygen delivery, is broken down to lactate. Using glycerol as a marker, Sollingard et al. [21] suggested that gut luminal microdialysis could serve as a valuable tool for surveillance not only during ischemia, but also after the ischemic insult.

These data support the idea that microdialysis could be a potentially useful method to monitor gut ischemia. However, even under investigational conditions, technical difficulties were reported in up to 15% of cases by either damage to the microdialysate membrane, dislocation of the probe, or incorrect placement [22].

SMALL INTESTINE

TESTS OF INTESTINAL ABSORPTION

Clinically, the recognition of malabsorption in the ICU is associated with a variety of signs and symptoms. On physical exam, abdominal distention, abdominal pain, and increased flatulence may be present. Isolated carbohydrate malabsorption may result in increased gas production, which can lead to flatulence, bloating, and abdominal distention. Likewise, diarrhea may indicate a problem with absorption of nutrients, but again it is nonspecific and other potential causes should be examined. Steatorrhea may indicate pancreatic insufficiency. It is also important to elicit the past medical history since it can provide useful information in regards to primary (i.e., lactose intolerance) or secondary (i.e., chronic pancreatitis) malabsorptive problems.

Malabsorption can be detected by a variety of tests. Stool analysis may provide information regarding carbohydrate and fat malabsorption. Bacterial fermentation of malabsorbed carbohydrates may result in an acidic fecal pH. Eherer and Fordtran [23] found that when diarrhea was caused by carbohydrate malabsorption (lactulose or sorbitol), the fecal fluid pH was always less than 5.6 and usually less than 5.3. Other causes of diarrhea rarely caused fecal pH to be as low as 5.6 and never caused a pH less than 5.3. Assuming than fecal osmolality is similar to that of

the serum, the fecal osmotic gap can be calculated. The sample is taken from the stool supernatant and if the value were greater than 50 to 100 mOsm, it would suggest the presence of an unmeasured solute. Although this solute may be a malabsorbed carbohydrate, other compounds, such as sorbitol, or ions, such as sulfates, may yield similar results.

Steatorrhea is defined as the presence of at least 7 g of fat in a 24-hour stool collection [24]. Sudan II stain is a simple screen testing and it is helpful to detect those patients with mild degrees of steatorrhea (7 to 20 g per 24 hours). The gold standard is represented by quantitative fecal fat analysis [25]. Stool is collected over 2 to 3 days while the patient ingests 75 to 100 g of fat within 24 hours. Normal values are less than 7 g per day. However, this test is laborious and may not help with differentiating diagnoses.

D-Xylose Uptake

The D-xylose test has been used in the diagnosis of malabsorption. This pentose sugar of vegetable origin is incompletely absorbed in the small intestine by a passive mechanism. The test consists in the ingestion of 25 g dose of D-xylose and the subsequent measurement of the levels on the serum or in urine. In normal individuals, a serum sample taken 1 to 2 hours after ingestion will reveal a level of 25mg per dL and a 5-hour urine collection will result in at least 4 g of this substance. Many entities such celiac disease, alterations in gastrointestinal motility, and impaired function of the pylorus will result in abnormal results. In the critically ill, renal function may be altered and may alter the results of the urine test. Chiolero et al. [26] studied the intestinal absorption of D-xylose in the critically ill patients that were tolerating enteral feeding. They introduced D-xylose to the stomach or the jejunum and found that although the levels in plasma in all patients in the study increased, indicating proper gastric emptying, in those receiving the compound in the stomach, the levels of D-xylose were lower than normal, indicating delays or depression in absorption. These results were similar to a prior study in trauma and septic patients. In this study, in both groups the D-xylose test showed abnormal results at the onset of the illness with resolution by 1 to 3 weeks after trauma or resolution of sepsis. Interestingly, enteral feedings were tolerated by these patients before the test results returned to normal [27]. As the patients in both studies were tolerating tube feeds even with abnormal D-xylose test results, Chiolero et al. [26] suggested that this test may not be a good indicator to determine the capacity of patients to tolerate enteral feeds. This does confirm that absorption of D-xylose stays depressed for a prolonged period of time in the critically ill.

Johnson et al. [28] also found decreased absorption in the septic population when compared with healthy individuals. They used an oral test solution that contained 5 g of lactulose, 1 g of L-rhamnose, 0.5 g of D-xylose, and 0.2 g of 3-O-methyl-D-glucose. L-rhamnose is absorbed by passive diffusion and therefore particularly sensitive to changes of the absorptive capacity of the gut when compared with D-xylose and 3-O-methyl-D-glucose, which depend on specific carrier mechanisms. The authors found that septic patients had decreased L-rhamnose/3-O-methyl-D-glucose ratios when compared with normal individuals, a result consistent with decrease absorptive capacity during sepsis. They also used the lactulose/L-rhamnose ratio to assess permeability of the gut. This group concluded that the changes in the absorptive capacities of the gut may contribute to the pathophysiology of sepsis.

Other Tests

The rapid absorption of acetaminophen at the jejunal level can also aid the assessment of the absorptive capacity of the gut. It has, however, been used more to assess gastric emptying [5] and tube feeding location for enteral feeding [29]. Details of this test were discussed in the motility section. From these data, it appears that either carbohydrate absorption tests or the acetaminophen test could be used to a monitor absorption in the critically ill. No correlation has been established between tolerating tube feeds and the degree of absorption. The role of this test may be to monitor improvement of absorptive function of the gastrointestinal tract after critical illness.

Breath tests are a simple and safe alternative to diagnose many gastrointestinal conditions including malabsorption. Most of the data are from gastroenterology literature and are used to diagnose specific gastrointestinal pathologies. However, it seems feasible to apply this test to the critically ill population. These tests are based on the appearance of a metabolite of a specific test substance in the breath [30]. Both hydrogen gas excretion and carbon dioxide appearance on breath test are available.

If carbohydrates are not absorbed in the small intestine, they are fermented in the colon by the colonic bacteria. This process results in the production of hydrogen. For example, in cases of lactase intolerance, this disaccharide will reach the colon and a peak on the end-expiratory hydrogen of more of 20 ppm over baseline by either gas chromatography or portable hydrogen analyzers at 2 to 3 hours indicates malabsorption for this carbohydrate [31]. A similar test using a nonabsorbable carbohydrate, such as lactulose, has been used for the diagnosis of bacterial overgrowth in which the peak of hydrogen occurs earlier but is less pronounced. The use of carbon dioxide that results from the fermentation of labeled substances has also been reported. The use of both radioactive ^{14}C and stable ^{13}C compounds has been described. However since the nonradioactive substances can be detected for mass spectrometry and do not involve radiation exposure, they seem to be preferred over the radioactive ones [31].

In critically ill patients ^{13}C-acetate has been studied to evaluate intestinal absorption [10]. Acetate possesses interesting properties that allow its use for absorption purposes since it is readily absorbed by the intestinal mucosa and it is metabolized through oxidative metabolism by nearly all body tissues. Acetate is converted into acetyl-CoA and then oxidized to CO_2. When marked acetate is provided, the $^{13}CO_2$ is then measured in the breath by mass spectometry. In this study, ^{13}C-acetate was provided by intravenous infusion and enterally at both gastric and jejunal levels. Surprisingly, the kinetics of all three routes was similar (the gastric group was delayed but probably secondary to the time for gastric emptying), indicating a rapid absorption and metabolism. The D-xylose absorption was delayed and all the patients were tolerating tube feeds. The authors concluded that further studies are needed in this area before this particular breath test can be used to assess tolerance of enteral feeding [13]. C-octanoic acid has been used to assess gastric emptying in the critically ill and was discussed in the motility section [3]. Other breath tests have been use to assess absorption anomalies [31]. In the case of bile acid malabsorption and bacterial overgrowth, cholylglycine (glycocholic acid) is not absorbed at the

ileum and the glycine is cleaved from the labeled cholylglycine by colonic bacteria. Glycine is then absorbed and metabolized into CO_2. The CO_2 can be detected in the breath and 4.5% of the radioactivity is seen in the breath over the subsequent 6 hours. To differentiate between bacterial overgrowth and bile acid malabsorption a stool collection is needed to detect bile acid losses.

For pancreatic insufficiency mixed triglycerides that are hydrolyzed to glycerol and fatty acid are then absorbed and finally metabolized in the liver where they release labeled CO_2. This test indirectly measures intraluminal fat digestion by pancreatic enzymes. Other substances such as triolein, hiolein, tripalmitin, and labeled starch have been use for this purpose but are not sensitive enough for patients with mild disease [31].

PANCREAS

Although the pancreas performs both endocrine and exocrine functions, only the functions affecting the digestive tract will be discussed here. Although diabetes mellitus may decrease gastric motility, the diagnosis and management of endocrine disorders can be found in Section 8 of Irwin RS, Rippe JM (eds): *Irwin and Rippe's Intensive Care Medicine.* 6th ed. Philadelphia, Lippincott, Williams & Wilkins, 2008.

FECAL FAT CONCENTRATION

As discussed in the digestion and absorption section, in the presence of pancreatic steatorrhea, fecal fat concentration is elevated [24,25]. Diarrhea resolves and fecal fat concentration abates once the individual is challenged with enzyme replacement therapy.

Amylase/Lipase

These simple blood tests are elevated in the presence of acute pancreatic inflammation. Although not indicative of the severity of injury, they do indicate that injury is present.

Secretin Test

The secretin test is a direct measurement of pancreatic exocrine function that measures the intraduodenal secretion of bicarbonate, amylase, and trypsin after exogenous administration of secretin. Generally, bicarbonate and amylase secretion will increase in adults, whereas the increase of bicarbonate, amylase, and trypsin will increase in children. In the presence of chronic pancreatitis, concentrations and quantity will be diminished; in contrast to pancreatic cancer, which presents with diminished volume but normal concentration. The maintenance of normal concentrations in pancreatic cancer is attributed to normal pancreatic function in the nonmalignant portions of the pancreas.

LIVER

Liver function includes vital functions of metabolism, synthesis, detoxification, and excretion. It is then, not surprising that patients with deteriorating liver function will have a more complex course during critical illness. Traditionally, tests related to measuring the products of liver synthesis have been use to assess liver function and damage in a static fashion, but as it will be discussed, tests that evaluate the liver function in a more dynamic fashion are also available.

TESTS OF LIVER INJURY AND STATIC FUNCTION

In the critically ill, different levels of dysfunction can be manifest ranging from mild elevation of the transaminases to profound hepatic failure. It is difficult to separate completely those tests that assess liver injury from those that are related to its function as some of them will suggest the insult to the organ as well as the alteration on its function, particularly in the acute setting. The tests described in this section are considered "static" and will reflect an injury that has occurred and changes on the liver's function, but they do not assess the current functionality particularly in the patient with chronic liver failure. However, in a critically ill patient with no prior liver problems these tests are helpful in detecting an ongoing morbid process on the liver.

Transaminases

Serum glutamic-oxaloacetic transaminase (SGOT), or aspartate aminotransferase (AST), and serum glutamate-pyruvate transaminase (SGPT), or alanine aminotransferase (ALT), are enzymes that are present in all the organism cells; however, they are found in highest concentration in the hepatocyte: SGPT in the cytoplasm and SGOT in the cytoplasm as well as the mitochondria. Therefore, as injury and necrosis of the hepatocyte occurs by microcirculatory failure and centrilobular necrosis (ischemia, sepsis), acetaminophen toxicity (by oxidation of key calcium regulation proteins causing hepatic necrosis), idiosyncratic drug reactions (isoniazid and phenytoin) viral hepatitis, parenteral nutrition, and other uncommon causes such as ingestion of the poisonous mushroom *Amanita phalloides* and halothane toxicity, the enzymes levels in the plasma will increase reflecting the damage to this organ. The rate and the level of the elevation are usually related to the onset of the dysfunction and its severity. For example, severe ischemic hepatitis is characterized by an acute elevation of the aminotransferases to at least 20 times the upper limit of normal [32].

Bilirubin

One of the main functions of the liver is to conjugate and excrete bilirubin, a product of erythrocyte breakdown. Therefore, either elevations of the bilirubin clinically (jaundice, icterus, dark urine) or by laboratory should raise the clinical suspicion of liver dysfunction or injury. It is possible to determine if the bilirubin has already been conjugated, and this helps in searching for the causes of the hyperbilirubinemia. Unconjugated (or indirect) hyperbilirubinemia is the result of excess production of bilirubin (e.g., hemolysis) or decreased hepatic uptake. Conjugated hyperbilirubinemia results when intrinsic parenchymal injury or biliary obstruction exists. Therefore, acute changes of the conjugated bilirubin levels are related to acute hepatocyte injury in situations such as viral hepatitis or ischemic hepatitis and will be related to the increase in the transaminases. This should alert the clinician of injury and dysfunction of the liver. Tests to study cholestasis are described in a separate section of this chapter. However, it should be remembered that biliary obstruction can also lead into hepatic dysfunction. Table 32-2 lists the causes of hyperbilirubinemia.

Lactate

The ability of the liver to clear lactate is profound. Greater than 99% of lactate is cleared by first pass metabolism by a healthy liver. Inability to clear the lactate may be an indicator of poor

TABLE 32-2. Causes of Hyperbilirubinemia

Bilirubinemia	Primary Cause	Differential Diagnosis
Unconjugated hyperbilirubinemia	Overproduction of bilirubin	Hemolysis
		Inefective erythopoiesis
		Massive blood transfusion
		Hematoma reabsorbtion
	Impaired hepatic uptake	Drugs (flavaspadic acid, rifampin, probenecid)
	Impaired bilirubin conjugation	Gilbert's syndrome
		Crigler-Najjar syndrome I and II
		Acquired deficiency of glucuronyltransferase
Conjugated hyperbilirubinemia	Hepatocellular dysfunction	Hepatitis (viral, ischemic)
		Hepatotoxic drugs
		TPN
		Shock and sepsis
	Biliary obstruction	Choledocholithiasis
		Biliary stricture
		Cholangiocarcinoma
		Pancreatic cancer

organ perfusion and anaerobic metabolism, and this metabolite can be used as a resuscitation parameter. If other indicators of resuscitation are optimized and the arterial lactate levels remain elevated, this may indicate severe liver dysfunction and injury, particularly in patients in shock.

Albumin

Liver function may also be evaluated by measuring its ability to synthesize a variety of proteins. Albumin is the most common protein measured when evaluating liver synthetic ability. Although hepatocellular dysfunction may be the cause of hypoalbuminemia, the protein concentration also varies in a variety of diseases/acute injury phases (e.g., burns, nephrotic syndrome, etc.) and can be nonspecific. It is a better marker to assess the degree of chronic hepatic failure than acute dysfunction and it does not reflect injury.

Coagulation Studies

More sensitive and specific measurements of hepatic function include evaluation of the coagulation cascade and the production of specific coagulation factors. If the prothrombin time (PT) is elevated, one of two conditions exists: vitamin K deficiency or deficiency in vitamin K dependent factors (II, VII, IX, and X). If vitamin K has been replaced and the PT remains elevated, this is very specific for liver dysfunction. This is not a sensitive test, as the PT remains normal as long as 20% of the liver remains intact. Far more sensitive, although more time consuming and costly, is the measurement of factor V levels. Factor V, produced in the liver, is not vitamin K dependent, and its deficiency is both sensitive and specific for hepatocellular synthetic dysfunction.

DYNAMIC OR QUALITATIVE TESTS OF LIVER FUNCTION

Although the tests discussed in the prior section are very important in detecting and helping the clinician assess liver dysfunction, they are not perfect as some are nonspecific (lactate, coagulation disorders, albumin levels) or reflect past damage (transaminases) in assessing the current state of liver functionality. Figg et al. [33] compared the Pugh's classification, which is based in clinical and laboratory data, with dynamic or qualitative methods of hepatic function and found that the Pugh's classification seemed to be a reliable indicator of the degree of chronic liver disease but could not replace qualitative metabolic markers particularly isozyme-specific markers. Although the quantitative tests may be more complicated to perform and more expensive than conventional tests, they may prove superior in monitoring the degree of liver dysfunction, by monitoring the liver's metabolic or clearance functions [34]. Therefore, different tests have been used in an attempt to have a dynamic or "real-time" assessment of the liver's metabolic or clearance functions and complement the information provided by the static tests. A discussion of some of these tests follows.

Monoethylglycinexylidide

The hepatic metabolism of lidocaine by sequential oxidative N-dealkylation by the cytochrome P450 system into its major metabolite; monoethylglycinexylidide (MEGX) is a dynamic liver function test [35]. Due to the high extraction ratio of lidocaine by the liver, this test not only evaluates liver metabolic capacity but also hepatic blood flow [36]. Detection of this metabolite can be accomplished by different techniques such as immunoassay based on the fluorescence polarization immunoassay technique, high performance liquid chromatography, and gas liquid chromatography [36]. Fluorescence polarization immunoassay technique may cross react with another metabolite (3-OH-MEGX). The other two tests are specific for MEGX.

This test has been useful in patients with end-stage liver disease in which a MEGX level at 15 or 30 minutes of less than 10 mg per L indicates poor 1-year survival. In liver transplant recipients, a change in the levels may indicate a deterioration of the graft function. In critically ill patients, a rapid decrease in MEGX test values have been associated not only with liver dysfunction but with the development of multisystem organ failure and an enhanced systemic inflammatory response [36]. McKindley et al. [37] reported on the pharmacokinetics of lidocaine and MEGX in a rat model of endotoxic shock. They found that the metabolism of both compounds was altered and attributed the results to both the reduced hepatic blood flow and altered function of the cytochrome P450 system, particularly cytochrome P450-3A4. Chandel et al. [38] also report the use of this test in an animal model of hypovolemic shock. They found that the MEGX levels were significantly lower in shocked animals. Once the animals were resuscitated with Ringer's lactate, the MEGX levels were higher but still lower than the control group. They concluded that shock produced significant depression of hepatocyte function and that MEGX seemed a suitable tool for clinical evaluation and therapeutic intervention after shock.

Dyes

Another dynamic test of liver function is related to the rate of elimination of dyes such as indocyanine green (ICG) and/or bromsulphthalein (BSP) [39]. Most of the data in the critically ill come from the use of ICG. This dye is a water-soluble inert compound that is injected intravenously. In the plasma it binds to albumin and is then selectively taken up by hepatocytes. The ICG is then excreted into the bile via an adenosine triphosphate (ATP)-dependent transport process. This compound is not metabolized and does not undergo enterohepatic recirculation. Therefore, the excretion rate of ICG into the bile reflects the hepatic excretory function and the hepatic energy status and justifies its use as a tool for assessment of liver function [40]. In a study comparing cirrhotic and noncirrhotic patients, Hashimoto and Watanabe [41] found that ICG clearance was proportional to liver parenchymal cell volume and is related to the hepatic dysfunction in cirrhotic patients. Traditionally, the ICG clearance has been measured by a series of blood samples and subsequent laboratory analysis. NIRS has also been used to measure hepatic ICG clearance with promising results in the assessment of hepatic parenchymal dysfunction [42].

Fortunately, bedside techniques have become available to measure the plasma disappearance rate (PDR) of ICG. Von Spiegel et al. [43] compared the clearance method of a transpulmonary indicator dilution technique with an arterial fiberoptic thermistor catheter that assessed the ICG circulating curve in patients undergoing liver transplantation. They found that both methods were effective in detecting onset and maintenance of graft function in these patients. Newer technology allows the use of assessment of ICG PDR transcutaneously. In two separate publications, Sakka et al. [44,45] suggested that this technology, when compared with invasive methods, reflected ICG blood clearance with sufficient accuracy in critically ill patients to be used as a surrogate. In contrast, in a model of hyperdynamic porcine endotoxemia the PDR ICG failed to accurately substitute for direct short-term measurements of ICG excretion [46]. The authors suggested that normal values of PDR of ICG should be interpreted with caution in early, acute inflammatory conditions. As mentioned before, ICG clearance also aids with the evaluation of the hepatic energy status since the excretion into bile is energy dependent. Chijiiwa et al. [47] correlated the biliary excretion of ICG with the ATP levels in liver samples obtained from patients with biliary obstruction, and in a second study they were able to correlate those variables with the biliary acid output [48]. They concluded that biliary bile acid output and ICG excretion are valuable parameters of hepatic energy status, which is essential for organ viability. ICG can be considered a valuable tool to assess liver function in patients after liver transplantation, at risk to develop, or with ongoing liver injury to assess damage and recovery and to assess the energy status of the liver.

Radiological Studies

Another method to assess functional liver reserve is with the use of technetium-99 diethylenetriamine pentaacetic acid galactosyl human serum albumin (99mTc-DTPA-GSA) clearance. Studies using hepatic scintigraphy and more recently single proton emission computer tomography (SPECT) scan have been described [49,50]. Hwang et al. [50] demonstrated the use of this test as a reflection of hepatic function and also suggested that predicting residual hepatic values was a good indicator of postoperative hepatic function and early prognosis after liver resection. Kira et al. [49] showed that using this test before and after transjugular intrahepatic portosystemic shunt was useful to evaluate changes in hepatic functional reserve and evaluate the degree of portosystemic shunt. At this time the test is mostly used as a predictor of liver function after liver resection and not used in the critically ill [51].

Breath Tests

The use of breath tests as qualitative measurement of liver function has also been described. The principle behind these tests is similar to the description of breaths tests used for monitoring of gut absorption described above. As the carbon marked compound is metabolized, the resulting marked carbon dioxide can be measured in the breath. As liver function declines, less of the marked CO_2 will be detected in the breath. In an animal model of hepatectomy, Ishii et al. [52] injected L-[1-(13)C] methionine and L-[1-(13)C] phenylalanine intravascularly and measured the exhaled $^{13}CO_2$ over 15 minutes. They concluded that this test could qualitatively evaluate hepatopathy. In a human study, Kobayashi et al. [53] demonstrated that the use of the ^{13}C phenylalanine test correlated well with ICG clearance test, Child Pugh's classification, and standard liver blood tests, suggesting that this test is a useful noninvasive method to determine liver functional reserve. In another study, Koeda et al. [54] studied the validity of the ^{13}C phenylalanine breath test in both chronic cirrhosis and acute hepatitis patients and concluded that in both groups this test allows the noninvasive evaluation of hepatic function. Hepatic dysfunction associated with obstructive jaundice in a rat model was also evaluated using this test. As similar results were achieved, the authors concluded that this test could be used to measure hepatic dysfunction associated with obstructive jaundice [55]. Reports of the use of other marked compounds to assess liver function utilizing the breath test principles, such as ^{13}C methacetin [56], L[1,2-13C] Ornithine [57], and 1-[1-130C] Alanine [58] have been described with promising results.

Other dynamic tests that are available include the antipyrine clearance test [33,34], the caffeine clearance test [34], and the pharmacokinetics of acetaminophen. Zapater et al. [59] reported a higher area under the curve concentration and lower clearance and higher elimination half-life in cirrhotics when compared with healthy volunteers.

Blood Flow Tests

Tests to determine hepatic blood flow are also useful. Xylocaine metabolism also evaluates hepatic blood flow [36]. The use of ICG has also been described for this purpose. The use of intravenous infusions of ICG seemed more reliable and accurate in evaluation of hepatic blood flow than with the use of boluses or intravenous injections of galactose [60]. Apparently with the use of boluses, extrahepatic accumulation of the dye occurs and alters the results [61]. More recently, pulse dye-densitometry (PDD) has been used in the critically ill patient instead of blood tests. Mizushima et al. [62] measured effective hepatic blood volume (EHBV) and cardiac output (CO) using ICG-PDD [62]. They found that in septic patients, the EHBF/CO ratio was lower than that of nonseptic patients, suggesting that inadequate splanchnic perfusion or metabolic changes occur in septic patients. In addition, the lower EHBF/CO ratio was related to a fatal outcome in septic patients. The authors concluded that PDD could be a clinically useful method of assessing splanchnic conditions in critically ill patients. Dysfunction in one of the components of the gastrointestinal system, in this case the liver, manifested by decreased metabolic [36–38] capacities or hepatic blood flow [37,62] are related to shock states and are probably an integral part of the multiorgan system failure (MOSF) cas-

cade, highlighting the relationship of the gastrointestinal system with immunity.

Tests of Cholestasis

In patients with conjugated hyperbilirubinemia but without other indicators of liver dysfunction or injury, biliary obstruction should be suspected. Alkaline phosphatase (AP), like SGOT and SGPT, is found in a variety of different organs, but has its highest concentration in the liver. As such, it is most often elevated in situations where cholestasis is present. AP is more specific than gamma glutamyl transpeptidase (GTT) for biliary tree inflammation, as GGT is sensitive to even mild liver inflammation and/or activation of the cytochrome P-450 enzymes.

Further workup may include radiological evaluation. Hepatic iminodiacetic acid (HIDA) scan may also prove valuable in differentiating the cause of cholestasis. The test reveals many facets of hepatic function with respect to its ability to conjugate bile: If the liver does not actively uptake tracer, than its ability to conjugate bile must be questioned. In addition, when conjugation is not an issue, definitive anatomic localization of biliary obstruction is possible. In addition, in the presence of a functional sphincter of Oddi, it is possible to diagnose acute cholecystitis. Further assessment of biliary architecture can be made with ultrasonography. Not only can one determine the architecture of the liver and gallbladder, but one can also determine the amount of intra- and extrahepatic biliary dilatation, further delineating the source of biliary obstruction.

CONCLUSIONS

Gastrointestinal function is of vital importance in the critically ill patient. These functions are not limited to the mere absorption of nutrients but are closely related with the immune system, particularly in the critically ill patient. Despite its importance, monitoring of intestinal function is limited, providing anatomic and physiologic information rather than an assessment of pathophysiologic change. However, assessment of absorption by sugar absorption tests and breath tests, of motility by manometry, and of ischemia by tonometry and microdialysis are promising modalities that may help monitor the functions of the gastrointestinal tract.

REFERENCES

1. Heyland DK, Cook DJ, Guyatt GH: Enteral nutrition in the critically ill patient: a critical review of the evidence. *Intensive Care Med* 19:435–442, 1993.
2. McClave SA, Lukan JK, Stafer JA, et al: Poor validity of residual volumes as a marker for risk of aspiration in critically ill patients. *Crit Care Med* 33:449–450, 2005.
3. Ritz MA, Frazer R, Edwards N, et al: Delayed gastric emptying in ventilated critically ill patients: measurement by 13 C-octanoic acid breath test. *Crit Care Med* 29:1744–1749, 2001.
4. Chang WK, McClave SA, Lee MS: Monitoring bolus nasogastric tube feeding by the Brix value determination and residual volume measurement of gastric contents. *J Parenter Enteral Nutr* 28:105–112, 2004.
5. Tarling MM, Toner CC, Withington PS, et al: A model of gastric emptying using paracetamol absorption in intensive care patients. *Intensive Care Med* 23:243–245, 1997.
6. Pastores SM, Katz DP, Kvetan V: Splanchnic ischemia and gut mucosal injury in sepsis and multisystem organ dysfunction syndrome. *Am J Gastroenterol* 91:1697–1710, 1996.
7. Heard SO: Gastric tonometry: the hemodynamic monitor of choice (Pro). *Chest* 123(469S): 469–474, 2003.
8. Elizalde JI, Heranndez C, Llach J, et al: Gastric intramucosal acidosis in mechanically ventilated patients: role of mucosal blood flow. *Crit Care Med* 26:827–832, 1998.
9. Morgan TJ, Venkatesh B, Endre ZH: Accuracy of intramucosal pH calculated from arterial bicarbonate and the Henderson-Hasselbach equation: assessment using simulated ischemia. *Crit Care Med* 27:2495–2499, 1999.

10. Schlichtig R, Mehta N, Gayowski TJ: Tissue arterial P_{CO_2} difference is a better marker of ischemia than intramural pH (Phi) or arterial pH-Phi difference. *J Crit Care* 11:51–56, 1996.

11. Kirton OC, Windsor J, Wedderburn R, et al: Failure of splanich resuscitation in the acutely injured trauma patient correlates with multiple organ system failure and length of stay in the ICU. *Chest* 113:1064–1069, 1998.

12. Maynard N, Bihari D, Bealae R, et al: Assessment of splanich oxygenation by gastric tonometry in patients with acute circulatory failure. *JAMA* 270:1203–1210, 1993.

13. Takala J, Parviainen I, Siloaho M, et al: Slaine P_{CO_2} is an important source of error in the assessment of gastric intramucosal pH. *Crit Care Med* 22:1877–1879, 1994.

14. Knichwitz G, Kuhmann M, Brodner G, et al: Gastric tonometry: precision and reliability are improved by a phosphate buffered solution. *Crit Care Med* 24:512–516, 1996.

15. Yuh-Chin TW: Monitoring oxygen delivery in the critically ill. *Chest* 128(S554):554–560, 2005.

16. Cohn SM, Crookes BA, Proctor KG: Near-infrared spectrometry in resuscitation. *J Trauma* 54:S199–S202, 2003.

17. Puyana JC, Soller BR, Zhang S, et al: Continuous measurement of gut pH with near-infrared spectroscopy during hemorrhagic shock. *J Trauma* 46:9–15, 1999.

18. Tenhunen JJ, Kosunen H, Alhava E, et al: Intestinal luminal microdialysis: a new approach to assess gut mucosal ischemia. *Anesthesiology* 91:1807–1815, 1999.

19. Sommer T, Larsen JF: Detection of intestinal ischemia using a microdialysis technique in an animal model. *World J Surg* 27:416–420, 2003.

20. Sommer T, Larsen JF: Intraperitoneal and intraluminal microdialysis in the detection of experimental regional intestinal ischaemia. *BJS* 91:855–861, 2004.

21. Sollingard E, Ingebjorg SJ, Bakkelund K, et al: Gut luminal microdialysis of glycerol as a marker of intestinal ischemic injury and recovery. *Crit Care Med* 33:2278–2285, 2005.

22. Sommer T, Larsen JF: Validation of intramural intestinal microdialysis as a detector of intestinal ischemia. *Scand J Gastroenterl* 39:493–499, 2004.

23. Eherer AJ, Fordtran JS: Fecal osmotic gap and pH in experimental diarrhea of various causes. *Gastroenterology* 103:545–551, 1992.

24. Weinstein WM, Hawkey CJ, Bosch JM (eds): *Clinical Gastroenterology and Hepatology.* Philadelphia, Elsevier, 2005.

25. Farrell JJ: Overview and diagnosis of malabsorption syndrome. *Semin Gastrointest Dis* 13:182–190, 2002.

26. Chiolero RL, Revelly JP, Berger MM: Labeled acetate to assess intestinal absorption in critically ill patients. *Crit Care Med* 31:853–857, 2003.

27. Singh G, Harkema JM Mayberry AJ: Severe depression of gut absorptive capacity in patients following trauma or sepsis. *J Trauma* 36:803–809, 1994.

28. Johnson JD, Harvey CJ, Menzies IS, et al: Gastrointestinal permeability and absorptive capacity in sepsis. *Crit Care Med* 24:1144–1149, 1996.

29. Berger MM, Werner D, Revelly JP: Serum paracetamol concentration: an alternative to x-rays to determine feeding tube location in the critically ill. *J Parenter Entreral Nutr* 27:151–155, 2003.

30. Swart GR, van den Berg JW: 13C breath test in gastroenterological practice. *Scand J Gastroenterol Suppl* 225:13–18, 1998.

31. Romagnuolo J, Schiller D, Bailey RJ: Using breath tests wisely in a gastroenterology practice: an evidence-based review if indications and pitfalls in interpretation. *Am J Gastroenterology* 97:1113–1116, 2002.

32. Seeto RK, Fenn B, Rockey DC: Ischemic hepatitis: clinical presentation and pathogenesis. *Am J Med* 109:109–113, 2000.

33. Figg WD, Dukes GE, Lesene HR, et al: Comparison of quantitative methods to assess hepatic function. Pugh's classification, indocyanine green, antipyrine and dextromorphan. *Pharmacotherapy* 15:693–700, 1995.

34. Burra P, Masier A: Dynamic tests to study liver function. *Eur Rev Med Pharmacol Sci* 8:19–21, 2004.

35. Tanaka E, Inomata S, Yasuhara H: The clinical importance of conventional and qualitative liver function test in liver transplantation. *J Clin Pharm Ther* 25:411–419, 2000.

36. Oellerich M, Amstrong VW: The MEGX test: a toll for real-time assessment of hepatic function. *Drug Monit* 23:81–92, 2001.

37. McKindley DS, Boulet J, Sachdeva K, et al: Endotoxic shock alters the pharmacokinetics of lidocaine and monoethylglycinexylidide. *Shock* 17:199–204, 2002.

38. Chandel B, Shapiro MJ, Kurtz M, et al: MEX (monoethylglycinexylidide): a novel in vivo test to measure early hepatic dysfunction after hypovolemic shock. *Shock* 3:51–53, 1995.

39. Tichy JA, Loucka M, Trefny ZM: The new clearance methods for hepatic diagnosis. *Prague Med Rep* 106:229–242, 2005.

40. Faybik P, Hetz H: Plasma disappearance rate of indocyanine green in liver dysfunction. *Transpl Proc* 38:801–802, 2006.

41. Hashimoto M, Watanabe G: Hepatic parenchymal cell volume and the indocyanine green tolerance test. *J Surg Res* 92:222–227, 2000.

42. El-Desoky A, Seifalian AM, Cope M, et al: Experimental study of liver dysfunction evaluated by direct indocyanine green clearance using near infrared spectroscopy. *Br J Surg* 86:1005–1011, 1999.

43. Von Spiegel T, Scholz M, Wietasch G, et al: Perioperative monitoring of indocyanine green clearance and plasma disappearance rate in patients undergoing liver transplantation. *Anaesthesist* 51:359–366, 2002.

44. Sakka SG, Reinhart K, Meir-Hellman A: Comparison of invasive and noninvasive measurements of indocyanine green plasma disappearance rate in critically ill patients with mechanical ventilation and stable hemodynamics. *Intensive Care Med* 26:1553–1556, 2000.

45. Sakka SG, van Hout N: Relation between indocyanine green (ICG) plasma disappearance rate and ICG blood clearance in critically ill patients. *Intensive Care Med* 32:766–769, 2006.

46. Stehr A, Ploner F, Traeger K: Plasma disappearance of indocyanine green: a marker for excretory liver function? *Intensive Care Med* 31:1719–1722, 2005.

47. Chijiiwa K, Watanabe M, Nakno K, et al: Biliary indocyanine green excretion as predictor of hepatic adenosine triphosphate levels in patients with obstructive jaundice. *Am J Surg* 179:161–169, 2000.

48. Chijiiwa K, Mizuta A, Ueda J, et al: Relation of biliary acid output to hepatic adenosine triphosphate level and biliary indocyanine green excretion in humans. *World J Surg* 26:457–461, 2002.

49. Kira T, Tomiguchi S, Kira M, et al: Quantitative evaluation of hepatic functional reserve using technetium 99 DTPA-galactosyl human serum albumin before and after transjugular intrahepatic portosystemic shunt. *Eur J Nucl Med* 24:1268–1272, 1997.

50. Hwang EH, Taki J, Shuke N, et al: Preoperative assessment of residual hepatic functional reserve using 99mTc-DTPA- galactosyl-human serum albumin dynamic SPECT. *J Nucl Med* 40:1644–1651, 1999.

51. Scheneider PD: Preoperative assessment of live function. *Surg Clin North Am* 84:355–373, 2004.

52. Ishii Y, Asai S, Kohno T, et al: (13) CO_2 peak value of L-[1-(13)C] phenylalanine breath test reflects hepatopathy. *J Surg Res* 86:130–135, 1999.

53. Kobayashi T, Kubota K, Imamura H, et al: Hepatic phenylalanine metabolism measured by the [13C] phenylalanine breath test. *Eur J Clin Invest* 31:356–361, 2001.

54. Koeda N, Iwai M, Kato A, et al: Validity of 13C-phenylalanine breath test to evaluate functional capacity of hepatocyte in patient with liver cirrhosis and acute hepatitis. *Aliment Parmacol Ther* 21:851–859, 2005.

55. Aoki M, Ishii Y, Ito A, et al: Phenylalanine breath test as a method to evaluate hepatic dysfunction in obstructive jaundice. *J Surg Res* 130:119–123, 2006.

56. Klatt S, Taut C, Mayer D, et al: Evaluation of the 13C-methacetin breath test for quantitative liver function testing. *Z Gastroenterol* 35:609–614, 1997.

57. Aoki M, Ishii Y, Asai S, et al: Ornithine breath test as a method to evaluate functional liver volume. *J Surg Res* 124:9–13, 2005.

58. Suzuki S, Ishii Y, Asai S, et al: 1-[1-(13)C] alanine is a useful substance for the evaluation of liver function. *J Surg Res* 103:13–18, 2002.

59. Zapater P, Lasso de la Vega MC, Horga JF: Pharmacokinetic variations of acetaminophen according to liver dysfunction and portal hypertension status. *Aliment Pharmacol Theo* 1:29–36, 2004.

60. Burczynski FJ, Greenway CV, Sitar DS: Hepatic blood flow: accuracy of estimation from infusions of indocyanine green in anaesthetized cats. *Br J Pharmacol* 91:651–659, 1987.

61. Burczynski FJ, Pushka KL, Sitar DS, et al: Hepatic plasma flow: accuracy of estimation from bolus injection of indocyanine green. *Am J Physiol* 252:H953–962, 1987.

62. Mizushima Y, Tohira H, Mizobata Y: Assessment of effective hepatic blood flow in critically ill patients by noninvasive pulse dye-densitometry. *Surg Today* 33:101–105, 2003.

Todd W. Sarge
Ray Ritz
Daniel Talmor

CHAPTER **33**

Respiratory Monitoring during Mechanical Ventilation

Respiratory function may be simply classified into ventilation and oxygenation, where ventilation and oxygenation are quantified by the ability of the respiratory system to eliminate carbon dioxide and form oxyhemoglobin, respectively. The goal of respiratory monitoring in any setting is to allow the clinician to ascertain the status of the patient's ventilation and oxygenation. The clinician must then use these data appropriately to correct the patient's abnormal respiratory physiology. As with all data, it is imperative to remember that interpretation and appropriate intervention are still the onus of the clinician, who must integrate these data with other pieces of information (i.e., history and physical exam) to make a final intervention. In the acutely ill patient, the principal intervention with regard to respiratory function and monitoring typically often involves the initiation, modification, or withdrawal of mechanical ventilatory support. This chapter will focus on respiratory monitoring for the mechanically ventilated patient.

Mechanical ventilation entails the unloading of the respiratory system via the application of positive pressure to achieve the goal of lung insufflation (i.e., inspiration) followed by the release of pressure to allow deflation (i.e., expiration). These simplified goals of mechanical ventilation are achieved in spite of complex and dynamic interactions of mechanical pressure with the physical properties of the respiratory system, namely elastance (E) and resistance (R). Furthermore, the patient's neurologic and muscular condition can also affect the goals of respiration, and they need to be monitored and evaluated as well. This chapter will focus on three specific areas in monitoring the mechanically ventilated patient: (a) the evaluation of gas exchange; (b) respiratory mechanics, and (c) respiratory neuromuscular function.

GAS EXCHANGE

BASIC PHYSICS OF GAS EXCHANGE

As mentioned, the primary function of the respiratory system is gas exchange (i.e., elimination of carbon dioxide while instilling oxygen to form oxyhemoglobin). Inadequate ventilation and oxygenation within the intensive care setting are typically caused by hypoventilation, diffusion impairment, or shunt and ventilation-perfusion mismatch.

Hypoventilation is defined as inadequate alveolar ventilation, and it is commonly caused by drugs, neurologic impairment, or muscle weakness/fatigue, which results in hypercarbia, according to the following equation:

$$P_aCO_2 = (\dot{V}_{CO_2}/\dot{V}_A) \times k,$$

where P_aCO_2 is the arterial partial pressure of carbon dioxide, $\dot{V}_{CO_2}$ is the production of carbon dioxide in the tissues, $\dot{V}_A$ is alveolar ventilation, and k is a constant. Fortunately, the institution of mechanical ventilatory support readily corrects hypoventilation while the underlying cause is determined and corrected.

Diffusion impairment results from inadequate time for the exchange of oxygen across the capillary-alveolar membrane. This may occur due to pathologic thickening of the membrane or high output cardiac states such as sepsis. However, the relative clinical significance of diffusion impairment in the intensive care unit (ICU) is debatable. This is because the hypoxemia that results from the acute exacerbation of diffusion impairment is usually corrected by supplemental oxygen therapy. Furthermore, P_aCO_2 is rarely affected by diffusion impairments because it is highly soluble and is eliminated in multiple forms, such as bicarbonate.

The most common cause of hypoxemia in the ICU is ventilation-perfusion ($\dot{V}/\dot{Q}$) mismatch. One manifestation of $\dot{V}/\dot{Q}$ mismatch is shunting. The true shunt fraction is the amount of cardiac output that results in venous blood mixing with end-arterial blood without participating in gas exchange. This has little effect on carbon dioxide tension; however, increases in shunt can lead to hypoxemia. The true shunt is expressed via the shunt equation as follows:

$$Q_s/Q_t = (C_c - C_a)/(C_c - C_v),$$

where Q_s and Q_t are the shunt and total blood flows, and C_c, C_a, and C_v represent the oxygen contents of end-capillary, arterial, and mixed venous blood, respectively. The concentration of mixed arterial and venous blood is calculated according to the oxygen content equation:

$$C_x = (1.34 \times Hb \times S_xO_2) + (PO_2 \times 0.003),$$

where C_x and S_xO_2 are the oxygen content and saturation of arterial and venous blood, respectively. The oxygen content of end-capillary blood is estimated by the alveolar gas equation as follows:

$$C_c = (P_{atm} - P_{H2O}) \times F_iO_2 + P_aCO_2/RQ,$$

345

where P_{atm} and P_{H2O} are the partial pressures of the atmosphere and water (typically 760 and 47 at sea level), respectively, while F_iO_2 is the concentration of inspired oxygen and RQ is the respiratory quotient. The significance of true shunt is the fact that it is not amenable to supplemental oxygen therapy. Shunted blood reenters the circulation and dilutes the blood that has been oxygenated by the lungs, resulting in a lower partial pressure of oxygen, PaO_2 in the arterial system. Increasing the F_iO_2 will not improve oxygenation since the blood does not meet alveolar gas.

Ventilation-perfusion ($\dot{V}/\dot{Q}$) mismatch is the result of inequality of the normal ventilation perfusion ratio within the lung. $\dot{V}/\dot{Q}$ mismatch is a spectrum of abnormal ratios signifying inadequate gas exchange at the alveolar level. It is possible with supplemental oxygen to overcome hypoxemia that is caused by an abnormal ratio of ventilation and perfusion, which differentiates this form of hypoxemia from true shunt. However, in the extreme, as the $\dot{V}/\dot{Q}$ ratio in any alveolus approaches zero (i.e., ventilation approaches zero), it approaches true shunt as described above. At the other end of the spectrum, as the ratio in any alveolus approaches infinity (i.e., as perfusion approaches zero), it becomes physiologic "dead space," which denotes alveoli that are ventilated but not perfused. Dead space will be described in greater detail later in this chapter.

DIRECT BLOOD GAS ANALYSIS

Monitors of gas exchange in the mechanically ventilated patient are typically directed at measurements of gas content and their gradients from the ventilator circuit to the alveolus and from the alveolus to the end-artery. As with most monitors, sources of error abound at many points as gases flow down their concentration gradients. The most accurate assessment of gas exchange is direct measurement from an arterial blood sample. This provides the partial pressures of carbon dioxide (P_aCO_2) and oxygen (P_aO_2) in the blood as well as the pH, base deficit, and cooximetry of other substances such as carboxyhemoglobin and methemoglobin. Advantages of arterial blood gas (ABG) analysis include the fact that it is a fairly exact representation of the current state of the patient with regard to acid-base status, oxygenation, and ventilation. However, the limitations of blood gas analysis as a tool for monitoring gas exchange are numerous, including the fact it is invasive, wasteful (blood), and noncontinuous (i.e., it is only a snapshot of the patient's condition at the time the ABG is drawn).

Central and peripheral venous blood gas sampling has been proposed as a surrogate to arterial blood for monitoring pH, PCO_2, and base deficit [1]. The obvious advantage is mitigation of the invasiveness (i.e., patients are not required to have arterial access or punctures), while the disadvantages are the need for correlation and inability to assess oxygenation. With the exception of patient's undergoing cardiopulmonary resuscitation [2], good correlation has been observed between arterial and venous pH and PCO_2 in patients with acute respiratory disease, with one author noting an average difference of 0.03 for pH and 5.8 for PCO_2 [1]. A recently published study in mechanically ventilated trauma patients also demonstrated good correlation between arterial and central venous pH, PCO_2, and base deficit; however, the authors concluded that the limits of agreement (−0.09 to 0.03 for pH and −2.2 to 10.9 for PCO_2) represented clinically significant ranges that could affect management and

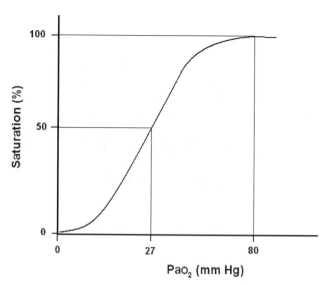

FIGURE 33-1. This is a schematic demonstrating a normal hemoglobin dissociation curve with 50% saturation at PaO_2 of 27 mm Hg and approaching 100% saturation at a PaO_2 of 80 mm Hg.

therefore should not be used in initial resuscitation efforts of trauma patients [3].

PULSE OXIMETRY

Without question, pulse oximetry has been the most significant advance in respiratory monitoring in the past three decades. Based on established oxyhemoglobin dissociation curve (Fig. 33-1), pulse oximetry allows for the continuous, noninvasive estimate of a patient's oxyhemoglobin and is expressed as a percentage of total hemoglobin [4–24]. A detailed explanation of pulse oximetry including the physics and limitations is provided in Chapter 27.

EXPIRED CARBON DIOXIDE MEASUREMENTS

Capnometry is the quantification of the carbon dioxide concentration in a sample of gas. Capnography is the continuous plotting of carbon dioxide over time to create a waveform (Fig. 33-2). When capnography is performed on continuous samples of gas from the airway circuit, a waveform is created whereby the plateau is reported as the maximum pressure in millimeters Hg and termed end-tidal carbon dioxide, or $P_{et}CO_2$. Although continuous capnography has limited usefulness in the ICU, capnometry has many clinical uses such as early detection of esophageal intubation [25–35]. For a detailed explanation of capnography and its uses, please refer to Chapter 27.

DEAD SPACE MEASUREMENTS

Dead space is defined as any space in the respiratory system that is ventilated but not perfused, such that no gas exchange can occur. Measurement of dead space is a marker of respiratory efficiency with regard to carbon dioxide elimination. Dead space can be subdivided into several categories including alveolar and anatomic. Anatomic dead space is the sum of the inspiratory volume that does not reach the alveoli and, therefore, participate in gas exchange. For mechanically ventilated patients, the anatomic dead space includes the proximal airways, trachea,

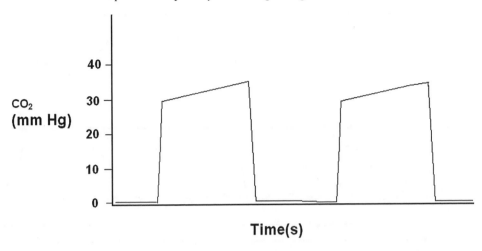

FIGURE 33-2. This is a schematic representation of a capnograph waveform with the expiratory plateau delineating the end-tidal CO_2 between 30 to 40 mm Hg.

endotracheal tube, and breathing circuit up to the Y-adapter. In normal human subjects, anatomic dead space is approximately 2 to 3 times the ideal body weight in kilograms, or 150 to 200 cc. Alveolar dead space is the conceptual sum of all alveoli that are ventilated but not participating in gas exchange, otherwise described as West Zone 1 [36]. Physiologic dead space (V_d) is the sum of anatomic and alveolar dead space and is usually expressed as a ratio of the total tidal volume (V_t) and can be calculated at the bed side using the Bohr equation:

$$V_d/V_t = P_aCO_2 - P_aCO_2/P_aCO_2 ,$$

where P_aCO_2 is the partial pressure of carbon dioxide and P_aCO_2 is the partial pressure of carbon dioxide in the alveoli. P_aCO_2 is often estimated as either end-tidal carbon dioxide, $P_{et}CO_2$ or more accurately as mixed expired carbon dioxide, P_eCO_2; however, the latter is more difficult to measure, often requiring metabolic monitors. *Volume capnography* is a novel and simple approach to estimating P_aCO_2, involving measurements of carbon dioxide at the Y-adapter, and has been shown to correlate with more complex methods of metabolic monitoring [37].

Physiologic dead space, V_d/V_t, is often increased in critical illnesses that cause respiratory failure, such as acute respiratory distress syndrome (ARDS) and chronic obstructive pulmonary disease (COPD). V_d/V_t can also increase with dynamic hyperinflation, or auto-PEEP, as well as overaggressive extrinsic PEEP due to overinflated alveoli impeding pulmonary artery blood flow, effectively increasing West Zone 1 volume. Serial measurements of V_d/V_t have been shown to correlate with outcome in ARDS [38] and have been used to monitor the degree of respiratory compromise in critically ill patients [39]. However, these data have not translated into changes in treatment and may only be prognostic for fibroproliferative ARDS, which is known to occur in a subset of these patients that fail standard treatment. Furthermore, Mohr et al. [40] found no appreciable difference in V_d/V_t while studying a series of post-tracheostomy patients successfully weaned from mechanical ventilation versus those who had failed weaning.

PULMONARY MECHANICS

Modern ventilators allow measurement of airway pressures (Paw), volumes (V), and flows ($\dot{V}$). Integration of these measurements allows assessment of the mechanical functions of the

respiratory system. These mechanical functions are influenced by various disease states, and understanding these relationships may allow delivery of more appropriate ventilator support.

Rapid airway occlusion during constant flow inflation in a relaxed, ventilator-dependent patient produces a typical picture as depicted in Figure 33-3 [41]. Rapid airway occlusion at end inflation results in a drop in Paw from the peak value (Ppeak) to a lower initial value (Pinit) and then a gradual decrease over the rest of the inspiratory period until a plateau (Pplat) is recorded. Pplat measured at the airway represents the static end-inspiratory recoil of the entire respiratory system [42]. Using an esophageal balloon catheter and measuring the pressure in the esophagus (Pes), it is possible to further partition all of these pressures into their lung (Ptp) and chest wall components (Ppl) using the equation:

$$Paw = Ptp + Pes.$$

These partitioned pressures are presented graphically in Figure 33-4.

COMPLIANCE AND ELASTANCE

The static compliance of the respiratory system and its reciprocal, elastance of the respiratory system, are measured clinically using the end-inspiratory airway occlusion method. The

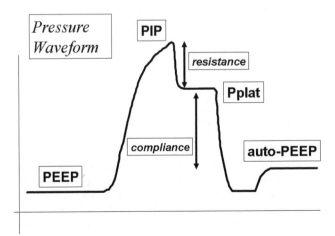

FIGURE 33-3. Schematic drawing of an airway pressure waveform delineating PEEP, auto-PEEP, Peak inspiratory pressure (PIP), plateau pressure (Pplat), resistance, and compliance.

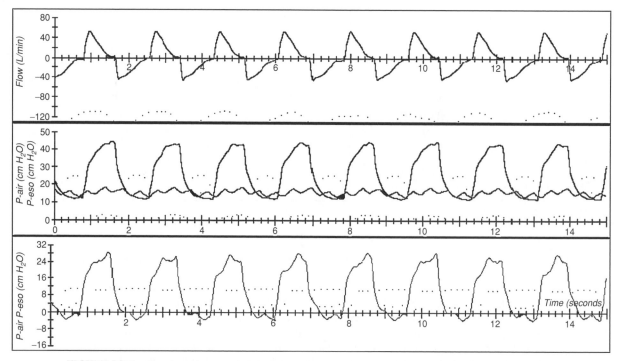

FIGURE 33-4. Esophageal pressure tracing (P-eso) can be seen super-imposed on the airway pressure tracing (P-air) during pressure control ventilation (PCV). Transpulmonary pressure has been estimated as the difference between these pressures with specific assumptions.

equation for elastance of the respiratory system (Est,rs) is based on the driving pressure between plateau pressure (Pplat) and the intrinsic PEEP (PEEPi). This number is then divided by V_t:

$$Est,rs = (Pplat - PEEPi)/V_t.$$

Est,rs may also be separated into its lung and chest wall components by applying this equation to the Ptp and Pes tracings obtained using Pes tracings (see Fig. 33-4). The relative contributions of the lung and chest wall to the total elastance may be dependant on the etiology of respiratory failure. By way of example, pulmonary edema, either cardiogenic or as a result of ARDS, will lead to an elevated lung Est and reduced compliance. ARDS of a nonpulmonary origin, sepsis as an example, may also lead to edema of the chest wall and abdominal distension. Both of these will lead to an additional increase in the Est,rs as a result of an increase in the elastance of the chest wall.

Dynamic Compliance

Effective dynamic compliance can be derived by dividing the ventilator-delivered V_t by [Ppeak – PEEP] [43]. Ppeak is influenced by all of the resistive and elastic pressure losses of the respiratory system and endotracheal tube and therefore cannot be considered a true measure of thoracic compliance. Alternatively, dynamic elastance of the respiratory system (Edyn,rs) can be obtained by dividing the difference in Paw at points of zero flow by the delivered V_t. Accordingly, Edyn,rs can be computed according to the formula:

$$Edyn,rs = Pinit - PEEPi/V_t.$$

Dynamic measurements of compliance and elastance have generally not been shown to be useful in predicting an individual patient's ability to breathe spontaneously [44].

Resistance

Airway resistance can be measured in ventilator-dependent patients by using the technique of rapid airway occlusion during constant flow inflation. The maximum resistance (Rmax) of the respiratory system is calculated by:

$$Rmax = [Ppeak - Pplat]/\dot{V}.$$

And the minimum resistance (Rmin) of the respiratory system can be computed by dividing

$$Rmin = [Ppeak - Pinit]/\dot{V}.$$

Rmin is considered to reflect ohmic airway resistance, while the difference between Rmax and Rmin (ΔR) reflects both the viscoelastic properties (stress relaxation) and time-constant inhomogeneities within the respiratory tissues (*pendelluft*).

PRESSURE VOLUME CURVES

Static Measurements of the Pressure-Volume Curve

The gold standard of pressure-volume (P-V) curve measurement is the super-syringe method. Using a large calibrated syringe, increments of volume of 50 ± 100 mL gas are used to inflate the lung up to a total volume of $1,000 \pm 2,000$ mL. After each increment, the static airway pressure is measured during a pause lasting a few seconds during which there is no flow, and the pressure is the same in the entire system from the super-syringe to the alveoli. The lung is then deflated in the same manner and the pressure at each increment of gas is recorded and the inspiratory and expiratory P-V curves are plotted. Continued oxygen uptake from the blood during this slow inflation-deflation cycle, coupled with equalization of the partial pressure of CO_2 in the blood and alveoli, will lead to a decrease in the deflation volume as compared to the inflation volume of gas. This artifact may appear to contribute to the phenomena of hysteresis. The more important mechanical cause of hysteresis is based on the slow inflation of the lung during the P-V curve maneuver. This slow inflation recruits or opens up areas of the lung with slow time constants and collapsed alveoli. This again will lead to a decreased expiratory volume and hysteresis.

Semistatic Measurements of the Pressure-Volume Curve

There are two methods for obtaining semistatic measurements of the P-V curve. These methods do not require the specialized skill and equipment needed for the super-syringe technique. The *multiple occlusion technique* uses a sequence of different-sized volume-controlled inflations with an end inspiratory pause [45,46]. Pressure and volume are plotted for each end inspiratory pause to form a static P-V curve. If expiratory interruptions are also done, the deflation limb of the P-V curve may also be plotted. This process may take several minutes to complete, but yields and the results are close to those obtained by static measurements. The second method is the *low-flow inflation technique*. This technique uses a very small constant inspiratory flow to generate a large total volume. The slope (compliance) of the curve is parallel with a static P-V curve only if airway resistance is constant throughout the inspiration. This is likely not the case as the low flow lessens airway resistance. The low flow also causes a minimal but recognizable pressure decrease over the endotracheal tube, which means that the dynamic inspiratory pressure volume curve will be shifted to the right [47,48]. The long duration of the inspiration produces the same artifacts as the super-syringe technique, which are represented as hysteresis. Another drawback of these static and semistatic methods is that they require stopping therapeutic ventilation while the maneuver is performed. The question has been raised, therefore, if these maneuvers are relevant in predicting the mechanical behavior of the lung under dynamic conditions, where resistance and compliance depend on volume, flow, and respiratory frequency.

Dynamic Measurements of the Pressure-Volume Curve

Dynamic measurement of the P-V curve allows continuous monitoring of the respiratory mechanics and in particular of the response to ventilator changes. These measurements are done with the patient on his or her therapeutic ventilator setting and therefore may reflect more accurately the complex interaction of patient, endotracheal tube, and ventilator. A continuous display of pressure may be obtained either proximal to the endotracheal tube (at the patient connector or from the ventilator itself) or distal to the endotracheal tube. This pressure may then be plotted against tidal volume to produce a dynamic P-V curve. Each of these methods has advantages; however, the more commonly used proximal method suffers from the disadvantage of being heavily influenced by the resistance of the endotracheal tube. Neither the peak pressure nor the end expiratory pressures are accurately recorded, and this will lead to an underestimation of compliance [45].

Clinical Use of the Pressure-Volume Curve

There is a characteristic shape to the static respiratory system P-V curve of patients with injured lungs. This shape includes an S-shaped inflation curve with an upper and lower inflection point (UIP and LIP respectively; Fig. 33-5), an increased recoil pressure at all lung volumes, and reduced compliance (Fig. 33-6), which is seen in the slope of the inflation curve between LIP and UIP. The LIP has often been considered the critical opening pressure of collapsed lung units and has been used as a method of setting the optimal PEEP in patients with acute lung injury. The pressure at UIP, in turn, was considered to indicate alveolar overdistension that should not be exceeded during mechanical ventilation [49]. These ideas have been challenged for multiple reasons. Accurate identification of the LIP and UIP is challenging even for experienced clinicians [50]. Additionally changes in the P-V curve are not specific for alveolar collapse and have been observed in saline-filled lungs, such as would be seen in patients with pulmonary edema [51,52]. When applied clinically to patients mechanically ventilated with ARDS, Amato et al. [53] demonstrated that use of the P-V curve and titration of PEEP to a level that exceeds the LIP may be part of a successful lung protective strategy. It is unclear from this study, however, what the relative importance of the higher levels of PEEP was in the context of the ventilatory strategy, which included delivery of low tidal volumes and the use of intermittent recruitment maneuvers. Subsequent trials have confirmed the survival benefit in patients ventilated using low TVs but not in those ventilated with a higher level of PEEP [54,55].

SEPARATING THE LUNG AND CHEST WALL COMPONENTS OF RESPIRATORY MECHANICS

Esophageal Pressure Monitoring

Ventilator-induced damage to the lungs arguably depends on the transpulmonary pressure ($P_{ao} - P_{pl}$), whereas current recommendations for management of ARDS specify limits for pressure applied across the whole respiratory system and are based

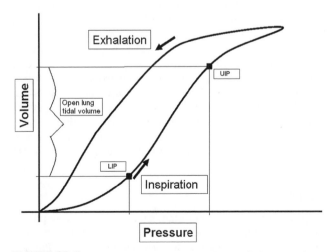

FIGURE 33-5. Schematic representation of normal pressure-volume curve (PV curve) with upper and lower inflection points (UIP and LIP, respectively) delineating the more compliant portion of the inspiratory limb and corresponding tidal volume that has been proposed as an "open lung" approach to ventilation in ARDS.

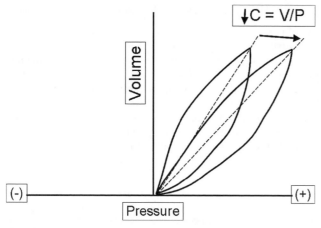

FIGURE 33-6.   Schematic representation of altered compliance (C) and the effect on the volume-pressure (V/P) curve as occurs with pulmonary edema.

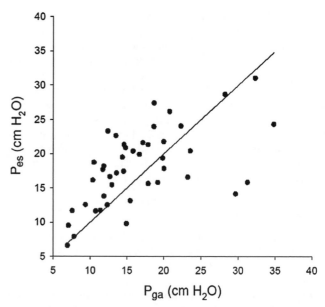

FIGURE 33-7.   This graph demonstrates the correlation between pressures measured in the esophagus (P_{es}) and gastric pressure (Pga).

on pressures measured at the airway. This approach could be seriously misleading if P_{pl} were to vary substantially among patients. In healthy subjects and upright spontaneously breathing patients, P_{pl} is often estimated by measuring esophageal pressure (P_{es}); however, this is rarely done in patients with acute injury, possibly because of a widespread, but untested, belief that artifacts make P_{es} unreliable as an estimate of P_{pl} [56]. Others have postulated the explicit assumption that P_{es}, corrected for a positional artifact, may reliably reflect an effective P_{pl} in critically ill patients as it does in healthy individuals [57].

Variations in P_{pl} may have contributed to inconsistent outcomes among clinical trials of ventilation strategies in ARDS. Whereas one large-scale randomized trial demonstrated a survival benefit from use of low tidal volume ventilation, results from other studies have been equivocal [54,58,59]. It is possible that in some patients with high P_{pl}, low tidal volume ventilation coupled with inadequate levels of PEEP results in cyclic alveolar collapse at end-expiration. In such cases, resulting atelectrauma might negate the benefit of limiting tidal volume. Similarly, higher levels of PEEP have been shown to be lung-protective in numerous animal models of ARDS but have demonstrated inconsistent benefit in clinical investigations [53,55]. This too may reflect failure to account for P_{pl}, leading to under- or over-application of PEEP in some patients as well as misinterpretation of high plateau airway pressures as evidence of lung overdistension [60,61]. Measuring P_{es} to estimate transpulmonary pressure may allow mechanical ventilator settings to be more appropriately customized to accommodate individual variations in lung and chest wall mechanical characteristics. Such an individual approach may reduce the risk of further lung injury in ARDS [56,60,62].

Gastric Pressure

Esophageal pressure monitoring is not a trivial task, requiring specialized equipment and experienced operators. Gastric pressure may provide a reasonable surrogate measure for Ppl. Recently, Talmor et al. [57] have demonstrated that there is a correlation between pressure measured in the esophagus and gastric pressures (Fig. 33-7). This relationship may be particularly important in patients suffering from ARDS with extrapulmonary

causes, where abdominal distension may contribute significantly to alveolar collapse.

Bladder Pressure

An alternative measurement of intraabdominal pressure may be obtained by measuring pressure in the urinary bladder [63]. Instilling 50 to 100 cc of sterile water through the Foley catheter, clamping the catheter and measuring the resulting bladder pressure has been shown to correlate well with intraabdominal pressure measured through a gastric tube [64]. These pressures have also been shown to correlate well with esophageal pressures [65]. Studies are still required to validate use of any of these measurements in the clinical care of patients with respiratory failure.

RESPIRATORY NEUROMUSCULAR FUNCTION

During mechanical ventilation, the goal of the clinician is to unload the patient's failing respiratory system and thereby reduce the work of breathing in the setting of respiratory failure [66]. Obviously, this goal is temporary with the later goal of weaning mechanical ventilation once the patient begins to recover from his or her disease process. To accomplish these goals, the clinician needs to have an understanding of the patient's respiratory function, which impacts each of these goals differently. For example, complete unloading of the respiratory system is common in the surgical operating room with general anesthesia, muscle relaxants, and controlled mechanical ventilation. However, the use of deep sedation and muscle relaxants for prolonged periods in the ICU has deleterious effects on the latter goal of ultimately preparing critically ill patients for extubation with several studies demonstrating increases in ventilator days, hospital length of stay, and associated costs [67–69]. Furthermore, assisted modes of ventilation with partial unloading have been surmised as beneficial for maintaining the conditioning of the diaphragm and reducing sedation requirements in the critical care setting [66,70]. No one has defined the ideal degree of unloading [66], which would presumably vary by individual and disease state. Nevertheless, it is helpful to understand and quantify the patient's neuromuscular function in order to facilitate unloading of the respiratory system, minimize patient-ventilator dyssynchrony, and ultimately wean the difficult patient from ventilatory support. This requires an understanding of respiratory neuromuscular physiology and how it cooperates with the ventilator. This relationship has been termed *patient-ventilator interaction.*

RESPIRATORY NEUROMUSCULAR ANATOMY

The respiratory system is involuntarily controlled by specialized neurons in the pons and medulla oblongata that control both inspiration and expiration. These neurons in the brainstem coordinate many inputs and feedback loops to control respiration and ensure adequate gas exchange. The specific types of feedback can be mechanical, chemical, reflex, and behavioral, all of which directly affect the neurons rate and intensity of neural firing [71]. Together these neurons and their feedback loops constitute the respiratory control center. Under normal resting conditions, neurons in the inspiratory center stimulate contraction of the diaphragm and intercostal muscles via the phrenic and spinal nerves, which creates a negative force in the chest cavity relative to the airway (i.e., a pressure gradient), thus allowing air to flow into the lungs (Fig. 33-8). Subsequent exhalation is typically passive, and air is exhaled as a consequence of lung and chest wall elastance. However, when the respiratory center is stimulated in the presence of carbon dioxide, acidosis, or hypoxemia, exhalation can be made more active by contraction of abdominal and chest wall muscles. The cerebral cortex has the ability to take control of the respiratory system by overriding the brainstem to change the frequency, depth, and rhythm of respirations. This is of minimal concern in the mechanically ventilated patient, whose cerebral cortex is sedated, either by medications or by illness, such that respiratory neuromuscular function is typically under the control of the brainstem as described above.

The muscular component of the respiratory system has been described as a pump that when stimulated creates a pressure, P_{mus} [71]. During assisted mechanical ventilation, this pressure can be added to a second pump, which is the airway pressure generated by the ventilator, P_{aw}. The sum of these two pressures, P_T provides the total driving pressure for inspiratory flow [71]. Although neglecting inertia, the equation for motion in the respiratory system states that P_T is dissipated while overcoming the elastive and resistive properties of the lungs as follows:

$$P_T = P_{mus} + P_{aw} = (E \times V) + (R \times \dot{V}), \qquad (1)$$

where the variables represent (E)lastance, (V)olume, (R)esistance, and Flow ($\dot{V}$) in the respiratory system [71]. Since the ventilator generated pressure, P_{aw} is intended to unload the patient's respiratory muscles, it should be synchronous with the neural impulses generated by the respiratory center and thus P_{mus}. To be synchronous with the patient's neural inspiration, the ventilator would need to initiate support simultaneously with the patient's neural firing at the onset of inspiration,

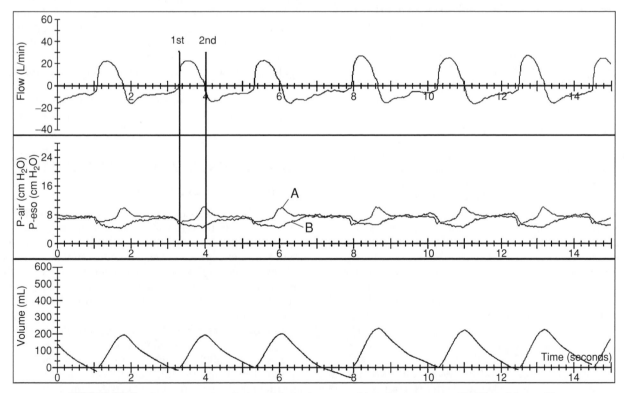

FIGURE 33-8. Spontaneous ventilation with continuous positive airway pressure (CPAP) at 7.5 mm Hg. Airway and esophageal pressure tracings are superimposed and marked as A and B, respectively. Note the onset of inspiration and flow, marked by the first vertical line, as esophageal (P-eso) and airway (P-air) pressures separate, creating a pressure gradient. Flow then ceases, as marked by the second vertical line, when the expiratory valve is opened on the ventilator and airway pressure quickly decreases.

continue this support throughout the neural firing, and stop support at the end of firing. In reality, this goal is virtually impossible, as at the present time there is no practical monitor for efferent motor neurons of the respiratory system. Rather than monitoring neural impulses, modern ventilators sense changes in pressure and flow within the circuit in an effort to match the patient's respiratory cycle. The variables that we will discuss in regard to the patient-ventilator interaction include ventilator triggering, cycling-off, and delivery of gas between these two events (i.e., the posttrigger phase). However, it is essential to first define some of the measures of respiratory drive and effort that are commonly used to assess patient-ventilator interaction and weaning such as work of breathing, pressure-time product, airway occlusion pressure, maximal inspiratory force, vital capacity, and rapid shallow breathing index.

WORK OF BREATHING

When considering patient respiratory effort, it is typically discussed and quantified via some measure of the patient's "work of breathing." *Work* is defined as the force acting on an object to cause displacement of that object. Therefore, mechanical "work of breathing" includes the measurement of a force required to create a change in volume of gas and is expressed in Joules per liter. However, measurements that are based on volume frequently fail to account for the work done by the diaphragm and respiratory muscles during isometric contraction against a closed valve [5], as occurs prior to triggering in some assisted modes of ventilation. The pressure-time product (PTP), which measures swings in intrathoracic pressure via an esophageal pressure monitor and correlates with oxygen requirements of breathing, is considered superior for quantifying a patient's effort and degree of unloading [66]. This is a calculation of the difference in the time integrals between esophageal pressure, P_{es} during assisted breathing and the recoil pressure of the chest wall during passive breathing at a similar tidal volume and flow [5].

AIRWAY OCCLUSION PRESSURE

Airway occlusion pressure at 0.1 seconds, $P_{0.1}$ is an indicator of respiratory drive and is determined by measuring the pressure in the airway a tenth of a second after the onset of inspiration beginning at functional residual capacity (FRC). This has been shown to correlate well with work of breathing during pressure support ventilation [5]. Therefore, several authors have advocated it use as a potential predictor for discontinuation of mechanical ventilation [72–75]. The threshold value for $P_{0.1}$ of 6 cm H_2O appeared to delineate success versus failure in one such study, although this value was variable among authors. Although the utility of this measurement is still debated, it has been incorporated into several commercially available ventilators.

MAXIMAL INSPIRATORY FORCE

Maximal inspiratory pressure (MIP), also known as negative inspiratory force (NIF), is another marker of respiratory muscle function and strength and is determined by measuring the maximum pressure that can be generated by the inspiratory muscles against an occluded airway beginning FRC. A normal value is considered to be approximately 80 cm H_2O, with respiratory compromise typically observed at values less than 40% of normal. The major disadvantage and limitation of this measurement is the fact that it is extremely effort dependent, which can make interpretation difficult in severely ill, sedated, and neurologically impaired patients.

VITAL CAPACITY

Vital capacity (VC) is the sum of tidal volume, inspiratory reserve volume, and expiratory reserve volume. Forced vital capacity (FVC) is measured by instructing a patient to inspire maximally to total lung capacity (TLC), followed by forced expiration while measuring the expired volume as the integral of the flow rate. FVC has also been used as an indicator of respiratory muscle function. However, similar to MIP, FVC is also effort dependent and therefore can lead to variable results. With limited success, it has been used to monitor trends in respiratory muscle strength in patients with neurologic impairment and muscle disorders such as cervical spine injury, myasthenia gravis, and Guillain Barre [76–78].

FREQUENCY/TIDAL VOLUME RATIO

Respiratory distress is typically marked by tachypnea and decreased tidal volumes, leading to inadequate ventilation and increases in P_aCO_2 secondary to disproportionate ventilation of anatomic dead space and inadequate alveolar ventilation. Therefore, the ratio of frequency to tidal volume, also known as the rapid shallow breathing index (RSBI), has been used to gauge respiratory distress and facilitate weaning and readiness for extubation [73,79–81]. As a criterion for extubation, the RSBI has had mixed success. Values of 100 to 105 breaths per minute per liter are typically used as a cutoff to predict extubation success from failure. The RSBI is limited by the fact that rapid and shallow breathing, although sensitive indicators of respiratory distress, are not specific. For example, pain and anxiety are also consistent with an abnormally high RSBI and are commonplace among critically ill patients weaning from mechanical ventilation.

PATIENT VENTILATOR INTERACTION

VENTILATOR TRIGGERING VARIABLE

During assisted modes of ventilation, the patient's inspiratory effort is sensed by the ventilator, which is then "triggered" to deliver support at a preset volume or pressure (Fig. 33-9). There are two distinct methods of triggering the ventilator—pressure and flow. *Pressure triggering* depends on patient inspiratory effort, creating a change in pressure that exceeds a preset requirement (typically –2 cm H_2O) to open the inspiratory valve on the ventilator and initiate ventilator support. Likewise, *flow triggering* depends on patient inspiratory effort, creating flow detected by a flow meter within the inspiratory limb that exceeds a preset threshold (typically 2 L per minute) for triggering the ventilator support. The significant difference between these two triggering criteria is the presence of a closed demand valve in the inspiratory limb in pressure-triggered ventilators. In general, flow triggering has been considered superior to pressure-triggered algorithms in that it is believed that the work of breathing is less in a system that does not require an initial inspiratory effort against

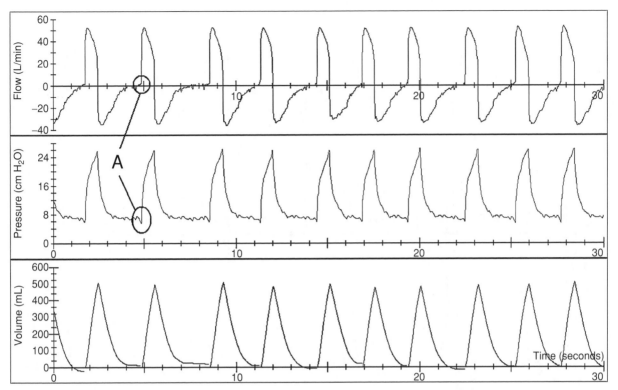

FIGURE 33-9. Normal triggering in assist-control ventilation. The circles marked A denote the pressure and flow that correspond to patient neural inspiration that is detected by the ventilator and leads to delivery of a mechanical breath.

this closed valve. Many studies have compared flow triggering and pressure triggering with respect to work of breathing with most showing significant advantages in favor of flow-triggered systems [82–84]. This is partially explained by the fact that flow triggering results in improved responsiveness with shorter delay between onset of diaphragm contraction and ventilator triggering [83].

The main variable that can be controlled on the ventilator with regard to triggering is termed *sensitivity*. Typical values for pressure triggering are 1 to 2 cm H_2O, while those for flow triggering are 2 to 3 L per minute. The sensitivity threshold is important because it is required to strike a balance between two main problems associated with triggering. First, if the sensitivity is set too low, patients may experience autotriggering, in which pressure and flow changes that occur from sources of artifact such as cardiac oscillations, water in the circuit, patient movement, or resonance with the system lead to irregular breathing patterns and dyssynchrony. Second, sensitivity settings that are too high will lead to ineffective triggering, which has the consequences of increased and wasted work and energy (Fig. 33-10). Ineffective triggering is also common in the setting of dynamic hyperinflation, as seen in obstructive disorders such as asthma and chronic obstructive pulmonary disease. In the setting of obstructive diseases, dynamic hyperinflation leads to elevations in the intrinsic PEEP (PEEP$_i$) above a critical threshold such that the patient's respiratory drive is insufficient to overcome the elastic recoil of the lung and chest wall and trigger the ventilator [66]. Clearly, this is also disadvantageous to the patient in terms of work of breathing and may contribute to ventilator dyssynchrony. Leung et al. [85] demonstrated that ineffective trigger attempts required 38% increases in patient effort as

compared to successfully triggered breaths. Obviously, autotriggering and ineffective triggering can create a challenge to the clinician when attempting to optimize the ventilator settings. In general, it is helpful to reduce the trigger threshold to a point where the delay between neural firing and ventilator support is minimized without allowing autotriggering to occur.

CYCLE-OFF VARIABLE

Neurons in the respiratory center continue firing beyond ventilator triggering and throughout inspiration. The cessation of firing is an important time point in the respiratory cycle and marks the beginning of expiration. The neural inspiratory time is often variable from breath to breath [66]. This can lead to considerable dyssynchrony in controlled modes of ventilation such as assisted-control, pressure-control, and intermittent mandatory ventilation, where "cycling-off" of the ventilator into expiration is a function of the inspiratory time (T$_i$) and is generally constant from one breath to the next. This can lead to increased sedation requirements, inconsistent with the goal of weaning the patient, as mentioned earlier. Ideally, the ventilator should be able to detect this event and react accordingly to halt the inspiratory pressure supplied. This is one of the goals and advantages of supportive modes of ventilation such as pressure support ventilation. That is, supportive modes of ventilation have the ability to detect patient expiration and stop ventilator inspiration such that the T$_i$ is variable. This can be accomplished by measuring flow or pressure changes within the circuit. As neural firing ceases and P$_{mus}$ decreases to baseline with muscle relaxation, total pressure and thus flow should decrease according to the elastive and resistive properties of the lung according

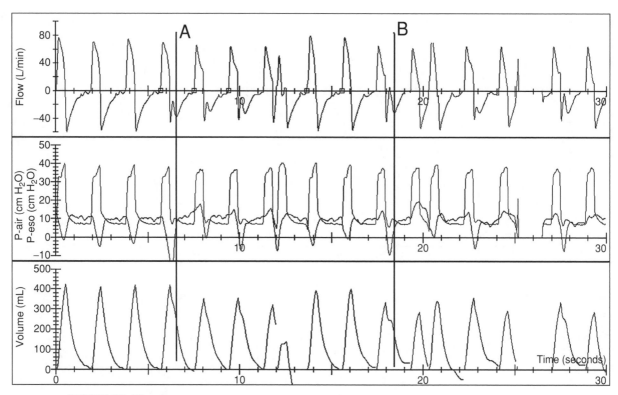

FIGURE 33-10. This pressure and flow tracing demonstrated failed trigger attempts that can be appreciated by the negative deflections in the expiratory limbs in the flow waveform and delineated by lines A and B.

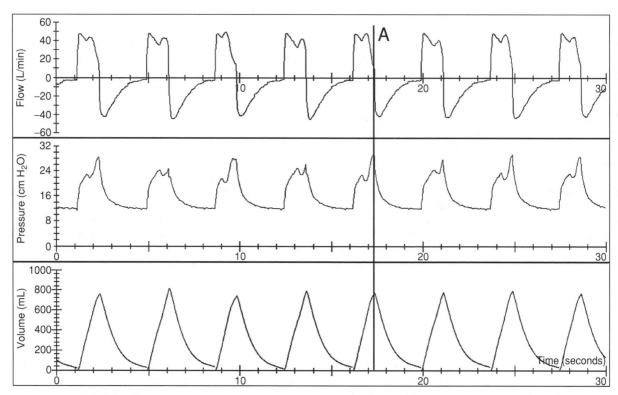

FIGURE 33-11. The pressure and flow waveforms demonstrate active recruitment of expiratory muscles to terminate ventilator inspiration. Note the time point marked by line A in which flow decreases rapidly corresponding to a sharp increase in the airway pressure due to active exhalation.

to equation (1). Typically, support modes have software that detects a preset decrement in flow, which in turn leads to cycling off the inspiratory support. This preset threshold can be an absolute value of flow or a percentage of maximum flow in the circuit, or both. Often, an increase in pressure that exceeds the programmed support level will also signal the ventilator to stop inspiration and open the expiratory valve as well.

Just as with triggering, the cycle-off variable can be a source of serious tribulations with the patient-ventilator interaction. For example, in the setting of decreased lung elastance, such as emphysematous lung disease, flow may not diminish enough to be detected properly despite a drop in P_{mus} at the end of neural inspiratory time. This can lead to patient discomfort and was studied by Jubran et al. [86], who noticed that 5 out of 12 patients with chronic obstructive pulmonary disease required active exhalation to cycle off the ventilator during pressure support ventilation at 20 cmH$_2$O. Active exhalation is counterproductive to both the primary goal of respiratory muscle unloading as well as ventilator synchrony (Fig. 33-11). Furthermore, active exhalation will increase transpulmonary pressure, which can lead to premature airway closure and increased intrinsic PEEP$_i$ as closing capacity increases.

INSPIRATORY FLOW VARIABLE

Inspiratory flow is now being recognized as an important parameter in assisted modes of ventilation. Critically ill patients in acute respiratory failure often have elevated respiratory drives that appear to demand greater flow to overcome the resistance of the failing respiratory system and ventilator breathing circuit [66]. Classically, this appears as a depression on the inspiratory limb of the airway pressure tracing and has been described by some practitioners as "flow hunger" (Fig. 33-12). Clinically, the response has been to increase flow, with typically ranges between 30 to 80 L per minute during assisted modes of mechanical ventilation in an effort to decrease the work of breathing and intrinsic PEEP in these situations. However, a recent series of studies has shown that this may in fact be counterproductive due to a phenomenon now recognized as "flow-associated tachypnea" [66]. Puddy and Younes [87] demonstrated this phenomenon by adjusting inspiratory flow in awake volunteers breathing on a volume-cycled ventilator in assist-control mode in which inspiratory T_i was variable. Laghi et al. [88] later delineated the contributions of flow, tidal volume, and inspiratory time in their study in which flow was increased from 60 to 90 L per minute and balanced with tidal volume settings of 1.0 and 1.5 L to maintain a constant inspiratory time, where frequency did not change. Furthermore, they were able to show that imposed ventilator inspiratory time during mechanical ventilation can determine frequency independently of delivered inspiratory flow and tidal volume. Therefore, the clinician must consider the counteracting variables of flow, tidal volume, and inspiratory time when attempting to ventilate patients with elevated respiratory drive in acute respiratory failure and how one may negatively influence the other.

SUMMARY

Respiratory monitoring is a complicated task in the critically ill patient who requires mechanical ventilation. The clinician must carefully balance a plethora of data acquired from studying

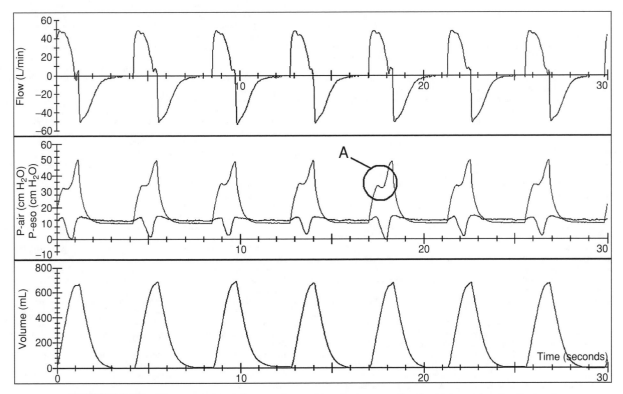

FIGURE 33-12. The pressure and flow waveforms above demonstrate the classic depressions on the inspiratory airway (P-air) pressure tracing in a patient with an elevated respiratory drive as highlighted by circle A. P$_{eso}$, esophageal pressure.

variables of gas exchange, pulmonary mechanics, neuromuscular function, and patient ventilator interactions. Skilled intensive care–trained personnel must then process this data so that a plan of respiratory support, often with mechanical ventilation, can be instituted. This plan must proceed in such a way that the patient is safely ventilated and oxygenated without imposing the undo harm that is associated with injurious modes of mechanical ventilation.

REFERENCES

1. Kelly AM, Kyle E, McAlpine R: Venous pco_2 and pH can be used to screen for significant hypercarbia in emergency patients with acute respiratory disease. *J Emerg Med* 22(1):15–19, 2002.
2. Weil MH, Rackow EC, Trevino R, et al: Difference in acid-base state between venous and arterial blood during cardiopulmonary resuscitation. *N Engl J Med* 315(3):153–156, 1986.
3. Malinoski DJ, Todd SR, Slone S, et al: Correlation of central venous and arterial blood gas measurements in mechanically ventilated trauma patients. *Arch Surg* 140(11):1122–1125, 2005.
4. American Society of Anesthesiologists: Standards for basic anesthetic monitoring. http://www.asahq.org.
5. Jubran A: Advances in respiratory monitoring during mechanical ventilation. *Chest* 116(5):1416–1425, Nov 1999.
6. Barker S MS, Bauder W: New pulse oximeter measures carboxyhemoglobin levels in human volunteers. Paper presented at: Annual Meeting of Society for Technology in Anesthesia, January 18–21, 2006. San Diego CA.
7. Lawless ST: Crying wolf: false alarms in a pediatric intensive care unit. *Crit Care Med* 22(6):981–985, 1994.
8. Wiklund L, Hok B, Stahl K, et al: Postanesthesia monitoring revisited: frequency of true and false alarms from different monitoring devices. *J Clin Anesth* 6(3):182–188, 1994.
9. Rheineck-Leyssius AT, Kalkman CJ: Advanced pulse oximeter signal processing technology compared to simple averaging. I. Effect on frequency of alarms in the operating room. *J Clin Anesth* 11(3):192–195, 1999.
10. Rheineck-Leyssius AT, Kalkman CJ: Advanced pulse oximeter signal processing technology compared to simple averaging. II. Effect on frequency of alarms in the postanesthesia care unit. *J Clin Anesth* 11(3):196–200, 1999.
11. Rheineck-Leyssius AT, Kalkman CJ: Influence of pulse oximeter settings on the frequency of alarms and detection of hypoxemia: theoretical effects of artifact rejection, alarm delay, averaging, median filtering or a lower setting of the alarm limit. *J Clin Monit Comput* 14(3):151–156, 1998.
12. Bohnhorst B, Peter CS, Poets CF: Pulse oximeters' reliability in detecting hypoxemia and bradycardia: comparison between a conventional and two new generation oximeters. *Crit Care Med* 28(5):1565–1568, 2000.
13. Malviya S, Reynolds PI, Voepel-Lewis T, et al: False alarms and sensitivity of conventional pulse oximetry versus the Masimo SET technology in the pediatric postanesthesia care unit. *Anesth Analg* 90(6):1336–1340, 2000.
14. Adler JN, Hughes LA, Vivilecchia R, et al: Effect of skin pigmentation on pulse oximetry accuracy in the emergency department. *Acad Emerg Med* 5(10):965–970, 1998.
15. Bothma PA, Joynt GM, Lipman J, et al: Accuracy of pulse oximetry in pigmented patients. *S Afr Med J* 86(5)[Suppl]:594–596, 1996;
16. Bickler PE, Feiner JR, Severinghaus JW: Effects of skin pigmentation on pulse oximeter accuracy at low saturation. *Anesthesiology* 102(4):715–719, 2005.
17. Cote CJ, Goldstein EA, Fuchsman WH, et al: The effect of nail polish on pulse oximetry. *Anesth Analg* 67(7):683–686, 1988.
18. Ralston AC, Webb RK, Runciman WB: Potential errors in pulse oximetry. III. Effects of interferences, dyes, dyshaemoglobins and other pigments. *Anaesthesia* 46(4):291–295, 1991.
19. Jay GD, Hughes L, Renzi FP: Pulse oximetry is accurate in acute anemia from hemorrhage. *Ann Emerg Med* 24(1):32–35, 1994.
20. Fitzgerald RK, Johnson A: Pulse oximetry in sickle cell anemia. *Crit Care Med* 29(9):1803–1806, 2001.
21. Kress JP, Pohlman AS, Hall JB: Determination of hemoglobin saturation in patients with acute sickle chest syndrome: a comparison of arterial blood gases and pulse oximetry. *Chest* 115(5):1316–1320, 1999.
22. Ortiz FO, Aldrich TK, Nagel RL, et al: Accuracy of pulse oximetry in sickle cell disease. *Am J Respir Crit Care Med* 159(2):447–451, 1999.
23. Blaisdell CJ, Goodman S, Clark K, et al: Pulse oximetry is a poor predictor of hypoxemia in stable children with sickle cell disease. *Arch Pediatr Adolesc Med* 154(9):900–903, 2000.
24. Pianosi P, Charge TD, Esseltine DW, et al: Pulse oximetry in sickle cell disease. *Arch Dis Child* 68(6):735–738, 1993.
25. McArthur CD: AARC clinical practice guideline. Capnography/capnometry during mechanical ventilation—2003 revision and update. *Respir Care* 48(5):534–539, 2003.
26. Goldberg JS, Rawle PR, Zehnder JL, et al: Colorimetric end-tidal carbon dioxide monitoring for tracheal intubation. *Anesth Analg* 70(2):191–194, 1990.
27. Knapp S, Kofler J, Stoiser B, et al: The assessment of four different methods to verify tracheal tube placement in the critical care setting. *Anesth Analg* 88(4):766–770, 1999.
28. Rabitsch W, Nikolic A, Schellongowski P, et al: Evaluation of an end-tidal portable $ETco_2$ colorimetric breath indicator (COLIBRI). *Am J Emerg Med* 22(1):4–9, 2004.
29. Bhende MS, LaCovey DC: End-tidal carbon dioxide monitoring in the prehospital setting. *Prehosp Emerg Care* 5(2):208–213, 2001.
30. Puntervoll SA, Soreide E, Jacewicz W, et al: Rapid detection of oesophageal intubation: take care when using colorimetric capnometry. *Acta Anaesthesiol Scand* 46(4):455–457, 2002.
31. Bhavani-Shankar K, Moseley H, Kumar AY, et al: Capnometry and anaesthesia. *Can J Anaesth* 39(6):617–632, 1992.
32. Russell GB, Graybeal JM: The arterial to end-tidal carbon dioxide difference in neurosurgical patients during craniotomy. *Anesth Analg* 81(4):806–810, 1995.
33. Russell GB, Graybeal JM: Reliability of the arterial to end-tidal carbon dioxide gradient in mechanically ventilated patients with multisystem trauma. *J Trauma* 36(3):317–322, 1994.
34. Russell GB, Graybeal JM, Strout JC: Stability of arterial to end-tidal carbon dioxide gradients during postoperative cardiorespiratory support. *Can J Anaesth* 37(5):560–566, 1990.
35. Prause G, Hetz H, Lauda P, et al: A comparison of the end-tidal-co_2 documented by capnometry and the arterial pco_2 in emergency patients. *Resuscitation* 35(2):145–148, 1997.
36. West JB, Dollery CT, Naimark A: Distribution of blood flow in isolated lung; relation to vascular and alveolar pressures. *J Appl Physiol* 19:713–724, 1964.
37. Kallet RH, Daniel BM, Garcia O, et al: Accuracy of physiologic dead space measurements in patients with acute respiratory distress syndrome using volumetric capnography: comparison with the metabolic monitor method. *Respir Care* 50(4):462–467, 2005.
38. Kallet RH, Alonso JA, Pittet JF, et al: Prognostic value of the pulmonary dead-space fraction during the first 6 days of acute respiratory distress syndrome. *Respir Care* 49(9):1008–1014, 2004.
39. Wathanasormsiri A, Preutthipan A, Chantarojanasiri T, et al: Dead space ventilation in volume controlled versus pressure controlled mode of mechanical ventilation. *J Med Assoc Thai* 85(4)[Suppl]:S1207–1212, 2002.
40. Mohr AM, Rutherford EJ, Cairns BA, et al: The role of dead space ventilation in predicting outcome of successful weaning from mechanical ventilation. *J Trauma* 51(5):843–848, 2001.
41. Bates JH, Rossi A, Milic-Emili J: Analysis of the behavior of the respiratory system with constant inspiratory flow. *J Appl Physiol* 58(6):1840–1848, 1985.
42. Polese G, Rossi A, Appendini L, et al: Partitioning of respiratory mechanics in mechanically ventilated patients. *J Appl Physiol* 71(6):2425–2433, 1991.
43. Rossi A, Polese G, Millic-Emili J: Monitoring respiratory mechanics in ventilator-dependant patients, in Tobin MJ (ed): *Principles and Practice of Intensive Care Monitoring.* New York, McGraw-Hill, 1998, pp 553–596.
44. Jubran A, Tobin MJ: Passive mechanics of lung and chest wall in patients who failed or succeeded in trials of weaning. *Am J Respir Crit Care Med* 155(3):916–921, 1997.
45. Stenqvist O: Practical assessment of respiratory mechanics. *Br J Anaesth* 91(1):92–105, 2003.
46. Iotti GA, Braschi A, Brunner JX, et al: Respiratory mechanics by least squares fitting in mechanically ventilated patients: applications during paralysis and during pressure support ventilation. *Intensive Care Med* May 21(5):406–413, 1995.
47. Lu Q, Vieira SR, Richecoeur J, et al: A simple automated method for measuring pressure-volume curves during mechanical ventilation. *Am J Respir Crit Care Med* 159(1):275–282, 1999.
48. Servillo G, Coppola M, Blasi F: The measurement of the pressure-volume curves with computerized methods. *Minerva Anestesiol* 66(5):381–385, 2000.
49. Roupie E, Dambrosio M, Servillo G, et al: Titration of tidal volume and induced hypercapnia in acute respiratory distress syndrome. *Am J Respir Crit Care Med* 152(1):121–128, 1995.
50. Harris RS, Hess DR, Venegas JG: An objective analysis of the pressure-volume curve in the acute respiratory distress syndrome. *Am J Respir Crit Care Med* 161(2 Pt 1):432–439, 2000;
51. Hubmayr RD: Perspective on lung injury and recruitment: a skeptical look at the opening and collapse story. *Am J Respir Crit Care Med* 165(12):1647–1653, 2002.
52. Martin-Lefevre L, Ricard JD, Roupie E, et al: Significance of the changes in the respiratory system pressure-volume curve during acute lung injury in rats. *Am J Respir Crit Care Med* 164(4):627–632, 2001.
53. Amato MB, Barbas CS, Medeiros DM, et al: Effect of a protective-ventilation strategy on mortality in the acute respiratory distress syndrome. *N Engl J Med* 338(6):347–354, 1998.
54. Ventilation with lower tidal volumes as compared with traditional tidal volumes for acute lung injury and the acute respiratory distress syndrome. The acute respiratory distress syndrome network. *N Engl J Med* 342(18):1301–1308, 2000.
55. Brower RG, Lanken PN, MacIntyre N, et al: Higher versus lower positive end-expiratory pressures in patients with the acute respiratory distress syndrome. *N Engl J Med* 351(4):327–336, 2004.
56. De Chazal I, Hubmayr RD: Novel aspects of pulmonary mechanics in intensive care. *Br J Anaesth* 91(1):81–91, 2003.
57. Talmor D, Sarge T, O'Donnell CR, et al: Esophageal and transpulmonary pressures in acute respiratory failure. *Crit Care Med* 34(5):1389–1394, 2006.
58. Brochard L, Roudot-Thoraval F, Roupie E, et al: Tidal volume reduction for prevention of ventilator-induced lung injury in acute respiratory distress syndrome. The Multicenter Trail Group on Tidal Volume reduction in ARDS. *Am J Respir Crit Care Med* 158(6):1831–1838, 1998.
59. Stewart TE, Meade MO, Cook DJ, et al: Evaluation of a ventilation strategy to prevent barotrauma in patients at high risk for acute respiratory distress syndrome. Pressure- and volume-limited ventilation strategy group. *N Engl J Med* 338(6):355–361, 1998.
60. Matthay MA, Bhattacharya S, Gaver D, et al: Ventilator-induced lung injury: in vivo and in vitro mechanisms. *Am J Physiol Lung Cell Mol Physiol* 283(4):L678–682, 2002;
61. Terragni PP, Rosboch GL, Lisi A, et al: How respiratory system mechanics may help in minimising ventilator-induced lung injury in ARDS patients. *Eur Respir J Suppl* 42:15S–21S, 2003.
62. Milic-Emili J, Mead J, Turner JM, et al: Improved technique for estimating pleural pressure from esophageal balloons. *J Appl Physiol* 19(2):207–211, 1964.
63. Malbrain ML: Abdominal pressure in the critically ill: measurement and clinical relevance. *Intensive Care Med* 25(12):1453–1458, 1999.
64. Collee GG, Lomax DM, Ferguson C, et al: Bedside measurement of intra-abdominal pressure (IAP) via an indwelling naso-gastric tube: clinical validation of the technique. *Intensive Care Med* 19(8):478–480, 1993.

65. Chieveley-Williams S, Dinner L, Puddicombe A, et al: Central venous and bladder pressure reflect transdiaphragmatic pressure during pressure support ventilation. *Chest* 121(2):533–538, 2002.

66. Tobin MJ, Jubran A, Laghi F: Patient-ventilator interaction. *Am J Respir Crit Care Med* 163(5):1059–1063, 2001.

67. Prielipp RC, Coursin DB, Wood KE, et al: Complications associated with sedative and neuromuscular blocking drugs in critically ill patients. *Crit Care Clin* 11(4):983–1003, 1995.

68. Carson SS, Kress JP, Rodgers JE, et al: A randomized trial of intermittent lorazepam versus propofol with daily interruption in mechanically ventilated patients. *Crit Care Med* 34(5):1326–1332, 2006.

69. Kress JP, Pohlman AS, O'Connor MF, et al: Daily interruption of sedative infusions in critically ill patients undergoing mechanical ventilation. *N Engl J Med* 342(20):1471–1477, 2000.

70. Le Bourdelles G, Viires N, Boczkowski J, et al: Effects of mechanical ventilation on diaphragmatic contractile properties in rats. *Am J Respir Crit Care Med* 149(6):1539–1544, 1994.

71. Kondili E, Prinianakis G, Georgopoulos D: Patient-ventilator interaction. *Br J Anaesth* 91(1):106–119, 2003.

72. Capdevila X, Perrigault PF, Ramonatxo M, et al: Changes in breathing pattern and respiratory muscle performance parameters during difficult weaning. *Crit Care Med* 26(1):79–87, 1998.

73. Sassoon CS, Mahutte CK: Airway occlusion pressure and breathing pattern as predictors of weaning outcome. *Am Rev Respir Dis* 148(4 Pt 1):860–866, 1993.

74. Sassoon CS, Te TT, Mahutte CK, et al: Airway occlusion pressure. An important indicator for successful weaning in patients with chronic obstructive pulmonary disease. *Am Rev Respir Dis* 135(1):107–113, 1987.

75. Murciano D, Boczkowski J, Lecocguic Y, et al: Tracheal occlusion pressure: a simple index to monitor respiratory muscle fatigue during acute respiratory failure in patients with chronic obstructive pulmonary disease. *Ann Intern Med* 108(6):800–805, 1988.

76. Rieder P, Louis M, Jolliet P, et al: The repeated measurement of vital capacity is a poor predictor of the need for mechanical ventilation in myasthenia gravis. *Intensive Care Med* 21(8):663–668, 1995.

77. Chevrolet JC, Deleamont P: Repeated vital capacity measurements as predictive parameters for mechanical ventilation need and weaning success in the Guillain-Barre syndrome. *Am Rev Respir Dis* 144(4):814–818, 1991.

78. Loveridge BM, Dubo HI: Breathing pattern in chronic quadriplegia. *Arch Phys Med Rehabil* 71(7):495–499, 1990.

79. Yang KL, Tobin MJ: A prospective study of indexes predicting the outcome of trials of weaning from mechanical ventilation. *N Engl J Med* 324(21):1445–1450, 1991.

80. Vallverdu I, Calaf N, Subirana M, et al: Clinical characteristics, respiratory functional parameters, and outcome of a two-hour T-piece trial in patients weaning from mechanical ventilation. *Am J Respir Crit Care Med* 158(6):1855–1862, 1998.

81. Krieger BP, Isber J, Breitenbucher A, et al: Serial measurements of the rapid-shallow-breathing index as a predictor of weaning outcome in elderly medical patients. *Chest* 112(4):1029–1034, 1997.

82. Barrera R, Melendez J, Ahdoot M, et al: Flow triggering added to pressure support ventilation improves comfort and reduces work of breathing in mechanically ventilated patients. *J Crit Care* 14(4):172–176, 1999.

83. Branson RD, Campbell RS, Davis K Jr, et al: Comparison of pressure and flow triggering systems during continuous positive airway pressure. *Chest* 106(2):540–544, 1994.

84. Aslanian P, El Atrous S, Isabey D, et al: Effects of flow triggering on breathing effort during partial ventilatory support. *Am J Respir Crit Care Med* 157(1):135–143, 1998.

85. Leung P, Jubran A, Tobin MJ: Comparison of assisted ventilator modes on triggering, patient effort, and dyspnea. *Am J Respir Crit Care Med* 155(6):1940–1948, 1997.

86. Jubran A, Van de Graaff WB, Tobin MJ: Variability of patient-ventilator interaction with pressure support ventilation in patients with chronic obstructive pulmonary disease. *Am J Respir Crit Care Med* 152(1):129–136, 1995.

87. Puddy A, Younes M: Effect of inspiratory flow rate on respiratory output in normal subjects. *Am Rev Respir Dis* 146(3):787–789, 1992.

88. Laghi F, Karamchandani K, Tobin MJ: Influence of ventilator settings in determining respiratory frequency during mechanical ventilation. *Am J Respir Crit Care Med* 160(5 Pt 1):1766–1770, 1999.

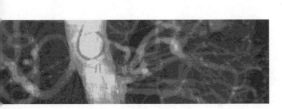

INDEX

INDEX